Annual Dues $8.00---Due January 1, 1938

THE JOURNAL

OF THE

OKLAHOMA STATE MEDICAL ASSOCIATION

VOLUME XXXI   McALESTER, OKLAHOMA, JANUARY, 1938   Number 1

Published Monthly at McAlester, Oklahoma, under direction of the Council.

THE JOURNAL
OF THE
OKLAHOMA STATE MEDICAL ASSOCIATION

| VOLUME XXXI | McALESTER, OKLAHOMA, JANUARY, 1938 | Number 1 |

Abortion—A National Health Problem*

GERTRUDE NIELSEN, M.D.

NORMAN, OKLA.

The publication three or four years ago of the reports on maternal mortality in New York and in 15 states made a great impression both upon the medical profession and upon laymen. It was appalling to learn that 375,000 women have died during the last 25 years in fulfilling their physiological function, as compared to 244,-000 soldiers killed in all the wars waged by this country. Many papers have been read at medical meetings on such causes of the high maternal mortality as toxemia, puerperal hemorrhage, and sepsis. However, it is only in the last year that we have begun to face one of the chief causes of our high maternal mortality, namely abortion. According to our best information, this cause alone is responsible for more than 25 per cent of all maternal deaths.

Abortion is not primarily a m e d i c a l problem. It is a public health problem closely linked with our social,. economic and religious life. However, it seems to me of importance that we as obstetricians and gynecologists study carefully the reliable data which have recently been furnished by various excellent surveys.

As far back as human records go there is evidence of the desire of the race to maintain some control over the number of offspring. Until the recent advent of con-* traception this was done by abortion and infanticide.

---

*Read before the Section of Obstetrics and Pediatrics, Annual Meeting, Oklahoma State Medical Association, Tulsa, May, 1937.

We find the first written prescriptions of abortifacient drugs as early as 2600 B.C. in China, and in the Ebert papyrus of Egypt the first list of abortion instruments was recorded. In Greece Plato and Aristotle on one side and Hippocrates on the other were having the same feud as sociologists and physicians of today. Hippocrates considered abortion an improper but necessary expedient. However, knowing about the injuries and sequelae of the practice, he was opposed to putting abortifacients into the hands of the laity.

A moral and religious attitude towards abortion appeared in the teaching of the Old Testament: "be fruitful and multiply." Nevertheless, the Jews permitted abortion within 40 days after conception. Only after the advent of Christianity was interruption of pregnancy designated as murder.

Some primitive peoples practiced abortion so extensively that the Paraguayans almost died out as a result of excessive abortions. Records show that some Indian women underwent as many as 33 abortions.

In the civilized world there is a steady rise in the frequency of abortions, the following factors being responsible according to Taussig: The secularization of thought, the increasing hedonism or pleasure philosophy, urbanization and the frantic desire to raise the economic standards of living, and last but not least, the slowness with which scientific contraceptive knowledge spreads.

Although as we have seen, the practice

very slow to come. In the meantime, we can greatly relieve the situation by helping to make contraceptives a v a i l a b l e to a larger part of the population.

REFERENCES

Taussig, F. J. Abortion, C. V. Mosby, 1936.
Litzenberg, J. C. he Challange of the Falling Birth Rate. Am. J. Obst. Gynec. 27:317, 1934.
    Kopp, Marie, Birth Control in Practice, McBride & Co., 1934.

Congenital Hypertrophic Pyloric Stenosis*

FRED A. GLASS, M.D.
TULSA, OKLA.

As to what causes this hypertrophy, much is to be said in theory but not much in facts. Hirschsprung believed there was hyperplasia of the muscle fibres of the pyloric muscle, which he called primary developmental hyperplasia. It is true that due to this hypertrophy there is a narrowing of the pyloric lumen. On the other hand a great many observers today do not believe that hypertrophy accounts for all the symptoms and that there is associated spasm with the hypertrophic condition. That the hypertrophy is primary is most likely, since it has been demonstrated at birth in some cases and the symptoms only appear when spasm occurs. One rarely ever sees bile in the vomitus, and from this it may be taken that the hypertrophy in itself may cause almost complete obstruction of the pylorus. The persistency of hypertrophy months after spontaneous recovery or years after a posterior gastroenterostomy proves, according to Sauer, that hypertrophy is not dependent on the spasm. The argument has been the question as to whether hypertrophy precedes the spasm or the spasm causes hypertrophy.

The familial occurence of this condition although unexplained is nevertheless interesting. The first case of congenital pyloric stenosis reported was by Armstrong in 1777 following autopsy findings, and was the third such case in the same family. Sauer reports two families in each of which there had been three cases, and twin boys in whom the condition was proved at autopsy. Fingelstein described four cases in one family and three in each of two other families. In my series I have seen two boys in the same family with congenital pyloric stenosis. Males are more frequently affected than females, the ratio being three or four to one. In my series of 26 cases all have been males.

The frequency of congenital hypertrophic pyloric stenosis is interesting. Hertz in 1916 reported that 2.7% of all children under one year of age showed this condition. Walls compares appendicitis with pyloric obstruction and says that in a clinic totalling 5,000 cases each year he found, during a five-year period, five cases of acute appendicitis compared with 30 cases of pyloric stenosis.

The diagnosis of this condition does not present much difficulty. The condition generally occurs in apparently normal infants in the second to fourth week of life; however, it may not show itself until the eighth to tenth week, and as said before, is usually in males. Projectile vomiting is an outstanding symptom, following the taking of milk or even water, associated with visible gastric peristalsis. Projectile vomiting usually occurs within a few minutes after nursing, and frequently with nursing, and practically never contains bile.

Constipation is marked and progressive, due to the lack of food, and is associated with progressive w e a k n e s s and loss of weight. With these symptoms or associated with them are usually cold extremities. The visible peristalsis after a few days becomes quite accentuated, and as the condition progresses; and frequently one sees the definite outline of the stomach, which becomes hypertrophied. Most observers

*Read before the Surgical Section, Annual Meeting, Oklahoma State Medical Association, Tulsa, May, 1937.

say that the presence of a palpable tumor at the pylorus is conclusive evidence in diagnosis of congenital hypertrophic pyloric stenosis. In regard to the palpable tumor I have never been able in my series of cases to regard this of much importance. I have never been able to positively convince myself I could detect a palpable mass at the pylorus. However, at operation a definite circular hypertrophy of the pylorus has always been demonstrated; but I do not feel that if a tumor mass cannot be demonstrated, it should in any way interfere with diagnosis if other cardinal symptoms are present.

Roentgenology, with b a r i u m meal of course, when showing obstructive evidence at the pylorus, is a positive diagnostic sign, but I do not feel that the use of X-ray examination is necessary for diagnosis, and in the past few years have not used this, due to the fact that if the case becomes operative, as many do, the retention of barium in the stomach interferes considerably with the operative procedure as well as post-operative convalescence.

As to the treatment, since there are so many theories regarding the etiology of the condition, there arises some question as to treatment, which may be medical or surgical. Medical treatment as a rule consists of the use of some atropine preparation with heavy gruel feedings. I do not feel that medical treatment should be prolonged unless there is noticeable and marked improvement, as medically treated cases frequently come to surgery for surgical interference, and if these infants have become m u c h undernourished and dehydrated, which they undoubtedly do, they make very poor surgical risks. While on the other hand if these infants are not too much undernourished and dehydrated, the mortality rate is not very high. In my series of 26 cases I have had two post-operative deaths.

In mild or questionable cases I feel that medical treatment is indicated; however, if the condition has gone on for four or five weeks, with marked dehydration and loss of weight, they should be treated medically to build up fluids; but with failure following this to gain weight, it is indeed indicated to use surgery. Blood transfusions are frequently helpful in severe cases.

The operation of c h o i c e today, is, of course, Rammstedt's operation. However in my earlier cases a gastro-enterostomy was done. In the Rammstedt operation an upper right rectus incision is made. Upon opening the peritoneum the stomach usually shows hypertrophy, and at the pyloric portion there is always found a circular band of tissue which feels firm. This is grasped between the thumb and index finger and an incision made through this tumor mass or hypertrophied area, longitudinally separating all fibres of the serosa and the muscular from the duodenal portion back along the pylorus. It is very essential to separate all muscle fibres, allowing the mucosa to bulge through the incision, of course using care not to open the mucosa. If this should happen it is quite essential to r e p a i r carefully to prevent leakage. I have always placed a small silk suture in each side of the incision, in order to hold this open to some extent, but I doubt very much if this is necessary.

Hemorrhage from the incision in the pylorus has never been of very much worry, excepting one occasionally meets with considerable oozing, making it necessary to delay operation in order to control this bleeding. After operation some three to four hours, water is started by mouth along with breast milk or barley water.

As to anesthesia, of choice I have always used ether, drop method. Some operators do this operation under local anesthesia, but I have always felt that the operative procedure was made easier under general anesthesia, such as ether. Practically always following operation the infant begins to retain nourishment and shows a noticeable gain in weight.

My last case operated March 11th, 1937, weighed at time of operation 6¼ pounds. He gained weight as follows:

1st postoperative day	7 lbs.	
2nd postoperative day	7 lbs.	7½ oz.
3rd postoperative day	7 lbs. 12	oz.
7th postoperative day	7 lbs. 13	oz.
9th postoperative day	7 lbs. 14½ oz.	
11th postoperative day	8 lbs. 1	oz.
12th postoperative day	8 lbs. 2	oz.

He was brought back to my office for observation six weeks following operation, and at that time weighed 10 pounds; his general condition was good and he was taking and handling all nourishment.

DISCUSSION

Dr. Horace Reed, Oklahoma City: I quite agree with the essayist and Dr. Long that when I have been able to feel a tumor, I think I have always overstrained my imagination. Another point in the diagnosis is that these children have a large abdomen in the upper half, and a very flat almost s c a p h o i d abdomen, very narrow, in the lower half. We have had the misfortune to be mistaken in certain cases even with careful study and consultation where we had evidence of obstruction in the stomach in which there was coexisting defect lower down. In one instance there was a terminal ileum which had never developed; it was just a narrow cord without an opening in it. In another case there was atresia of the pelvic bowel. In both of these cases

there was distention below the stomach. Then a point about the operation which I have found very valuable. I use the method as suggested by Dr. Solomon, local anesthesia until we get to the peritoneum or through it, then a whiff of ether. The point I have found most valuable is making a rather short incision, making it as high as possible, and when you have made it you have nothing but the liver in view when you first open the peritoneum. This acts as a valve and you do not have any extrusion of the viscera if the patient happens to cough or strain. Then when you are through, again the liver drops back down and acts as a valve to prevent the extrusion that you might have if you make a low incision and one that is too long.

Dr. Glass: I am very glad to have these discussions. As for Dr. Solomon's point, I have always had that opinion myself.

———————o———————

CLINICAL LABYRINTHITIS

THEODORE G. WAILS
OKLAHOMA CITY, OKLA.

Labyrinthitis may be classified in many ways; some are important and some are not. For instance, there often is a retrograde infection of the labyrinth from a contagious meningitis, and the entire inner ear may become filled with exudate and be completely lost. This would not be important clinically since one could do no more about it than if it had not become infected. On the other hand, it may be ascending from the middle ear; then it becomes very important clinically, since there is possibility of stopping it before it becomes a purulent meningitis.

A classification as to bacteria is not very practical because in old cases there is always mixed infection, and in acute cases the patient must show some signs of resistance or you can do very little.

A classification that tells us whether the l e s i o n is circumscribed or diffuse, and whether it is serous or purulent will en-

able us to tell whether it is possible to be of any help. Also we must know whether it is affecting only the bony wall of the vestibule and irritating the endothelial membrane, or whether it is actually inside the labyrinth, destroying the membrane. Also whether it is limited to a canal, invading the entire vestibular part, whether the cochlea is involved and whether the meninges are also being irritated or actually infected through the endolymphatic duct, the cochlear or vestibular ducts and the internal auditory meatus. Whether the petrous pyramid and tip are also being destroyed, and whether there is a basilar meningitis developing, or a circumscribed extra dural or subarachnoid abscess developing. All these things, we should try to ascertain, in order to treat an ear correctly where the lesion has gone further than the middle ear and mastoid.

In the first place a patient coming in with vertigo does not necessarily have a labyrinthitis at all, particularly if there is no tinnitis, nystagmus or impaired hearing. One may have a giddiness as a reflex from eye strain, generally due to astigmatism slightly off the 90° axis.

However, if the patient has spontaneous nystagmus, or impaired hearing, or marked tinnitis in either ear, with a history of vertigo on sudden change of position, then a careful, complete ear examination is indicated.

I

Circumscribed labyrinthitis m a y b e traumatic, serous or purulent; and may affect only the bony capsule and irritate the endothelial membrane, or it may have actually invaded the canal and still be limited to one area.

Case Report: A white boy, age five, entered University Hospital because of having a nail stuck into the left ear canal. There had been profuse bleeding through the drum. He had begun immediately to be so dizzy he could not stand and vomited all food, had spontaneous nystagmus, but could hear perfectly. He did not look sick and had no fever. Spinal punctures after several days showed normal spinal fluid. He evidently had a puncture into the vestibule with blood and serum thrown out into the vestibular portion and the cochlea unaffected, and no infection followed. The treatment was expectant and he made an uneventful recovery, the puncture wound healing without infection or fistula.

Circumscribed labyrinthitis, purulent in type, from an erosion of the canal or vestibule in chronic otitis media, may be very serious. If the infection is inside the canal any attempt at treatment may start a diffuse purulent condition. However, if it is limited only to the bony canal and is irritating the membrane, then radical mastoidectomy is indicated.

If the condition follows acute mastoidectomy, it may be an induced type (Ruttin's classification) and a simple mastoidectomy will suffice.

Case Report: Mrs. C., female, white, age about 40, first seen two years previous, with occasional attacks of vertigo. Large s u p e r i o r posterior perforation, slightly moist. Spontaneous nystagmus present, caloric showed normally functioning canals, fistula test questionable. Radical mastoidectomy suggested and refused. Two years later symptoms had progressed until patient was unable to turn in bed or even t u r n her eyes without violent dizziness ending in vomiting. There was no lessening of symptoms with time, as in latent purulent labyrinthitis, showing it was an irritative lesion rather than destructive. Fistula test now s t r o n g l y positive, and hearing good for whisper and no signs of intracranial lesion. Radical mastoid operation done and erosion found in Trautman's triangle, including the posterior canal. All dead bone removed around this area. Patient made uninterrupted recovery, and two months later is living a normal life with dry ear, no vertigo, and hearing not so good because of skin over oval window.

Another case of circumscribed purulent perilabyrinthitis; i.e., irritative lesion. Mr. E., railroad engineer, about 48 years old, began having so many dizzy attacks he could not run his train. Examination showed spontaneous nystagmus and tinnitis, but hearing fairly good. Moist, old drum perforation close to oval window. Fistula test positive. X-ray showed chronic mastoiditis. Caloric showed good labyrinth function, and patient incapacitated for work.

Radical mastoidectomy done and drum and membrane around oval window carefully removed, and this region was allowed to cover with granulation tissue and later be covered with skin, thus burying the sensitive vestibule. In about one month, patient had dry ear; no dizziness, and has now been running his train since that time with no more attacks, though hearing has not been so good due to covering up the oval window; however, he can now work where previously he could not.

One must be careful in these cases to not curette the lesion and turn an irritative lesion into a purulent destructive one.

II

Diffuse labyrinthitis may be serous or purulent. In the serous type there is a sudden effusion of blood or serum into the vestibular portion and produces (or it may be induced from an acute middle ear infection) the typical signs of Meniere's syndrome, and the cochlea may or may not be affected. These will usually clear up with time, relieving the cause, generally high blood pressure, nephritis, or focal infection, middle ear infection and occasionally toxic conditions, such as produced by quinine and tobacco. Large doses of ammonium chloride, grains eight, six times daily should be given.

Diffuse purulent labyrinthitis, however, is rarer and more interesting. It may come through the round, or oval window, from an acute middle ear infection; it may come as the result of traumatic opening of the labyrinth; or from a chronic circumscribed purulent labyrinthitis which has been walled off in a canal; or it may come from an irritative perilabyrinthitis which has been activated by operation.

Ruttin also makes a classification as to whether it is primary or induced from the middle ear.

During the first few days the condition is manifest because the membranes have not died and the infection irritates different portions of the vestibular apparatus and cochlea. Therefore, the patient is sick, has spontaneous syntagmus, nausea, vomiting, tinnitis, impaired hearing, falling and past pointing, and usually shows some cerebral symptoms, such as headaches, pressure signs and cranial nerve palsies.

The spontaneous syntagmus may be toward the lesion or away from it, and has no regularity at first. However, as pus develops and destruction occurs, then the function of the opposite ear becomes dominant and pulls the eyes slowly toward the affected ear. The cerebrum then quickly pulls the eyes back, producing the quick or cerebral component, which will thus always be toward the good ear when the lesion is destructive.

If the lesion remains serous and is induced from an acute tympanum, then a simple mastoidectomy will cure it. If it is secondary to a chronic mastoiditis and is still serous, then a radical mastoidectomy will cure it. If it is secondary to a chronic mastoiditis that has or has not had a radical mastoid operation, and destruction of the membrane in the vestibule takes place as shown by all the above related symptoms being present, plus inability to stimulate the vestibule by the caloric method and with syntagmus present toward the

good ear, then opening the labyrinth is indicated after the radical mastoid operation.

If hearing is present, the cochlea may not be opened, but if all gone then the cochlea should also be opened. No one can tell for sure in the first few days of a labyrinthitis whether it is diffuse serous or diffuse purulent, except by checking the spinal fluid frequently.

A purulent condition will always show some irritation of the meninges, shown by cloudy fluid with the predominating cell polymorphonuclears, sugar reduced or absent, globulin increased and the spinal pressure up. There may or may not be organisms in the fluid.

Organism may be present and the condition can still become circumscribed and subject to treatment. So if on repeated spinal taps the total count decreases, the percentage of polys. decrease and the lymphocytes increase, the bacteria disappear and the sugar returns, then there has been a circumscribed meningitis formed, and it is indicated to do a labyrinth operation, either a Newman, Hinsberg Richards, or Eagleton, depending on whether the cochlea is involved and whether the petrous tip is involved.

Case Report: A negro girl, age six, came into University Hospital, stuperous, spontaneous syntagmus, both ears draining profusely, swelling over both mastoids, both eyes turned in, chocked disc, increased reflexes, no hearing and inability to stimulate either labyrinth. Diagnosis of double, acute mastoiditis, double labyrinthitis, double petrositis and basilar meningitis was made. Spinal puncture done and cloudy fluid found but no organisms. Patient died before operation was performed. Autopsy showed mastoiditis, labyrinthitis, petrositis and basilar meningitis on each side. One or two days earlier, this could possibly have been treated, as she did not have a general diffuse purulent meningitis.

Case Report: Mrs. S., female, white, age about 47, came into University Hospital, with chronic otitis media and mastoiditis with recent exacerbation and involvement of the seventh nerve. Radical mastoid operation was performed by one of the staff. About one week later, she became dizzy, had spontaneous syntagmus, at first in any direction. She fell and past pointed toward the affected ear. Could not hear with affected ear, vomited and developed somewhat dull cerebration. Optic nerves showed some swelling. Spinal puncture showed about 3,000 white blood cells, mostly polys. and a gram negative bacillus, resembling colon bacillus.

On daily spinal punctures the cell count dropped, the percentage of polys. dropped, the lymphocytis increased to 50 per cent, sugar returned and the colon bacillus could not be found again. About this time, the sixth nerve became impaired, and the right fifth also, and she lost conjugate movement of both eyes to the right, showing pressure on the cerebral peduncles. Diagnosis increased to acute diffuse purulent manifest labyrinthitis, petrositis and circumscribed meningitis.

Neuman labyrinth operation was done, opening both vestibule and cochlea. Then unlocking of the petrous pyramid according to Eagleston and dura pushed away above and in front of the internal auditory meatus to the tip. Adhesions encountered and some pus extra dural; attempt made to perforate the tip with hook, unsuccessful. Wound was then enlarged downward to the tip through the cochlea in front of the nerve. Drains placed and supportive treatment. Four days later, spinal cell count still dropping, no organism found, patient brighter mentally and seems to not have general meningitis. Drain being kept between dura and petrous tip which we expect will prevent the tip from rupturing into the dura.

―――――o―――――

Insulin Shock Therapy
Results to Date

G. WILSE ROBINSON, JR., M.D.
KANSAS CITY, MO.

At frequent intervals there appears in the world of medicine a new discovery, some apparently new principle or chemical isolation which revolutionizes not only the treatment but frequently the entire concept of some condition hitherto considered either s o l v e d or understood only through unprovable theories. The most recent of these advances in medicine is the insulin shock therapy for schizophrenia. Results to date have shown definitely that this therapeutic procedure is a great advance in the treatment of a condition which previously could not be specifically treated.

However, it is not as yet perfect or completely specific. There are many patients who will not respond, and many who relapse as soon as the treatment is terminated. Much must be learned and much must be done before we can say that it is the perfectly understood treatment. It may be that some day it will be abandoned for something better, which is either perfect, or which approaches perfection. But at

this time it is the best, and should be given to every patient as early as possible.

To the latter statement, however, there is one dissenting view-point. Metrazol and camphor convulsions have been used by several investigators as long as insulin therapy. Many of these, especially Meduna[8], who first standardized the treatment, and Anggal and Gyarfas[10], consider this treatment equal to insulin therapy. This conclusion may be based upon the concept that insulin shock accomplishes its results through a pre-conclusive or convulsive mechanism alone (Wortis[11]). If this is true, the treatment should give the same results. It does not, however, and the percentage of remissions is smaller and more transitory. Of course, metrazol is more easily controlled and does not produce complications or death except in an infinitesimal percentage of cases. Therefore, if we may adopt for a comparison of results between insulin and metrazol the method of arriving at cancer statistics through the comparison of surgery and radiation, we find the same considerations. Radiation and metrazol do not cause death. Surgery and insulin do, occasionally. While the former have lower percentages of results, the two methods of approach may give almost equal results when we take mortality rates into consideration. The important question of cost also should be borne in mind. Metrazol treatments are much less expensive b e c a u s e they are quickly given, the entire procedure being over in 15 to 20 minutes, making prolonged special nursing care unnecessary. In insulin therapy, special nurses are required for at least six hours every day that a treatment is given.

It was approximately three years ago that Sakel[1] began to use the treatment and make his first reports. The use of the treatment soon spread to surrounding territories., then to this country. The pioneers who have carried on the work and made frequent reports are Muller[2], Ross[3], Glueck[4], Wortis[5], Young[6], and others. Wilson[7] made the most comprehensive report ever attempted in English, and today the psychiatrists all over the world have settled down to the steady use of this treatment on all cases where it is indicated. A complete scientific investigation by every possible means of the reactions of the patients before, during and after treatment has been and is being made in order to solve the many practical and theoretical problems presented.

The treatment is proved. The good effects are known. That it is an improvement over every other form or previously used therapy is brought out conclusively by Whitehead[9]. In a review of the prognosis in dementia praecox cases, he reviewed the work with this type of case at the Utica State Hospital. He concludes from record study that insulin shock therapy is twice as efficient as older forms of treatment. Analysis of cases of schizophrenia admitted before i n s u l i n shock t h e r a p y was available, treated by the older methods, lead him to these conclusions. This has been the experience of all psychiatrists.

Occupational, p s y c h o- and suggestive therapy always seemed to bring about a more or less complete remission in approx-

imately 25 per cent of all cases. An additional 25 per cent showed marked clinical improvement. The percentage of relapses in these cases, however, was probably greater than that of those treated by newer methods.

In evaluating results from insulin shock therapy, we must take several factors into consideration: first, the duration of the illness; secondly, the type of manifestations of the disease; thirdly, the expected mortality and complications. These criteria are very similar to those used by the American Cancer Committee to evaluate the various treatment procedures used in the therapy of various cancerous conditions.

DURATION

So many factors enter into this aspect of the case that it is difficult to interpret properly each individual case. No one is justified in approaching the individual case in a dogmatic attitude as to prognosis, type of reactions desired, or duration of treatment. Every case is still an experimental problem which must be reviewed each day so that needed changes in approach can be made as necessary. Since duration is the governing factor in prognosticating, it is important that we should always know the exact duration of symptoms. The only exact source of information is the patient, and these patients are notorious for their reticence about themselves. Usually the patient must be forced to come to the physician for advice and treatment. American families usually do not force their relatives until the situation has become so intolerable that the patient cannot be controlled at home. If we date onset at the period of onset of uncontrollability we fall into pitfalls, because the patient may have had symptoms for months or even years before the family became aware of them. One of our cases had had auditory hallucinations for five y e a r s before anyone realized it except the patient. She told nobody about them, and it was only after they disappeared under insulin treatment that she discussed them with us and the true story came out. The onset of acute mania, agitation and severely abnormal behavior may not be the onset of the disease at all, but rather a further progression of a condition which has been present for a long time.

Everyone makes the same report. Cases of less than six months' duration, if properly treated, have an 85 per cent chance for improvement or remission. Our personal results, however, cause us to feel that if it were possible to date onset exactly, many of our tables of results would have to be changed, and that every case which has been having symptoms for less than six months would show a complete remission if properly treated.

TYPES OF MANIFESTATIONS

The type of case must enter into the above theoretical concept. Sakel divides his cases into three groups: stuporous, paranoid, and katatonic. Stuporous (depressed) cases are treated by termination of the daily treatment in the state of precomatose excitement. This frequently leads to a reversal of the picture, the development of mania and increased psychomotor activity, suggesting Kraeplin's mixed type of manic-depressive psychosis. The patient is then given prolonged precomatose somnolence, and the remission may be expected very shortly after the change has occurred.

Paranoid cases are carried into complete coma, with the hope that convulsions may develop. Katatonic cases are given either coma or prolonged pre-comatose somnolence by repeated injections of i n s u l i n during the day. Thus, we see that the dosage of insulin and the management of the patient must be changed frequently, perhaps daily, to meet indications. In all cases, a reversal of the previous abnormal picture is desired, and where that is accomplished remission can be expected. Stuporous cases that develop increased, even abnormal, psychomotor activity are well on the road to recovery, although the apparent increased severity of the disease may discourage the inexperienced staff, and terrify the relatives. Katatonic cases give us the best prognosis, because their insulin reactions can be made to force them into increased activity. Frequently, however, we find that the katatonic becomes a paranoid under treatment. This is unfortunate, because paranoid trends are more difficult to remove. On the other

hand, they are more favorable than simple stupor.

Hebephrenic mannerisms disappear, the patient clears quickly, usually, but is not as stable in recovery as the paranoid and katatonic types.

Therefore, we may list our symptoms in order of prognostic favorability as follows: katatonia, hebephrenia, paranoia and depression. Agitation and increased psychomotor activity always resolve although, perhaps, only temporarily, to return when treatment is terminated. The patient must be relieved of all symptoms, and if the correction of behavior abnormalities, which are the dramatic admission s y m p t o m s, leaves an apparently new picture of fixed ideation and reaction abnormalities, the prognosis must be revised, because fixed delusions and schizophrenic reaction mechanisms do not respond as well as behavior motor abnormalities.

We can say that while the type of manifestations and the duration may lead us to make a rather exact prognosis, it must be carefully explained to the family that developments in the individual case may alter the prognosis completely. This reversal may take a pleasant turn, as in a recent case admitted for treatment. After study we predicted that six to eight weeks of intensive treatment might be required. She returned to normal after her second shock, and has remained so ever since.

COMPLICATIONS AND MORTALITY

When we give a patient insulin shock we are inducing upon him a serious physical and functional illness, and doing it from four to seven times a week. The condition is so theoretically dangerous that in the early days of insulin and diabetes many precautions were taken to prevent the slightest reaction. Intravenous glucose owes much of its widespread use in many conditions to the fact that it was first commercially introduced and made widely available as part of these precautions.

Complications, of course, can be expected. Some are serious, some are not. As our experience grows, something we now try to avoid may be induced. Convulsions have passed through this sequence, and today some men are actually producing convulsions at the proper stage of insulin shock. Types of complications and their treatment are not in the scope of this paper.

We may say that alertness, experience and preparedness are the best safeguards. Alertness is vital in order to comprehend a complication in its earliest stage, even at times almost before it begins to develop. Temperature, pulse, blood pressure and respiration are taken every 15 minutes. Any change, no matter how minor, is recorded and the patient is observed constantly by trained physicians and nurses. Experience is necessary to interpret the above observations so that the treatment may be interrupted before any dangerous conditions can develop. Preparedness, by having at the bedside of the individual every possible medicinal aid on the individual shock trays, frequently means the difference between life and death. A second's delay or a second's neglect may turn the balance against the patient.

Complete laboratory and X-ray studies must be made. Laboratory investigations should be carried on to interpret progress, protect the patient, and investigate scientifically the treatment by the accumulation of data. X-rays may be of value only rarely to check upon a pneumonic process, but when they are needed they are important. Improper or incomplete preliminary studies may mean a great difference.

All of these precautions do not eliminate danger, and deaths do occur. But competent practitioners report large series, running into thousands, of individual shocks with no mortalities. The percentage of deaths is lower than the expected mortality rates in any form of major surgery.

CONCLUSIONS

1. Insulin shock is a vast improvement over previous methods of treating schizophrenia and, at the present time, it is probably the treatment of choice.

2. An exact prognosis cannot be made. Therefore, every suspected case should be treated so as to give the patient the only opportunity available.

3. Early treatment gives the best results.

4. The treatment is dangerous, but not as dangerous as major surgery. Proper precautions eliminate almost all dangers.

BIBLIOGRAPHY

1. Sakel, Manfred: Schizophreniebehandlung mittels Insulin-Hypoglykamie sowie hypoglykamischer Schocks. Wien. med. Wochnschr., 84:1211, Nov. 3; 1265, Nov. 17, 1299, Nov. 24; 1326, Dec. 1; 1353, Dec. 8; 1383, Dec. 15; 1401, Dec. 22, 1934.

2. Muller, M.: Hypoglycamie-Behandlung der Schizophrenie. Schweiz. med. Wschr., 66:929-935, 1936.

3. Ross, John R.: Report of the Hypoglycemic Treatment in New York State Hospitals. The American Journal of Psychiatry, Vol. 94, No. 1, July, 1937.

4. Glueck, Bernard: The Effect of the Hypoglycemic Therapy on the Psychotic Process. The American Journal of Psychiatry, Vol. 94, No. 1, July, 1937.

5. Wortis, Joseph: On the Response of Schizophrenic Subjects to hypoglycemic Insulin Shock. Journal of Nervous and Mental Diseases, 84:497, November, 1936.

6. Young, G. Alexander, et al.: Experiences with the Hypoglycemic Shock Treatment of Schizophrenia. The American Journal of Psychiatry, Vol. 94, No. 1, July, 1937.

7. Wilson, Isabel G. H.: A Study of Hypoglycaemic Shock Treatment in Schizophrenia. London, 1937.

8. Meduna, L. von: Zeitschrift fur die gesamte Neurologie und Psychiatrie, February 21, 1935.

9. Whitehead, Duncan: Prognosis in Dementia Praecox. The Psychiatric Quarterly, 11:383, (July) 1937.

10. Angyal and Gyarfas: Arch. f. Psychiat. 106:1, 1936.

11. Wortis, Joseph: Metrazol Versus Insulin in the Treatment of Schizophrenia. The Journal of the American Medical Association, Vol. 109, No. 18: C-1470, October 30, 1937.

---o---

Fractures of the Lower End of the Humerus in Children*

JOHN E. McDONALD, M.D.
TULSA, OKLA.

These injuries furnish an important problem in juvenile fractures. A thorough study of my own cases plus a study of reports of a large series of cases by Speed,

*Read before the Section on Surgery, Annual Meeting, Oklahoma State Medical Association, Tulsa, May, 1937.

Eliason, Wilson and others furnished the information for discussion in this paper. It was learned that about 82 per cent of these injuries occur in young people under 20 years of age and 62 per cent under the age of ten. From this study it is gratifying to see the results which follow early and proper handling in contrast to the disappointing and unfortunate complications which too often follow their improper management. Recent years have seen rapid progress in the number of good results. Formerly, it was considered to be the rule to have some deformity, while now we expect to have good anatomical and functional results.

To better understand the problem of handling fractures in this area, it is essential to have an accurate knowledge of the anatomy around the elbow joint. The lower end of the humerus is composed of four separate epiphyses; the capitellum, the internal epicondyle, the trochlea, and the external epicondyle which occur in the order named. The capitellum appears from the sixth to the twelfth month in life, the internal epicondyle about the sixth year, the trochlear about the tenth year, and the external condyle during the twelfth year. Except for the internal epicondyle, the remaining epiphyses are united by the thirteenth year. The entire lower epiphyses is firmly united to the diaphysis during the sixteenth and seventeenth years. Ossification of the lower end of the humerus is complete about the twenty-second year of life.

In many children the elbow joint may normally be hyperextended, the average range of extension being about 186 degrees. The forearm does not extend in a straight line with the arm, therefore, we have what is known as a carrying angle of the forearm. The intercondylar line is at right angles to the axis of the humerus but is oblique to the axis of the forearm. This angle is about 170 degrees in boys and about 168 in girls, the difference being in the wider pelvis of the female. When the arms are hanging free at the sides, the external condyles are on an anterior plane to the internal condyles. If the forearm is acutely flexed by carrying the hand to the corresponding shoulder, the natural relationship has not changed. If, however, the flexed forearm is carried across the chest, the arm being moved forward in front of the body, the internal condyle will be rotated approximately 20 degrees. This is an important anatomical fact and is responsible for cubitus varus or "gun stock"

deformity so often seen in supracondylar fractures.

The bony landmarks at the elbow are the internal, the external condyles and the olecranon process of the ulna. With the forearm in extension, the t h r e e prominences are on a straight line when it is in the flexed position, they form a triangle with the intercondylar notch as the base. When the forearm is at right angles to the humerus, these three points are on the same plane with it.

The capsule of the elbow joint is attached to the h u m e r u s above the epiphyseal line and a great many fractures in this region pass into the joint space which is a factor in the production of extreme swelling often seen in fractures around the elbow.

The actual structure of the bone itself in the lower end of the humerus makes it susceptible to fracture. The change in shape from a triangular shaft to a thin flat one makes it weaker and more easily broken. The forward angulation of the distal end, the change from compact to cancellous bone, and the attachment of powerful muscles are also factors to be considered. The frequency with which the elbow is exposed to trauma is another reason.

The types of fractures to be considered in this paper are supracondylar, dicondylar, condylar with either internal or external condyles and internal epicondyle.

The supracondylar fracture occurs across the lower humerus above the olecranon fossa and is extra capsular. This fracture usually produces a definite deformity with posterior, upward, and occasionally outward displacement of the distal fragment. Swelling is an early and important sign in these injuries. It is the result of tearing of a rich plexus of veins around the lower extremity of the humerus and the adjacent soft parts. Bleb formation is frequently seen in the skin from these injuries.

If they are diagnosed early and are reasonably well reduced, union takes place rapidly with little or no limitation of motion in the joint or disturbance with future growth.

Immobilization in acute flexion with the arm supported at the side of the body is the method of choice. Turning the arm across the chest is dangerous. Diligent observation for normal circulation is essential. This position is maintained for approximately ten days, when the forearm is brought down to a right angle and passive motion begun. As soon as X-ray evidence of bony union is found, the splint may be removed and active motion instituted.

The dicondylar injury, being only slightly lower, involves the olecranon fossa and extends into the joint capsul. The same problems of treatment are encountered as in the previous type.

True condylar types occur almost entirely in children. They are divided into the internal condyle and external condyle with the epicondyle, capitellum, and trochlea occurring with the latter. Both condyles are the attachment of strong groups of muscles. From the lateral, arise the extensors and supinators and from the medial, the flexors and pronators. A goodly number of these fractured fragments are pulled down and rotated while some are only moderately displaced.

In these fractures, experience has taught us that we are facing a much more serious situation. Non-unions and mal-unions are common and end with various complications. Imperfect reductions in this area result in increasing deformity and distortion of the elbow. Due to failure of the affected fragment to develop and because of disturbed epiphyseal growth, cubitus valgus and varus result. This condition produces unstable and painful joints with frequent disturbance of the ulnar nerve. Limited motion is another likely complication.

These complications may be avoided by early and accurate reduction. If no marked displacement has occurred, a closed reduction is possible. If good apposition is not obtained, open reduction should be done as early as possible with accurate replacement of the fragment and good internal fixation. I have used the wire nail with good results. It is easily removed later under local anaesthesia.

In the delayed cases further trouble arises. I believe the fragments should be replaced by open reduction and internal fixation. Usually good bony union may be expected in anatomical position. Definite

distortion of the epiphyseal growth results with a decreased size and irregularity of the condyle, premature ossification of the epiphysis, and varying degrees of varus and valgus deformity. Permanent limitation of motion is usual.

Avulsion of the internal epicondyle, being an epiphyseal injury, is also to be considered. It results when lateral strain is placed on the strong flexor group of muscles. There is usually considerable displacement and closed reduction is difficult due to muscle pull. Best end results are obtained when an open reduction is done with internal fixation.

When not properly reduced, limitation of extension results due to blocking of the olecranon. Pain and tenderness are present over the affected area. Ulnar neuritis may occur.

The usual complications of these fractures may be classified as deformity with continuous or recurrent pain, limitation of motion and instability, nerve injuries or delayed neuritis; Volkmann's contracture; and traumatic myositis ossificans.

Wedge supracondylar osteotomies will frequently correct the varus and valgus deformities when the fracture has already united and there is satisfactory motion. Condyles must not be removed in children. Frequently a displaced external condyle continues to grow and furnishes stability to the head of the radius. These may unite if the ends are freshened and internal fixation is established.

Arthroplasty is definitely contra-indicated in children and may not be used to relieve limitation of motion.

Acute nerve injuries, such as impingement, stretching, or actual severence, are uncommon but do occur in fractures in this area. The ulnar and radial are most frequently involved. Care should be taken to observe their condition before treatment is begun. Frequently, after reduction, the tension is relieved and the condition improves. Neurological consultation combined with electrical reactions may avoid considerable future trouble. Delayed ulnar neuritis may be relieved by anterior transplantation.

One of the most damaging complications,

Volkmann's contracture, is easily prevented by proper care. The position of acute flexion with interference of circulation is often associated with this lesion. Occasionally, sufficient swelling may occur in the elbow to affect normal circulation without any external fixation. The acute flexed position without replacing the fragments may also produce it.

Pain is the warning symptom and usually becomes severe about two hours before the onset of this condition. The circulation must be watched most carefully. In the presence of this danger signal, the bandage should be released as fractures in good position seldom produce severe pain. If the condition is allowed to progress, a hopelessly crippled arm results.

Traumatic myositis ossificans or ossified hematoma may result from these fractures. I believe it best to delay removal for a few weeks so as to lessen its possible recurrence.

SUMMARY

(1) Accurate knowledge of anatomical details around the elbow is essential for physicians handling these fractures.

(2) Early diagnosis and accurate reduction is essential to obtain good anatomical and functional results.

(3) Neglected cases produce serious and often irreparable deformities with markedly disturbed function.

* * * *

DISCUSSION

Dr. O'Donoghue: In my opinion, there is one point which deserves emphasis in the consideration of elbow fractures, and that is, that, in the child, the X-ray plate shows only the bone. Very often the center of ossification of the fragment may be so small that it appears on the X-ray film as a very small shadow. This small center may not appear to be displaced. If this factor is not recognized, the injury may be minimized and not treated adequately until later developments reveal the true condition. Careful examination and interpretation of X-ray films, in conjunction with clinical findings, will demonstrate this condition in its true light.

---------o---------

Abdominal Pain During Pregnancy*

MILTON J. SERWER, A.B., M.D.
OKLAHOMA CITY, OKLA.

Abdominal pain is one of the most common symptoms complained of during pregnancy. In a series of 300 consecutive cases taken from office files over 95 per cent of the patients complained of some form of abdominal pain. While some of these conditions existed previously, the majority had their onset during gestation. This pain was influenced by many factors and was variable both as to character and severity.

I shall attempt to discuss only those conditions associated with, or related to, pregnancy. Almost any condition may occur or be aggravated by pregnancy. Those re-

*Read before the Section on Obstetrics and Pediatrics, Annual Meeting, Oklahoma State Medical Association, Oklahoma City, May, 1935.

lieved by it, and temporarily—as dysmenorrhea, visceroptosis, and ptosis of the kidney—are relatively few. Since most women have their threshold for pain lowered during this period, many conditions formerly not noticed are suddenly brought into prominence. De Lee once stated, "Women are three-quarters nervous system," and it is this three-quarters that physicians so consistently ignore. In general, it may be said that the neurotic and the asthenic, tall, slender type of women are much more sensitive to, and complain of more of all types of abdominal pain, especially that of the abdominal wall.

PAIN IN THE ABDOMINAL WALL

The most frequent location of abdominal

wall pain is across the anterior portion of the lower abdomen. At times this may be just a tingling or numbness, but usually it is a marked aching or shooting pain sufficient to limit the activity of the woman. It is first noticed about the fifth month of pregnancy and increases in severity until the eighth month, at which time it decreases. Though the condition is due to pressure from within the abdomen, as in pressure from the foetus when the woman has been too active, or in pressure from over distension of the uterus, as in multiple pregnancy, polyhydramnios, or hydatidiform mole, tenderness can be demonstrated to be in the abdominal wall. By gently stroking the hand over the lower abdomen, tenderness, often severe, can be obtained. The symptom can be readily relieved by bed rest and an abdominal support.

Pain across the upper abdomen is most pronounced after the sixth month and is due to the same factors causing pain in the lower abdominal wall. The condition is further aggravated by a flaring of the lower chest wall due to the growth of the uterus. The condition may be relieved by Fowler's position when resting or by the erect posture. The flaring recedes following delivery.

Pain about the navel occurs most frequently in the latter months of pregnancy in multipara who have had frequent pregnancies. The abdominal wall in this region becomes very thin and is painful and tender. Beneath the thin skin wall the uterus can be made out. Slight touch of the skin elicits pain. The condition is relieved by the application of adhesive strips. The pain does not recur after parturition.

I have frequently noticed pain over the region of a fibroid. I believe this to be due to the pressure of the tumor against the abdominal wall with irritation of the wall resulting, rather than a referred symptom, since the tenderness is localized directly over the tumor.

Hernias of the abdominal wall may cause intense pain and tenderness. The condition is not aggravated by the pregnancy but, on the contrary, is relieved by it and usually is self-limited. This is especially true of inguinal, femoral, and umbilical hernias. The growth of the uterus grad-

ually pushes the intestines and omentum to the upper abdomen, sealing over temporarily the hernial opening with relief of symptoms.

Pain complained of in the posterior quadrants of the abdomen on close examination will usually be found to be due to a pathological condition of the non-demonstrative areas of the peritoneal cavity and not in the abdominal wall.

I have never noticed any aggravation of pain in an abdominal incision during pregnancy. On the contrary, it is seldom complained of when most expected.

PAIN IN THE PERITONEAL CAVITY

Pain in the peritoneal cavity is almost always a secondary process. To better understand the mechanism of the localization of the pain one must first understand the innervation of the peritoneum.

For practical purposes it is very useful to divide the abdominal parietal lining into demonstrative and non-demonstrative areas. The demonstrative area is the larger and includes all the lining of the abdominal cavity except the pelvis and the central and inferior part of the posterior abdominal wall. The non-demonstrative or silent area comprises the pelvis and that part of the posterior abdominal wall bounded roughly by the ascending colon, the descending colon, and the transverse mesocolon. The distinction is a clinical one, but has an anatomical basis in a relatively free or meager afferent nerve supply. The non-demonstrative area is probably supplied chiefly via the sympathetic system, the demonstrative area, from the main somatic nerves. In the renal region there are more nerves in the connective tissue behind the kidneys than in the peritoneum in front of these organs, indeed, the latter region should be included in the non-demonstrative areas.

The manifestations of pain produced depend partly on the nature of the irritant. Since normal parietal peritoneum is almost insensitive to touch, though the deeper tissues are more so, clear non-infective and non-toxic fluids, serous ascites, or sanguinous fluid resulting from the rupture of a gestational sac, do not cause any irritation other than the mere mechanical effect of the pressure or sudden flooding. Quite different is that resulting from bacterial or toxic irritation, as from appendicitis, salpingitis, necrosing fibroids, infected ectopic gestation sacs, twisted ovarian tumors, etc. In these the peritoneum is painful, tender, and congested.

The local pain due to parietal irritation varies according to the part affected. The non-demonstrative areas furnish little localizing indication of acute irritation. Thus it is possible for the most serious pathological process to be proceeding within the pelvis or against some parts of the posterior abdominal wall without there being any spontaneous, definite, localizing symptoms. The sensitivity is greatest in the anterior part of the abdominal cavity. .

Adhesions when present may c a u s e sharp pains, often knife-like, and described by the woman as a pulling sensation. This is due to traction as a result of the growth of the uterus and adnexae. The pain continues throughout the entire pregnancy and is relieved only at parturition. Indeed, due to the subsequent relaxation, the pain from adhesions may be entirely relieved. When the uterus is incarcerated, abortion is the usual termination.

PAIN FROM THE GENITAL TRACT

Extra-uterine pain. The most common uterine pain complained of is that localized over the pubis. It is frequently described as being a soreness or aching across the entire lower abdomen and is due to the jarring of the presenting part. It usually occurs in cephalic presentations, but may be present in a breech presentation when the breech is hyperactive. The pain usually occurs about the seventh month and subsides when the presenting part engages. It can be relieved by an abdominal support.

Retroverted uterus is the cause of frequent backache during the second and third months. The condition is self-limited after the latter months due to the uterus growing out of the pelvis. Attempts at correction by means of pessaries are not usually advised due to the frequency of abortion. In cases of incarceration the pain is great and the patient acutely ill. Abortion at the third or fourth month is the rule. The condition is markedly aggravated by urinary retention and an associated overflow of the bladder with incontinence resulting. The disturbance is partly caused by pressure on the neck of the bladder and urethra by the cervix, resulting in mechanical interference with urination, and partly to pressure by the cervix on the veins of the b l a d d e r producing congestion and oedema.

In much the same manner suspension of the uterus causes distress, except that the pain persists as a rule throughout the entire pregnancy, and the tendency to abort is increased. This is especially true in any operative procedure which plicates the round ligaments and less likely when the round ligaments are pulled through the inguinal canal.

Braxton-Hicks contractions u s u a l l y cause little discomfort. Occasionally in the nervous, asthenic type of woman the pain may become very noticeable. This is especially true at the time when the menses would be due. On one occasion I have seen morphine required.

Abruptio placenta, with its occasional sequela the Couvelaire uterus, is perhaps one of the most serious of all conditions causing acute pain in the uterine wall. The pain usually comes on suddenly, is sharp and knife-like, and can be localized over the attachment of the placenta. As the disease progresses the entire uterine wall may be involved, with resulting board-like rigidity, sharp, severe pain and marked tenderness over the entire uterine wall, followed by a dull aching pain, nausea and vomiting, and signs of hemorrhage and shock.

Interstitial and intra-uterine angular pregnancies are characterized by pain of varying severity, coming on in the first months of pregnancy. The pain is well localized to the horn of the uterus and the region is tender. Should the pregnancy develop into the uterine cavity the subsequent course is normal. Should it extend into the tube the course is that of an ectopic pregnancy.

Another common cause of pain is uterine fibroids. Since they are frequently symptomless they are much more common than is usually believed. Those giving trouble fall into three groups:

a. The subserous, pedunculated fibroid

that may give rise to various mechanical changes, so causing sudden, sharp, severe pain. The proper course I believe to be to treat the symptoms conservatively, and this failing, to resort to surgery. Leslie Williams, however, recommends operative removal in all cases because of the danger of twisting of the pedicle, causing acute abdominal symptoms with danger of miscarriage; also, because of the slight danger of miscarriage when operated on in the quiescent stage.

b. The interstitial fibroids which cause distortion of the uterus and pressure symptoms. These should be treated conservatively because of the danger of miscarriage.

c. The fibroid may be of variable size, single or multiple, and may undergo degeneration with symptoms of sudden pain and tenderness, vomiting, fever, etc. Conservative treatment is usually recommended as laparotomy and myomectomy are prone to cause abortion. The diagnosis is established by the occurrence of a sudden tenderness in a fibroid which has been previously known as a painless tumor. There is no added liability to abortion. The symptoms seldom last over a few days following bed rest.

Rupture of the uterus, though rare, is of sufficient seriousness to warrant its mention. The condition usually occurs in the scars of a previous Cesarean section (of which about four per cent rupture), and may be partial or complete. It is characterized by sudden uterine pain with vomiting, followed by symptoms of hemorrhage and shock. Treatment usually consists of immediate operative procedures.

Intra-uterine pain. Rapid stretching of the uterus, as in acute polyhydramnios, hydatidiform mole, or multiple pregnancy, is a frequent cause of severe pain. The sudded increase of amniotic fluid is an uncommon condition, but simple as to diagnosis, as it is usually sudden, and is associated with an albuminuria and other signs of toxemia. The pain due to chronic polyhydramnios, multiple pregnancy, or mole, is much less severe since the onset of the condition is more gradual.

As described above, the presentation of the foetus, as breech or transverse, may cause localized pain within the uterus.

Disease of the decidua is an important factor in the causation of intra-uterine pain. The role of abruptio placenta has already been discussed.

Endometritis is an occasional cause of intra-uterine pain. The uterus is tender and contractions may be extremely painful. This is called "rheumatism of the uterus," and may be associated with hyperemesis. When acute, there may be fever, malaise, and a bloody discharge. Foetal death with abortion may result, or the ovum may be transformed into a hydatidiform mole.

Submucous fibroids usually do not cause pain. Acting as a foreign body with associated pressure symptoms, uterine contractions are frequently initiated, with abortion the rule.

Pain in the Adnexae. One of the common pains in pregnancy is that due to stretching of the round ligaments. It is often severe. The pain may begin as early as the fourth month and continue throughout the course of gestation. It is complained of over the regions of the attachments of the ligaments in the groins, and on either side of the uterus. It may be felt only at one site of attachment or only on one side. Palpation of the round ligaments over the regions of pain are usually quite tender. Torsion of the uterus has been suggested as the cause of unilateral pain. A corset so designed as to support the lower abdomen and to lift the uterus will frequently give relief.

Ectopic pregnancy is the most important cause of adnexal pain. The acute pain is caused by the erosion of the chorionic villi into the blood vessels with the addition of pressure on the adjacent areas. Though several terminations are possible, the most common is that in which the patient suffers for some time with abdominal uneasiness, pain, occasional faintness, and hemorrhagic vaginal discharges. Rupture, though uncommon, is a serious complication and should be treated as an emergency. This occurs usually between the sixth and tenth weeks. There is a history of sudden onset of violent pain, a feeling of something giving way, accompanied by faintness, vomiting, pallor, unexpectedly rapid pulse, collapse, and uterine bleeding.

Oophoritis or salpingitis rarely flare up during pregnancy. However, when this does occur the situation is usually serious and may entail surgical intervention.

The most common cause of pain in the ovary is that due to an ovarian cyst in which there has occurred (a) twisting of the pedicle (in about 15 per cent), (b) pressure, or (c) degeneration. The pain occurring in a twisted pedicle is acute, severe, and is followed by signs of shock and collapse. Treatment is usually surgical. Eskridge states that torsion of the pedicle occurs most frequently before the fifth month and during the puerperium, rarely in the interval.

Rupture of a cyst is usually devoid of pain and may be associated only with a feeling of uneasiness and a rise of temperature.

The pain coming from degeneration is usually mild, since the condition is chronic and is followed by signs and symptoms of toxemia.

Sclerosis of the tunica albuginea is believed to be an occasional cause of ovarian pain, since during pregnancy oedema, vascularization, and decidua-like formations tend to cause an enlargement of the ovary. This is hindered by the sclerotic capsule.

Varicosities of the broad ligaments occasionally are a cause of abdominal pain. The condition increases in frequency with the number of pregnancies. The pain is complained of as a dull aching sensation in either or both lower abdominal quadrants. However, it is more common on the left. This is believed to be due to the more frequent torsion of the uterus to the right. Examination elicits tenderness over the broad ligament region. The pain usually increases in severity as the pregnancy progresses. Diagnosis is aided by the presence of varicosities elsewhere, the presence of a uterine bruit on the affected side, and the difference in tenderness during pelvic examination when lying down or standing upright. Relief from pain can be elicited often by placing the patient on the affected side, thus relieving the congestion and tenseness. The knee-chest position gives relief when both sides are involved.

PAIN IN THE URINARY TRACT

Pyelitis of pregnancy is a frequent cause of abdominal pain. The condition has a predilection for the right side. This is believed by some to be due to pressure of the uterus on the ureters, especially the right, since torsion is more frequent on that side. However, the most accepted belief is that the uterus does not cause obstruction by direct pressure but by causing a twist in the ureter during the enlargement of the uterus. Leslie Williams suggests that the ureteral obstruction is probably due to diminution of the lumen of the fibrous ureteral canal deep to the uterine vessels in the loose tissue of the broad ligament. This can be demonstrated during a Wertheim operation to be due to the increased vascularity of the pelvic organs during pregnancy. The condition is more common in a prolapsed kidney. The end result, in any case, is stagnation in the renal pelvis.

The same author groups pyelitis under three headings:

1. The renal type, in which pain is localized to the back and loin, usually the right, with associated fever, chills, headaches, and tenderness in the costo-phrenic angle.

2. The abdominal type, with acute abdominal pain of such severity that the differential diagnosis is often difficult.

3. The generalized type, in which abdominal pain is slight and the patient presents the picture of a generalized sepsis.

Associated with pyelitis is a ureteritis. Pain, often sharp and knife-like, is complained of along the course of the ureter and referred down the inner side of the thigh. There is tenderness along the course of the ureter which at times may be palpated vaginally. Blakely states that pain referred to either side of the umbilicus is diagnostic of urinary pathology. This has not been my experience.

Pain in the bladder is occasionally met with. It may be due to pressure, previously mentioned, or to infection. The pain is sharp, knife-like, and is well localized over the bladder aread. A mild non-septic inflammation of the trigone is common in the early months of pregnancy and induces a frequency of urination with no further symptoms. When the cystitis is severe the pain is intense with frequent burning on urination, pain following emptying of the bladder, and malaise, chills, and fever.

PAIN IN THE GASTRO-INTESTINAL TRACT

The most common conditions complained of in the intestinal tract during pregnancy are constipation, intestinal colic, and flatulence.

Pain due to gaseous distension is frequently complained of over the upper abdomen along the course of the transverse c o l o n and occurs usually between the fourth and sixth months, seldom later.

Pain is frequently complained of over the caecum. This is a region of frequent low-grade colitis and chronic irritation of the appendix, brought into prominence by the lowered threshold of pain existing during pregnancy. A diagnosis of chronic appendicitis is frequently made. The condition is seldom present after the fourth month.

The most serious causes of acute epigastric pain are the toxemias of pregnancy and cardiac decompensation. That it is located in the liver can be demonstrated by Murphy percussion which causes tenderness. Lane-Roberts suggests the pain in a toxemia may be due to the production of areas of focal necrosis in the liver. Acute epigastric pain in the presence of a toxemia should make for a guarded prognosis.

An attack of severe coughing or vomiting may evoke sharp upper abdominal pain through irritation of the diaphragm. It is frequently referred to the subscapular and intrascapular areas, because of the reflex innervation.

Pain in the right upper quadrant, demonstrated on Murphy percussion to be in the liver, is often complained of in the two latter months of gestation in a right breech presentation. It is due to direct pressure of the head against the liver.

Constipation usually causes little pain, if any, in the sigmoid colon or rectum. However, it may cause a proctitis by formation of hemorrhoids, resulting in an a c u t e, sharp pain in that region.

CONCLUSION

In concluding let me stress the importance of the proper evaluation of pain, not only from the standpoint of symptoms and physical findings, but also with regard to the mental state of the woman. A due consideration of the latter, so frequently disregarded by the physician, is often of infinite help in directing proper treatment; thus building up within the woman's mind confidence in the physician under whose care she may be.

BIBLIOGRAPHY

1. Adair and Stieglitz: Obstetric Medicine, first edition, Lea and Febriger, Philadelphia, 1934.

2. Blakely, S. B.: Abdominal Pain in Pregnancy, J.A.M.A. 101:970, 1933.

3. Cope, Zachary: Clinical Research in Acute Abdominal Disease, second edition, Oxford University Press, London, 1927.

4. De Lee, Joseph B.: Principles and Practice of Obstetrics, sixth edition, W. B. Saunders Company, Philadelphia, 1933.

5. Kerr, Ferguson, Young, Hendry: Obstetrics and Gynecology, second edition, William Wood and Company, Baltimore, 1933.

6. Lane-Roberts, C. S.: Abdominal Pain in Pregnancy, The Lancet 215:1288-1290 (December 22) 1928.

7. Williams, Leslie: Abdominal Pain in Pregnancy, Clinical Journal 55:463-466, 1926.

———————O———————

1938 American Medical Association Meeting, San Francisco

When San Francisco was selected as the host city for the 1938 Annual Session of The American Medical Association, the profession of this Golden Gate metropolis promptly initiated plans for the comfort, pleasure and entertainment of all who come to that national meeting. A local executive committee on arrangements composed of five members with Dr. Howard Morrow as general chairman and Dr. Frederick C. Warnshuis as general secretary, and 18 sub-committees have been busy since July in developing plans and local arrangement details. Their objectives are the biggest, best, and most memorable annual session in the history of the American Medical association.

Atlantic City, Kansas City, Cleveland, Detroit, with their known facilities and attractions have been host cities in recent years, and have justified their selection as meeting places. However, and without disparagement, none of them possess the background, the setting, the resources, the history and romance, or the facilities that are found in San Francisco and in the great state of California —the Golden Bear Empire of the Pacific Coast. To reveal these, to extend California's and San Francisco's noted hospitality, and to cause those who plan to attend the 1938 session to experience ten days of profit and pleasure midst the environs of the annual meeting city, is the goal toward which the local profession is pointing.

The local committee on arrangements cordially invites the profession of the country to be San Francisco's guests this coming June. Decide now to attend the 1938 American Medical Association Meeting and plan accordingly. During the coming months an insight to some of the feature functions will be disclosed, but the final details and program of events will not be revealed until you arrive. You will long regret it if you fail to attend the coming national meeting. Talk it over tonight with the good wife and your professional associates, and join the party of your state members that is coming to San Francisco—June 12th to 17th, 1938.

THE JOURNAL
OF THE
Oklahoma State Medical Association
Issued Monthly at McAlester, Oklahoma, under direction of the Council.

| Vol. XXXI | JANUARY, 1938 | Number 1 |

DR. L. S. WILLOUR..................................Editor-in-Chief
McAlester, Oklahoma

DR. T. H. McCARLEY..................................Associate Editor
McAlester, Oklahoma

Entered at the Post Office at McAlester, Oklahoma, as second-class matter under the act of March 3rd, 1879.

This is the official Journal of the Oklahoma State Medical Association. All communications should be addressed to The Journal of the Oklahoma State Medical Association, McAlester Clinic, McAlester, Oklahoma. $4.00 per year; 40c per copy.

The editorial department is not responsible for the opinions expressed in the original articles of contributors.

Reprints of original articles will be supplied at actual cost provided request for them is attached to manuscripts or made in sufficient time before publication.

Articles sent this Journal for publication and all those read at the annual meetings of the State Association are the sole property of this Journal. The Journal relies on each individual contributor's strict adherence to this well-known rule of medical journalism. In the event an article sent this Journal for publication is published before appearance in The Journal the manuscript will be returned to the writer.

Failure to receive The Journal should call for immediate notification of the Editor, McAlester Clinic, McAlester, Oklahoma.

Local news of possible interest to the medical profession, notes on removals, changes of addresses, births, deaths and weddings will be gratefully received.

Advertising of articles, drugs or compounds unapproved by the Council on Pharmacy of the A. M. A., will not be accepted.

Advertising rates will be supplied on application.

It is suggested that wherever possible members of the State Association should patronize our advertisers in preference to others as a matter of fair reciprocity.

Printed by News-Capital Company, McAlester.

EDITORIAL

UNCLE SAM . . . DOCTOR

The medical and political worlds have been deeply stirred by proposals to put the government in the doctoring business. The American Medical Association bitterly opposes any such inroads, but the federal government is continuing to experiment on the side with "state medicine" in various forms.

A new experiment has just been started under the very eaves of the national capitol. And already a controversy is rumbling. This latest venture into mass-production medical practice has just completed its first month. It is called the group health association and offers to employes of the home owners loan corporation a definite amount of hospitalization and medical care in return for a regular monthly fee. The benefits are limited at present to the 2,000 HOLC employes in Washington and to date about half of them have signed up.

Here's how it works:

If the employe wants medical and hospital care for himself alone he pays $2.20 a month. An employe wanting care for himself and members of his family pays $3.30.

In return they get necessary hospitalization up to 21 days a year and medical attention from five physicians, including all varieties of surgery and medicine except treatment for certain prolonged diseases, such as cancer and advanced tuberculosis, where extensive confinement in an institution is required. Dental service is not included.

The federal part in the program came when the HOLC advanced $20,000 to finance establishment of a clinic and pledged $20,000 more for next year.

All members are urged to go at once to the clinic for a comprehensive physical examination since disease prevention is emphasized as a major purpose of the association.

But with 1,000 salaried potential patients taken from them, with a degree of federal assistance, it is perhaps not especially remarkable that the physicians in the district are disturbed.

The first protest is that the $40,000 contributed by the HOLC was an unauthorized contribution to "socialized m e d i c i n e." HOLC officials replied that sickness cost the Washington office $100,000 a year in lost time and that if increased medical attention would reduce the loss, the cost would be offset.

The second protest is that group medical practice will remove healthful competition among physicians and allow medicine to go stale, will reduce physicians' income to a minimum, will attract only second rate physicians and, in the end, will leave few but the poor and jobless to be treated by doctors in private practice. Moreover, physicians are worried over the prospect of extending membership to all federal employes in Washington (about 115,000), making Washington a medical desert for private practitioners.

Just what may come of it all is problematic. If the plan actually works out to effect a real saving to the HOLC and at the same time materially reduces the cost to the individual of medical attention without lowering the class of attention he receives, then "socialized medicine" may be here to stay.

But it won't come without a fight from the doctors who are left on the outside— and they certainly will represent a vast majority of practicing physicians of the country. And it's far too early to tell whether this "buy - a - club - membership-and-stay-well" plan will or can prove at all satisfactory—*Editorial from the Muskogee Daily Phoenix, December.*

* * * *

The above editorial is copied verbatim from a recent issue of the Muskogee Daily Phoenix and indicates exactly the reaction of the lay press to the matter of medical service for HOLC employes. This is not a threat of socialized medicine but IS socialized medicine sustained by both the moral and financial support of the federal government. The doctors that have been employed to do this work in Washington are not members of the District of Columbia Medical Society and I am informed they have had great difficulty in obtaining hospitalization for their patients as the standardized hospitals of Washington, D. C., refused to give these practitioners membership on the hospital staff.

There seems to be no limitation as to how far this proposition may be extended to employes of the federal government and can be made to include all federal employes throughout the United States. Should it be extended to include the employes in the city of Washington, and if the employes a c c e p t e d the proposition there would be very few left to be served by the regular practitioners of that city.

The Council has instructed the Secretary to write all of our congressional delegates in opposition to this $20,000.00 a year appropriation. Of course this appropriation has not been authorized by congress for this particular purpose, but it has been used without the consent of congress for the use of the HOLC socialized medical plan.

Any members of our State Association who are sufficiently interested should give this matter careful consideration and if you are opposed to this plan it might be well for you to communicate with your respective representatives in congress and let them know exactly your attitude in the matter before it grows to uncontrollable magnitude.

———o———

Editorial Notes—Personal and General

DR. T. J. McGRATH, Sayre, has been appointed County Health Superintendent of Beckham County, effective December 4, 1937, to succeed Dr. H. K. Speed, Jr., resigned.

———o———

News of the County Medical Societies

MURRAY County Medical Society held its annual meeting for election of officers on December 10, 1937. The following were elected: P. C. Annadown, president; Byron B. Brown, vice-president; Richard M. Burke, secretary-treasurer; C. W. Sprouse, delegate; A. Fowler, Jr., alternate delegate, and the councillors are George W. Slover, F. E. Sadler and P. V. Annadown. All of the above named reside at Sulphur, except Byron B. Brown, who lives in Davis.

———

PUSHMATAHA County Medical Society met January 3, 1938, at Antlers, for their first meeting of the year and election of officers, as follows: President, Dr. E. S. Patterson, Antlers; Secretary, Dr. D. W. Connally, Antlers; Drs. B. M. Huckabay, Antlers, and John S. Lawson, Clayton, were elected delegate and alternate, respectively, for the 1938 meeting.

———

CHOCTAW County Medical Society officers for 1938 are as follows: President, Dr. G. E. Harris, Hugo; secretary, Dr. F. L. Waters, Hugo.

———o———

RESOLUTIONS

Whereas Dr. G. W. Crawford was an active member of the Washington County Medical Society for several years—during which time he was a conscientious and tireless worker for the good of the Washington County Medical Society and for the medical profession as a whole—his contacts and association with us were of a most pleasant nature and we feel that we have lost a gifted and useful member of our profession.

BE IT RESOLVED that we express to his wife— his father, mother and other relatives our appreciation of his great worth, while living; and great loss in his death, and that we extend to his family an expression of deep sympathy which we individually and collectively feel in his death.

Committee: Dr. J. V. Athey,
Dr. J. P. Vansant,
Dec. 3, 1937.   Dr. L. D. Hudson.

ABSTRACTS : REVIEWS : COMMENTS
and CORRESPONDENCE

EYE, EAR, NOSE AND THROAT
Edited by Marvin D. Henley, M.D.
911 Medical Arts Building, Tulsa

Glaucoma at the Wills Hospital. Louis Lehrfeld, M.D., and Jacob Reber, M.D., Philadelphia. Archives of Ophthalmology, November, 1937.

Glaucoma is a rather broad term which includes all conditions in relation to the eyes which pathologically cause an increased intra-ocular tension. This lengthy paper is an analysis of case records at this hospital of glaucoma from 1926-1935. This report contains numerous tables in its classifications. The reading is interesting. The author's summary and conclusions are as follows:

"The records for 1,876 patients with glaucoma seen at the Wills Hospital during the ten years from 1926 to 1935 were examined and analyzed. This represents an incidence of glaucoma of 0.78 per cent in the patients with ocular conditions.

In the group, 413 cases of secondary glaucoma were found—22 per cent of the total series of cases.

Trauma and syphilis were the two most prominent factors in the causation of secondary glaucoma.

The development of a secondary rise in tension in any given ocular lesion is of grave significance; in 34 per cent of the cases of secondary glaucoma the condition ended in serious visual impairment.

Twenty-eight cases of congenital, and 20 cases of juvenile, glaucoma are reported.

One thousand, four hundred and fifteen cases of primary glaucoma are reported, 27.7 per cent cases of the congestive type and 72.3 per cent cases of the non-congestive type. These are analyzed on the basis of age, sex, refractive error, race, previous treatment, duration of symptoms and other factors.

The average age of the males in the series was 59.9 years, and that of the females, 59.7 years.

There appears to be no evidence for the theory that the Jewish race is more susceptible to glaucoma than other races.

There is evidence for the belief that acute attacks of glaucoma tend to occur during periods of colder, more unstable weather.

The results of the follow-up study and field work carried out among the patients living in Philadelphia are reported.

The results of treatment for the various types of glaucoma are presented from the standpoint of reduction of the intra-ocular tension during the period of observation, ranging from two to ten years.

It would appear that the Elliot trephine operation is the most efficient form of operative treatment.

A small control group of patients receiving no treatment is presented to show the ultimate ocular damage in untreated patients.

From the standpoint of public health, the most significant finding is the fact that 784 eyes had vision already reduced below 6/60 when the patients first presented themselves at the hospital. This is a commentary on the state of ignorance of the early signs and symptoms of glaucoma existent among patients, to some extent among family physicians and certainly among non-medical ocular practitioners.

Herpes Zoster Oticus. Dr. Durwin Hall Brownell, Ann Arbor, Mich. The Laryngoscope, November, 1937.

This is a clinical entity known variously as Hunt's syndrome, zona of the Greeks, cingula of the Romans and shingles by the lay English speaking people. 1835 gave the first published good description of herpes zoster. The lesion is in the sensory ganglia on the posterior spinal roots. It usually applies to a specific infectious disease. The term herpes zoster Oticus was first used by Koerner in 1904 and Gradenigo in 1907.

According to Hunt herpes zoster of the auricle was seen twice among 47,000 cases at the Manhattan Eye & Ear Hospital in ten years. It was seen once in 15,000 cases at the Brooklyn Eye & Ear Hospital in five years. In the Massachusetts Eye & Ear Infirmary there were 65,000 patients seen in a ten year period with 33 diagnosed cases of herpes zoster oticus. The disease is induced by a filtrable virus, which commonly inhabits the nasopharynx. Harvey Cushing's work of 1904, on areas of anaesthesia resulting from section of the proximal roots of the Gasserian ganglion and the upper cervical roots, is discussed. Also J. Ramsay Hunt's work on peripheral distribution of the sensory root of the seventh cranial nerve is reviewed. Herpes zoster oticus is occasionally associated with similar involvement of the ganglia of the fifth, eighth, ninth and tenth cranial nerves.

The disease is self limited; there is an indefinite prodromal period, which is characterized by malaise, mild gastrointestinal upset, occasionally fever, and localized hyperesthesia which later becomes painful. This stage usually lasts from two to five days. Pain which is the more constant symptom, is deep-seated in the ear and may be radiating, pulsating, lancinating, boring and prostrating in character. After a day or two the external auditory canal and auricle assume an indurated and edematous appearance; characteristic herpetic vesicles appear in the concha, over the antitragus, posterior canal wall and, occasionally on the tympanic membrane. These vesicles usually disappear in ten to 14 days with the gradual subsidence of pain which has persisted through this period. Hyperesthesia of the region may be present for six months or longer. Sometimes there occurs a facial palsy at about the time of the appearance of the eruption.

Treatment is entirely symptomatic. Suitable measures are used to prevent a secondary infection in the vesicles, i.e. dry open treatment, non-irritating powders, quickly drying antiseptics, etc. Hypnotics and narcotics are used to help control the pain.

Recovery is usually complete. There is no tendency to recurrence.

Chronic Sinusitis. W. Raymond McKenzie, M.D., F.A.C.S., Baltimore, Md. Southern Medical Journal, November, 1937.

The author makes a point that has probably occurred to every rhinologist. He says: "While one group is reporting good results from conservative, non-operative treatment, another group is reporting similar results accomplished by surgery — both groups equally sincere and honest in their opinions and deductions."

Mechanical obstructions to ventilation and drainage, such as, septal deviations, true hyperplasia or polypoid formations, can only be removed by surgery. In such cases, drops, sprays, douches, suction, medicated tampons, ionization, diathermy, irradiation, vaccines, non-specific protein therapy, etc., are ineffective. Where there is good ventilation and drainage and no abnormal tissue condition present, cases of so called chronic sinusitis, can be cleared up by some of the above mentioned means at least symptomatically, for years.

The author says that if the patient is properly examined and studied, and that if the operation best suited for that particular case is done by a competent surgeon, that the percentage of good results from "sinus surgery" will be equivalent to that of surgery in any other part of the body.

The author's operation is a combined intranasal, trans-antro-ethmo-sphenoidal one; done under general anaesthesia; time for a bilateral operation— two to four hours. His technic is briefly as follows: morphine and atropine pre-operative; a special type of airway that eliminates respiratory embarrassment; a gauze sponge in pharynx; epinephrine pack both nares; if the septum is deflected enough to interfere with the operation, a submucous resection is done; displacement of the middle turbinate away from the lateral wall and opening of the ethmoid cells; opening the antrum through the canine fossa; exeneration of antral contents including mucous membrane; removal of nasal wall of antrum beneath inferior turbinate (¼ x ½ in.); removal of anterior ethmoid cells via posterior antral wall; retract, with deep killian nasal speculum, middle turbinate inward away from outer wall; removed ethmoid cells under middle turbinate—this exposes entire ethmoid labyrinth; now looking straight through you see the exposed anterior wall of the sphenoid, which is opened. The ethmoids, sphenoid and maxillary antrum are thus converted into one large, smooth cavity, protected by the middle and inferior turbinates but opened well for drainage. Silk cheek stitches are removed in seven days. Gauze packs are removed in 24 hours and saline irrigations are started in 48 hours. Hospitalization lasts ten days. Treatments are continued eight to 12 weeks. Two hundred consecutive cases furnish data for this report. There were three deaths (one as a result of operation); 107 were classified as cured: 84 were improved, and six were unimproved.

The Pathology and Treatment of Carcinoma of the Bronchus. F. C. Ormerod, London. The Journal of Laryngology and Otology, November, 1937.

The result of 100 consecutive cases is summarized. In each case a portion of the growth was removed through the bronchoscope and proven histologically. They cover a period of about five and a half years. The average age was 51.7 years. There were 92 men and eight women. There were 58 on the right side and 42 on the left side. All tumors had an intrabronchial portion, varying in size from a nodule to a cauliflower-like mass occluding the main bronchus. In many the extrabronchial portion was the larger. In normal cases and in the presence of a neoplasm, after proper cocainization, passage of the bronchoscope produces very little tendency to cough. In the presence of inflammation such as lung abscess or bronchiectasis, it is much harder to do away with the cough reflex.

The differential diagnosis includes bronchiectasis, lung abscess, gumma, mediastinal tumour and benign tumour of the bronchus. An X-ray after lipiodol introduction makes obvious a bronchiectasis. In lung abscess it is harder to differentiate; the X-ray helps some by showing the amount of displacement of the mediastinum and the trachea; bronchoscopic examination shows presence or absence of tumor (granulation tissues may require histological examination); usually in lung abscess there is a flow of pus and the characteristic odor of broken down lung tissue. In the gumma you have the histological examination of the tissue, Wasserman and rapid disappearance of the growth under treatment. The author cautions not to overlook the possibility of a malignant growth even in the presence of a positive Wasserman. The appearance of the bronchus helps to differentiate the mediastinal growth. History usually helps in the benign and malignant growth.

The pathology of the tumours is discussed at length. Many microphotographs accompany the discussion.

The majority of these cases were too far advanced for a successful lobectomy or pneumonectomy. They were treated by insertion of either a container with radon in it or the implantation of seeds. Both methods have certain advantages. The difficulty with the use of the tube is keeping it in place and also the radon is concentrated at one point which is liable to produce a stenosis of the bronchus afterwards. In the use of the seeds, usually a series of six to eight seeds, each representing two millicuries of radon is used (number varies with size of tumour). Probably at the end of two months and again at five months this is repeated depending on the result obtained. X-rays are taken following treatments.

About half of the seeds implanted were coughed up. Sometimes the remainder were found to have migrated into the mediastinum, pleural cavity or on the upper surface of the diaphragm. They cause no untoward symptoms as they become inert after 14 days.

It is difficult to tell how long a patient has had the tumour. The majority gave a history of symptoms of from four to nine months. The object of the treatment is to destroy the growth and to open up the bronchus and drain and aerate the lung distal to the obstruction. Sixty-seven cases were treated with radon. There were a number of these strikingly succesful. Twenty-eight cases for different reasons were untreated. Their average life was 3.5 months. The average life of the treated case was 7.8 months. As the author states, averages many times give a false impression. Some of the treated cases were able to resume their work and live comfortably for 12, 18, 30 or 50 months. The benefit of opening the bronchus and aeration of the lung is soon seen.

It is the author's opinion that unless the patient is obviously in a dying condition and surgery is not practical, that radon treatment should always be carried out.

PLASTIC SURGERY

Edited by

GEO. H. KIMBALL, M.D., F.A.C.S.
404 Medical Arts Building, Oklahoma City

Ptosis and Its Surgical Correction. Edmond B. Spaeth, M.D., Philadelphia, A.M.A. Journal, December 4, 1937.

The author divides blepharoptosis, commonly spoken of ophthalmologically as ptosis, into groups: Ptosis may be (1) congenital, (2) traumatic, (3) residuals of an inflammatory condition of the orbit or (4) may be a part of a complete or incomplete external ophthalmoplegia, either central or peripheral in origin. Surgical ptosis should be considered as any one of these cases which is stationary, which cannot be corrected by any medical treatment and which impairs vision. The author makes a plea for diversified surgery in the correction of ptosis. He quotes Terson as saying that "it is only with precise appreciation of the peculiarities of the individual case that one may hope to succeed in this delicate and special surgery of the lid."

Three muscles are of importance in a surgical consideration of ptosis. (1) Levator palpebrae superioris. (2) Occipital frontalis. (3) Superior rectus.

The author points out that some cases of ptosis as may result from an intracranial neoplasm may not be considered surgical so far as ptosis is concerned. Also ptosis from myasthenia gravis in which surgery is contra-indicated.

Four general procedures are available in the correction of ptosis: (1) Shortening of the lid. (2) Advancement with the resection of the levator. (3) Replacement of the levator by the occipitofrontalis. (4) Utilization of the superior rectus.

The author illustrates his article by some unusually fine drawings. The procedures indicated for ptosis are outlined in the following chart:

Procedures Indicated for Ptosis

Condition Present	Unilateral	Bilateral
A.—Infants up to 3 years.	Crutch glasses.	Crutch glasses
B.—Children, 3 to 5.	Hunt-Tansley, utiilzation occipitofrontalis.	1.—Hunt-Tansley, utilization of occipitofrontalis. 2.—Modification of Motais.
C.—Children 5 to 15.	1.—Blakovics if levator action is present. 2.—Hunt-Tansley Blaskovics or some modification of a levator advancement.	1.—Blaskovics. 2.—Modification of the Motais.
D.—Adults, uncomplicated and with levator action present.	Blaskovics or some modification of a levator advancement.	1.—Modification of Motais. 2.—Blaskovics of some modification of a levator advancement.
E.—Adults, bilateral without levator action but with superior rectus intact.		1.—Modification of the Motais. 2.—Resection with advancement of the levator (see Lindner's statement).
F.—Adults, unilateral without superior rectus or levator action of any degree; acquired paralysis.	1.—Use of fascial sling, utilization of occipitofrontalis. 2.—Hess, direct anchorage to occipitofrontalis. 3.—Hunt-Tansley.	
G.—Adults, bilateral without superior rectus or levator action of any degree; acquired paralysis.		1.—Resection with advancement of the levator (see Lindner's statement). 2.—Use of fascial slings. 3.—Bilateral Hess.
H.—Trachomatous ptosis.	1.—Tarsus and culdesac resection with advancement of the levator.	1.—Tarsus and culdesac resection with advancement of the levator.
I.—Children acquired paralysis and without uncorrected or accompanying external ophthalmoplegia; correction depends on the degree of involvement.	1.—Utilization of sutures which form permanent cicatricial tracts. 2.—Hunt-Tansley. 3.—Hess, all occipitofrontalis action.	1.—Utilization of sutures which form permanent cicatricial tracts. 2.—Hunt-Tansley operation. 3.—Bilateral Hess.
J.—Adults with conditions as in I (correction depends on degree of involvement): (complete third nerve paralysis. See L.)	1.—Utilization of sutures which form permanent cicatricial tracts. 2.—Utilization of fascial slings. 3.—Hess. 4.—Muscle surgery with superior oblique.	1. Utilization of sutures which form permanent cicatricial tracts. 2.—Utilization of fascial slings. 3.—Bilateral Hess.
K.—Ptosis with incomplete external ophthalmoplegia.	1.—Utilization of sutures which form permanent cicatricial tracts. 2.—Crutch glasses. 3.—Hess operation.	1.—Utilization of sutures which form permanent cicatricial tracts. 2.—Crutch glasses. 3.—Bilateral Hess.
L.—Ptosis with complete external ophthalmoplegia.	Crutch glasses.	Crutch glasses.
M.—Cicatricial ptosis.	1.—Scar resection and suture. 2.—Lid shortening oper. Everbusch operation.	
N.—Ptosis following long standing enucleations.	1.—Blaskovics or some similar levator muscle procedure. 2.—Lid shortening oper. (Everbush oper.) also a levator procedure. 3.—Tarsus resection.	
O.—Ptosis with neurofibromatosis.	1.—Tumor resection. 2.—Hunt-Tansley with resection of the redundant tissue. 3.—Hess operation.	

Comment: Dr. Spaeth had an exhibit at Atlantic City last spring with accompanying charts as an outline of his work on ptosis. In my judgment it is a most comprehensive one and the most common sense plan that I have ever seen.

My own experience has included the use of the Hunt-Tansley procedure, the use of the fascial sling and the utilization of skin grafts in traumatic cases. This type of surgery calls for considerable detail and careful follow up work.

I agree with the author that improvements can be made in this branch of surgery if each case is carefully studied and a reasonable operation carried out.

In order to do this one must have at his finger tips the possibilities that have been outlined by the author.

————————o————————

ORTHOPAEDIC SURGERY
Edited by Earl D. McBride, M.D., F.A.C.S.
717 North Robinson Street, Oklahoma City

Acute Bone Atrophy (Die akute Knochenatrophie) W. Rieder, Deutsche Ztschr. f. Chir., 936, 248:269.

The author points out there are three types of acute bone atrophy: (1) the peripheral, which develops because of some external source of irritation; (2) the nervous, which is due to damage of the peripheral neurons from the posterior spinal ganglia, downwards; and (3) the thrombotic, due to thrombosis of the femoral vein. All these forms have in common the alteration of the circulation of the blood and of the qualitative nutrition. Numerous experimental researches were undertaken by various authors to study the effect of the nerve-section on bone. Their results were not uniform, however, in large part because of inflammatory lesions and, frequently, quite early ulcers.

Acute bone atrophy was first pointed out by Sudeck. It may be more appropriately called "trophic disturbance of the extremities," developing after trauma or inflammation, near or distant to the site of activity, and may show atrophic spots throughout the bone at a very early date.

The researches of the author are concerned with the pathologico-anatomical changes, not studied until now, with the systematic histological demonstration of the acute form of spotty bone atrophy, and further, with the histological researches of experimentally produced acute bone atrophy. A series of typical findings were picked from a large group; the most important data were taken from the clinical histories such as fractures, gun-shot wounds, osteomyelitis, tuberculosis, and whitlows, supplemented by roentgen films and histological illustrations. The experimental observations were reported in a similar manner. From all these researches the results were correlated in the following way:

A marked hyperemia of the bone blood vessels could be found even in the early phases of bone atrophy. The resorption of bone in this stage is brought about by narrow, spindle-shaped osteoclasts. Even after only two or three weeks a very much more marked apposition and resorption is established. In spite of widespread and often piled-up chains of osteoblasts, the calcification of the wide, osteoid trabecular borders is deficient. The pathologico-anatomical changes, particularly the failure of calcification, are the expression of a qualitative defective new bone formation or dystrophy. Clinically, one finds in the stage of acute bone atrophy of the involved extremity a hyperemia and hypertrophy of the skin; edema; cyanosis; diminu-

tion of tissue ability to react; delayed appearance and disappearance of reactive erythema on stimulation by cold; pathological changes in the microscopic picture of the capillaries.

Bone atrophy is also produced by immobilization, although in this type vasomotor and trophic disturbances are absent. Arterial ligation has no influence upon bone structure. Four to six weeks after thrombosis of the femoral vein, a typical picture of acute spotty atrophy occurs; this could not be reproduced in animal experiments by ligation of the larger veins. Determination of the alkali reserve by the Van Slyke method gave no uniform elevation of CO_2 in venous blood; just as seldom was there a uniform change in the blood lactic acid. By venous blood perfusion of an isolated area of living blood, an elevation of the calcium level of the venous blood is demonstrable, although the calcium level remains the same during the normal circulation of mixed arterial and venous blood. In experimentally produced bone atrophy the determination of the calcium level peripheral to the site of diseased bone shows a reduction of calcium. Exclusion of vessel constrictors in animal experiments tends to restrain the development of bone atrophy. Accordingly, cases in which the limp dystrophy has not been of too long duration may be cured by ramisection. The separate parietal layers of the medullary matter are interspersed by a thick network of nerves. There exists a uniform localization and correlation with the vessel damage in the bones. Occasionally, after the subsidence of the original stimulus of the dystrophic symptom-complex, an independent disease of the peripheral vasomotor system may persist. Common to all forms of acute bone atrophy is the damage to the circulation and local metabolism. It forms the basis for the subsequent development of bone dystrophy. The damage to circulation and metabolism leads to a disturbance of equilibrium, particularly of bone apposition and resorption, so that resorption predominates. The same stimulating factors which dilate the vessels lead to an increase of osteoclasts. The irritating factors, which directly or indirectly attack the terminal vessel bed, are also responsible for the development of traumatically produced extremity dystrophy. This dystrophy may persist after the exclusion of the original cause. A great number of damaging factors may influence the development of atrophy due to inflammatory extremity dystrophy. In the necrotic form the disturbance of circulation occurs because of direct nerve influence. The existence of the thrombotic form of atrophy is bound up with the optimum acidity. The foremost principle of treatment aims at the eradication of the underlying disease, the improvement of circulation, and thereby the improvement of local metabolism.

In difficult and refractory dystrophies of the extremity ramisection may bring cure, and even progressive improvement may be noted after its use in cases of several years' duration.

————————

Further Report on Osteomyelitis at the Massachusetts General Hospital, R. H. Miller and M. N. Smith-Petersen, New Eng. J. Med. 1937, 216:827.

This is a report of 90 cases of osteotomyelitis over a period of two years. Although this is a short time to draw definite conclusions, the authors have a tendency to become more and more conservative in the treatment of acute cases. They make the patient as comfortable as possible and then attack the local condition.

Sub-periosteal abscesses should be drained and if they suspect pus being present to a definite degree, a few holes are drilled in the bone, but nothing more. In cases with a streptococcus septicemia immunotransfusions should be done, and in those with a staphylococcus septicemia an antitoxin should be tried.

The most discouraging cases are those involving the femur; of 23, only five are completely healed and 12 are being followed. Three amputations were done to save life; two patients died; and one patient was lost from observation. Osteomyelitis of the tibia is less discouraging because the bone is more superficial.

Any bone cavity should be uncovered thoroughly. The wound may then be packed, and the packing changed every few days under an anesthetic, if necessary; or the wound may be closed with glass cannules, such as devised by Smith-Petersen, sewed in at each end. A constant stream of Dakin's solution is then kept running through the depths of the wound. In several cases this last procedure resulted in satisfactory healing in a shorter time.

Abstractor's Note: Frequently there are articles written regarding osteomyelitis. It is interesting to note that men of authority like Smith-Petersen still adhere to the old method of drilling early holes in the bone and treating the wound with continuous Dakin's solution. The Orr method has replaced this form of treatment in the hands of a great many competent orthopedic surgeons, and the final results, as seen through the crippled children's clinics held throughout Oklahoma, are convincing that the uniformity of result proves definitely the Orr method is better than the washing of wounds and frequent dressings as recommended in the above article.

Earl D. McBride, M.D., F.A.C.S.

SURGERY AND GYNECOLOGY
Abstracts, Reviews and Comments from
LeRoy Long Clinic
714 Medical Arts Building, Oklahoma City

Cancer of the Breast. Charles C. Lund, Boston, Mass. Surgery, Gynecology & Obstetrics, December, 1937.

The material from which this paper was written was obtained from work done under the direction of Dr. Robert B. Greenough at the Huntington Memorial Hospital and at the Massachusetts General Hospital in Boston. Dr. Greenough had a wide experience with carcinoma of the breast. Although Dr. Greenough has now passed on, his work is being carried forward by Dr. Grantley Taylor, Ernest Daland and others including Charles Lund, the latter being the author of this article.

There has been a great amount of discussion as to the necessity for and results of preoperative or postoperative radiation. The conclusions that follow will therefore be of value since they are the result of open minded, careful work by one of the great leaders in cancer therapy in one of the great medical centers of the world.

The conclusions of this article (which are essentially those of Dr. Greenough in fact) are as follows:

"1. Patients with suspected cancer of the breast should be very carefully studied before the course of treatment is decided upon. This study includes complete history, physical examination, and X-ray examination of the chest, spine, pelvis and skull.

"2. Following this study the patients should be separated into two classes: (1) those with a chance of cure; (2) those without a chance of cure.

"3. The former should u n d e r g o radical procedures, without previous radiation treatment. Post-

operative X-ray treatment is not a necessary part of the routine for all patients.

"4. The patients classed as incurable should be given powerful doses of X-ray, and no surgery and usually no radium."

I interpret this to mean that if a surgeon knows how to do an adequate radical operation and if the patient under consideration has, in his judgment, a possibility of cure, there is no obligation on his part to use radiation of any kind before or after the operation.

LeRoy D. Long.

Uterine Prolapse

The three following abstracts are particularly interesting in relation to treatment of advanced stages of procidentia and vaginal herniation in older women. There is also an interesting unanimity of opinion about procedures to be employed in prolapse in younger women where partial or total preservation of function is essential.

An Efficient Composite Operation for Uterine Prolapse and Associated Pathology. Edward H. Richardson, Baltimore, Maryland. American Journal of Obstetrics and Gynecology, November, 1937.

Richardson has attempted to devise an operative procedure for advanced grade genital prolapse largely because recent follow-up studies at John Hopkins Hospital reveal the fact that total vaginal hysterectomy for the treatment of advanced grade vaginal hernias failed to achieve complete anatomic success in 30 per cent of the cases, whereas only four per cent of failures occurred following the interposition operation.

This operation is not devised for employment in the younger age group where the surgical problems presented are relatively simple. In the younger age group treatment includes conservative therapy to a damaged and infected cervix, plastic repair of the fascial bladder and urethral support, reconstruction of the pelvic floor, and recto-vaginal septum, together with an efficient suspension of the uterus by the abdominal route.

This operation has been devised for the more complex problems associated with advanced stages of vaginal hernias frequently encountered in elderly women. The advanced grades of uterine prolapse are commonly encountered in association with "hypertrophy, elongation and chronic infection of the cervix, benign disease of the corpus, pronounced descent of the bladder or cystocele, impairment of the vesical sphincter, urethrocele, a broken down perineum and pelvic floor, rectocele and enterocele."

The most widely employed procedures for the treatment of this condition are: (1) Total vaginal hysterectomy. (2) Watkins Wertheime inter-position operation. (3) Manchester-Fothergill procedures. (4) Curtis advancement operation. (5) Partial (Le Fort) colpocleisis; and (6) total colpectomy.

There are certain inherent defects chargeable to each of the more popular procedures, when one considers the primary purpose as complete elimination of both actual and potential disease and restoration with permanent stabilization of normal anatomic relationships.

"Judged by this standard both colpocleisis and total colpectomy, while possessing undoubted merit, must be regarded as last resort measures which, even if objectively efficient, are both subjectively and anatomicaly far from ideal. The entire group of transposition operations are open to the objection that they leave the uterus as a potential source of later benign or malignant disease. In total vaginal hysterectomy the most dependable supporting structures are first partly devitalized by the application of crushing clamps, division and ligation with constricting sutures; these same impaired structures are then relied upon to furnish the central and main support of the entire reconstruction plan."

"Now the composite operation here offered avoids the objections to the commonly used procedure noted above. By utilization of the time honored high amputation of the cervix coupled with subtotal vaginal hysterectomy, it eliminates existing and potential uterine disease, thereby also relieving the supporting structures of considerable dead weight; by preserving intact that segment of the cervix to which are normally attached the cardinal and the uterosacral ligaments together with the sturdy pubocervical fascia, ideal conditions are created for adaptation of the most dependable features of the several transposition operations; plication of the vesical sphincter is easily executed; accurate identification and dissection of the pubocervical fascia permits imbrication of this valuable unit beneath the bladder neck and urethra in accordance with the established principles of hernioplasty; suture of the round ligaments into the angles of the cervical stump provides additional lift and support; adequate circulation to the cervical stump and attached structures is assured through preservation of the adjacent main trunks of the uterine vessels and their branches; the ureters are not endangered by any step of the operation; obliteration of the culdesac and plication of the uterosacral ligaments for associated enterocele are readily effected; and, finally, reinforcement of the rectovaginal fascia together with reconstruction of the pelvic floor and perineum completes the operation with accurate restoration of normal anatomical relationships having been achieved. Attention is again called to the fact that every important step of the operation is borrowed from an already well established procedure in the treatment of vaginal herniae. Immediate results in the small series of cases thus far dealt with by this method, totaling about 25, have been completely satisfactory."

The operative technic is very carefully described and illustrated.

Prolapse of the Uterus-Shifting Trends in Treatment. Joseph L. Baer, Ralph A. Reis & Robert M. Laemle, Chicago, Ill. American Journal of Obstetrics and Gynecology, November, 1937.

These authors report a recent review of the operative results in 220 instances of prolapse of the uterus. Of these, 17 patients had a first degree prolapse, 76 had a second degree prolapse, and 123 had a third degree prolapse. Ten types of operation were employed. Based upon the immediate and remote results these authors considered three of these as well suited to meet particular indications, namely the interposition operation, the LeFort vaginal occlusion operation, and the Mayo vaginal hysterectomy.

"The interposition operation was completely successful in 56 out of 64 (87.5 per cent) in the series previously published. In the present series, the interposition operation was successful in 17 out of 19 (89.5 per cent). Vaginal hysterectomy, to which we turned in order to improve our results and the results of which were followed in 65 women, was successful in only 46 instances (70.7 per cent). The patients in both series were operated upon by the same group of gynecologists. Since it may be assumed that these operators were equally competent in both types of operation, the results obtained em-

phasize the superiority of the interposition operation over vaginal hysterectomy in our hands."

They therefore believe that the interposition operation should take precedence over vaginal hysterectomy whenever the conditions for its election are met. They also feel that vaginal hysterectomy should be restricted to prolapse in which the pathology of the uterus itself carries the indication for hysterectomy.

They too, feel that Gilliam suspension operation, combined with vaginal reconstruction, is best suited for third degree prolapse in the child bearing group.

Procidentia: A New Operation for Cure of Fourth Degree Prolapse. Rafe C. Chaffin, Los Angeles, Calif. The American Journal of Surgery, August, 1937.

The operation described in this article embodies many of the principles employed by Richardson in his so-called composite procedure. A vaginal subtotal hysterectomy is performed. The round and broad ligaments are sutured to the posterior surface of the cervix. The cervical stump is interposed between vagina and bladder, and an anterior colpoplasty performed over the stump of the uterus. He does not speak about amputation of the cervix.

COMMENT

Comment on the three previous articles concerning the treatment of procidentia:

Complete uterine prolapse with the many associated pathological conditions is a very common condition. Because of the admitted incidence of both partial and complete anatomic failure with the operative procedures usually employed and because of the rapid succession of articles upon this subject in gynecological literature, it is quite evident that improvement should be sought in the operative approach. It is equally evident that, regardless of the operative procedure, no one plan can be used in every instance and the proper procedure must be applied to each individual patient.

There is much to be said in favor of the composite operation as devised by Richardson and Chaffin. They should both receive recognition in patients where there is pronounced benign pathology of the uterine fundus.

It is also an interesting circumstance to observe the recurring popularity of the interposition operation, following so closely upon the rather widespread condemnation which it has received in the past five years. I continue to consider it as an ideal operation in a selected group of patients with large cystocele, uterine body that is neither too large nor too small, absence of gross adnexal pathology, and in women past the menopause.

The essential difference between complete vaginal hysterectomy and the operation devised by Richardson and Chaffin lies in allowing the cervix, all or in part, to remain and in interposing the cervix or its healthy remnant between the bladder and the vaginal wall as in the average interposition operation where the fundus is so placed. One can easily recognize merit in this type of variation from the usual vaginal hysterectomy in certain types of patients.

The principal objection to this variation lies in the fact that potentially diseased cervical tissue may be left in situ to cause subsequent trouble. However, if the uterine tissue is not the location of actual pathology, removal of the uterus in part or entirely should be determined upon the basis of whether or not the uterus would be valuable tissue employed in the reconstruction of the vagina.

Wendell Long.

Ileocecal Lymphadenitis in Children. Arthur E. Brown, M.B., B.Ch., F.R.A.C.S., Colac., Cictoria, Australia. Surgery, Gynecology and Obstetrics, December, 1937.

The article is introduced by this statement: "It is now generally recognized that there exists in children and young adolescents, an acute abdominal condition, in which the symptoms are very similar to those of appendicitis, but in which the predominant findings at operation, and presumably the principal pathological basis, consists only of an inflammatory enlargement of the mesenteric and retroperitoneal lymph glands draining from the ileocecal angle."

The statement is made that the condition is common, that it usually comes under the observation of surgeons, that the diagnosis is nearly always appendicitis.

The author believes that a preoperative diagnosis is possible in a reasonable proportion of cases.

The author says: "The general picture of such a case is as follows: The patient is between the ages of 3 and 18 years. He is seized with abdominal pain which is of varying severity and can generally be traced to the right lower abdomen. During that attack there is evidence of definite toxicity. The attacks subside as a rule, and the child has intervals of weeks or months during which he is apparently perfectly well; but the attacks recur and will continue to recur, until the operation of appendectomy is performed, after which he will be free from symptoms. In English the standard and probably best known descriptions of the condition are those of Fraser in his book 'The Surgery of Childhood,' and of Braithwaite in the British Journal of Surgery of 1925."

Fraser is quoted as saying: "There is considerable general disturbance and fever. The symptoms rarely last for more than 24 to 48 hours and abate with characteristic suddenness. The pain is local from the start, never referred. The tongue remains clean." And he emphasizes a little later, "The attack subsides with characteristic rapidity."

The author, based upon his experience, divides the patients into two groups. The first group presents very acute symptoms, the second group milder symptoms.

Illustrative of the first group, the following history is recorded: "Frank A., age 14 years, male. First symptoms occurred six days prior to examination when he became ill with what his parents described as 'influenza.' He was feverish for two days, immediately after which he had severe abdominal pain with fairly severe retching. The pains persisted, being more or less severe in degree, and was said to be definitely worse after taking food. The day before examination he had an attack of shivering, and that evening the pain became localized in the lower right side of the abdomen. His bowels were described as being 'inclined to constipation.' During the past two years he had had repeated attacks of general abdominal pain, these being less in evidence during the last 12 months. On examination: Tongue was found to be dry and dirty; the temperature 102; pulse, 112; respiration, 20; leucocytosis, 18,000. The abdomen was flat. There was tenderness in the right iliac region, overlying a tender mass felt beneath the abdominal wall. The mass was dull to percussion, and lay higher and rather more internally than the usual position of an appendiceal abscess. The urine showed a cloud of albumin. A diagnosis was made of ileocecal adenitis, and operation was withheld for a period of observation. The blood picture on the succeeding four days is shown in the table

which follows: (the table shows W.B.C. from 18,000 to 11,000 over a period of three days).

On the fourth day the mass felt appeared to be more extensive in an upward direction, and his temperature was 103.2. Operation was performed. The appendix was normal in appearance, though with a slight degree of congestion in the serosa. It was neither inflamed nor edematous. There was a large mass of retroperitoneal glands acutely inflamed, the largest and reddest being in the ileocecal angle, smaller and less inflamed along the common iliac vessels and toward the root of the mesentery, becoming smaller as they went centrally. The temperature became normal within 24 hours of the operation and remained so. The albumin disappeared from the urine, and six days after the operation the blood picture was: Leucocytes 12,800, polymorphonuclears 57.5, eosinophiles 4.5, lymphocytes 33, monocytes 5.

"His health has been uniformly good since the operation, with no attacks of pain."

The subacute or recurrent cases are illustrated by the following report: "George P., aged 13 years, male. First symptom appeared two days before examination. The boy had an attack of pain in the abdomen in the afternoon while going to work. He did not vomit, but felt sick. He had his evening meal and slept well all that night. The pain was still present the next morning, and he stayed away from school, but had all his meals. There was an interval at mid-day free from pain, but they recurred in the afternoon. He slept all night, but found the pains still present on waking the following morning. The bowels were open normally throughout. The pain was always located below and to the right of the navel. In the previous six months there had been three attacks of pain similar in nature, and lasting from half a day to a day. On examination, the tongue was found to be dirty; the temperature was 99.6 degrees; pulse, 112; respiration rate, 20. The urine showed no abnormality. Blood examination showed a leucocyte count of 20,000, the differential count being: Polymorphonuclear leucocytes 44.5 and mature in type; eosinophiles, 6.5; lymphocytes, 46; monocytes, 3 per cent. The abdomen was tender just below and to the right of the umbilicus, not at McBurney's point. There was no rigidity, but a feeling of slight mass under the pressure of the fingers. A diagnosis of ileocecal adenitis was made, and operation fixed for the following day. On the next morning the blood count was repeated, and showed a strikingly different picture. The total leucocyte count was 29,600, with 86 per cent polymorphonuclear cells, well matured, and only 10.5 per cent lymphocytes. The eosinophiles had disappeared altogether. At the operation the appendix was found to be large and bulky, with some congestion in its appearance, but neither edematous nor inflamed. The retrocecal glands of the ileocecal angle, those of the mesoappendix, and those in the mesentery of the terminal six inches of the ileum, were enlarged and hard, but quite discrete. The temperature fell to normal immediately following the operation and remained at a normal level throughout a normal convalescence. He had no recurrence in his intermittent pains since his operation."

In a rather lengthy discussion, there is an attempt to make an analysis of the symptoms in the cases reported.

With reference to the etiology, the statement is made: "It remains the most likely possibility that the condition is caused by an infection with an organism in the ileocecal area, which has a slight local effect, but a marked secondary effect on glands in the draining area."

Apparently, the author has concluded that appendicectomy is the proper treatment for ileocecal lymphadenitis in children. In his summary the statement is made: "I have drawn from them the conclusion that if the operation is not done the attacks of pain will continue to occur intermittently, but that the removal of the appendix will bring about complete and permanent cure."

COMMENT

Notwithstanding the rather dogmatic statements and the apparent enthusiasm of the author, this article does not appear to be either very satisfactory or enlightening.

An attempt is made to show that there are certain characteristic symptoms and signs in ileocecal lymphadenitis that are not present in appendicitis. At the same time, the author makes the definite statement that ileocecal lymphadenitis is cured by an appendicectomy.

When one reads the article with care one is impressed with the significant fact that all the cases reported could reasonably fall into the group which surgeons have recognized for a long time as recurrent appendicitis.

Altogether, the article is a striking paradox.

LeRoy Long.

UROLOGY

Edited by D. W. Branham, M. D.
514 Medical Arts Building, Oklahoma City

The Criteria of Cure of Gonococcal Infections in Women. Lawrence R. Wharton, M.D., Baltimore, Md. American Journal of Syphilis, Gonorrhea, and Venereal Diseases, November, 1937.

The author states he was induced to make this study because of the lack of general knowledge among both physician and the laiety as regards the permanent cure of gonorrhea in women. He has taken for material the case records of 75 patients as a basis for this investigation. Several of these patients were induced to return for a complete follow-up examination in an attempt to see whether evidence of infection still persists after a number of years.

The author writes informally and freely of his views in regard to many phases of diagnosis and treatment of this disease. He uses for treatment in gonococcal vaginitis in children a combination of both local applications of mercurochrome in conjunction with amniotin suppositories. He is of the opinion that his results are satisfactory with such treatment, but he emphasizes a follow-up program extending for at least a year after apparent cure.

As regards the value of smears in the determination of cure he feels their importance is over-rated. To be of much value they should be repeated many times. He is of the opinion cultures would be a more reliable method of determining whether a cure has been completed.

His criteria of cure is based on the following:

1. Long observation of the patient with repeated follow-up examinations for signs of infection.

2. Repeated negative smears.

3. Continually negative history of infection both personal and marital.

He briefly records his impression of the various physical methods of treatment, namely, the Elliott treatment, diathermy and fever therapy as being rather disappointing so far as producing more than a symptomatic cure. He specificially mentions fever therapy as being too radical for the average gonococcal infection and recites of a catastrophe in his experience in which a fatality occurred with this treatment.

His conclusions were briefly that no swift, simple, easy test is available that will indicate the presence or absence of gonorrhea. Only continuous observation over a long period of time will indicate freedom from the disease. Of the patients studied by his criteria of cure 90 per cent were proven to be well and he feels on the basis of his experience gonorrhea in women can be permanently cured.

Traumatic Ruptures of the Bladder. A. R. Stevens, Chicago, Illinois, and W. R. Delzell, New York. Journal of Urology, November, 1937.

The authors discuss this most important urological emergency using for study 27 such cases. They state the etiological factors for such conditions rests in most instances on the fact that the bladder previous to rupture is distended and vulnerable to injury. Blows over the lower abdomen with complicating fracture of the pelvic bone are the most frequent direct cause for rupture and resultant extravasation. Oftimes other viscus are seriously injured.

The diagnosis is based on evidence of shock with the presence of blood in the urine. Catheterization is a particularly fallacious method for determining the presence of rupture as not infrequently urine will be aspirated from the abdominal cavity or the rent in the bladder wall may be temporarily sealed by omentum or blood clot. They believe that cystoscopy is a safe and more reliable method of diagnosis. Cystograms using the retrograde method with air or contrast media are also an excellent diagnostic procedure. They do not feel the intravenous method in obtaining cystograms is very conclusive.

They discuss the treatment emphasizing early surgical intervention and providing supra-pubic drainage, at the same time repairing the tear. Adequate extra vesicle drainage is essential and at times it may be necessary in the presence of perineal extravasation to place a drain in this region.

In their series of cases they encountered 37 per cent mortality. In 14 intraperitoneal ruptures there were eight deaths, but only two deaths occurred in 13 cases of extraperitoneal rupture. In their summary they stressed that rupture must be differentiated from perforation as the mortality is higher in the former. Early diagnosis and prompt surgical treatment are vitally important.

Comment: A thoroughly timely and practical article on a condition that is becoming more prevalent in this day of excessive beer drinking with resultant diruresis and automobile accidents. I disagree with them as regards the safety of catheterization and cystoscopy and feel that these instruments hold a potential danger in favoring infection. Intravenous urography has been an invaluable aid in the diagnosis and I feel that this is the first diagnostic procedure to be made in every instance of suspected bladder rupture.

Some Observation on the Renal Capsule. Harry C. Holnick, Chicago, Illinois. Journal of Urology, 1937.

An anatomic-physiological study of the renal capsule, a structure that has been somewhat neglected but nevertheless is important in various ways.

The author remarks of the elasticity of the fibrous capsule of the kidney which allows the organ to expand and contract as it changes its intrarenal tension. It also protects the parenchyma of the kidney from injury by its elasticity as well as a barrier to extension of infection from the perirenal tissue.

In a series of observations made on dogs in which he performed decapsulation he found the newly formed capsule lacked the normal elasticity and had a tendency to contract and compress the kidney. He believes decapsulation is harmful to the kidney and may result in interference with its function, therefore should never be done routinely in renal operations.

The Effect of pH of the Urine On Concentration Of Free and Conjugated Sulfanilamide Necessary For Bactericidal Action. Staff Meetings of Mayo Clinic, Rochester, Minnesota, H. F. Helmholz and A. E. Osterberg, October 20, 1937.

The authors have previously reported on the effect of urinary reaction or bactericidal effect of sulfanilamide. It was found that the bactericidal action of sulfanilamide for suseptible organisms was decidedly enhanced when the urine was rendered alkaline.

Their conclusions were that sulfanilamide probably is most effective bactericidally in the free form and rather low concentration of the drug 25 to 30 milligrams per 100 c. c. when excreted in a highly alkaline urine will inhibit the growth of bacteria. The conjugated form when excreted in the urine is of lesser value so far as bacteriostatic power is concerned. They are of the opinion that this needs further observation

COMMENT

A practical bit of knowledge regarding a drug that is receiving a considerable proportion of the profession's interest at the present time. Administration of alkalies in conjunction with sulfanilamide should be productive of better therapeutic results.

What Every Woman Doesn't Know—How to Give Cod Liver Oil

Some authorities recommend that cod liver oil be given in the morning and at bedtime when the stomach is empty, while others prefer to give it after meals in order not to retard gastric secretion. If the mother will place the very young baby on her lap and hold the child's mouth open by gently pressing the cheeks together between her thumb and fingers while she administers the oil, all of it will be taken. The infant soon becomes accustomed to taking the oil without having its mouth held open. It is most important that the mother administer the oil in a matter-of-fact manner, without apology or expression of symphty.

If given cold, cod liver oil has little taste, for the cold tends to paralyze momentarily the gustatory nerves. As any "taste" is largely a metallic one from the silver or silverplated spoon (particularly if the plating is worn), a glass spoon has an advantage.

On account of its higher potency in Vitamins A and D, Mead's Cod Liver Oil Fortified With Percomorph Liver Oil may be given in one-third the ordinary cod liver oil dosage, and is particularly desirable in cases of fat intolerance.

Pneumococcic Research
State Medical School Asks Cooperation of State Doctors

Under the direction of Dr. H. D. Moor, the Bacteriology Department of the Oklahoma University, School of Medicine, is investigating the prevalence of the various types of pneumococcic pneumonia in the state. This is being undertaken purely as a research problem and is definitely not intended as a diagnostic service. Results of this research will be given to the profession, in published articles, as the work progresses.

The doctors are asked to cooperate in this work by supplying material for examination. Please send to the Bacteriology Department specimens of sputum from any cases of pneumonia, either lobar or broncho-pneumonia, which you may have. The department will gladly send a messenger for the specimens in Oklahoma City or will mail out containers to those out of the city, who will kindly assist in this research.

Roentgen Therapy of Lobar Pneumonia

In January, 1933, Eugene V. Powell, Temple Texas (Journal A. M. A., Jan. 1, 1938), employed roentgen therapy on a patient who was ill with lobar pneumonia. Unable to find any references in the literature on dosage, he used a technic which had proved valuable in the treatment of carbuncles. However, he increased the filtration and skin-target distance, so as to irradiate more homogeneously the large mass of tissue that is involved in a consolidated pulmonary lobe. Within a few hours after the treatment the patient was relieved of much of his distress, and within 24 hours his temperature dropped by crisis. He then pursued an uneventful and complete convalescence. Since then he has used roentgen radiation in the treatment of 104 cases of acute lobar pneumonia and in 30 cases of bronchopneumonia. Only five of the patients with lobar pneumonia died, and those with bronchopneumonia showed a reduction in mortality from 30 per cent to 13 per cent. From 250 to 350 roentgens of 0.3 angstrom unit of effective radiation (135 kilovolts with 3 mm. of aluminum filter) is given anteriorly or posteriorly over an area a little larger than the involved portion of the lung. If the temperature and white blood cell count have not dropped to normal within 36 to 48 hours, a second roentgen treatment is given to an opposite field. Usually within two or three hours after the first treatment the patients report feeling much better. Clinically, too, they look less sick. Within 36 hours, frequently during the first 12 hours, their temperature drops to normal. The pulse rate, the respiration rate and the white blood cell count drop also, but usually not quite so rapidly as the temperature. A secondary rise in temperature, not very high and lasting only a few hours, is not uncommon. It is only when the leukocyte count stays high or when the temperature remains elevated that the additional treatment is given. The resolution of the pulmonary consolidation practically always lags behind the other evidences of recovery. A few patients with pneumonia of mixed infection have received a third or fourth treatment, but then successively smaller doses were given so as to avoid any cutaneous reactions. Except in the treatment of three patients, two of whom died, serum was not used in this series. Bronchopneumonia seems to be more variable and as a whole less favorably influenced than lobar pneumonia. There is no definitely proved explanation as to why patients with pneumonia respond as favorably as they do to roentgen treatment, but the improvement seems to be associated with the destruction of the infiltrating leukocytes. Roentgen therapy appears to be the preferred method in the treatment of pneumonias. So far the only contraindication seems to be definite leukopenia, such as is encountered occasionally in patients with postinfluenzal pneumonia.

OFFICERS OKLAHOMA STATE MEDICAL ASSOCIATION

President, Dr. Sam A. McKeel, Ada.
President-Elect, Dr. H. K. Speed, Sayre.
Secretary-Treasurer-Editor, Dr. L. S. Willour, McAlester.
Speaker, House of Delegates, Dr. J. D. Osborn, Jr., Frederick.
Vice Speaker, House of Delegates, Dr. P. P. Nesbitt, Medical Arts Building, Tulsa.
Delegates to the A. M. A., Dr. W. Albert Cook, Medical Arts Building, Tulsa, 1937-1938; Dr. Horace Reed, 1200 North Walker, Oklahoma City, 1937-1938; Dr. McLain Rogers, Clinton, 1938-1939.
Meeting Place, Muskogee, May, 1938.

SPECIAL COMMITTEES

Annual Meeting: Dr. Sam A. McKeel, Ada; Dr. H. K. Speed, Sayre; Dr. L. S. Willour, McAlester.

Conservation of Hearing: Dr. J. A. Morrow, Chairman, Sallisaw; Dr. Howard Brown, Ponca City; Dr. E. A. Hale, Alva.

Conservation of Vision: Dr. Milton K. Thompson, Chairman, Muskogee; Dr. William F. Klotz, McAlester; Dr. O. H. Miller, Ada.

Crippled Children: Dr. D. H. O'Donoghue, Chairman, Oklahoma City; Dr. George S. Baxter, Shawnee; Dr. Ray Lindsey, Pauls Valley.

Industrial Service and Traumatic Surgery: Dr. Earl McBride, Chairman, Oklahoma City; Dr. J. F. Park, McAlester; Dr. G. H. Stagner, Erick.

Maternity and Infancy: Dr. John A. Haynie, Chairman, Durant; Dr. Edward P. Allen, Oklahoma City; Dr. Marvin B. Glismann, Okmulgee.

Necrology: Dr. C. E. Williams, Chairman, Woodward; Dr. James L. Shuler, Durant; Dr. E. P. Green, Westville.

Post Graduate Medical Teaching: Dr. Henry H. Turner, Chairman, Oklahoma City; Dr. H. C. Weber, Bartlesville; Dr. T. H. McCarley, McAlester.

Study and Control of Cancer: Dr. Wendell Long, Chairman, Oklahoma City; Dr. Paul B. Champlin, Enid; Dr. Ralph McGill, Tulsa.

Study and Control of Tuberculosis: Dr. Carl Puckett, Chairman, Oklahoma City; Dr. Will C. Wait, Clinton; Dr. L. J. Moorman, Oklahoma City.

STANDING COMMITTEES

Medical Defense: Dr. L. C. Kuyrkendall, Chairman, McAlester; Dr. O. E. Templin, Alva; Dr. W. A. Howard, Chelsea.

Medical Economics: Dr. Rex Bolend, Chairman, Oklahoma City; Dr. E. M. Gullatt, Ada; Dr. R. B. Gibson, Ponca City.

Medical Education and Hospitals: Dr. Robert U. Patterson, Chairman, Oklahoma City; Dr. W. P. Longmire, Sapulpa; Dr. LeRoy Long, Oklahoma City.

Public Policy and Legislation: Dr. J. M. Byrum, Chairman, Shawnee; Dr. Sam A. McKeel, Ada; Dr. H. K. Speed, Sayre; Dr. W. P. Neilson, Enid; Dr. R. C. Pigford, Tulsa.

Scientific Exhibits: Dr. Halsell Fite, Chairman, Muskogee, Dr. Curt Von Wedel, Oklahoma City; Dr. E. Rankin Denny, Tulsa.

Scientific Work: Dr. W. G. Husband, Chairman, Hollis; Dr. C. Stevens, Seminole; Dr. W. N. Johns, Hugo.

SCIENTIFIC SECTIONS

General Surgery: Dr. Stratton E. Kernodle, Chairman, 635 First National Building, Oklahoma City; Dr. H. G. Crawford, Vice-Chairman, Bartlesville; Dr. E. P. Nesbitt, Secretary, Medical Arts Building, Tulsa.

General Medicine: Dr. Minard F. Jacobs, Chairman, Medical Arts Building, Oklahoma City; Dr. Frank Nelson, Vice-Chairman, Medical Arts Building, Tulsa; Dr. Milam F. McKinney, Secretary, Oklahoma City.

Eye, Ear, Nose and Throat: Dr. Chester McHenry, Chairman, Medical Arts Building, Oklahoma City; Dr. A. H. Davis, Vice-Chairman, Medical Arts Building, Tulsa; Dr. Edwin H. Coachman, Secretary, Manhattan Building, Muskogee.

Obstetrics and Pediatrics: Dr. M. B. Glismann, Chairman, Okmulgee; Dr. C. W. Arrndell, Vice-Chairman, Ponca City; Dr. C. E. White, Secretary, Muskogee.

Genito-Urinary Diseases and Syphilology: Dr. Chas. B. Taylor, Chairman, Medical Arts Building, Oklahoma City; Dr. D. W. Branham, Vice-Chairman, Medical Arts Building, Oklahoma City; Dr. Shade Neely, Secretary, Commercial National Building, Muskogee.

Dermatology and Radiology: Dr. L. S. McAlister, Chairman, Barnes Building, Muskogee; Dr. M. M. Wickham, Vice-Chairman, Norman; Dr. John H. Lamb, Secretary, Medical Arts Building, Oklahoma City.

STATE BOARD OF MEDICAL EXAMINERS

Dr. Thos. McElroy, Ponca City, President; Dr. C. E. Bradley, Tulsa, Vice-President; Dr. J. D. Osborn, Jr., Frederick, Secretary; Dr. L. E. Emanuel, Chickasha; Dr. W. T. Ray, Gould; Dr. G. L. Johnson, Pauls Valley; Dr. W. W. Osgood, Muskogee.

STATE COMMISSIONER OF HEALTH

Dr. Chas. M. Pearce, Oklahoma City.

COUNCILORS AND THEIR COUNTIES

District No. 1: Texas, Beaver, Cimarron, Harper, Ellis, Woods, Woodward, Alfalfa, Major, Dewey—Dr. O. E. Templin, Alva. (Term expires 1937.)

District No. 2: Roger Mills, Beckham, Greer, Harmon, Washita, Kiowa, Custer, Jackson, Tillman—Dr. V. C. Tisdal, Elk City. (Term expires 1939.)

District No. 3: Grant, Kay, Garfield, Noble, Payne, Pawnee—Dr. A. S. Risser, Blackwell. (Term expires 1938.)

District No. 4: Blaine, Kingfisher, Canadian, Logan, Oklahoma, Cleveland—Dr. Philip M. McNeill, Oklahoma City. (Term expires 1938.)

District No. 5: Caddo, Comanche, Cotton, Grady, Love, Stephens, Jefferson, Carter, Murray—Dr. W. H. Livermore, Chickasha. (Term expires 1938.)

District No. 6: Osage, Creek, Washington, Nowata, Rogers, Tulsa—Dr. W. A. Howard, Chelsea. (Term expires 1938.)

District No. 7: Lincoln, Pontotoc, Pottawatomie, Okfuskee, Seminole, McClain, Garvin, Hughes—Dr. J. A. Walker, Shawnee. (Term expires 1939.)

District No. 8: Craig, Ottawa, Mayes, Delaware, Wagoner, Adair, Cherokee, Sequoyah, Okmulgee, Muskogee—Dr. E. A. Aisenstadt, Picher. (Term expires 1939.)

District No. 9: Pittsburg, Haskell, Latimer, LeFlore, McIntosh—Dr. L. C. Kuyrkendall, McAlester. (Term expires 1939.)

District No. 10: Johnson, Marshall, Coal, Atoka, Bryan, Choctaw, Pushmataha, McCurtain—Dr. J. S. Fulton, Atoka. (Term expires 1939.)

CLASSIFIED ADVERTISEMENTS

THE JOURNAL
OF THE
OKLAHOMA STATE MEDICAL ASSOCIATION

| VOLUME XXXI | McALESTER, OKLAHOMA, FEBRUARY, 1938 | Number 2 |

Treatment of Urethral Fistula*

BASIL A. HAYES, M.D.
OKLAHOMA CITY, OKLAHOMA

Definition: Urethral fistula may be defined as an abnormal opening from the urethra to the outer surface of the body or to another hollow organ; for example, the rectum. The management and cure of this condition is somewhat difficult and all those who have served internships in charity hospitals are familiar with the fact that such cases often lie around the wards of the hospitals for months, awaiting the time when some of the staff surgeons take an interest in them and finally cause them to be healed up. A few years ago it was my experience to have three or four of these cases suddenly assigned to me in University Hospital so that I was forced to study out the necessary procedures which caused them to recover. Since that time I have maintained a keen interest in urethral fistulae and wish to present today some guiding principles by which they can be managed.

CLASSIFICATION

A convenient classification, according to location and origin, is as follows:

1. Simple urethrol fistula, occurring either on the under surface of the shaft of the penis or in the perineum. In this the opening is merely a straight channel leading from the urethra to the outside of the body. In some cases it is single and in others it is multiple, having several openings widely scattered over the perineum but all leading to a single opening in the

*Read before the Section on Genito-Urinary Diseases and Syphilology, Annual Meeting, Oklahoma State Medical Association, Tulsa, May, 1937.

urethra. It is commonly seen following urinary extravasation.

2. Urethrorectal fistula; that is, an opening from the urethra leading into the ampulla of the rectum. The commonest cause is injury to the rectum while doing perineal prostatectomy.

3. Urethrorectoperineal fistula; that is, an opening leading from the urethra into the rectum and also to the outside of the perineum. Sometimes numbers two or three are complicated by other channels running laterally or upward on either side of or through the scrotum.

4. Prostatic fistula; that is, there occurs a leak in the prostate which extends downward and backward, surrounding the rectum.

ETIOLOGY

The causes of urethral fistula may be summed up under three general headings:

A. *Trauma*, of which there are four types:

1. Direct blows on the perineum, rupturing the urethra and causing urinary extravasation with abscess formation. This is usually followed by necrosis or incision of the perineal tissues, thus causing the fistula.

2. Fractures of the pubic arch, causing a spicule of bone to penetrate the urethra with the same result as in (1).

3. Operative sequellae, as w h e n the urethra or both urethra and rectum are

opened while doing perineal prostatectomy or other surgery of this region.

4. Instrumental accidents, as when the urethra is torn while passing a sound or other instrument through it.

B. *Infection*, such as periurethral or prostatic a b s c e s s, occurring during the course of a gonorrheal urethritis. Occasionally such abscesses are non-specific and are seen in old or debilitated individuals.

C. *Syphilis, cancer, or tuberculosis.*

PATHOLOGICAL PROCESS

It is well known that there are layers of dense fascia in the perineum and surrounding the penis. Buck's fascia is the name given to the layer of fascia which surrounds the penis and extends backward as far as the scrotum. Colles' fascia covers the entire scrotum and extends backward around the urethral bulb up to the membranous urethra and sphincter ani. If a diseased process starts within the urethra and ruptures out through the mucosa and muscular coats of this tube, the first arresting structure is Buck's fascia, providing the process is along the shaft of the penis. Here it meets a resistance which lasts for some time, allowing the infection to spread up and down the length of the penis for a distance, thereby creating an abscessed cavity inside Buck's fascia and outside of the urethra. Eventually the swelling becomes great enough that it is either opened by the physician or ruptures spontaneously and thus is left a fusiform channel, small on the outside and small in the urethral wall but large in the middle. If the process begins in the membranous urethra, practically the same thing occurs except that the spread in the midline tissues is brought about by the resistance of Colles' fascia instead of Buck's fascia and the abscess forms and spreads through and around the bulb of the urethra. If the process begins in Cowper's gland or in the prostate, it is not confined by Colles' fascia but distends the tissues behind and below this structure and appears alongside the anus or sometimes spreads and goes on both sides of this, thus pointing in one or both ischio-rectal fossae. In some cases of prostatic abscess or of abscess of Cowper's gland where undue traumatism is

employed or where the infection is extremely violent, there may be so much tension on the wall of the rectum that it becomes gangrenous and an opening appears in it as well as in the urethra. I have seen one such case where there was an opening into the rectum, thence into the urethra, as well as a lateral channel which went around the penile structures. One could put a sound into the opening in the rectum and pass it all the way up to the skin just inside the right anterior superior spine.

TREATMENT

The processes used in the treatment of these fistulae may be summed up as follows:

1. Be sure that the urethra is wide open; that is, that all strictures have been dilated.

2. Divert the urinary flow either by a retention catheter or by a supra-pubic drain (preferably the latter).

3. Open all channels down to the one urethral opening in the perineum. If a channel passes through the scrotum, pass a probe through it and open the skin on each side up to the point of entry into the scrotal tissues. This will allow all the urethral drainage to come from one central point, and the tract beyond this will heal.

4. Saucerize the fistulous tract.

5. If the fistula is rectourethral, dissect the perineum, close the opening in the rectum, and leave a large rubber tube coming out through the r e c t a l sphincter for a period of about ten days so that all gas will pass out without distending the n e w l y made suture line, thus allowing it to heal.

In carrying out these procedures, if the fistula is on the under side of the penis, it is merely necessary to remove the epithelialized lining and sew up the urethra as well as the skin on the outside. If this is done and a retention catheter left in the bladder or a suprapubic drain placed, the fistulous opening will usually heal without difficulty providing the patient will cooperate and will not allow the wound to become infected or unduly irritated by attempting to pass urine through the urethra. If the opening is in the perineum and is a simple urethral fistula, all that is necessary is to saucerize the skin and superficial fascia so that the wound is an inverted cone instead of a fusiform cavity. Usually in such cases the fistula will heal without further trouble even though the urine is not diverted. In case such a procedure does not bring about healing, the proper thing to do would be to drain the bladder suprapubically, repeating the saucerizing process. The wound will then heal. In the case of a rectourethral fistula, Young's transverse perineal incision s h o u l d be used, dissecting down to the opening and closing the rectal mucosa by ordinary chromic catgut sutures. The sphincter should be then dilated and a one inch rubber tube about six inches long placed in the rectum and fastened with a suture to the skin of the anus. A second layer of muscular tissue is then brought together over the rectal opening and a suprapubic cystostomy is done, allowing the urethra to remain at rest while the rectum heals. This usually takes about ten days. In one case I sewed up a large opening and it healed nicely until the rectal tube came out. Healing then ceased, leaving a very small opening instead of the large one as before. I then dilated the rectal sphincter greatly and sewed the opening together from inside the rectum with a small needle holder and needle. The tube was again placed and the patient made an uneventful recovery. Two weeks later I passed a sound into the urethra and found it slightly strictured but it dilated without difficulty. In another case I had a perineal fistula with several openings, one of which ran forward from the bulbous urethra through the scrotum and opened on the anterior side of the scrotum. I passed a probe through the opening and felt it subcutaneously on the posterior side of the scrotum, cut across it, then opened the channel from there on into the urethra. Meanwhile I left a silk suture running through the scrotum until the skin of the perineum had healed posterior to it. I then removed this suture and the scrotum healed spontaneously because it was not being fed by a discharge of pus or urine from the original tract. The cases of combined rectal and perineal fistulae may be handled in identically the same manner: that is, dissecting the perineum by Young's transverse incision, closing the rectum, leaving a tube in it to carry off the gas while the incision heals, and diverting the urine either by a retention catheter or suprapubic drain. These fistulae usually take about three or four weeks to heal. During the first week the patient should be given no food; during the second week only liquids or concentrated foods which leave little residue. After ten days, the tube can be removed and a daily warm soda enema given.

---o---

Low Back Pain in Relation to Urology*

STANLEY F. WILDMAN, M.D.
OKLAHOMA CITY, OKLAHOMA

On January 14, 1937, there appeared in the Daily Oklahoman a column entitled "Aches." The writer discussed backache which he termed "Sacro-iliac." Some of the statements he made are: (quote)

"Sacro-iliac is an ailment of the back and the beauty of it is that it doesn't show. When a workman applies for compensation b e c a u s e of this ailment insurance companies can't prove that he doesn't have it—even the X-ray won't tell.

"A blow, strain or twist may injure the sensitive muscles around the joint and the only evidence of the ailment is the victim's statement of pain.

"Records of the state industrial commission show an average of 125 back injury claims filed a month and insurance companies estimate about 75 per cent of these are "Sacro-iliac" claims—about 95

*Read before the Section on Genito-Urinary Diseases and Syphilology, Annual Meeting, Oklahoma State Medical Association, Tulsa, May, 1937.

cases per month. Oil field workers and truck drivers are the most common victims." [1]

It is the purpose of this paper to show that backache is seldom due to injury, but more often due to some genito-urinary tract pathology.

Anatomically the sacro-iliac joints are not true joints. They consist of two irregular, congruous joint surfaces. The congruity tends to increase their stability.

They are very large and very firm, and are held together by powerful ligaments and *not by muscles,* thus possessing but very little motion. They are kept securely in place by the "grip" due to the irregularity of the opposed surfaces of the two sacro-iliac articulations. Therefore, the human pelvis presents a mechanism the principal requirement of which is stability and not movement. [2-3-4-5-6]

The sacro-iliac joint is considered the strongest joint in the body, not only bearing the weight of the individual but great loads imposed upon it.

Sometimes before old age the joint is replaced by bone. If great force is applied to the pelvis and strain is placed upon the posterior sacro-iliac ligament they *may* rupture, but are more likely to withstand the violence and there be produced a tearing away of a portion of the bone into which the ligament is inserted.

Marked ecchymosis, swelling and tenderness over the sacro-iliac region are evidence of the tearing of the ligaments, or the fracture of the bones.

The sacro-iliac ligaments derive their innervation from the first and second sacral nerves—hence, referred pain from a sacroiliac lesion is distributed over the gluteal r e g i o n, posterior thigh, posterio-lateral calf and lateral border of the foot. This distribution of pain is commonly referred to as "sciatica" and is present in the great majority of cases of lesions of the sacroiliac joint. [7-8]

The genito-urinary tract plays a great role in the etiology of back pain. In fact, it is one of the most common complaints for which patients consult the physician.

There is often present a combination of *urological, gynecological, psychogenic* and *orthopedic conditions.*

The most frequent direct cause of "low back pain" in women is pelvic congestion, and any pathology within the pelvis producing this condition is the causative factor in 85 per cent of all gynecological cases. [10-11-12]

According to Crossen [13] pain across the sacral region is a common accompaniment of genital lesions; any inflammation or growth involving the pelvic connective tissue or causing intra-pelvic pressure may cause persistent, severe backache.

Folsom [14] calls attention to low backache in women due to reflex pain from the urethra.

The psychogenic factor plays a large part in low back pain. Kelly [15] claims a large group with neuresthenic or a pure neurotic basis may account for the whole complaint or at least for the exaggeration and protraction of symptoms from some trifling injury. The somewhat puzzling group labeled coccydinia probably f a l l s into this class.

The psychogenic origin is also sighted by Clancy [16] showing cases in which removal of the neurosis results in recovery.

Allison [17] sums up the causes of backache from the standpoint of the orthopedist, listing general debility, mental and physical fatigue first; gynecological and genito-urinary lesion second; and strain and injury fifth, in a list of 15 causes.

The majority of patients with genito-urinary lesions refer to their disability as a "backache" and not a back pain. These conditions, according to Kutzmann [18] are grouped in four types, namely; (a) localized, (b) radiating, (c) referred and (d) metastatic.

Localized pain is confined to the region of origin. In this type is found the true kidney pain; it is located particularly in the flank, usually at the level of the first to third lumbar vertebra. Radiation does not usually accompany a true kidney lesion, since there is no path of transmission. Exceptions have been noted as in the case of reno-renal reflex where the pain is referred to the opposite kidney. Renal pain is of a dual character, due to the fact the capsule of the kidney and the pelvis have separate innervations. [18-19-29-21-22]

The characteristics of a radiating pain is spasmodic and colicky. This type of back pain is caused by the alternate distention and muscular spasm of the ureter and kidney pelvis, beginning in the lumbar region and radiating downward and anteriorly into the groin, and genitalia, occasionally as far as the knee.

The principal causes are: calculi, blood clots, kinking of the ureter and particles of new growth. [18-23-24-25]

Referred pains ordinarily have no localizing or radiating character from the point of origin, but are felt at a distance in various regions along the course of the nerve fibers.

This type of pain is intermittent or continuous and may present a dull dragging or an aching sensation. [26-27-28-29]

Metastatic type of pain usually has its origin as a focal infection in the genito-urinary tract. In the sacral region the most frequent cause is a prostato-seminal vesiculitis, and the relationship of this to some orthopedic problem is c o m m o n. Namely; involvement of one or more joints with the prostate as a focus of infection. [30-31-32]

Any one who keeps the genito-urinary tract in mind when attempting to find the cause of backache knows that it is one of the chief sources, if not the most common, cause of backache. Inflammatory changes in the prostate and vesicles is the cause of backache in many cases. The complaint in practically every case is sacral disability. The pain is often referred down the course of the sciatic nerve, occasionally to the feet. [33] Pain may follow the pudendal n e r v e s in the back along the perineal branches, thus affecting the sacrum, buttox and perineum. This is *frequent* because of the close relation of the roots of these nerves to the sacral and lumbar plexuses.

This diffuse distribution allows pains caused by disease of the prostate and seminal vesicles to be referred to any part of the body below the diaphragm. [34]

We must continually bear in mind that branches of the nerves that supply the sacro-iliac joint also extend to the prostate and seminal vesicles, namely; the tenth, eleventh and twelfth dorsal; fifth lumbar and first, second and third sacral supply these areas.

In view of the development of compensation laws, infection of the prostate and seminal vesicles is assuming increasing importance, particularly so in reference to the "sprained back."

Pain in the back and groins is a common complaint, as pointed out by. Wesson [35] and is often diagnosed as sprained back, and recorded as such, instead of prostato-seminal vesiculitis and its sequela.

Pugh, [36] states that he believes there are millions being paid in compensation insurance for gonococcal infection of the prostate and seminal vesicles.

The injured back holds an enviable record as refuge for malingerers. The so-called sacro-iliac sprain which causes so much litigation in industrial injuries is a problem with which we are continuously confronted. Does backache really exist, and if so, is it the result of injury?

Many patients may say, and honestly conclude, that the backache of today was caused from the injury or the work of yesterday.

Numerous writers have stated that backache is curable and belongs in the domain of orthopedics, gynecology or i n t e r n a l medicine, overlooking that of urology. McBee states that a great per cent of backache is of urological nature, both as to cause and cure. [37]

According to Hoffman, "When searching for localization of focal infection in the male, every male beyond the age of 16 must be considered a potential candidate for prostatitis, and no case of suspected focal infection in the male can be said to have a thorough and proper consideration of all possible foci of infection until the prostate and seminal vesicles have proven themselves innocent or guilty." [38]

Treatment: Much can be done for the patient with the backache. Above all he should be assured the protection of a definite diagnosis. Those due to toxemias yield readily to the treatment of the focus, plus general measures. Little things such as flat feet should not be overlooked. [39]

Orthopedic and gynecological conditions can in most cases be relieved by those measures.

Genito-urinary c o n d i t i o n s are now known to cause about 75 per cent of backaches. The other 25 per cent are gynecologic, orthopedic or psychogenic. This is definitely proven by the relief secured when genito-urinary treatments are applied. Many chronic backaches have been relieved by dilatation of the ureter. Many have been relieved by dilatation of strictures of the urethra in both sexes. Prostatic massage, systematically done, is very frequently followed by prompt relief from backache — the small, firm but smooth gland often harbors the most virulent infection, which can only be diagnosed by a study of the expressed fluid.

From this it will be seen that the physician must seriously consider the entire genito-urinary tract in studying back pain, especially those uncertain dull backaches which superficially appear to be without apparent cause.

CONCLUSIONS

1. The sacro-iliac joint is the strongest joint in the body. So strong are the ligaments that bind it together that the bone gives way before the joint itself opens.

2. Branches of the same nerves that supply the sacro-iliac supplies the prostate, seminal vesicles and rectum. Often this accounts for referred pain to the joint if either is effected.

3. In men 75 per cent of backache is genito-urinary. In women 50 per cent of backache is gynecological—the remainder falling in the fields of orthopedic and psychogenic.

4. There are many drawing compensation for alleged sacro-iliac sprain who have only a prostato-seminal vesiculitis.

5. Psychic conditions are frequently to be considered.

6. Modern diagnostic m e t h o d s have brought the a c c u r a c y of diagnosis of genito-urinary tract lesions to such a degree that in general one can prove or disprove these organs as being the cause of backache.

REFERENCES

1. Parr, Ray: Daily Oklahoman. January 14, 1937, Vol. 45, No. 7.

2. Jones-Lovett: Orthopedic Surgery, PP 194, Wm. Wood and Company.

3. Grays Anatomy, P. 302, Leo & Febiger.

4. Cunningham: Text Book of Anatomy, PP 335, Wm. Wood and Company.

5. Spalteholz, Werner: Hand Atlas of Human Anatomy, Vol. I, PP 210. J. B. Lippencott & Company.

6. Piersol, George A.: Human Anatomy. J. B. Lippencott & Company.

7. Christopher, Frederich: Text Book of Surgery, P. 421. W. B. Saunders Company.

8. Jepson, Paul N.: Backache, Traumatic, Vol. 101, PP 1778-1782. Journal of American Medical Association.

9. Goldthwait, Joel E.: Backache, Vol. 209, 1933, PP 722-729. New England Journal of Medicine.

10. Ward, George G.: Backache from the Standpoint of the Gynecologist. American Journal of Surgery, Vol. 2, 1937, PP 257-260.

11. Dicks, John F.: Gyn. Aspects of Low Back Pain, Vol. 88, PP 554-556. New Orleans Medical Surgery Journal. July, 1935.

12. Stumdorf, Arnold: Gynopathic Backache Surgery—Gyn. Obstet. Vol. 53, 1931, PP 209-215.

13. Crossen, Harry S.: Diseases of Women, P. 196. C. V. Mosby Company.

14. Folsom, A. I.: Abstract Discussion, Vol. 99, 1932, PP 2237-2241. Journal of American Medical Association.

15. Kelly, Howard A.: Gynecology, P. 469. D. Appleton Company.

16. Clancy, Frank J.: Urol & Cut Revue. Oct. 1933, PP 703.

17. Allison, Nathaniel: Backache from the Standpoint of the Orthopedist. American Journal of Surgery, Vol. 2, 1927, PP 261-265.

18. Kutzmann, Adolph A.: Back Pain of Urologic Origin. Urol & Cut Revue, July, 1931, PP 454.

19. Wright, Samson: Applied Physiology. Oxford Medical Publishing Co., PP 550.

20. Ball and Evans: Diseases of the Kidney. P. Blackstons Son & Company, PP 15.

21. Starling: Human Physiology. Leo & Febiger, PP 329.

22. Kuntz, Albert: Autonomic Nervous System. Leo & Febiger, PP 306-307.

23. Wildman, Stanley F.: The Ureter in Relation to Urology. Urol & Cut Revue, Vol. XL, No. 8, 1936.

24. Jones, Fay H. and Brown, T. Duel: Backache from the Urological Viewpoint. Urol & Cut Revue, June, 1935, PP 402.

25. Seng, M. L: Significance of Backache in Genito-Urinary Diseases. Canada, J. A. J., 28-283-285, March, 33.

26. Wallace, W. J.: Abstract Discussion Urological Backache. Journal of American Medical Association. Vol. 99, 1932, PP 2237-2241.

27. Keyser, Linwood D.: Pain Syndromes in the Upper Urinary Tract. Southern Medical Journal, Oct. 1936, Vol. 29, PP 953-963.

28. Reed, W. A.: Symptomatic Relation of Urinary Disturbances to Diseases of the Intestinal Tract. Southern Medical Journal, Vol. 20, 1936, PP 1099-1101.

29. Behan, Richard J.: Pain. D. Appleton & Company, P. 95.

30. Duncan, Wallace S.: The Relation of the Prostate Gland to Orthopedic Problems. Journal of Bone & Joint Surgery. Jan. 1936, PP 101-104.

31. Pratt, John G.: Urological Aspects of Low Back Pain. New Orleans Medical & Surgical Journal. Vol. 88, PP 556-558. 1935-36.

32. Margo, E.: Journal Oklahoma Medical Association. Vol. 24, PP 16-19, 1931.

33. Smith, Clinton K.: Facts and Fallacies Regarding the Prostate Gland. Medical Herald-Physical Therapy, July, 1930.

34. Himan, Frank: Urology, P. 266. W. B. Saunders & Company.

35. Wesson, M. B.: Quoted by W. Scott Pugh, P. 309, Seminal Vesiculitis. Urol & Cut Revue, May, 1929.

36. Pugh, Winfield Scott: Seminal Vesiculitis. Urol & Cut Revue, PP 309-312, May, 1929.

37. McBee, Jud T.: Backache in Relation to Urology. Vol. 32. Urol & Cut Revue, PP 230-232, April, 1929.

38. Hoffman, Claude G.: Prostate & Seminal Vesicles as Foci of Infection. Urologic & Cut Revue, PP 230-232, April, 1929.

39. Harting, Edward F.: Low Back Pain. N. Y. State Journal of Medicine. 36, 979-1936.

40. Culver, Harry: Chronic Prostatitis, Vol. XXVI, PP 401-406. The Journal of Urology, September, 1931.

Cancer of the Stomach*

D. D. Paulus, M.D., and J. H. Robinson, M.D.
OKLAHOMA CITY, OKLAHOMA

THE DIAGNOSIS: It seems to me that one of the important problems in cancer of the stomach is the early recognition of the condition. A problem which has been emphasized time and again, but very little progress has been made in the past decade as compared with the previous two decades. If we are to increase the number of cases that are operable when first seen, then the clinician must b e c o m e more cancer-conscious. The so-called typical textbook type of case of cancer of the stomach is all too frequently still the mental picture of cancer of the stomach in the eyes of most laymen and also many members of the profession.

The symptoms of early cancer of the stomach depend to a great extent on its location, its size and whether it interferes with the motility of the stomach. A carcinoma at the pyloric end will cause early interference with motility; whereas if it is located in pars media it may remain silent for a considerable time. This is especially true if it happens to be located on the anterior or posterior margin of pars media or on the greater curvature. A cancer located close to the cardiac orifice will soon interfere with the entrance of food into the stomach.

We must remember that most of the cases of cancer of the stomach occur in a previously well male i n d i v i d u a l, with practically no previous digestive disturbance. Any digestive disturbance coming in a patient at or past middle life, which persists for one or two months in spite of the usual m e d i c a t i o n, should have a thorough investigation. The symptoms may often mimic ulcer early in the case. The patient complains of a gnawing sensation coming on at variable periods after a meal, usually several hours, and is relieved to a considerable extent by additional food intake. Later the gnawing dis-

tress comes sooner after meals and is more or less persistent all the time. If this is associated with loss of appetite and weight, and progressive pallor, it calls for complete laboratory investigation of the case. The clinician should not wait until he finds a questionably palpable tumor mass or a definitely palpable mass to verify his suspicions. In other cases a progressively increasing pallor and weakness or easy fatigue, without scarcely any digestive disturbance, may be the only early complaint.

In known ulcer cases of long standing a change in the symptomatology, such as persistency of distress in spite of good ulcer therapy, and especially if this is associated with loss of appetite, increasing pallor and weakness, should awaken the clinician's interest and suspect a beginning cancer. Unfortunately in a certain number of cases, especially those located in pars media or the greater curvature, a palpable tumor mass may be the first thing that calls the attention of the patient to the fact that something radically wrong exists. He may have enjoyed fairly good health up to this time, so far as any digestive disturbance is concerned.

Of the various laboratory procedures the X-ray gives us the most valuable help. Gastric analysis, as a rule, does not help us very much as carcinoma may be present when free hydrochloric acid is found. Persistent findings of blood, with positive test for occult blood in the stool, of course gives corroborative evidence.

The X-ray is not alone valuable in locating the lesion but also gives us some idea of its size. The most frequent finding in early cases is the carcinomatous ulcer. The niche, when longer than 2.5 centimeters, is generally to be strongly suspected as a carcinomatous ulcer but must be evaluated in the case, taking into consideration the history and other findings. It is more frequent to mistake a carcinamotous ulcer for benign ulcer than it is to

*Read at Seminole County Medical Society in March, 1936, and at Comanche County Society at Lawton in November, 1936.

call it a carcinoma when actually it is benign. A very large benign ulcer with considerable infiltration in the surrounding area is practically impossible to differentiate and may cause the surgeon to be doubtful, even when he has the lesion exposed and can palpate the same.

In the cases that are more advanced and show considerable filling defect the important question to decide is the extent and location of the lesion, to see if the case might be amenable to surgery. There is no question that the average clinician has taken too gloomy and pessimistic a view of the situation and all too often the case is turned down as hopeless, when an exploratory operation may show the lesion is still localized to the stomach, except perhaps for some palpable lymph nodes along the lesser curvature. These lymph nodes may or may not be carcinomatous and may on microscopic examination prove only to be inflammatory in nature.

All cases in which exploratory operation is decided upon should have adequate preoperative perparation, so that extensive resection of the stomach can be undertaken if the surgeon finds it feasible from a technical standpoint to do so.

THE SURGERY

In connection with gastric carcinoma, it is my impression that there are two definite shortcomings in this immediate area.

No. 1. When a diagnosis of carcinoma of the stomach is made, we are too quick to admit that the patient is incurable and we too often fail to offer relief by way of exploration and resection.

No. 2. When operating these weakened patients, we too often fail to sustain them while the operation is in progress. Most of these patients are frail, toxic and weak. They are poor operative risks. While on the table, they should be receiving intravenously glucose, acacia, or b l o o d. If their blood pressures are falling and they are going into shock during the operation, the operation should, as a rule not be hurried, but should be *stopped*, and the patient revived by work of the anesthetist in forcing CO_2 and oxygen, and by the giving of intravenous fluids mentioned; i.e., glucose, acacia and blood. I wish to place much emphasis on this point.

Patients with carcinoma of the stomach

are entitled to an exploration if they can be made operable. Upon opening the abdomen, a review of the stomach itself should be made, then the surrounding tissue should be studied in search for metastases. The lymph nodes about the pylorus, the gastro-colic mesentery, the amount of fixation of the tumor, and then a search is made in the liver. If there is evidence of metastases beyond what can be removed, then, of course, only a gastroenterostomy, in the event of pyloric obstruction, should be undertaken. On the other hand, if it seems reasonably sure that a resection is possible, the p a t i e n t is entitled to this chance, which of course, is his only hope of recovery. When a roomy incision is made and we avoid pulling on the mesentery, I find this operation is no more shocking than any other intra-abdominal operation lasting the same period of time. When a patient recovers from this operation, his health is functionally restored.

After getting into the problem of cancer of the stomach, I have concluded that the operative technique is by no means as complicated as I have formerly thought. Many of the little features which add to the confusion of a gastric resection are not necessary. The principle is the same as when laid down by Billroth in the eighties. That is, we do an end to end, stomach to duodenum, when we resect only a small amount of the stomach. This is known as the Billroth I procedure; and the modifications which I have adopted for use are being sketched hereunder.

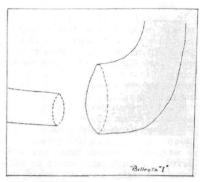

The Billroth I type of Partial Gastrectomy. Billroth of Vienna reported the first case of partial gastrectomy done in 1881. He united the stomach to the duodenum.

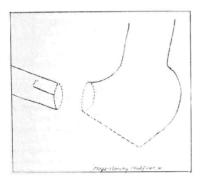

The method of increasing the caliber of the duodenum by splitting its wall back a varying distance was advocated by C. H. Mayo. Horsley advocates closing the lower half of the cut end of the stomach by a purse string suture. This leaves the open portion next to the lesser curvature for anastomosis to the duodenum.

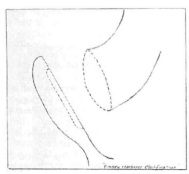

This is merely an anastomosis of the end of the stomach to the side of the duodenum after closure of the end of the duodenum. This can be done only in cases which have a long duodenal mesentery.

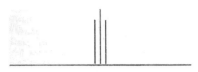

When a large portion of the stomach is being removed, as for an advanced carcinoma, an end to side, stomach to jejunum anastomosis is necessary. This is known as the Billroth II procedure.

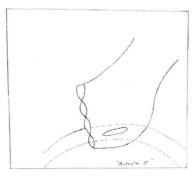

This method is recommended where a large portion of the stomach is removed. The ends of the stomach and duodenum are closed, then a standard posterior gastrojejunostomy is done.

For the sake of simplicity, we have adopted for our use the modifications you will find s k e t c h e d hereunder. These methods are relatively simple, but adequate for most of the cases of cancer of the stomach encountered. No originality is claimed for any of these procedures selected.

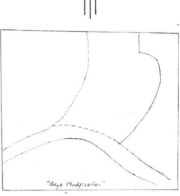

This method is popular. It entails the anastomosis of the open end of the stomach to the side of the jejunum, through the colonic mesentery.

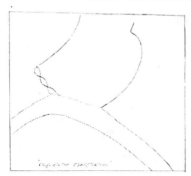

In certain cases the open end of the stomach is very large. Hofmeister, for these cases, advocates closing a portion of this next to the lesser curvature by use of a purse string suture. Anastomosis end to side, stomach to jejunum is then done.

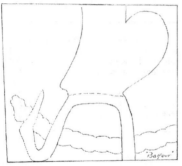

This is merely the Polya or the Hofmesiter done by throwing the jejunum up over the colon, for the anastomosis to the stomach, rather than doing the operation through the colonic mesentery.

POST-OPERATIVE MANAGEMENT

The patient must be treated about the same as any other patient convalescing from a major operation, except that the stomach is put at rest. For a normal-sized adult, we usually give around 3.000 cc of fluid each day, and a practical way to do this is to administer a hypodermoclysis of 1,000 cc of normal saline and give 500 cc of 10 per cent glucose in the vein morning and evening. This is kept up a few days until the patient is taking fluids by mouth. Sedation is, of course, required and a choice among the more frequently used opiates is made. After 48 hours, the dosage is reduced. If the convalescence is smooth, we start water by mouth in one-ounce quantities at two to four hour intervals, about the fourth to the sixth day. Next day, the patient is given a choice between water and milk in two-ounce quantities at two hour intervals. By the end of the first post-operative week, the patient is taking cooked cereal or some thin gruel of his choice in two-ounce quantities at intervals of two to four hours. In the early post-operative period, we do not hesitate to use the nasal suction apparatus for the purpose of gastric lavage if we have vomiting, distension, or other reason for washing out the stomach. Care must be taken, of course, to throw no strain on the stomach. This can be done by allowing only a small amount of water to be used at a time in the lavage and that to run in by gravity.

Nowhere in surgery does the principle of "suturing without tension" a p p ly more sharply than in stomach work. If the jejunum is anastomosed to the stomach in such a way as to create a pull on the suture line somewhere, a leak can be expected. The swelling subsides on about the fourth day. For this reason, the fourth or fifth post-operative day may be considered the most dangerous from the standpoint of leakage. This justifies a very cautious and slow increase in dietary intake. However, many patients who have had two-thirds of the stomach removed are taking as much as a standard soft diet in ten to 14 days. It seems advisable for these patients to take nourishment at about four hour intervals from the time they begin taking soft diet to the end of a three or four months period. After this, they eat three times a day and have no difficulty. The quantity of stomach removed pretty well prognosticates the future for the patient. The patients who have so much as one-third of the stomach left are pretty likely to get along well. Those who have one-fourth or less must be watched carefully after a year, for the onset of pernicious anemia. As a rule, when a patient has a gastric resection, if there are no metastases, and metastases are often late in gastric cancer, his health is restored.

Diagnosis and Treatment of Maxillary Sinusitis*

W. L. ALSPACH, M.D.

TULSA, OKLAHOMA

The maxillary antrum, or sinus, is generally the one most frequently involved and probably the most frequently overlooked of any sinusitis. This paper will not go into the anatomy or physiology of the antrum, nor will it discuss any definite surgical procedure except to indicate when surgery is necessary and the type of operation required.

In treating diseases of the antrum, the object in view is to provide ventilation, drainage and to allow proper moisture with the least possible trauma or injury to the sinuses and mucus membrane. Briefly maxillary sinusitis falls into three types, acute, sub-acute and chronic.

It is generally agreed that the antrum is usually infected by direct extension to the maxillary ostium. The principal causes of infection are the common head cold, grippe, influenza, or direct infection from another sinus. However, one must remember that infected teeth, neoplasms, or osteomyelitis of the m a x i l l a can also be responsible for an infected antrum.

The symptoms of an acute antrum are varied. There may be pain, fullness or throbbing of the cheek, pain over the eye on the infected side, pain in the cheek when w a l k i n g, and particularly when coming down on the heel, and there are usually complaints of frontal headaches. Fever as a rule is present but it may be absent. The patient appears toxic and complains of the nose being stopped up, with or without a nasal discharge. Quite frequently a patient with an infected antrum has a larynxal cough, which disappears in about the same ratio as the infection in the antrum clears up. Trans-illumination does not seem to be of much assistance in diagnosing an acute antrum unless it is positive. Quite frequently an infected antrum gives a negative trans-illumina-

*Read before the Eye, Ear, Nose and Throat Section, Annual Meeting, Oklahoma State Medical Association, Tulsa, May, 1937

tion. X-ray may be of some help but clinical findings in the nose plus the symptoms, are generally sufficient for a diagnosis. In the nose one finds an inflamed mucus membrane with hypertrophied turbinates. After shrinking the nose with ephedrine three per cent and cocaine one per cent pus may or may not be found in the middle meatus, depending on whether the ostium is open or not. If the ostium is open and pus escaping, the patient does not suffer so much from pain and fullness in cheek or systemic symptoms as when the ostium is closed.

The treatment for acute antrum is chiefly systemic. The patient should be put to bed, given large amounts of fruit juices, with a light diet and have the infra red lamp or its equivalent applied over the antrum for about 20 to 30 minutes daily. Care must be taken not to apply too much heat to an acute antrum since the resulting hyperemia might shut off the o s t i u m, thereby preventing ventilation and drainage. The nose should be shrunk with a nasal pack of ephedrine and cocaine. The correct placing of the pack is very important. It should be inserted well into the middle meatus as near as possible to the ostium of the maxillary sinus and left there from 20 to 30 minutes. This p a c k i n g should be done daily and the infra red treatment may be given while the pack is in the nose.

After five to seven days of this treatment, the majority of the patients recover. If, however, the symptoms continue to persist, it is probably advisable to do an antrum puncture for irrigation.

Speaking of antrum punctures, it is well known that there is considerable difference of opinion among rhinologists in regard to the various ways of entering the antrum. The natural opening has its advantages and it appears to be the most logical method, but due to anatomical reasons, it is impossible to pass a probe through the opening in 50 per cent of the average cases. In the average chronic case, not complicated by polyps, hypertrophied or hyperplastic mucus membrane, entrance through the natural ostium is indicated. Antrum puncture through the middle meatus is a very dangerous procedure because of the possibility of entering the orbit. It appears then, that the route through the inferior meatus below the inferior turbinate and through the maxillary process is the most efficient and desirable.

Due to the fact that cocaine causes a systemic or general reaction in so many patients it is advisable to discard its use. In many cases a patient has suffered more from the cocaine reaction than from the actual antrum puncture and this has had a tendency to bring the antrum puncture into disrepute. Pontocaine two per cent, or larocaine 10 per cent will give the same local anesthetic action but without the dangerous reaction which c o c a i n e may give.

The acute antrum is irrigated with about a pint of normal saline solution every four to five days until the thick pus is eliminated. Normal s a l i n e solution is used rather than a strong antiseptic or astringent because if there should be a mishap and the fluid be injected into the tissues there would be no dangerous r e s u l t s. Strong antiseptic solutions also have a tendency to injure the tissues and inhibit the action of the cilia, which would hinder the recovery.

After the puncture and irrigation, before the needle is withdrawn, an injection of five to six cc of ephedrine one per cent in normal saline solution is put into the antrum and left there. It has been found that ephedrine at this strength (one per cent) does not injure the cilia or mucus membrane and instead, when left in the antrum is distinctly beneficial in keeping the ostium open. It has been noticed that when after one or two irrigations the pus begins to clump and to take on a rusty color, one can reasonably assume that the antrum will recover shortly.

Before leaving the acute a n t r u m, it might be mentioned that, if possible, an antrum is never punctured during the vascular stage of an acute attack. It may,

however, be necessary in some cases to make a window into the antrum below the inferior turbinate if the antrum puncture does not relieve the acute condition readily.

To diagnose the sub-acute stage of sinusitis is slightly more difficult than the acute. There is generally a history of head colds, a stopped up nose at times, and the patient is troubled with headaches, as a rule frontal. He also complains of a postnasal drip and of blowing out large quantities of pus from the nose. There may be a cough or hoarseness and in general the patient feels below par and can not snap out of his cold. On examination of the nose, one finds the mucus membrane congested and the turbinates, particularly the inferior turbinate, hypertrophied. There may or may not be a slight discharge of pus in the middle meatus, depending on the potency of the ostium and the amount of pus in the antrum. In most case there is a considerable amount of pus in the middle meatus. Posterior rhinoscopy will reveal pus more often than the anterior view. A routine trans-illumination and X-ray of the sinuses is always made in these cases.

An antrum puncture is done and the character and cytology of the pus, if any, is noted. If the patient finds that the antrum puncture, followed by the injection of normal saline ephedrine solution has given him relief, then the next time he returns for treatment, the Proetz displacement method is used with normal saline in one per cent ephedrine for the displacing fluid. He is given about five such' treatments, one every other day, and then for the next two displacement treatments an iodized oil, diluted with light mineral oil three to one, is used for the displacing fluid. Patients seem to prefer the iodized mineral oil to the ephedrine saline solution, probably because the dried mucus membrane is lubricated and it is soothing to the general soreness of the nose.

If the first antrum puncture with irrigation does not give much relief, the puncture should be repeated every four to five days, using saline solution until relief is obtained, always leaving the normal saline ephedrine solution in the antrum after irrigation. If, after five to seven washings and a good systemic and supportive treatment, there is no clearing up of the antrum infection, an internasal operation is indicated. This operation gives very little discomfort to the patient and may be done in a clinic or in the office. The patient does not lose more than one to three days from work and the convalescence is much speedier than repeated antrum lavages.

There is one type of sub-acute antrum that is always a problem. In these cases, the lining of the antrum is very thick, hyperemic and edematous. Even weeks after the onset of the sinusitis the patient still complains of headaches, fullness in cheek and general run down condition. The natural ostium is closed by the edema or swelling of the mucus membrane, and it is practically impossible to shrink with ephdrine or other solutions. An antrum puncture is unsuccessful because the needle either pushes the m u c u s membrane in front of it or the needle becomes embedded in it. It is impossible to inject even small quantities of air or fluid into the antrum. It is also not possible to withdraw fluid from this antrum even with a small glass syringe.

In these cases, a window made in the nasal antrum wall with no further operative procedure seems to give the most satisfactory results. Due to the fact that the mucus membrane of the antrum is particularly sensitive, a general anesthetic is advisable. After the window is made, the mucus membrane seems to shrink, and the antrum may be irrigated through the window. An internasal or Cadwell-luc operation may be necessary later, but the majority of cases clear up with ventilation and drainage. If not, then the Proetz displacement method very often helps this type of case after the window has been made.

In the chronic antrum the first consideration is to remove the source of infection and then p r o v i d e ventilation and drainage. The chronic antrum may be d i v i d e d into the suppurative and non-suppurative types. With our clinical findings, trans-i l l u m i n a t i o n and X-ray, a chronic maxillary sinus that has large quantities of pus should not be difficult to diagnose. The symptoms are varied. The patient complains of frequent colds following one another closely, or of a post-nasal discharge, irritated pharynx, cough and

hoarseness. Others have a slight headache and some complain of loss of sense of smell, which may be partial or complete. Still others complain of quantities of pus and mucus discharged from the nose at intermittent intervals. A few chronic sinuses have no local symptoms whatever, and are discovered only when checking up the sinus for a focal point of infection. On the objective examinations, the nose may or may not show abnormalities. The mucus membrane may appear normal or one may find pathological conditions in the nose such as polypoid-degeneration of the turbinates, hypertrophies and hperplasias of the turbinates and polyps. The amount of pus in the middle meatus varies. At times in the same patient one may see pus escaping and at other times it may be entirely clear. Pus in the 'middle meatus, of course, does not always originate in the antrum and may be due to infection of the frontal or anterior ethmoid sinus. If the pus is wiped away and reappears immediately, in all probability it is due to either a frontal or ethmoid sinus. It may be remarked here that finding pus in the antrum does not necessarily mean that the antrum is infected. It may be acting as a reservoir for pus that has been discharged from the frontal or ethmoid sinus.

Posterior rhinoscopy frequently shows us more than the anterior, most likely because the inferior turbinate slopes downward and back; this allows drainage into the throat from both the maxillary and accessory ostiums. In treating the chronic antrum, irrigations every five to seven days are given either through the maxillary ostium or by puncture through the inferior meatus. Normal saline only is used as the irrigating medium. If the pus continues to have a fetid or foul odor after two or three washings, it is wise to think of the infection as possibly dental or neoplastic in origin. If the antrum clears up fairly well with irrigations, we switch over to the Proetz displacement method, using normal saline with ephedrine.

Frequently the anterior portion of the middle turbinate is enlarged, either hypertrophied or hyperplastic, shutting off the ostium of the antrum. In these cases, it is better to amputate the anterior part of the middle turbinate in order to allow ventilation and drainage. A sub-mucus resection may be also required so that the nose will have proper ventilation and that there will be no obstruction.

If after a month's irrigation and no gross pathology has been demonstrated, the antrum has not cleared up entirely, an internasal or Caldwell-luc operation is advisable. When an internasal o p e r a t i o n is done, it is performed under local anesthetic. The internasal wall is removed and the floor of the nose is lowered to the level of the antrum and any polyps or hypertrophied mucus membrane curretted. With the antrum that has polypoid degeneration of the mucus membrane, polyps or cysts, or ulcerations, a Caldwell-luc operation is advised. To diagnose a chronic antrum without suppuration, an X-ray is taken. If the presence of polyps, cysts, hypertrophies or hyperplasia is suspected, another X-ray is taken after an injection of iodized oil in the antrum. The oil may be injected by canula through the natural o s t i u m through the inferior meatus by puncture or by the displacement method. When X-rays are negative, with and without the iodized oil, and the objective examination

of the nose reveals nothing, a sterile antrum puncture through the inferior meatus is often very helpful. The nasal wall is anesthetized and an antiseptic applied to the wall. The puncture is made with the patient in a prone position and about five cc of sterile normal saline solution is injected into the antrum with the patient's head turned toward the infected or suspected side. The sterile saline solution is then withdrawn and transferred to a test tube for examination. Three or four syringe fulls are generally used. It is surprising the amount of mucus and pus that is found in a seemingly negative antrum by this simple procedure. These washings may then be used for bacteriological examination and for culture for vaccine.

With youngsters that have running noses and a pussy discharge, this sterile puncture gives us much information about the antrum and the pus may be used for culture for vaccine. Speaking of vaccines, there have been very good results obtained from vaccines. These v a c c i n e s are only of benefit in those cases where we do not have any greatly manifested pathological condition of the mucus membrane.

Shall We Destroy Medical Protection For Selfish Gain?

L. H. RITZHAUPT, M.D.
GUTHRIE, OKLAHOMA

To understand the magnitude of the healing art, it is well that we consider the chronological steps of m e d i c a l science which is as old as mankind yet more modern than any invention.

From the day that man sinned and disobeyed the laws of God, disease has attacked the human family. Primitive man forgot the cause of his suffering and his philosophy of life's problems was founded on mystery and magic. Driven from the Garden of Eden, he became a roving savage, facing a hostile world, hunting his food by day and hiding for protection at

night. The agony of disease and the injuries which befell him caused him to crawl to his lair to die. This primitive man, though savage, was nevertheless, intelligent and reasoned on abstract matters. Those things for which he could not find a tangible form were credited as supernatural. Into this category he placed disease and so it remained for centuries, with its chief treatment practiced through mystery and magic.

Today we can trace the development of practice from the earliest times — when the medicine man dressed in his bizarre and fantastic costume, pretending, by his weird chant, continuous stomp and the laying on of hands, to drive away the evil spirit. On through the early days of civilization, Egyptian, Babylonian and Jewish, we can see rising almost imperceptibly above the morass of mystery and magic the beginning of rational medical practices. In time, mystery and magic gave place to religion. The Jewish people developed a very sound and rational code of hygiene; sanitation at their hands became a religious precept with the rabbis as sanitary police.

It was among the ancient Greeks that the principles of modern scientific medicine were formulated. They separated it from religion, removed mystery from medicine and made it a practice, not of magic, not of religion, but of common sense, observation and logical deduction.

Hippocrates 2,300 years ago gave us the nucleus of science and medicine. It is he whom we revere as the father of modern medicine; his philosophy and ethics have been a guiding i n f l u e n c e to this day. Dioscarides, a Greek army surgeon, originated the Materia Medica, and recorded the use of mandragora wine as an anesthesia for surgical operations. The great Roman physician, Galen, enlarged upon the medical knowledge practiced by the conquered Greek physicians. Rome ruled the world, built cities with paved streets, aqueducts and sewers and instituted the principles of public health.

In the years between the days of Hippocrates and the rise of the modern period, civilization was to decline, and with it medicine. Science and civilization rose and fell many times with very little progress in either. Speculation and dogmatism entered the field of medicine to displace observation and clear reasoning. Rival schools sprang into existence; the men of these s c h o o l s were more interested in making additions to their dogmas than they were in carrying on unsullied the great principles that Hippocrates had outlined. This type of thinking, and the rivalry established led to quackery and was the mother of many of the healing cults and fads of today. It was a difficult path that Hippocrates pointed out for medicine to follow — one that involved intellectual honesty. Only the highest type of men

have the intelligence, the independence, the integrity and the courage to admit their errors and seek after the truth without bias. It is men of this type that have given us modern medicine.

John Hunter, who correlated surgical procedures with the physiology and pathology of the diseased part, along with Lister who modernized asepsis, did more to elevate surgery to a specialty than any other men. Edward Jenner founded the principle of preventive medicine and gave us vaccination, the most valuable of all prophylactic measures. It is by the application of this principle that smallpox, typhoid and typhus fever, diphtheria, tetanus and many other diseases have ceased to terrorize the human family.

Phillippe Pinal demonstrated that the mentally deranged were ill, thus opening the way for adequate care of the insane and for modern psychiatry.

The center of medical education shifted from Leyden and Paris to Vienna and Edinburg during the 18th c e n t u r y and scientific medicine was at a stand-still. As the 19th century began, we recognize the turning point—years filled with knowledge of cellular pathology, bacterial cause of infection and disease, revolutionary discoveries as that of anesthesia, asepsis and the application of chemistry and physics to physiological problems. During this century such names as Marton, Long, Wells, Pasteur, Koch, Lister, Ephrian, McDowell, Richard Bright, James Parkinson, Carl Basedow, William Stokes, Thomas Addison, Edward Squibbs, and many other physician-scientists who have altered our way of living, our ways of thinking more profoundly than the warriors, the traders, and even the philosophers of all ages w e r e written on the pages of history never to be erased.

Any fair-minded individual can easily recognize that the progress by scientists and the medical profession have been responsible for the rapid and progressive development of the healing art. It has meant years of hard work, with the cost of countless lives well spent, from the first primitive efforts which were made to allay human suffering to the present day operating room with its great sterilizing machines, its immaculate linens, its gleaming instruments for every need, and its efficient anesthesia, all administered and supervised by a corps of men and women, trained to the f i n e s t detail, who have consecrated their lives for the relief of human suffering, never willing to discard from their ethics the religious sacrifice of self for the good of others, principles older than science. T h i s technical development has reached far into the new world. By means of the laboratory we trace down the cause of nearly every disease. The wonders of diagnosis and the efficiency of therapy cannot be too greatly emphasized because through this route has come the science of m o d e r n medicine. But no matter how glorious are its potential benefits, or how great its contributions, it is not of itself medicine complete. As long as human beings remain human beings, and there exists the freedom of thought and the privilege of individual contacts, personality must remain an integral part of the practice of medicine. It is not to the great laboratory technicians nor yet to the centers of industrial medicine that we turn when in pain, but to the family physician, the man of the individual's choice, the man in whom the sick p e r s o n has implicit confidence. This family physician, this personality, aided by science and industry, stands as a peer among men, at the helm of one of the ships of civilization, with its cargo of diseased human beings, guiding it through the troubled days of pain and suffering into the harbor of recovery, or to a painless and less troubled death.

Each physician maintains and operates an office which is open to the public and in which the public is given service and for which the public compensates the physician. The hospital, however, which is the workshop of the doctor, and corresponds to the court house, which is the workshop for the lawyer, in many instances, is maintained by a doctor, a group of doctors or some philanthropic society or organization.

Hospitals, dealing with life and death, must of necessity forget the economical basis of maintenance and think primarily of efficiency, accuracy and the end results. This efficient s e r v i c e rendered necessitates the outlay of more money than is required to run the ordinary type of business

and, in turn, the compensation fee required by the hospital may be higher than the average individual expects.

Certain organizations led by dissatisfied, uninformed persons with a desire to increase the financial gain of a few individuals, professing to be ethical practioners of medicine, are attempting to break down all the safeguards of this noble profession, by changing the medical practice act of the state. In order to maintain a hospital, they are offering in glowing terms cheap hospital rates, and selling professional service, depriving the individual who enters into contract the privilege of being served by the physician of his choice.

The medical profession of the state of Oklahoma offers no opposition to establishment of cooperative hospitals. Few, if any, physicians would be unwilling to transfer their hospitals to an organization if they would be maintained efficiently and ethically, to protect the lives of those who must needs be treated therein, but every doctor who has embedded in his heart and mind the principle upon which the healing art has made its progress—and of this type there are the greatest number — resents the interference of any group or organization who, for its own advantage and selfish interests, attempts to break down the medical practice act of the state. If we allow an organization, whether it be a group of farmers or doctors, under the guise of church or cult, to organize for the purpose of sending out "cappers and steerers," men and women to sell the professional services of those who have, through years of contact with the people of the state, built up enviable reputations as internists or surgeons, then we are reverting to the age of mystery and magic and commercializing the sacred profession which can only be classed as the healing hand of Christ.

The present Cooperative Hospital plan, as outlined by its sponsors, provides that a farm family that can p u r c h a s e $50.00 worth of stock and is able to pay a definite annual fee, is eligible for membership. The thrifty farmer who has had considerable illness sees in this plan a chance to save money. High-powered salesmen are sent out to make unwarranted statements as to the hospital and medical service offered, and lead thoughtless individuals to purchase stock. The whole plan, as set out, is to provide hospital and medical attention for the families who are in the middle and upper financial classes, while no provision is made for the poor man and his family. Hospitalization cannot be offered to them unless the institution is compensated for the services rendered, whether by the county or state. The consequences are that private institutions o w n e d by other organizations or individuals m u s t bear the brunt of the financial burden and render service to the poor man and his family. It is evident that such individually owned hospitals cannot o p e r a t e unless those who are financially able to pay for medical and hospital service also come. Therefore, without paying p a t i e n t s, it would be necessary for such hospitals to close their doors and the local community would be without proper hospitalization. The very principle upon which this cooperative plan is suggested is definitely undemocratic.

The last legislature recognized the trend of sentiment in Western Oklahoma and attempted to provide for the poor by setting aside $175,000.00, or that portion necessary, for the purchase of an institution whereby people who are not financially able to pay for hospitalization and medical care could receive proper attention at the expense of the state.

The idea of establishing hospitals under group or board management is not new. During more prosperous former years, doctors and laymen have organized similar enterprises to make money, but with contrary results. Their financial reserve exhausted, the buildings and equipment were sold or turned to some benevolent organization. The operation of a hospital is a highly specialized business, demanding a consecration of time and thought that few are willing to give. The Catholic Sisterhoods, with their quiet, congenial manner and self-sacrificing spirit, c o u p l e d with long years of hospital management, are accepted as criterions in this field, and any other hospital organized may well follow their competitive example as to services and fees.

Why is a cooperative hospital established? Is it to secure cheaper hospital service? If so, is there any reason to believe that a group without experience in such management or even a faint idea of what is needed in the way of service to the sick, can operate a hospital more economically and efficiently than those who have made a life study of it? The actual expense of sickness must either be paid by the one who is ill or proportioned out among many lay members, stockholders and members of the controlling organization. If distribution of cost is desirable, it would be far wiser to take a policy in one of the many hospital insurance companies. Such reliable companies pay the prevailing prices for hospitalization, and in addition each member has the right to choose the hospital he feels will give the best service and meet his particular needs. The patient can select the physician or s u r g e o n in whom he has confidence — few people would have the necessary confidence in a man hired by the state to take care of whomever was sent to him. T h e r e is something touching and sacred in the admiration and respect and confidence of an individual for his own doctor, a feeling not replaced by man-made laws designating whom shall serve in hours of need.

Under the plan that has been submitted for cooperative hospitals in Oklahoma, not only is hospitalization offered, but medical, dental and surgical services as well. This is nothing more than a feeble attempt to offer hospital and sickness insurance, capitalizing on the services rendered.

Such sickness insurance is now compulsory for employees of railroads and various other large corporations; some European countries have forms of sickness insurance, foremost among them being England, who passed the National Health Insurance Act in 1911. Since that time the capitation fee has increased until it is now nearly three times the original cost and, in spite of this increase in cost, the service rendered is far from adequate. The Social Insurance Law of Germany includes sickness, and the ever-increasing cost of this phase is giving the government considerable worry. Denmark, Switzerland, France and the Scandinavian countries have some form of sickness insurance, but not controlled by lay management. In these countries there is marked disagreement as to the quality of the medical service. It is generally admitted that there is a tendency towards superficial diagnosis, over-medication and excessive hospitalization.

The financial aspect of medical care is the only reason given by promoters for changing the present system—certainly no one questions the advancement of the type and manner of treatment. There is a distinct tendency to lose sight of the relationship of this question to the general family budget and to national expenditures. Non-governmental medical services represent about 2.4 per cent of our national income. Governmental expenditures, raised by taxation for medical and institutional care, bring the sum total to three per cent.

Comparing the cost of medical services required for the average family to the cost of luxuries for the same family, will prove that sickness requires an expenditure of $65.00 per year, while the non-essentials which are directly under the family control, as tobacco, candy, soft drinks, jewelry, perfumes, sports, alcoholic beverages, etc., amount to the sum of $450.00 per year.

The total of the nations' bills for sickness is only about one-thirteenth of the national income, and the source of complaint seems not so much the amount as the manner of distribution. Sickness bills differ from nearly all other expenditures in the family budget because they occur unexpectedly and in varying amounts. Approximately half of the total expenditure falls to about one-sixth of the families. Any type of health insurance will be advantageous to this one-sixth of the families, yet the greater portion of the expense will be borne by the other five-sixths.

There should be a united effort by all the thinking people of Oklahoma to defeat Initiative Petition No. 166, which attempts to destroy present medical program and provide that the board of medical examiners shall be composed of seven members, two from the school of homeopathy, two from the eclectics and three from the regulars. It states that no school shall have a majority of members of the board, however, it allows the five per cent belonging to the schools of homeopathy and eclectics to have four members on the board

of examiners against three members from the regular physicians who represent 95 per cent of those practicing in the state. The schools of homeopathy and eclectics are fast joining the regulars or closing their own doors and before this petition would function there will not be more than one school teaching either homeopathy or eclecticism. However, the attempt of non-professional men to control the board of examiners of the medical profession is not the worst feature of this petition. It further provides that any group, either farmers, religious organization or charitable institution, can organize a cooperative hospital and legalize the sending out of "cappers and steerers" to secure members, offering not only hospitalization but the services of dentists, nurses and physicians. It makes no provision that a group of doctors may organize for the same purpose. This part of the petition places a stigma upon the doctors and insinuates that a profession which has rendered service to humanity for more than a thousand years and has elevated the healing art from the category of mystery and magic to the peak of scientific knowledge, would not have a right to compete with some organization that cannot possibly have the interest of the people at heart or know anything about the innermost workings of combating bodily ills. The medical profession in this state, and in fact in all states, has continued to live in a false dignity and stand aloof in a halo of medical ethics, and has allowed certain grasping individuals to enter into the realm and seize the reins of medical government. During years of economic depression, these outsiders have attempted to hoodwink those who have felt the sting of hunger and pain into the belief that they were being offered a sanctuary of medical protection. For four years, I have implored the physicians of this state to shake from them the mantle of reserve and the false ego that "I am mightier than thou." In this question of idealism versus realism, we must control some form of socialized or state medicine, hospitalization and medical care for those who cannot pay at all and offer to low-wage earners the best of medical and hospital service at a cost which they can pay.

The desire of the medical profession is

not to destroy but to build, to make new progress, and hold the advancement that has been made. The search for means to alleviate h u m a n suffering has stirred man's very souls. Theirs has not been a task for remuneration, for worldly glory, for fine buildings, but a service that found its compensation in resulting good for both rich and poor, regardless of color or creed. Shall the result of centuries of work and study, that each physician might to the best of his ability serve his fellowmen, be swallowed up by a few money-seekers? Shall individuals be forced to call upon someone not personally interested in their illness? Shall the respect and confidence earned by years of faithful service be exchanged for a mere scrap of paper bought at a specific price?

Professions, to be worthy of the name, must ever have higher standards than business. From the first cry of the infant to the sunset of life necessarily come many times when human bodies and emotions need the helping hand of a trained physician. Let us maintain the high standards of our calling—let us serve our fellowmen as helpers of The Great Physician who ministered to all. Ours is an obligation that cannot but increase our proper pride and our determination to carry forward what has been so well begun by our colleagues. The extent of human need is appalling—everywhere there are individuals who need our help. The mass of God's people will never be released from sickness and despair by passing laws to protect a few who are able to pay while others suffer. This is not a time for us to quibble over quotas that are to be levied or false goals set up and professional reserve advanced, but rather for an awakening of a spirit that will give renewed courage in the heart of every professional man in the state of Oklahoma.

This awakening should be now!

"Tomorrow you will live, you always cry;
In what far country does this morrow lie,
That 'tis so mighty long ere it arrive?
'Tis so far fetched, this morrow that I fear
'Twill be both very old and very dear.
Tomorrow I will live, the fool does say;
Today itselfs' too late—the wise lived yesterday."

(Procrastination, by Martialis.)

American Board of Ophthalmology

The American B o a r d of Ophthalmology announces that in 1938 it will hold examinations in:

San Francisco, June 13th, during the American Medical Association; Washington, D. C., Oct. 8th, during the American Academy of O. and O.L.; Oklahoma City, Nov. 14th, during the Southern Medical Association.

Up to the end of 1937, the Board has held 56 examinations and had certified 1,498 ophthalmologists. The Board on January 1st, 1938, issued a new and complete list of physicians certificated to date, arranged geographically. This list was mailed gratis to all certificated persons and to over 250 hospitals and institutions.

During 1937, examinations were held at Los Angeles on January 23rd, at Philadelphia on June 7th, and at Chicago on October 8th and 9th. At these examinations, 25, 71 and 84 candidates respectively were examined; of whom 19, 42 and 56 respectively were passed; 3, 17 and 25 respectively were conditioned; and 3, 2 and 1 respectively failed.

The American Board of Ophthalmology has established a Preparatory Group of prospective candidates for its certificate. The purpose of this Group is to furnish such information and advice to physicians who are studying or about to study ophthalmology as may render them acceptable for examination and certification after they have fulfilled the necessary requirements. Any graduate or undergraduate of an approved medical school may make application for membership in this Group. Upon acceptance of the application, information will be sent concerning the ethical and educational requirements, and advice to members of the Group will be available through preceptors who are members or associates of the Board. Members of the Group will be required to submit annually a summarized record of their activities.

The fee for membership in the Preparatory Group is ten dollars, but this amount will be deducted from the fifty dollars ultimately required of every candidate for examination and certification. For sufficient reason, a member of the Preparatory Group may be dropped by vote of the Board.

In future issues of the directory of the American Medical Association certificated ophthalmologists will be so designated in their listing.

Applications should be filed immediately. Required number of case reports must be filed at least 60 days prior to date of examination. Application blanks can be procured from: Dr. John Green, 3720 Washington Ave., St. Louis, Mo.

———o———

Spring Medico-Military Symposium

The annual Spring Medico-Military Symposium, sponsored by the Kansas City Southwest Clinical Society in conjunction with the medical department Seventh Corps Area, will be presented in Kansas City, Missouri, March 28, 29, 1938. This is a meeting devoted to medical subjects of military interests to which the entire medical profession is invited.

Medical reserve officers will gain information which will be of value in event of war, a not impossible eventuality; much that will be of value in his practice as well as being given credits which will apply on his advancement.

Guest speakers will include Dr. J. Albert Key, professor of clinical orthopedic surgery, Washington University Medical School, St. Louis, and Dr. Ovid O. Meyer, professor of medicine, University of Wisconsin, Madison.

The Kansas City Southwest Clinical Society invites the physicians of the Southwest to reserve March 28th and 29th to attend this meeting.

THE JOURNAL
OF THE
Oklahoma State Medical Association
Issued Monthly at McAlester, Oklahoma, under direction of the Council.

Copyright, 1938, by Oklahoma State Medical Association, McAlester, Oklahoma.

| Vol. XXXI | FEBRUARY, 1938 | Number 2 |

DR. L. S. WILLOUR..............................Editor-in-Chief
McAlester, Oklahoma

DR. T. H. McCARLEY......................Associate Editor
McAlester, Oklahoma

Entered at the Post Office at McAlester, Oklahoma, as second-class matter under the act of March 3rd, 1879.

This is the official Journal of the Oklahoma State Medical Association. All communications should be addressed to The Journal of the Oklahoma State Medical Association, McAlester Clinic, McAlester, Oklahoma. $4.00 per year; 40c per copy.

The editorial department is not responsible for the opinions expressed in the original articles of contributors.

Reprints of original articles will be supplied at actual cost provided request for them is attached to manuscripts or made in sufficient time before publication.

Articles sent this Journal for publication and all those read at the annual meetings of the State Association are the sole property of this Journal. The Journal relies on each individual contributor's strict adherence to this well-known rule of medical journalism. In the event an article sent this Journal for publication is published before appearance in The Journal the manuscript will be returned to the writer.

Failure to receive The Journal should call for immediate notification of the Editor, McAlester Clinic, McAlester, Oklahoma.

Local news of possible interest to the medical profession, notes on removals, changes of addresses, births, deaths and weddings will be gratefully received.

Advertising of articles, drugs or compounds unapproved by the Council on Pharmacy of the A. M. A., will not be accepted.

Advertising rates will be supplied on application.

It is suggested that wherever possible members of the State Association should patronize our advertisers in preference to others as a matter of fair reciprocity.

Printed by News-Capital Company, McAlester.

EDITORIAL

POST GRADUATE MEDICAL TEACHING

The Committee on Post Graduate Medical Teaching of the State Medical Association is rapidly completing the plans for post graduate medical teaching in obstetrics to be held throughout the state during the next two years. This work is under the auspices of the State Medical Association; however, the Commonwealth Fund of New York City is placing in the hands of this committee considerable money to assist in the expense of this undertaking. Also the Oklahoma state health department is cooperating financially in this matter.

The plan is to bring to this state a full time instructor in obstetrics and he will give in each locality a ten weeks intensive course in the handling of obstetrical cases. The plan is, that he will spend an entire day in each town in the circuit; that he will see patients in consultation; that he will make talks before civic clubs, women's clubs and other organizations and that he will carry on a well planned post graduate course.

There will be a director employed who will arrange these courses in advance. He will enroll members and collect a small fee for this post graduate teaching. This plan will be entirely perfected within the next few weeks and it is hoped that in the next issue of the Journal the profession of the state will be given all of the particulars as to how this work is to be carried out.

This is a most forward step in post graduate medical teaching and is similar to the work that is being done at this time in Tennessee under the direction of our old friend, Mr. L. W. Kibler.

Let the profession of the state be prepared to accept this wonderful opportunity.

---o---

1938 ANNUAL MEETING

Arrangements are r a p i d l y perfecting themselves for the Annual Meeting which will be held in Muskogee, May 9, 10, 11, 1938.

The local Committee on Arrangements have perfected their plans so that all Sections will be comfortably and conveniently housed. The entire basement of the Hotel Severs will be revamped for our registration booth, the commercial and scientific exhibits.

We have been fortunate indeed in procuring t h r e e outstanding men for our guest speakers: Frank Neff, Kansas City, pediatrics; Edward Wm. Alton Ochsner, New Orleans, surgery; Wm. S. Middleton, Madison, Wis., internal medicine.

It is not too early for you to begin to make your plans to attend this meeting and make your individual contribution to see that this meeting is an outstanding success.

THE SOUTHERN MEDICAL ASSOCIATION

At the meeting of the Southern Medical Association held in New Orleans last fall, Oklahoma was honored by having this year's meeting placed in Oklahoma City.

This meeting was placed in Oklahoma upon the combined invitation of the profession of Oklahoma City and the State Medical Association and we must all thoroughly cooperate in order to make this meeting the success that the members have every reason to expect.

The medical profession of Oklahoma City has perfected its Committees and Dr. Henry H. Turner has been elected as General Chairman. The names of the Vice-Chairmen include Dr. L. J. Moorman, Dr. W. K. West, Dr. Lea A. Riley, Dr. W. W. Rucks, Dr. E. S. Lain and Dr. C. J. Fishman. Dr. John F. Burton will be convention secretary.

Honorary vice-chairmen include Dr. Robert U. Patterson, Dr. Geo. A. LaMotte, Dr. Chas. M. Pearce, Dr. E. S. Ferguson, Dr. Horace Reed, Dr. LeRoy Long, Dr. H. K. Speed, Dr. William Taylor, Dr. A. W. White, Dr. R. J. Howard, Dr. C. E. Barker, Dr. J. T. Martin and Dr. John F. Kuhn.

Sub-committee chairmen are: Finance, Dr. Wendell Long; Program and Clinic, Dr. H. Dale Collins; Entertainment, Dr. Rex Bolend; Membership, Dr. E. S. Lain; Hotels, Dr. P. M. McNeill; Publicity, Dr. Basil A. Hayes; Alumni Reunions and Fraternity Luncheons, Dr. D. H. O'Donoghue; Scientific Exhibits, Dr. W. W. Rucks, Jr.; Information, Dr. W. F. Keller; Transportation, Dr. E. R. Musick; Golf, Dr. L. Chester McHenry; Trap-shooting, Dr. Theodore G. Wails; Women Physicians, Dr. Leila E. Andrews: Ladies' Entertainment, Mrs. L. J. Moorman.

The State Organization wishes at this time to offer the medical profession of Oklahoma City any assistance that we may be able to render and we feel sure that the individual members of the Association will be very glad to give freely of their services when called upon.

Opportunity for Physicians to Tour America En Route to the Convention

The thought that the forthcoming A.M.A. Convention in San Francisco, June 13th to the 17th, is a splendid opportunity for a tour of the United States both going out and coming back, has inspired definite action. The cooperation of more than 25 state medical societies has made it possible to arrange a special train tour which will include such outstanding highlights of the North American continent as the Indian Detour, the Grand Canyon, Los Angeles, Riverside and Santa Catalina Island—on the way out to San Francisco. A choice of two return routes is possible, one of which visits the charming cities of Portland, Seattle, Victoria and Vancouver and the beautiful scenic spots of the Canadian Rockies; the second route travels via Yellowstone National Park, Salt Lake City, Royal Gorge, Colorado Springs, and Denver.

There is an all-inclusive price for this tour which includes transportation from home-town to home-town, though the tour starts officially at Chicago on Monday, June 6th, from which point an American Express escort joins the group, as this travel company has been appointed transportation agent and the business details of the trip are in their capable hands.

Let us take a preview of the tour. The first day out of Chicago, racing across the broad, wheat-growing face of Kansas, we become acquainted with our traveling companions, physicians from other states, their families and friends, and find ourselves among congenial, like-minded traveling companions. We first leave our train at Lamy, New Mexico, to enter the Indian Pueblo district by motor-coach. We spend a whole day exploring the traces left by a vanished civilization on this continent, visiting Santa Fe, Tesuque, Puye and Santa Clara Pueblo.

The next morning's arrival at the Grand Canyon will remain in our memories forever. The vast chasm, four to 18 miles wide from rim to rim gives us stupendous vistas of awe-inspiring beauty, unparalleled the world over. We drive over the famous Hermit Rim Road, skirting the edge of the chasm in the morning, and in the afternoon over Desert View Road through the Tusayan National Forest and along the Canyon's rim, stopping at Yavapai Point Observation Station for a short, interesting lecture by the park naturalist. This drive ends at the Watch Tower, a recreation of the ancient towers erected by the prehistoric inhabitants of the southwest.

The golden, amazing city of Los Angeles is next on our itinerary, and our sightseeing trips acquaint us with its Spanish Quarter and Chinatown, as well as its beautiful environs, including flowering Pasadena. Riverside and its orange empire, its lemon and grapefruit orchards and its famous Mission Inn, is another destination; and then, on our third day in California we sail to beautiful Santa Catalina Island, playground of this land of the sun. And in this delightful manner, a week after leaving Chicago we arrive at San Francisco in time for the Convention. We shall not discuss the interesting time that awaits us at our conclaves, as the object of this article is to describe the pre- and post-convention tour. So we turn again to our itinerary after the Convention.

Supposing we had chosen Return Route No. 1. We shall visit Portland, Oregon, famed as the city of roses, and enjoy as well a drive along the noted Columbia River Highway. Seattle is next, and here we also cover all the points of interest, including both the Lake and Sound districts. Now the Canadian part of our journey begins, and we sail by comfortable steamer to the cities of Victoria and

Vancouver, where we do sightseeing. Now a train takes us into the enchanting scenic regions of the Canadian Rockies, and we stop at Chateau Lake Louise, at the lake of the same name—a gem of exquisite color, surrounded by green forests and snowy peaks. Our drives through the heart of the Rockies takes us to Moraine Lake, the Valley of Ten Peaks, Johnson Canyon and finally to Banff, where we make another stopover. After additional sightseeing around Banff, we entrain for Chicago.

Return Route No. 2 takes us to Chicago in a more southerly route. A 3½-day tour of Yellowstone National Park is one of the highlights of this tour. Ranger naturalists conduct our party to the geysers and hot pools, and we feast our eyes on Old Faithful in its hourly eruption. We also see the Grand Canyon of the Yellowstone and Mammoth Hot Springs. Salt Lake City is on our itinerary, which gives us an opportunity to visit Saltair Beach on Great Salt Lake, also the Great Copper Mills and Smelters. Our next call is at Colorado Springs, the noted health and pleasure resort. Our travels in the Rockies take us up to the summit of Pikes Peak. to the Garden of the Gods, to Seven Falls, and finally to Denver. This lovely city is a center for outings in the Rockies, and we are soon off on a 65-mile tour of Denver Mountain Parks, including Memorial Museum and Tomb of Buffalo Bill of western fame. From Denver we travel to Chicago.

The above is barely a glimpse of the outline of the tours, but it is hoped that some idea has been given of the enjoyable travel awaiting those physicians and their families and friends, who wish to combine attendance at the Convention with an interesting journey and a happy vacation.

————o————

Editorial Notes—Personal and General

SOUTHEASTERN Oklahoma Medical Association met in McAlester, December 9, 1937, at the Aldridge Hotel and the following program was heard: Traumatic Injuries—First Aid and Office Treatment, Dr. M. L. Henry, Heavener, Okla.; X-Ray Therapy in the Treatment of Carcinoma of the Breast and of the Cervix, Dr. Edward Greenberger, McAlester, Okla.; business session; luncheon—12:15 Aldridge Hotel. Program resumed 1:15 p.m.: Invocation, Rev. S. R. Braden, pastor, First Presbyterian church, McAlester, Okla.; welcome address, Dr. C. E. Lively, president Pittsburg County Medical Society, McAlester, Okla.; response to welcome address, Dr. H. B. Fuston, Bokchito, Okla.; Present Status of the Medical Profession in Oklahoma, Dr. Sam A. McKeel, president, Oklahoma State Medical Association; The Pathology of Fractures, Dr. L. S. Willour, member and district chairman, Oklahoma Regional Fracture Committee, American College of Surgeons, McAlester, Okla.; The Management of Fractures — Demonstrated with Motion Pictures, Dr. Earl D. McBride, general chairman, Oklahoma Regional Fracture Committe, American College of Surgeons, Oklahoma City, Okla.; The Treatment of Fractures of the Bones of the Hand and of the Feet, Dr. Pat Fite, member Oklahoma Regional Fracture Committee, American College of Surgeons, McAlester, Okla.

Officers elected for 1938 were: Dr. E. H. Shuller, president, McAlester; Dr. W. Keller Haynie, vicepresident, Durant; Dr. John A. Haynie, secretarytreasurer, Durant.

DR. HUSTON K. SPANGLER, former assistant Superintendent of the Worcester, Mass., City Hospital, has been appointed Superintendent of Valley View Hospital, Ada, upon its completion. Dr.

Spangler is a graduate of the University of Pennsylvania Graduate School of Medicine, and was engaged in general practice in Philadelphia, associated with the Nanticoke Hospital in Pennsylvania, before going to Worcester in 1934.

————

DR. R. H. LYNCH, Hollis, has been appointed County Health Superintendent of Harmon County.

————

DR. FOWLER BORDER, Mangum, has announced his candidacy for governor.

————

DR. JAMES D. OSBORN, Frederick, who was injured in an automobile accident in December is reported much improved.

————

DR. B. J. CORDONNIER, Okeene, is taking post graduate work at the Augustana Hospital, Chicago.

————

DR. E. S. KILPATRICK, Elk City, announces his removal to Leedey, where he will establish a private practice and hospital.

————

DR. W. R. BLACK, Seminole, is reported ill from an acute heart attack.

————

DR. and MRS. F. B. ERWIN, Oklahoma City, spent three weeks in California, vacationing, in January.

————

DR. J. M. PEMBERTON, Oklahoma City, announces his removal to Okemah.

————o————

News of the County Medical Societies

TULSA County Medical Society launched its activities for 1938 at the first meeting of the year, January 10th, with the employment of an executive secretary and the installation of the new officers for the year.

Dr. M. J. Searle, who served the past year as president-elect, assumed the president's chair and the following officers were elected: Dr. A. Ray Wiley, president-elect; Dr. P. P. Nesbitt, vice president and Dr. Roy L. Smith as secretary-treasurer. Dr. A. W. Pigford was elected to the board of trustees which is composed of Drs. Henry S. Brown, W. Albert Cook, Charles H. Haralson, Ned R. Smith, Searle and Wiley. The board of censors for the coming year will be Drs. Nesbitt, G. A. Wall and V. K. Allen. Delegates are Drs. G. R. Osborn, J. Stevensoon, R. C. Pigford, W. Albert Cook, M. D. Henley, W. S. Larabee, Ned R. Smith, M. J. Searle and A. Ray Wiley. Alternates are Drs. Haralson, Roy W. Dunlap and J. C. Brogden.

Lloyd Stone, advertising man and former secretary of the Tulsa Junior Chamber of Commerce, was elected executive secretary of the organization. Stone has lived in Tulsa since 1914. He attended the University of Oklahoma and since that time he has been engaged in newspaper, advertising and public relations work, with the exception of four years when he was secretary of the Junior Chamber which was the largest in the United States during his terms of office.

With the society's objective of a greater influence in medical work in Tulsa County, Stone will leave immediately to study the organization set-ups in Detroit, Chicago and Wichita. The work of the Tulsa organization will be along the lines followed in these other cities.

PAYNE County Medical Society elected the following officers for 1938, at their meeting held December 16, 1937: Doctors E. M. Harris, Cushing, president; P. M. Richardson, Cushing, vice-president; John W. Martin, Cushing, secretary-treasurer.

HUGHES County Medical Society elected the following officers for 1938 at their meeting in December: President, Dr. W. L. Taylor, Holdenville; vice-president, Dr. R. B. Ford, Holdenville; secretary-treasurer, Dr. Imogene Mayfield, Holdenville.

PITTSBURG County Medical Society met at the Aldridge Hotel, McAlester, January 25th for their first program of the year. Drs. Wann Langston and Harry Wilkins, Oklahoma City, spoke on "Coronary and Heart Diseases" and "Injuries of the Spinal Cord," respectively. New officers for the year are: President, Dr. Allen R. Russell; Vice President, Dr. Floyd T. Bartheld; Secretary, Dr. E. D. Greenberger, all of McAlester.

WOODS County Medical Society met at the Bell Hotel, Alva, January 25th for the following program and election of officers: Dinner at 7:30; Film, "Sterility"; Paper, "Bowel Surgery," Dr. Green K. Dickson, Oklahoma City; Paper, "Skin Diseases in Children," John H. Lamb, Oklahoma City.
Dr. Arthur E. Hale, Alva, president; Dr. O. E. Templin, Alva, secretary.

MUSKOGEE County Medical Society met December 20th, for election of officers for 1938: President, Dr. Finis W. Ewing; vice-president, Dr. Ira C. Wolfe; secretary-treasurer, Dr. Shade D. Neely; board of censors, Drs. W. D. Berry, Chairman, Geo. T. Kaiser and Joel T. Woodburn, all of Muskogee.

MUSKOGEE County Medical Society met January 17th at the Baptist Hospital for the following program: "Pathology, Special Reference to Autopsy," Dr. I. A. Nelson, Tulsa; "Breast Tumors," Dr. Walter Larrabee, Tulsa.

---o---

Recent Deaths

DR. JOHN HAMMER, Kiowa, Kansas, January 3, 1938.

DR. H. A. HARRIS, McAlester, January, 1938.

DR. CHARLES CATON, Wynona, January 3, 1938.

---o---

Books Received and Reviewed

PSYCHIATRIC NURSING, By William S. Sadler, M.D., Chief Psychiatrist and Director, The Chicago Institute of Research and Diagnosis; Consulting Psychiatrist to Columbia Hospital. IN COLLABORATION WITH Lena K. Sadler, M.D., Associate Director, The Chicago Institute of Research and Diagnosis; Medical Director, The Northside Rest Home; Attending Physician, Columbus Hospital and the Women and Children's Hospital. WITH Anna B. Kellogg, R.N., Member American Nurse Assiciation; Chief of Nurses, The Psychiatric Clinic of the Chicago Institute and Diagnosis; Instructor of Psychiatric Nursing, The North Side Rest Home. The C. V. Mosby Company, St. Louis, 1937.

This book has been written to meet the requirements of the recently enlarged courses in psychiatric nursing, which have been adopted by the majority of American schools of nursing. The book endeavors to give the nurse a broad but comprehensive view of the approach to mental hygiene, the technic of dealing with human beings as a whole and the nursing care of the different psychiatric diseases. It is divided into four parts: General Considerations, the Neuroses, the Psychoses, and Psychotherapeutics.

CRIPPLED CHILDREN, Their Treatment and Orthopedic Nursing, by Earl D. McBride, B.S., M.D., F.A.C.S., Assistant Professor of Orthopedic Surgery, University of Oklahoma, School of Medicine; Attending Orthopedic Surgeon to St. Anthony Hospital; Associate Orthopedic Surgeon to Oklahoma City General and Wesley Hospitals; Visiting Surgeon to W. J. Bryan School for Crippled Children; Chief of Staff to Reconstruction Hospital, Oklahoma City, Oklahoma; Member of American Academy of Orthopedic Surgeons. IN COLLABORATION WITH Winifred R. Sink, A.B., R.N., Educational Director, Grace Hospital School of Nursing, Detroit, Michigan; Formerly Head Nurse of James Whitcomb Riley Hospital of the Indiana University Group; Instructor of Nurses, Indiana University School of Nursing; Educational Director, General Hospital, Mansfield, Ohio. Second Edition. Cloth, Price $3.50. C. V. Mosby Company, St. Louis, 1937.

The organization for work among crippled children is far advanced in practically all of the states of the Union. Not only are physicians interested in this work, but many civic clubs, women's organizations, et cetera, have given of their time and money toward the advancement of the care of these unfortunate children. This book gives information that will be of value to the orthopedic surgeon, general practitioner, nurse and social worker, and by their education is the only hope of preventing many crippling conditions, especially following poliomyelitis.

Dr. McBride's extensive experience in this work makes him a very capable authority and in this work he has placed his materials in such a fashion that it is readily accessible and contains all of the procedures useful in the prophylactic as well as curative treatment of the crippled child. Its wide application bespeaks for it an extensive circulation and it is hoped that those interested will avail themselves of this wonderful book.

THE PHYSICIAN'S BUSINESS, Practical and Economic Aspects of Medicine, By George D. Wolfe, M.D., Attending Otolaryngologist, Sydenham Hospital, New York City; Attending Laryngologist, Riverside, New York City; Fellow, New York Academy of Medicine; Fellow, American Medical Association, etc. Foreword By Harol Rypins, A.B., M.D., F.A.C.P. Fifty-seven Illustrations; Cloth. J B. Lippincott Company, Philadelphia.

The Physician's Business is a very exhaustive treatise of value primarily for young physicians just entering the profession. In my opinion it tries to cover too much territory and the name "Physician's Business" is misleading, if not a misnomer. The author is not satisfied in confining himself to the business end of physicians problems, which though are thoroughly, and I believe well covered, but includes numerous suggestions as to treatment such as giving in detail the antedotes for poisons, advice on diets, et cetera, et cetera, even to mentioning such suggestions as "that babies shouldn't be allowed to suck their thumbs."

ABSTRACTS : REVIEWS : COMMENTS
and CORRESPONDENCE

SURGERY AND GYNECOLOGY
Abstracts, Reviews and Comments from
LeRoy Long Clinic
714 Medical Arts Building, Oklahoma City

The Role of Liver Damage in the Mortality of Surgical Diseases. By Frederick Fitzherbert Boyce and Elizabeth M. McFetridge, New Orleans, La. Southern Medical Journal, January, 1938, Page 35.

Directing attention to the importance of liver function which the authors believe has been too lightly regarded, there is a reference to liver damage in connection with infectious processes, such damage being regarded as a secondary "and often a terminal phenomenon." While this is regarded as being of importance, there is no discussion of that type of damage—that is, terminal damage due to infection, it being the obvious purpose to consider two other types of liver insufficiency.

In the first group there is hyperpyrexia which overwhelms the patient within the first 48 hours, notwithstanding clinical evidences of having been a good surgical risk before the operation. Autopsy in this group discloses degeneration or actual necrosis in the liver.

In the second group the patient may live from seven to 14 days after operation but finally dies "with uremic symptoms dominating the picture." Here, too, "these same findings are present (degeneration and necrosis), plus similar changes in the convoluted tubules of the kidneys."

Heyd is given credit for first describing the so-called liver or liver-kidney death in 1924, the reference in the bibliography showing that it was published in the Journal of the American Medical Association in 1931, Volume 97, page 1847.

It is believed that unrecognized liver insufficiency is always a tremendously important predisposing cause of degeneration in the liver after surgical operations in which there is no definite infection, the immediate cause being an overwhelming toxemia with hyperpyrexia due to absorption from the degenerating areas.

In this connection, the authors make a contrast between the difficulties following stab wounds of the liver and crushing wounds of the liver. In the latter there is rapid necrosis, accompanied by hyperpyrexia, while, in the former, necrosis of the liver and hyperpyrexia are not nearly so common.

It is indicated that the same type of liver damage may be associated with intestinal obstruction and toxic thyroid disease. Speaking of the liver damage in toxic thyroid disease the statement is made, "The possible association has been noted since 1865, though it was not considered anything but accidental until well into the present century, and the relationship has been studied intensively only within the last few years."

In connection with diseases of the biliary tract, the following statement is made: "Our theory as to the cause of death in such cases resembles that advanced by Helwig. Briefly, we believe that the damaged livers of some patients with biliary tract disease, while they can withstand the strain of normal life, cannot withstand the added strain of surgery and its concomitant trauma and changes."

There is a rather enthusiastic reference to the value of the Quick hippuric acid test of liver function in which the authors apparently have great faith. The references in the bibliography show articles by McFetridge and Boyce. The articles have not been published, but are in press.

The authors have been surprised by the indication of low liver function as shown by the test, particularly in connection with toxic thyroid disease. In addition to that, they have been astonished at finding, by this test, evidences of great hepatic insufficiency even in young and apparently vigorous persons used as controls. In this class comparatively simple and ordinary operative procedures, like appendicectomy and hernioplasty may be followed by dangerous symptoms.

A rather striking statement is this: "Under ethylene anesthesia it (presumably liver function) fell 21 per cent on the first postoperative day, under ether it fell 25 per cent, and under spinal it fell 49 per cent." While it is not perfectly clear, it appears that the statements about the effect of anesthesia upon the liver function were based upon observations in the cases of those who had preoperative evidences of low liver function as determined by the Quick hippuric acid test.

LeRoy Long.

Effect of Certain Gynecologic Lesions on the Upper Urinary Tract. By Kretschmer and Kanter. Journal of the American Medical Association, Oct. 2, 1937, Bol. 109, Page 1097.

In previous studies by Kretschmer and Heaney it was demonstrated that dilation of the ureters and kidney pelves occured in 100 per cent of their cases of pregnancy and that there was a recovery to normal within 12 weeks following delivery.

With this in mind, the present study was organized to determine changes in the upper urinary tract from lesions of the pelvic genitalia in non-pregnant women. They desired answers to the following questions:

"1. Do changes in the upper urinary tract occur in association with lesions of the pelvic organs in women?

"2. How frequently do they occur?

"3. Is there any definite relation between the type of disorder in the pelvis and the lesions in the upper urinary tract?

"4. In what way, if any, do the changes resemble changes found during pregnancy?

"5. Do these changes completely disappear after the pelvic disorder has been corrected by the appropriate surgical measures?"

They selected only patients with no urinary symptoms and with normal urine examination. They excluded instances of carcinoma of the cervix because of the almost universal involvement of the ureters and because the lesion could not be satisfactorily eradicated for the purposes of the present study.

Intravenous pyelograms were employed routinely both before and after operation.

Fifty-one patients were so studied with the intravenous pyelogram supplemented by retrograde pyelogram when the intravenous was not satisfactory. Of these cases 35 were fibroid tumors, 11 ovarian cysts, 4 uterine prolapse and 1 tubo-ovarian abscess.

They found secondary changes in the upper urinary tract in association with these gynecological disorders in the following percentages. For the entire series of 51 cases 64.7 per cent, for the group of fibroids changes were found in 65.7 per cent, in ovarian cysts 81.9 per cent, in the uterine prolapse patients 25 per cent, and in the one case of tubo-ovarian abscess there was no change in the upper urinary tract.

Following appropriate surgical procedures there was a return to normal in 72.5 per cent of the patients. Most of these examinations postoperatively were done soon after operation and the authors feel that after a longer time has intervened there will be a slightly higher recovery rate to normal.

They feel that the failure to appreciate the frequency with which these lesions occur, is due to the fact that there has been no routine preoperative study of the urinary tract in the group of patients who do not present urinary symptoms or urinary signs.

Comment: Instances of the effect of gynecological lesions on the urinary tract are common and can be readily understood. Where patients have urinary symptoms and signs leading to the proper investigation of the urinary tract and also have gynecological lesions, proper correction of the gynecological disease, by surgery or other means, materially assists in the treatment of the urological disease and the return of the urinary tract to normal.

This study, by careful reputable urologists, directs our attention to the changes which frequently occur in the upper urinary tract from pelvic lesions even in the individuals who do not have symptoms. Since it also demonstrates the therapeutic effects of correction of the gynecological lesions upon the urinary tract changes, the conclusion can quite evidently be drawn that patients with upper urinary tract disease deserve pelvic investigation and indicated treatment.

Wendell Long.

Endometriosis of the Colon and Rectum with Intestinal Obstruction. By Richard B. Cattell. New England Journal of Medicine, Vol. 217, No. 1, P. 9-16, July 1, 1937.

Cattell again emphasizes the fact that endometriosis involving the pelvic organs is quite common and that with increased familiarity of the disease, it is being recognized more frequently.

In a series of 104 patients with endometriosis whom they have treated at the Lahey Clinic, 17 have had involvement of the sigmoid colon or rectum while four showed endometriosis of the appendix. It is upon this group of 17 patients that he bases the discussion in this article. "Any female patient with abnormal menstruation and positive pelvic findings, and with a long standing history of bowel symptoms suggesting an obstruction but without loss of weight must be suspected of having endometriosis. This diagnosis may be fur-

ther supported by the relation of the obstructive symptoms to menstruation."

He emphasizes the importance of carefully studying the recto-vaginal septum region in such suspects. The differential diagnosis lies largely between carcinoma of the sigmoid and rectum and endometriosis. Sigmoidoscopic examination, if possible, is helpful in that there is rarely gross bleeding or ulceration and that the only positive finding will be that of narrowing of the lumen with congestion of the mucosa. Biopsy has not been practical for the mucosa is not extensively involved and only negative results will be obtained. Barium enema has been of help but diffuse endometrial lesions cannot be differentiated in this way from diverticulitis or spasm. "In the four patients with endometriosis of the sigmoid involving the entire wall, a preoperative diagnosis of malignancy was made in every instance."

Their treatment of cases involving the recto-sigmoid and rectum due to extensive endometriosis in the pelvis has been radical in so far as the uterus, tubes and ovaries were concerned. In the presence of an intestinal obstruction that is not severe it is safe to remove the ovaries without resecting the bowel. It is Cattell's opinion that resection should be carried out in patients where carcinoma cannot be excluded but that frozen section should always be done. He again points out that the results of surgical treatment of endometriosis are, and should be, satisfactory.

Case reports are given to demonstrate the various types of involvement of the recto-sigmoid and rectum.

"The diagnosis is seldom made preoperatively, but this condition should be suspected when the obstruction is long-standing and worse at the time of menstruation, when there are associated pelvic findings, and when the local lesion on examination by the sigmoidoscope and barium enema is not typical of carcinoma of the colon or rectum. The condition can be recognized at operation."

Comment: Endometriosis (adenomyosis, chocolate cysts of Sampson, hemorrhagic pelvic cysts) is not uncommon and the relative rarity of the diagnosis depends largely upon the lack of familiarity with the disease. The instances of endometriosis, carefully proven by microscopic examination, are becoming increasingly frequent.

Positive preoperative diagnosis is exceedingly difficult, unless a positive biopsy of the tissue from the recto-vaginal septum has been possible. Proper diagnosis and thereupon the indicated treatment lies primarily in recognition of the disease at operation. In patients where there is diffuse involvement of the pelvis, recognition is a relatively simple matter. However, the endometrial implants frequently occur in bizarre patterns, with the major involvement lying principally in one or another of the organs within or near the pelvis.

In a great many respects, endometriosis can be likened to neoplastic disease but it is definitely not malignant. It is the only condition of which I know in which there is an uncontrolled extensive growth of cellular tissue and is yet not malignant.

Removal of all ovarian tissue produces a positive cure of the disease and yet conservative surgery, with the salvage of ovarian tissue, may be satisfactorily employed where the endometrial implants are so located that the disease can be entirely removed without sacrifice of all ovarian tissue. As the disease commonly occurs in reasonably young women, conservative surgery should be employed wherever possible, with the understanding in mind that complete castration may be an early necessity if the disease is not adequately controlled and removed.

Wendell Long.

Recurrent and Continuing Hyperthyroidism. By Thomas O. Young, Duluth, Minnesota. The American Journal of Surgery, January, 1938.

Tracing the history of "therapeutic excision of the thyroid gland" which was first done by Theodore Kocher in 1878; referring to the important work of Charles H. Mayo and William H. Halstead; and directing particular attention to the value of the "epoch-making treatment of this disease with compound iodine solution" advocated by Plummer in 1921, there is a quotation of statistics which seem to indicate that the percentage of recurrent or continuing hyperthyroidism after operative treatment is unnecessarily too high.

The author believes that "such a large group of so-called recurrences may be due to one of several factors:

"1. Incomplete or insufficient operation due to inexperience on the part of the operator.

"2. Anatomical variations not recognized at the time of operation. These would include aberrant thyroid tissue, pyramidal lobes, superior accessory lobes, retro-tracheal, lateral and inferior extensions, or substernal lobes.

"3. Improper preparation and follow-up of these cases."

In connection with these statements the inference is drawn that during recent years too many operations have been undertaken by those whose knowledge of the pathology, the necessary surgical technique, and of the indispensable collateral information touching the treatment of thyroid disease is defective.

A review of the literature discloses, according to the author, that the question of recurrence or persistence of goiter has been considered almost altogether in connection with diffuse toxic goiter. However, his investigations lead him to believe that there is a large percentage of recurrences in connection with the nodular type of goiter.

It is the belief of the author that, "Next to insufficient surgery, the outstanding neglect is the failure to properly follow-up and study these cases postoperatively. Frequent post-operative examinations with metabolic studies, plus the constant saturation of the gland with iodine over a period of several months, seems to be the best insurance against recurrence.

"It would seem that from the results of this study a warning to the general practitioner or the occasional operator of goiter would not be out of place. It is not unreasonable to assume that if a real thyroidectomy is not done, the number of cases of 'continuing goiter' will be on the increase. The surgeon must be on the lookout for extraneous contiguous anatomical variations. The thyroidectomy must be sufficiently complete to definitely interrupt the course of the disease, and the extreme importance of protection of the recurrent laryngeal nerves and parathyroid glands must be constantly kept in mind."

The following is the summary of the article:

"1. That a much larger percentage of recurrence of goiter than was formerly suspected is found in the group of nodular goiters.

"2. That the number of cases of true recurrences and 'continuing goiter' is on the increase, due to the fact that this disease is being treated more generally by the profession as a whole, and that fewer cases are being handled by surgeons who have made a particular study of this disease.

"3. That an unreasonably large percentage of the cases of diffuse toxic goiter coming to second operation are not recurrent, but are cases of 'continuing goiter,' due chiefly to an inadequate operation plus insufficient post-operative follow-up care."

LeRoy Long.

The Conservative Treatment of Gall Bladder Disease. Harry E. Mock, C. F. G. Brown and Ralph E. Dolkart. Surgery, Gynecology and Obstetrics, January, 1938, Page 79.

Critical survey of present day surgical and medical management of gall bladder disease convinces one that it is inadequate. "From the surgeon's point of view the concensus is that if there is any evidence of pathological changes in the gall bladder, the structure should be immediately removed. From the internist's point of view, the use of the low fat, low cholesterol diet in conjunction with catharsis comprises the average conception of the medical management of gall bladder disease and has remained unchanged as the treatment of choice for the past three or four decades."

The authors do not concur with either of these generally accepted ideas of gall bladder management. Cholecystectomy, which for two decades has been the most popular form of surgical treatment, is not always indicated when surgery is performed; neither has it relieved the symptoms in a reasonable proportion of the cases in which it was used. Cholecystostomy has a more definite place in gall bladder surgery than recent trends would indicate. It seems that most have disregarded the fact that roentgenologically functioning gall bladders can be demonstrated after surgical drainage. They believe that most patients with "low grade right upper quadrant symptoms" can be as completely or more completely relieved by proper medical management than by surgery.

"The inadequacy of the present popular medical treatment accounts for the dominance of surgical treatment. Medical treatment, however, based upon the physiological principles of the biliary tract will relieve symptoms and can restore to normal roentgenological functioning, gall bladders which gave pathological findings on previous examination."

The stated object of this study was to correlate conservative surgical ideas with medical opinion guided by recent advances in the knowledge of the physiology of the biliary tract.

The available data indicates quite definitely that approximately one-third of all patients subjected to biliary tract surgery show little or no improvement after operation. Two conclusions become apparent: first, there is a definite need for a more careful selection of cases for operation; second, adequate medical management is a problem of paramount importance. Apparently the best subjective results are obtained in patients subjected to surgery who give histories of repeated colic, common duct stone or chronic pancreatitis; poorest results in patients in whom cholecystitis existed without cholelithiasis.

Fundamental conditions requiring consideration in the medical and surgical management of the diseased gall bladder are: (1) Stasis in the biliary tract. (2) Infection of the gall bladder. (3) The varying degrees of hepatitis and liver damage accompanying the changes in the gall bladder. (4) Pericholecystitis with adhesions to adjacent viscera. (5) Accompanying pancreatitis, the result of stasis or blocking of the sphincter of Oddi.

Lyon's duodenal drainage therapy was based on the attempt to eliminate or at least palliate bile stasis. This form of treatment has been largely abandoned because the results are too inconstant. Many cholagogues have been employed. Magnesium sulphate has been used because of its action in relaxing the sphincter of Oddi. It has been proved that magnesium sulphate is not as effective as egg yolks and cream or olive oil and oleic acid. If stasis is to be overcome the most physiological method is to place fat in the duodenum. Also magnesium sulphate creates an irritable bowel with accompanying reflex pylorospasm.

There is no conclusive evidence that there is any increase in cholesterol in the blood of patients with gall stones (provided there is no hypothyroidism or obstructive jaundice). Numerous investigators have showed that the feeding of cholesterol has no relation to either the blood or bile levels.

Gall bladder "disinfectants" such as salicylates and hexamines have been employed to cope with the factors of primary infection and reinfection. These substances irritate the stomach outlet. Besides, it does not appear that infection plays an especially significant part.

The authors have become convinced that many patients (with and without stones) can become relatively symptom free and ultimately have a roentgenologically normal gall bladder under the form of medical management employed by them. However, the gall bladders with calculi did not show the roentgen improvement that was obtained in those without stone.

The medical plan they have adopted as best (after trying several) consists in simultaneously administering: (1) Ketocholanic acids (Ketochol, supplied to them by G. D. Searle and Co., Chicago) to stimulate the flow of hepatic bile; (2) hourly feedings of milk and cream to induce contracting and emptying of the gall bladder at intervals; antispasmodic medication (tincture of belladonna M VIII, elixir of phenobarbital gr. ½, t.i.d.) to diminish the irritability of the gastro-intestinal tract, thereby alleviating stasis due to hypertonicity. In severe cases bed rest was necessary at the time this form of management was started.

The choice of ketocholanic acids for the purpose of stimulating the secretion of bile was based upon experimental work on animals. Their studies indicated that greater choleresis with less toxic manifestations could be obtained using this preparation of bile acids.

In the absence of other indications they believe that there are three groups of gall bladder disease which will respond to physiological medical treatment: (1) The gall bladder dyskinesias; (2) Chronic cholecystitus where no calculi are present; (3) Chronic cholecystitis with large soft calculi, few in number, and with which the patients have no, or very infrequent, colic-like attacks.

They give the following indications (in their order of frequency together with their opinion as to when to operate) for operation in gall bladder disease:—

(1) Cholelithiasis giving definite gall stone colic.

(2) Empyema of the gall bladder.

(3) Obstructed cystic duct with a markedly dilated gall bladder.

(4) Obstructive jaundice.

(5) Subacute or chronic pancreatitis, usually accompany a cholecystitis, provided the "psyiological medical management" has been ineffective.

(6) Cholecystitis, only after medical failure.

(7) Gangrenous gall bladder.

The authors also carefully describe the conditions under which they think that the gall bladder should be drained or removed. They are definitely opposed to routine cholecystectomy. One point strongly emphasized is that when drainage operation is done that many times prolonged drainage for six to 12 weeks is preferable to the usual few days to two weeks.

Conclusions of the authors:—

(1) They believe that the present conceptions of the medical management of gall bladder disease, using low fat, low cholesterol diets in conjunction with saline purgatives have no sound physiological basis.

(2) On basis of studies of 120 patients with chronic gall bladder disease, they have found that the use of hourly feedings of milk and cream to induce contraction and emptying of the gall bladder, ketocholanic acids to stimulate the flow of hepatic bile, and antispasmodic medication to diminish the irritability of the gastro-intestinal tract, effectively relieve symptoms and reduce the incidence of colic in the majority of cases.

(3) Statistical data indicate the persistence of morbidity in patients with gall bladder disease following approximately one-third of all operations upon the biliary tract. In a large number of patients, therefore, an adequate program of medical management would be preferable to surgery.

(4) Removal of the gall bladder does not necessarily bring relief to patients with chronic gall bladder disease, especially if associated with pancreatitis unless colic and intermittent obstruction has been the predominant clinical picture. In their opinion, routine cholecystectomy is an unwarranted procedure and in many cases surgical drainage would be preferable.

(5) There should be a definite revision of ideas as to what constitutes adequate medical management and what constitutes indications for surgery in patients with chronic gall bladder disease.

LeRoy Downing Long.

————o————

EYE, EAR, NOSE AND THROAT

Edited by Marvin D. Henley, M.D.
911 Medical Arts Building, Tulsa

Chancre of the Upper Eyelid in an Infant Two Months of Age. Alfred Appelbaum, M.D., New York. Archives of Ophthalmology, December, 1937.

The rarities of this case are the site of occurrence and the age of the individual. The author's review of literature on the subject shows Marin reported chancres on the vulva of a child age 11 months; a case of chancre of the upper lip of a two-year-old child; chancre of the gums, reported by Foveau de Courmelles, in an infant; chancre of the upper eyelid, girl age eight years, by Bertin, Christin and Lesenne; chancre of the upper eyelid on a colored man eight weeks after a fight, by Fox and Machlis; simultaneous chancre on the penis and upper eyelid in a Chinese, age 43, by T'ang and Hu; chancre of internal angle of eyelids in a man, age 26, by Gate and Genet.

Bulkley, Muncheimer and Scheuer classified respectively 9,058, 10,265 and 14,590 cases and found that the eyelids and conjunctiva were involved in four per cent of the cases.

The case reported is that of a male infant, age two months. There occurred a swelling on the right upper lid, which increased in size and became an "open sore." The preauricular glands on the affected side were involved. A point of diagnostic importance at this time was that the dark field examination was negative. The following day another dark field examination was positive for spirochetes. The Wasserman was four pus. The physical examination was otherwise negative.

Treatment was with emulsion of bismuth subsalicylate and mepharsen, intramuscularly, for 15 weeks. At this time the chancre was completely healed but the Wasserman remained the same.

Differentiation of the lesion from gumma was unnecessary because of the age of the patient.

The source of the infection was the moot question. The author states that the incubation period for a chancre may be as long as 90 days; that secondary lesions are infectious only when situated on surfaces of mucous membranes with proper fields for growth. His opinion is that the infection occurred from a secondary lesion in the mother's birth canal at the time the child was born.

The family history showed the father and mother had syphilis, for which they had had some treatment, before the pregnancy occurred. Her Wasserman about midterm was negative. She gave birth to a normal, healthy-appearing infant, weighing seven pounds, five ounces, whose Wasserman from the cord at birth was negative. A checkup three weeks after the birth of this child showed nothing abnormal. A month after the child was born, the mother had a generalized cutaneous e r u p t i o n, which was diagnosed as a "late secondary."

The child evidently profited from the antisyphilitic treatment of the mother in that he had a negative Wasserman at the time of birth.

Eye Changes in the Management of Hypertensive Toxemia of Pregnancy. Alton V. Hallum, M.D. Atlanta, Georgia. Southern Medical Journal, January, 1938.

According to McCord "study of the eyegrounds by an experienced individual gives the most information as to the course of the various toxemias of pregnancy." Increase in blood pressure usually means a more severe toxemia. Eyeground changes correspond to the severity of hypertension more uniformly than any other single laboratory or clinical sign.

The first change noted is usually a slight generalized constriction or narrowing of a single artery or branch. Arterial constrictions are usually spastic in nature, which vary in degree and amount from day to day. If the blood pressure is lowered the arteries resume their normal caliber (unless the arterial walls have become sclerotic).

The ratio of vein to artery diameter is approximately three to two. In the presence of a severe toxemia and hypertension this ratio may be as high as five or six to one.

Edema of the retina shows first at the upper and lower poles of the disc, spreading along the course of the retinal vessels. The retina appears swollen, fluffy, grayish or milky in color, and tends to envelop the retinal vessels.

Hemorrhages and exudates appear last. They are usually flame-shaped. The posterior third of the fundus is where they are most liable to occur. Cotton-wool exudates have a similar l o c a t i o n. Rarely do star-shaped exudates occur in the macular region. If present there is a marked arteriosclerosis or a diffuse retinitis.

Retinal detachment occurs rarely. If present is usually bilateral; reattaches 10 to 14 days after the uterus is emptied. Operative procedures are not necessary.

The author states that if nephritis is allowed to develop during pregnancy it probably means that the mother's life has been shortened several years.

To substantiate this he cites Stander's statistics, who found in the follow-up of 800 toxic cases that 35 per cent had chronic nephritis, and that 40 per cent of those with chronic nephritis were dead in five to seven years. One hundred and thirty-two of the 800 mothers died prematurely.

Various phases of retinitis, toxemias of pregnancy and hypertension are discussed. The author's conclusions are:

"During the course of every case of hypertensive toxemia of pregnancy, the advisability of abortion must be kept in mind, and it requires the most discriminative judgment. As H e r r i c k suggests, if nephritis is present abortion must be more seriously considered than if the toxemia is of vascular origin. The obstetrician will find that a study of the eyegrounds, when considered with the other signs and symptoms of toxemia, will be a real aid, probably the most consistently reliable single guide in determining when pregnancy should be terminated. When hypertension or other evidence of toxemia develops during pregnancy a frequent examination of the fundus oculi should be made, and when in spite of conservative medical treatment the eyeground changes continue to become more severe, abortion should be done. This is especially true if severe eye changes appear before the 28th week, for then there is only one chance in five of obtaining a live baby, and severe damage to the mother's cardiovasculorenal system will result if pregnancy is allowed to continue.

We should endeavor to terminate pregnancy before retinitis appears, surely as soon as the first hemorrhage or exudate is seen. A better plan would be routinely to examine the eyes early in pregnancy before toxemia develops, in order to interpret accurately the changes that may appear if toxemia develops later in pregnancy.

Finally, the obstetrician should learn to use the ophthalmoscope well enough to do his own eyeground study. This can be accomplished with a reasonable amount of practice, especially if he at first receives some help from his fellow ophthalmologist. The value received is worth the effort required, for the eyegrounds give valuable information in the management of every case of hypertensive toxemia of pregnancy. This information is very available and it can be learned quickly and economically.

The Function of the Tonsils and Their Relation to the Aetiology and Treatment of Nasal Catarrh. Ivor Griffiths, (London). (Lancet, September 25th, 1937, ccxxxiii, 5952.) Abstracted by Douglas Guthrie. Published in the Journal of Laryngology and Otology, December, 1937.

The operation of tonsillectomy has been practised somewhat indiscriminately in many cases. A study of 4,500 children sent to hospital for tonsillectomy showed that in 31 per cent of the cases there were no symptoms, the tonsils having been discovered to be slightly enlarged on routine examination. Apparently the observer had overlooked the fact that physiological enlargement of the tonsil is found between the ages of four and six years and again at puberty, and that temporary enlargement is an accompaniment of the common cold.

There is a widespread notion, unsupported by observation, that tonsillectomy prevents otitis media. Tonsillectomy is also recommended, on insufficient evidence, as a treatment for nasal catarrh. The writer has observed 385 cases in nearly all of which the catarrh was worse after operation than before. He suggests that an explanation for this should be sought in the accessory nasal sinuses. In the 385 cases under his care, nasal sinus disease was present, usually in the maxillary sinus, but in the ethmoidal cells in 15 and in the frontal sinus in three children. He conducted a number of experiments on animals and found that Indian ink, introduced into the nasal sinuses, appeared in the tonsil. From this he argues that the tonsillar enlargement may be the result rather than the cause of nasal catarrh. He found that sinusitis was actually commoner in children who had undergone tonsillectomy than in those whose tonsils were intact. He admits that removal of adenoids alone is justified in nasal catarrh, but he regards the removal of tonsils for nasal catarrh as illogical.

Mild cases of nasal catarrh in children may be treated by the instillation of five to 15 per cent argyrol, attention to nutrition and general hygiene, and breathing exercises in the open air. For more severe cases puncture and lavage of the maxillary sinuses is necessary, and this may be performed under local anaesthesia. The results of antrostomy in children are bad, as the opening often closes and an area of scar tissue devoid of ciliated epithelium is created.

Differential Diagnosis Between Thrombosis of the Lateral Sinus and Acute Bacterial Endocarditis. Harry Rosenwasser, M.D., New York. Archives of Otolaryngology, December, 1937.

Five cases are reported from Mount Sinai Hospital which required a differential diagnosis between thrombosis of the lateral sinus and acute bacterial endocarditis.

The prognosis in sinus thrombosis is grave, while acute endocarditis presents a practically hopeless prognosis. Mortality statistics of sinus thrombosis varies in different clinics. The treatment is usually surgical. Although spontaneous cures are reported. Surgery has no place in the treatment of acute bacterial endocarditis.

This paper stresses certain criteria which aid in the differentiation of those cases which may have either one or both conditions above mentioned present.

The cases are presented in detail with postmortem findings, when there was a postmortem done.

There is a discussion of:

1. Bacteriology in the differential diagnosis between thrombosis of the lateral sinus and acute endocarditis.

2. Direct evidences of involvement of the endocardium as aids in the differential diagnosis between thrombosis of the lateral sinus and acute endocarditis.

3. Embolic phenomena in the differential diagnosis between thrombosis of the lateral sinus and acute endocarditis.

4. Changes in the fundi in the differential diagnosis between thrombosis of the lateral sinus and acute endocarditis.

5. Aural Findings and other aids in the Differential Diagnosis between Thrombosis of the Lateral Sinus and Acute Endocarditis.

The author's summary follows:

Certain diagnostic features which aided in making the correct differential diagnosis between thrombosis of the lateral sinus and acute bacterial endocarditis have been stressed. When the Ottenberg differential blood culture indicates large numbers of colonies in the cultures of blood from the jugular vein and a peripheral vein in the arm, it points to endocarditis as the cause, whereas a large number of colonies in one or both jugular veins and many fewer colonies in the arm point to sinus thrombosis. Correlation of the bacteriologic character-

istics of the aural discharge and the pus from the mastoid with blood cultures, as described by Libman and Celler, Ottenberg and Friesner, is helpful. Important in the differential diagnosis is the fact that none of the pneumococci with the exception of the type 111 pneumococcus cause sinus thrombosis. The significance of the embolic phenomena should be emphasized again because of their diagnostic importance. Cutaneous embolic lesions, petechiae, have never been observed by me in a case of sinus thrombosis uncomplicated by bacterial endocarditis. Changes of the fundi, varying from slight blurring of the margins of the disks to four diopters of papilledema, occurred in 16 per cent of the cases of sinus thrombosis which my associates and I have observed. It is uncommon in a case of acute endocarditis to note any change in the fundi other than embolic lesions or their manifestations, namely, petechiae, Roth spots or Doherty-Trubeck lesions. The changing character of the cardiac murmurs from day to day is significant of endocardial involvement. A definite history of aural disease, mastoiditis and a tender gland at the angle of the jaw associated with corroborative local evidences of venous involvement are additional factors in determining the correct diagnosis. In conclusion, it must be apparent that these cases of serious borderline conditions require the closest cooperation between the otologist, the internist and the bacteriologist for their proper solution.

---o---

PLASTIC SURGERY
Edited by
GEO. H. KIMBALL, M.D., F.A.C.S.
404 Medical Arts Building, Oklahoma City

Tendoplastic Amputation Through the Femur at the Knee. Further Studies. C. Latimer Callander, M.D., San Francisco, Calif. A.M.A. Journal, January 8, 1938.

The author introduced this type of operation in the Journal 1½ years ago. He has recently completed additional studies and made some refinements in technique.

Synopsis: Briefly, the operation is performed as follows: The anterior flap is fashioned from the soft tissues of the upper part of the leg as far distally as the level of the tibial tuberosity; the posterior flap is longer than the anterior, and it extends well down on the gastrocnemius muscle. The popliteal vessels and nerves are ligated through an amuscular and avascular cleavage plane on the medial aspect of the lower part of the thigh. All the hamstring muscles are severed at their tendinous insertions on the tibia, and the femur is sectioned in the condylar flare just proximal to the adductor tubercle. The patella is dissected from the anterior flap from the joint side, leaving the rectus femoris tendon in the floor of the patellar fossa to act as an end-bearing buffer for the femur. No coapting primary sutures are used, save from four to six skin clips or sutures to hold the flaps roughly in position.

As the edges of the flaps unite, the posterior flap retracts gradually but extensively until the femur occupies the patellar fossa snugly, and the suture line is located well up behind the stump end.

Description of Operation: The patient is placed in the dorsal decubitus position, the knee of the affected extremity is flexed slightly and the leg is elevated a little above horizontal on one or two sandbags. No tourniquet is applied. The surgeon stands on the side opposite the affected extremity and faces the medial aspect of the thigh and knee to be operated on. He maintains this position throughout the operation, because the essential steps are directed through a medial approach to the popliteal space. The operative work on the lateral aspect of the lower part of the thigh and knee is accomplished readily by rotating the knee medially.

The incisions in the skin outlining the slightly unequal anterior and posterior flaps coincide with the incisions that cover all the deeper soft parts. The incision on the medial aspect of the thigh begins at a point three finger breadths proximal to the most prominent part of the medial femoral condyle and runs horizontally distally in the palpable groove between the vastus medialis and the sartorius muscles. With the knee in partial flexion this groove can be defined readily. After the incision has been deepened to the enveloping or deep fascia of the thigh, the adductor tubercle of the medial femoral condyle, sweeps forward and crosses the anterior surface of the tibia at the anterior tibial tuberosity, the point of insertion of the quadriceps extensor tendon. The thigh then is rotated medially (toward the surgeon). The incision on the lateral aspect of the leg begins at a point three fingerbreadths proximal to the lateral femoral condyle in the palpable groove between the tendon of the tensor fascia latae (iliotibial tract) and the biceps femoral muscles. This incision must overlie and split the tensor facsiae latae tendon in order to avoid the muscle fibers of the biceps. Continuing distally over the lateral epicondyle, the incision extends forward to meet the medial incision at the anterior tibial tuberosity, thus outlining the anterior flap of the amputation.

Corresponding incisions from each femoral epicondyle are carried obliquely posteriorly and inferiorly until they meet on the calf of the leg at a point considerably inferior to the level of the anterior tibial tuberosity, at about the midpoint of the belly of the gastrocnemius muscle. This incision for the posterior flap is deepened to the fascia on the gastrocnemius muscle. Thus are outlined two long amputation flaps, the posterior a little longer than the anterior. Each flap partakes not only of the soft parts of the lower thigh but of a considerable portion of the soft parts of the leg.

Attention is then centered again on the medial aspect of the thigh and knee. The horizontal portion of the medial incision, common to the two flaps (i.e., that portion lying between the vastus medialis and the sartorius muscles) is deepened through the deep fascia of the thigh. Division of this powerful fascial layer, which is the only strong structure in the medial wall of the popliteal fossa at this level, affords ingress to the popliteal space. The left forefinger, now inserted into the superficial popliteal space, by blunt dissection frees the medial hamstring tendons as far as their tibial insertions. At this juncture these tendons are divided in the order named: sartorius, gracilis, semimembranosus and semitendinosus. During this dissection, no fleshy portion of any of the medial hamstring muscles nor any part of the vastus medialis muscle need be exposed, much less severed. The severed hamstring tendons retract at once into the aponeurotic and areolar tissue of the posterior flap and are not dealt with again. Further exposure is gained by severing the tendon of the adductor magnus muscle at its attachment to the adductor tubercle. Free access to the vasculoneural contents of the popliteal space thus is afforded. Moderate flexion of the knee relaxes the popliteal vessels and nerves and favors their manipulation. With a finger now inserted more deeply into the popliteal space and kept close to the posterior surface of the femur, the popliteal artery and vein are

withdrawn easily to the level flush with, or even outside of, the incision in the skin. Here they are clamped, ligated and divided as far distally in the popliteal space as possible. The tibial (internal popliteal) and common peroneal nerves are then drawn readily into the wound as one trunk and are anesthetized, ligated and divided. Each of the components of the nerve bundle then is injected with absolute alcohol to prevent formation of neuroma, and the stump is allowed to retract into the proximal recess of the popliteal space. Ligation of these three essential structures low down in the popliteal space prevents unnecessary separation of the posterior flap from the femur and minimizes formation of dead space.

The partly flexed knee then is rotated toward the operator, and the lateral longitudinal incision is deepened through the more posterior fibers of the tensor fasciae latae tendon. This incision is carried inferiorly as far as the insertion of the biceps muscle on the head of the fibula, where the biceps tendon then is severed. At this stage of the operation the popliteal space may be opened widely from side to side, since the essential structures have been divided. Deepening of the incision outlining the posterior flap down to the gastrocnemius aponeurosis, and clearing from it the areoloadipose debris, free the posterior flap. It is advantageous to leave as much as possible of the fibro-areolar tissue of the popliteal space in contact with the femur as far distally as the level of the adductor tubercle in order that there may be but little dead space between the posterior flap and the femur.

The knee then is extended and the incision marking the distal portion of the anterior flap is deepened through the capsule of the knee joint down to the femoral condyles and to the tibia, thereby severing the quadriceps tendon at its insertion into the tibial tuberosity. The anterior flap, containing the patella, is dissected upward off the infrapatellar fat pad and drawn upward on the thigh until the superior synovial recesses of the subquadriceps space are seen. The patella is dissected from the apex to the base from its sesamoid position in the quadriceps tendon, care being taken to preserve the longitudinally disposed tendon of the rectus femoris muscle, which runs over it. Preservation of this tendon adds materially to the end-bearing capacity of the stump after the cut end of the femur is fitted into the socket from which the patella has been removed. The synovia on the anterior flap and on the femur proximal to the condyles is not excised. The femur now is sawed through its cancellous portion just proximal to the adductor tubercle. At this level the shaft of the femur corresponds in size to the patellar socket in the quadriceps tendon. The cut end of the femur is rounded with a bone-cutting forceps and a rasp until no sharp surfaces and no fringes of periosteum remain.

The two large flaps are inspected for small bleeding points. These can be ascertained best by sluicing the surfaces of both flaps with large quantities of warm salt solution. The flushing has the additional advantage of washing away soft tissue or bone debris. Many small bleeding points may require ligation after this procedure. Inspection of the body of the posterior flap shows no muscle fibers. It does show areolo-adipose tissue and the cut ends of the hamstring tendons which already are retracted into their aponeurotic beds and scarcely are visible. The flaps now are allowed to fall loosely together.

The coaptation suturing during the operation is limited to the placing of six or eight clips or sutures at such intervals as to keep the flaps in fair apposition. When the edges of the skin are approximated, the aponeurotic edges also lie in contact; mere apposition is sufficient to produce firm union. None of the tendons or aponeuroses of the anterior flap are sutured to the corresponding structures of the posterior flap. In this way no structure is under any tension, and the trauma and consequent pressure necroses which result from suture of these deeper structures cannot occur. The flaps appear exceedingly long and extend one or more inches beyond the end of the femur immediately after they are fashioned. To the surgeon accustomed to the routine type of amputation in the lower third of the femur, the flaps appear excessively redundant and clumsy and arouse suspicion that a bulbous stump end and large dead spaces will result. When he notes how wobbly the femur lies between the flaps, he questions whether the end will gain contact with the patellar socket and fuse there. As early as the second or third postoperative day and sometimes even within a few hours after the operation, the reason for leaving these flaps under no tension becomes apparent, as the hamstring muscles, severed only at their distal attachment, contract to the degree that the cutaneous suture line lies posteriorly at about the level of the stump end, and the femur is felt in the patellar fossa.

Convalescent: There is no indication for limiting the patient's activity during the early convalescent period. The routine of having the patient sitting up in bed on the day of the operation and in a wheel chair on the day after the operation reduces the postoperative complications. The short posterior splint used to close dead spaces does not interfere with activity and actually steadies the stump. Freedom from tension at the end of the stump allows free and comparatively p a i n l e s s movement.

Mortality: I have recorded 80 cases of amputation according to this method; 32 are my own and my associates', and the remainder were reported to us from about the country. By far the majority of the patients were over 65 years of age; 11 have died, a mortality of 13 per cent.

Comment: It has been my privilege to do two amputations using the Callandar method. One case for a diabetic gangrene of the foot and another for an extensive crushing injury about the foot. The diabetic case terminated fatally a few months after the operation.

In this city I have seen the operation performed by other men. The technique in this operation should be kept in mind by surgeons doing amputations of the leg. I believe it is a distinct advance in this field of surgery. The operations require at least for me a little more care at operation. The post-operaitve care is simpler.

The author points out that he had had a lower incidence of gas bacillus infection when using the tendoplastic amputation.

---o---

ORTHOPAEDIC SURGERY

Edited by Earl D. McBride, M.D., F.A.C.S.
717 North Robinson Street, Oklahoma City

A Review of Synovectomy, Paul P. Swett, Jr. Bone & Joint Surg. Vol. XX, No. 1, January, 1938.

Synovectomy is an operation for the removal of diseased synovial membrane from a joint which is the seat of an inflammatory reaction. Ordinarily the operation is applicable to any joint of the extremities. Its use has been limited largely to the knee. Its purpose is to remove inflammatory membrane which may add to the damage to the joint, or to increase the efficiency in function of the joint, and influence the patient's general health.

In 1925 Key reported that the synovia could be removed completely and a new membrane develop which was essentially normal in its function. Theoretical considerations upon which the operation was originally applied are:

1. The possibility of promoting the resumption of joint function by the operative removal of the organized inflammatory exudate and of preventing such further joint damage as would result from the continued presence of unabsorbed exudate.

2. The possibility of assisting the local and general recovery of the patient by eliminating the metastatic foci of infection in the joints themselves. This point probably should not be stressed.

3. This was based on the s t i m u l a t i o n of the metabolism and the decrease in the suboxidation processes with lowered sugar tolerance which Pemberton had found to accompany arthritis, improvement in which might be expected to follow the restoration of joint function.

Of the three theoretical considerations which originally led up to this operation, the first and third seem to be valid.

The definite indications for synovectomy cannot be given categorically and they should not be dogmatically stated. The original purpose of the operation was directed t o w a r d the treatment of chronic atrophic arthritis on the grounds listed above, and the validity of these considerations seem to be substantiated by the author's experience, as well as by the reports of others. A synovial membrane which shows signs of subacute synovitis, that is, local tenderness, pain on motion and stiffness of the joint, and an excess of synovial fluid is the type for which synovectomy is indicated. While synovectomy is most frequently performed on the knee, it may be used with effect on other joints, especially in multiple arthritis.

The author reviews carefully the literature of the past 15 years and the operation seems advisable in the following types of joint disease. That in which there is extensive induration and fibrosis of a capsule, enlargement of the synovial villi, and persistent increase of joint fluid. Such a joint may be caused by:

1. Chronic atrophic arthritis.
2. Traumatic arthritis.
3. Benign tumors.
4. Osteochondromatosis.
5. Syphilitic arthritis.
6. Intermittent hydrarthrosis.
7. Synovitis ossificans.
8. Hypertrophic arthritis.
9. Synovial tuberculosis.
10. Synovitis caused by foreign-body irritation.

Synovectomy is a useful prevention of joint deformity, but it is not considered an operation to correct deformity. It is urged that those interested in treating this type of case make further study of synovectomy in that it is relatively seldom used but is a very valuable procedure in many cases and can bring freedom from pain and increase in joint motion in from 65 to 90 per cent of the cases in which it is used.

Tears of the Supraspinatus Tendon, Tom A. Outland and Walter F. Shepherd, Annals of Surgery, Vol. 107, January, 1938.

The authors point out that Codman has written a wonderful monograph on this injury, but they also have noted that medical literature is rather scarce in listing this injury. It seems that the injury is noticed and found more often when it is looked for. Anatomically it is mentioned that the tendinous insertion of the supraspinatus, together with the infraspinatus, teres major and teres minor, is closely attached to the capsule of the shoulder joint, reinforcing the latter in its upper half. The supraspinatus and infraspinatus both intimately blend and insert into the greater tuberosity. The function is to pull the greater tuberosity under the acromion, fix the humeral head in the glenoid, and abduct the shoulder through the first few degrees.

The cause of ruptured supraspinatus tendon is traumatic in origin. However, there are predisposing factors. The injury occurs in one of two ways—either by the patient falling and abducting his arm in an attempt to break the fall, the rupture occurring during the movement before the shoulder struck the ground, or by a direct blow (or fall) in which the back of the shoulder received the blow, and in which there was forward displacement of the humeral head. Dislocation may be only momentary, followed by spontaneous replacement. The tendon may have been previously weakened by defects left as a result of so-called calcified deposits; necrosis of the tendon or other diffuse pathologic processes similar to arthritis in other joints; or by attrition. Age may be considered a predisposing factor since it is commonly seen around or beyond the fifth decade.

Pathology—The site of the rupture is usually very close to, or at the greater tuberosity.

The following signs are considered of greatest importance:

1. Diminution or loss of the power to abduct.
2. Tenderness over the greater tuberosity.
3. Undue prominence of the greater tuberosity due to the fact that its tendinous covering is absent.
4. Crepitus of a fine nature, palpable over the tuberosity as it moves under the acromion.
5. A negative roentgenogram.

Treatment.—In cases where the injury is incomplete, it is entirely possible to rest the patient in abduction for a few weeks until the crepitus disappears. In the series of cases of the authors they have treated some cases this way and have obtained very satisfactory results. However, they feel that open operation would have speeded the recovery. For the complete tear, operative repair is the only logical treatment. The retracted tendon ends are approximated to the greater tuberosity and held with heavy silk mattress sutures. It may be necessary to make drill holes in the tuberosity in order to obtain firm fixation. The arm is immobilized with an axillary pad, sling and bandage. Physical therapy is begun as soon as the wound is healed and dry.

Summary.—"This lesion is considered common. It occurs most frequently in laboring men over 40. The lesion presents a characteristic history with well defined physical findings. Continued shoulder disability following any trauma should be considered a general indication of rupture. Complete separation of the tendon demands surgical repair."

(The above articles were abstracted by: Howard B. Shorbe, M.D.)

---o---

UROLOGY

Edited by D. W. Branham, M. D.
514 Medical Arts Building, Oklahoma City

Transurethral Diverticulotomy. Roger W. Barnes, M.D., Russell T. Bergman, Los Angeles, California. Urologic and Cutaneous Review, January, 1937.

The authors present a new surgical procedure for the treatment of diverticulum of the bladder. Radical removal of a bladder diverticulum is a rather hazardous procedure especially in the age group in which it is most often found. They felt that by improving the drainage from these sacs to the bladder proper through enlarging the orifice communicating between the diverticulum and bladder, relief to the patient could be obtained. By means of the regular McCarthy electrotone or Collings knife they excised by the high frequency cutting current the inferior portion of the orifice. Because this complication is associated with prostatic hypertrophy, an electro resection of the bladder neck can be performed before this is done and usually at one sitting.

Thirty cases had such an operation performed and by preoperative and post-operative study they concluded the results were very satisfactory. Diverticuli that failed to drain before operation showed almost complete emptying following the procedure. No complications were encountered in performing the operation and they state that if it is carefully done the risk is negligible.

Comment: This is an interesting article detailing a relatively simple procedure for a rather frequent complication of prostatism. I have found, however, that many times a diverticulum of the bladder often shows marked improvement following relief of the badder neck obstruction. It seems to me that rather than risk the hazard of perforating a bladder wall by such a procedure it would be better judgment to wait and see what prostatic resection accomplishes in improving bladder drainage.

Sexual Debility and Marriage. Winfield Scott Pugh, New York, N. Y. Urologic and Cutaneous Review, January, 1937.

The author describes his paper as a brief resume of the most common bars to domestic felicity. In his own inimitable style he informally discusses several phases of the problem of sexual incompatibility. He prefaces his remark with the statement that nothing contributes to the mutual well being of the male and female as a well regulated sexual life.

From his experience of many years he has selected examples of several common conditions responsible for much sexual disability in marriage. He considers premature ejaculation not only the most common bar to a satisfactory sex life, but a rather prevalant condition in men in general (60 per cent). By premature ejaculation he defines as an inability to prevent ejaculation within five minutes after insertion of the penis in the vagina. The etiological factor responsible for this disturbance is masturbation in which the individual has conditioned himself by autoeroticism to reach the climax as quickly as possible. He states premature ejaculation often follows the practice of withdrawal which many men do for the purpose of contraception. The latter condition results in a chain of symptoms due to the excess congestion induced by this habit. He has often found premature ejaculation may result from infectious conditions of the prostate and vesicles.

His treatment of such conditions is first advising a period of sexual rest following an examination to determine whether organic pathology is present. Prostatitis and seminal vesiculitis are treated by appropriate therapeutic measures, and last but not least, the re-education of the patient, in the correct method of performing sexual intercourse, in order that not only he but his partner may obtain greatest benefit from the act. He details the correct technique for intercourse which he states many men are deficient, despite an egotistical pride to the contrary.

———o———

INTERNAL MEDICINE

Edited by C. E. Bradley, M.D., Medical Arts Building,
Tulsa; Hugh Jeter, M.D., 1200 North Walker,
Oklahoma City

HUGH JETER, M.D., F.A.C.P., A.S.C.P.

Hematological Observations on Bone Marrow Obtained by Sternal Puncture. Peter Vogel, Lowell A. Erf and Nathan Rosenthal. From the Medical Department and the Laboratories of the Mt. Sinai Hospital, New York, N. Y. Vol. 7, No. 6, November, 1937. American Journal of Clinical Pathology.

The authors in this paper, their second on the hematological observations on bone marrow obtained by sternal puncture, present the findings of the marrow (aspirated by Arinkin's technique) in 246 cases. They find the material obtained by the simple puncture method to be nearly identical with those made by biopsy. However, they point out the following disadvantages encountered with the simple puncture method: (1) there is a loss of histological structure of the marrow and the distribution of megakaryocytes and fat cells is altered. (2) Evaluation of the degree of hyperplasia or hypoplasia is at times difficult. (3) Rarely the sternal puncture is unsuccessful due to thickening of the sternal plate or marrow fibrosis. (4) There is an admixture of blood when large amounts are withdrawn. This is overcome, however, by withdrawing only 0.1 to 0.2 ccs. of marrow fluid. The authors feel that simplicity of this technique outweighs the disadvantages and state that the procedure is adaptable for ward, clinic, home or office use and no special permission is required for a biopsy. Repeated punctures may be readily and easily done.

The authors discuss the cellular findings in various diseases and classify them as to (a) sternal puncture of diagnostic importance, (b) sternal puncture of confirmatory value and (c) sternal punctures of little or no aid. Gaucher's disease, myeloma, leishmaniasis, malaria, leukemia and in certain cases of carcinoma where there is general bone metastasis are considered by the authors to be diseases in which the sternal puncture is of diagnostic importance. Leukemia, leukopenic infectious monocytosis, agranulocytosis, pernicious anemia, spure, hemolytic jaundice, polycythemia and apastic anemia are diseases in which the sternal puncture is of confirmatory value. Agranulocytosis is felt by the author to be a most interesting disease from the standpoint of blood and marrow findings and they believe that much information will be gained from marrow studies during the disease process.

The authors of this paper conclude that the aspiration of the sternal marrow by the simple puncture technique is of diagnostic, prognostic and corroborative value in certain diseases.

The Etiology and Pathology of Agranulocytic Angina. Present-Day Findings and Hypotheses. Thomas Fitz-Hugh, Jr., Philadelphia, Pa. Vol. 7, No. 6, November, 1937. American Journal of Clinical Pathology.

The author outlines a brief history of the status of agranulocytic angina since its original description 15 years ago. In addition he outlines by means of a graphic chart the chief components of the present day view of the etiology and pathologic

physiology of the disorder. The author believes that the disease is a distinct entity and that it does not involve the red cells or platelets or the coagulation factors of the blood. He reports a case that recovered and shows a very interesting graph with a tabulation of the white blood count, total granulocytes and total myelocytes during the course of the disease.

According to the author the pathological findings are (1) maturation arrest of the myeloid series of leucocytes at the myeloblast-myelocyte level; (2) arrest or partial non-migration into the blood stream of the other leucocytes; (3) maintenance of normal red cell and platelet structure and function; (4) oropharyngeal and other mucosal and cutaneous ulceration and necrosis with complete or nearly complete absence of polymorphonuclear infiltration; (5) invasion by "opportunist bacteria" with various types of ensuing sepsis (pneumonia, septicemia, osteomyelitis of the jaw, perforation of the nasal septum, nephritis, intestinal ulceration and necrosis, phlegmonous angina with neighborhood adenitis, endarteritis, acute splenic tumor, acute hepatitis with or without jaundice and finally necrosis of the bone marrow, lymph nodes, adrenals, etc.); (6) recovery initiated by myelocytic hyperplasia of the bone marrow, a myelocyte crisis in the peripheral blood (with extreme left-shift in the neutrophile formula which here is a happy omen), sometimes a monocytosis as well, and then a return of normal polymorphonuclear and other white cells to the circulation and tissues with ensuing tissue recovery (provided some septic or necrotic process has not already gone beyond repair).

Dr. Fitz-Hugh discusses the therapy and compares his mortality rate to others. He concludes that the earlier the diagnosis is established and the earlier the offending drug is stopped, the better the outlook. Furthermore, the author predicts that the benzol-ring sulphonamid compounds may sooner or later be added to this group of drugs which may cause the syndrome of agranulocytic angina. However, he feels that their theoretical danger is outweighed by their value in combating the hemolytic streptococcus.

———

Observations on the One Hour Two Dose Dextrose Tolerance Test. J. Shirley Sweeney, J. J. Muirhead and Louie E. Allday, Dallas, Texas. American Journal of Clinical Pathology. Vol. 7, No. 6, November, 1937.

The authors report a study of the effect of extreme and abnormal antecedent diets on the one-hour, two-dose dextrose tolerance test of Exton and Rose. This test consists of the administration of two doses of glucose 30 minutes apart, on the assumption that the first dose activates the insulin glycogen mechanism. The authors believe that this one-hour two-dose test has been thoroughly proved and that it eliminates many abnormal tolerance curves. They feel that the simplicity of this procedure will make it a more dependable means of differentiating suspected and renal diabetes from true diabetes. They emphasize the fact that the test is less time consuming and less disturbing to the patient.

This study of the one-hour two-dose dextrose tolerance test was made to determine the effects of extremely abnormal antecedent diets. Normal healthy young adults were used in the study. Some of the subjects abstained from all food for 48 hours, some ate only fats, some consumed only protein, while others received only sugars preceding the tolerance test. The blood sugar determinations were done by Folin-Wu technique.

Interesting graphs with tables are shown with

the average figures for each group. In another table and graph the figures for the controls are shown. The controls consisted of those subjects eating normally preceding the test.

The authors conclude from this study that the antecedent diet has a very marked effect on the tolerance test. Furthermore, they find from this study that the graphic curves were typically those of a diabetic in the individuals who had fasted and who had been on high fat diets. In addition they found that the average curve of each group in general was considerably lower at the end of two hours than it was following the single dose tolerance test. They conclude that this is due to the two dose of dextrose ingested at 30 minute intervals. The authors conclude that the one-hour two-dose test will show definite changes in individuals who have been on ordinary diets preceding the test and it is their opinion that the test will serve as a valuable differential diagnostic procedure.

-----o-----

The New Orleans Graduate Medical Assembly

The second annual New Orleans Graduate Medical Assembly will be held at the Roosevelt Hotel in New Orleans on March 7, 8, 9 and 10, 1938.

For over 100 years, New Orleans has been recognized as one of the nation's greatest medical centers. During that century it has been growing progressively greater in importance. Being the second port of the United States its geographic situation has made it a crossroad of the shipping of the western hemisphere. As a consequence, while its general health is second to none in the United States, it was but a natural sequence that an opportunity would be afforded to see a variety of disease conditions only possible in a port of its size. An additional reason has been the fact that Charity Hospital has always been a mecca to which have come sufferers as well as students of medicine. Those who were ill have realized that in this medical center the facilities for relief would be found. Physicians and students in a like manner have always known it as a center of medical knowledge with unsurpassed clinical material.

For 104 years New Orleans has been the home of the School of Medicine of Tulane University, whose graduates have taken their places in the medical profession all over the world. Many of them have made medical history by their scientific achievements and many have become distinguished teachers in medical schools in New Orleans and elsewhere.

Just a few years ago there came into existence the Louisiana State University Medical Center, which has made amazing progress in these few years so that New Orleans now has two well organized, equipped and staffed medical schools.

The success of the New Orleans Graduate Medical Assembly at its initial meeting last year exceeded the most optimistic expectations of its sponsors. This year 18 physicians of national and international reputation, representing the principal branches of medicine, have accepted invitations to be the guest speakers. They will be as follows:

Dr. Warren T. Vaughan, Richmond, allergy.

Dr. Udo J. Wile, Ann Arbor, dermatology.

Dr. Charles Mazer, Philadelphia, endocrinology.

Dr. Burril B. Crohn, New York City, gastroenterology.

Dr. Norman F. Miller, Ann Arbor, gynecology.

Dr. Richard P. Strong, Boston, medicine.

Dr. Sydney R. Miller, Baltimore, medicine.

Dr. Temple S. Fay, Baltimore, neurology.

Dr. William C. Danforth, Chicago, obstetrics.

Dr. Algernon B. Reese, New York City, ophthalmology.

Dr. Philip D. Wilson, New York City, orthopedics.

Dr. Frank R. Spencer, Denver, otolaryngology.

Dr. Fred W. Stewart, New York City, pathology.

Dr. A. Graeme Mitchell, Cincinnati, pediatrics.

Dr. Frederick M. Hodges, Richmond, radiology.

Dr. Arthur E. Hertzler, Halstead, Kans., surgery.

Dr. Harvey B. Stone, Baltimore, surgery.

Dr. William E. Lower, Cleveland, urology.

A cordial invitation is extended to the physicians of the state of Oklahoma to attend the assembly.

Report of Licenses Granted to Practice Medicine

NAME	Year of Birth	Place of Birth	School of Graduation	Year of Graduation	Permanent or Present Address
Brown, Forest Reed	1913	Hannah, Okla.	Oklahoma Univ.	1936	Ancon, Panama C. Z.
Kennedy, Louis James	1910	Purcell, Okla.	Oklahoma Univ.	1936	St. Louis, Mo.
Swanson, Homer S.	1910	Kansas City, Mo.	Oklahoma Univ.	1936	Nashville, Tenn.
Olson, Virginia Claire (F.)	1913	Guthrie, Okla.	Oklahoma Univ.	1936	Des Moines, Iowa
Prosser, Moorman P.	1910		Oklahoma Univ.	1935	Norman, Okla.
Tupper, Walter Richard	1908	Springfield, Mo.	Oklahoma Univ.	1936	Cleveland, Ohio
Cameron, Paul Broomhall	1907	St. Louis, Mo.	University Kansas	1930	Tulsa, Okla.
Coots, William Norvel (col.)	1906	Richmond, Va.	Meharry Medical	1936	Tulsa, Okla.
Felts, Clifton	1906	Marion, Ill.	University Illinois	1932	Seminole, Okla.
Finley, Gravelly E. (col.)	1909	..........., Ark.	Meharry Medical	1935	Oklahoma City, Okla.
Forry, Willis Wendell	1905	Muskogee, Okla.	Univ. Tennessee	1935	Bixby, Okla.
Gaede, Eva Marie (F.)	1908	Weatherford, Okla.	Medical Evangelist	1937	Weatherford, Okla.
Heiss, John Ernest	1884	Morrison, Ill.	Loyola University	1916	Orlando, Okla.
Johnson, Obbo William	1894	Dubuque, Iowa	University Kansas	1927	Kansas City, Mo.
Lytle, William Rowland	1911	Fredericktown, Mo.	Univ. Tennessee	1935	Oklahoma City, Okla.
Markland, James David	1894	Kokomo, Ind.	Univ. Tennessee	1936	Tulsa, Okla.
Mahon, George Savage	1908	Humboldt, Tenn.	Univ. Tennessee	1932	Ada, Okla.
Melvin, James Henry	1908	Winona, Miss.	Univ. Tennessee	1933	Oklahoma City, Okla.
Morton, William Ambrose (col.)	1908	Richmond, Va.	Meharry Medical	1936	Tulsa, Okla.
Pigford, Charles Alfred	1907	Mobile, Ala.	Univ. Tennessee	1932	Tulsa, Okla.
Pittman, Cole Dilling	1908	Sweatman, Miss.	Univ. Tennessee	1933	Tulsa, Okla.
Stough, Austin Robert	1910	Geary, Okla.	Univ. Tennessee	1936	Oklahoma City, Okla.
Walker, John Hicks	1904	Atlanta, Ga.	Harvard Medical	1930	Muskogee, Okla.
Waters, Gregory Roy	1901	Constantinople, Tur.	Loyola University	1932	Wright City, Okla.
Wright, Jack McLellan	1912	Canton, Miss.	L.S.U. Med. Center	1936	New Orleans, La.
Yandell, Hays Richmond	1907	Seattle, Wash.	Harvard Medical	1934	Ponca City, Okla.
Young, Clarence Calhoun	1895	Nashville, Tenn.	Univ. Tennessee	1932	Shawnee, Okla.
Baker, Roscoe Conkling	1882	Clarksdale, Mo.	Ensworth Medical	1904	Enid, Okla.
Ketchersid, John W.	1878	Martin, Ga.	Vanderbilt Medical	1898	Mannsville, Okla.
Lowther, Robert Dow	1868	Hollywood, Ark.	Ky. School of Med.	1893	Norman, Okla.
Snelson, Seaborn C. (col.)	1867	Andersonville, Ga.	Howard Medical	1890	Oklahoma City, Okla.
Welch, A. J.	1853	Columbus, Ohio	Starling Medical	1881	McAlester, Okla.
Wolff, Elewullyn Gilmer	1868	Shawnee Mound, Mo.	Missouri Medical	1899	Okarche, Okla.
Thompson, Wildridge Clark, Jr.	1903	Union Springs, Ala.	John Hopkins	1930	Stillwater, Okla.
Bradfield, Eldon O.	1912	Elk City, Okla.	Oklahoma Univ.	1936	Temple, Texas
Sizemore, Oliver Paul	1909	..........., Mo.	University Arkansas	1934	DeQueen, Ark.

THE JOURNAL
OF THE
OKLAHOMA STATE MEDICAL ASSOCIATION

| VOLUME XXXI | McALESTER, OKLAHOMA, MARCH, 1938 | Number 3 |

Facial Paralysis in Mastoiditis*

WELBORN W. SANGER, M.D.
PONCA CITY, OKLAHOMA

My attention has been attracted to this subject because of the pitiful, depressing, permanent disfigurement. This subject should not only be discussed, but every effort made to *manage* it properly. The loss of function of this nerve handicaps one to the extent of tragedy. For a person to go through life with one-half of his face motionless and expressionless, his occupation, his social life, and his attitude toward himself and his external world are made much less pleasant, prosperous, and happy.

Until a few years ago only a moderate amount of work had been done to alleviate this distressing condition. Many methods have been advanced, but most of these have been only to inspire hope for the return of facial movements. We still have no perfect treatment. The medical treatment consists of massage, electrical stimulation, and waiting. The surgical treatment will be considered later.

I do not wish to consider mastoiditis from any relationship other than with facial paralysis or vice versa; that is, paralysis due to nuclear origin in the brain, or from toxins, cerebral hemorrhage, Lues, or any other reason. I shall consider only the causes due to trauma, contused, torn, or completely severed nerve at time of operation, and those due to too tight packing, or fracturing inward of the' fallopian canal during operative procedure.

I have been unable to find much data on

*Read before the Eye, Ear, Nose and Throat Section, Annual Meeting, Oklahoma State Medical Association, Tulsa, Okla., May, 1937.

the number and case percentage of facial paralysis in relation to mastoiditis, either pre or post-operative. I have only to quote the number of mastoid operations done in the Baltimore Eye and Ear Hospital during the year of 1933-34. There were a total of 70 cases—63 simple and s e v e n radicals. Two cases of facial paralysis developed from the simple mastoids, coming on immediately, and to date one has remained permanent, the other clearing up to about 85 per cent return of f u n c t i o n in five months. No case of paralysis developed in any of the seven cases of radical mastoidectomies. In Ancker Hospital, St. Paul, 66 mastoidectomies, one radical, were done during the year 1934-1935 with no cases of facial paralysis. In the last 10 years there have been three cases of facial paralysis at the Ponca City Hospital in 110 cases— only one remains paralyzed.

I have also been unable to find any data on the percentage of cases of acute mastoiditis with facial paralysis before operation who clear up either with, or without, operation. I have seen a few of these cases and all have cleared up in a few days, or a few weeks, post-operative. Some men are of the opinion that all or most of these cases would clear up just as quickly without operation. I do not believe this to be true. Jackson and Coates, and most other textbooks, give facial paralysis in mastoiditis as one of the cases when immediate mastoidectomy should be performed.

The diagnosis of this distressful condition is so easy that it almost "hits you in the face." Following a mastoid operation the paralyzed side of the face has no motion or movement, and the lines of the face are so obliterated as to look like a "curtain of tissue" hung on that side of the face. The patient is unable to wrinkle the forehead or close the eye, and care must be taken to avoid dryness of the cornea and ulceration. When the patient laughs, cries, or shows the teeth, the face is pulled toward the opposite side; the paralyzed side remains motionless and expressionless. In the interest of relief for these unfortunate people this paper deals with repair of the facial nerve.

Taste is sometimes interfered with when the chorda tympani has been severed, and occasionally the patient has t r o u b l e in chewing the food properly because he cannot keep the cheek moving on that side. As the seventh nerve is p u r e l y motor there is no anesthesia or hyperasthesia of the face.

To briefly r e v i e w the anatomy: The fibres of the facial nerve spring from a nucleus of cells in the lower part of the pons. It enters the internal auditory canal in company with the auditory nerve and the glosso-palatine (or chorda tympani) nerve. At the outer end of the meatus the trunk pierces the arachnoid and dura and enters the facial canal (Fallopian canal).

In its course through the temporal bone the nerve traverses three separate routes:

I. *Labyrinthine segment:* — e n t e r s through the internal auditory canal from the posterior cranial fossa, running outward between cochlea and vestibule in a horizontal plane. Here it is not accessible to injury during the mastoid operation unless petrositis has developed. It makes a right angle turn posteriorly at the knee and goes into the—

II. *Tympanic portion* — here it runs backward along the medial wall of the middle ear, just above the oval window and b e l o w the horizontal semi-circular canal. It enters the middle ear just above and slightly posterior to the point where the ligament of the tensor tympani muscle is given off for its attachment to the handle of the malleus. This ligament is a reliable guide to the position of the nerve during the radical mastoid. In this middle ear the

bone is very thin covering the nerve, and in this portion the nerve is injured more frequently during the radical mastoid. This tympanic p o r t i o n makes another right angle turn downward to form the mastoid division of the nerve.

III. *Mastoid division* — runs directly downward in the vertical plane along the bottom of the posterior canal wall, leaving the temporal bone t h r o u g h the stylomastoid foramen at the mastoid tip. The average adult canal measures about 25 mm.

SURGICAL INJURY

The *vertical* (mastoid) and tympanic sections are m o s t commonly injured in surgical intervention. The mastoid portion is often injured in searching *too low* for the antrum, fracture of the tip with rongeurs or chiseling the posterior canal wall at too acute an angle during the radical mastoid.

The *tympanic* (horizontal) portion is injured by:

1. The injudicious use of the curet in the auditus.
2. Breaking off of the bridge too violently with the gouge.
3. As the nerve is covered by a very thin bone, undue pressure may cause definite compression.

As the radical operation constitutes a small percentage of the total number of mastoid operations, the *vertical portion of the nerve is most often injured.* In many cases the patients recover when trauma and bruising have not been too great—and in those in whom the nerve exposed by caries and cholesteatoma lies bare and is compressed by too tight packing. These usually do not show a complete paralysis on recovering from the anesthetic. The patients showing complete paralysis have had the nerve cut or bruised usually beyond Nature's repair.

Injury to the facial nerve occurs either from the c a r e l e s s manipulation of the chisel, curet or rongeur forceps during the excavation of the bone while performing the radical mastoid operation, or because of dehiscences or defects in its bony covering which have resulted from necrosis.

In extensive necrosis of the temporal bone the nerve trunk is prone to become exposed at some point, and this is so especially along the floor or the inner wall of the aditus ad antrum. When thus exposed, unless great care is exercised, the nerve trunk may be severely injured or completely severed during the operation. Furthermore, the nerve may be injured at any point in its course in the fallopian canal, and, when the excavation of the cells and necrosed bone at the mastoid tip requires the exposure of the digastric muscle, there is considerable danger of injuring the facial nerve at its exit from the fallopian canal. The latter form of injury is more liable to occur while operating upon infants and young children. Effusion into the fallopian canal and u n d u e pressure upon an exposed facial nerve by instruments or packing are less serious; nevertheless, they are usually of sufficient severity to induce temporary paralysis of the muscles supplied by this nerve. Anomalies in the course of the facial nerve in rare instances are accountable for operation injuries.

Facial paralysis e i t h e r temporary or permanent is the deplorable result of injury to the facial nerve. The paralysis is temporary when caused by an injury which does not sever or otherwise destroy the nerve trunk, when resulting from pressure upon an exposed section of the nerve, or when due to inflammatory effusion into the fallopian canal.

Permanent facial paralysis o c c u r s in cases where the n e r v e trunk has been severed, when a segment had been cut away, or when destroyed at some point by the purulent inflammatory process. In the latter class of cases the facial paralysis is complete; its advent is sudden and sometimes apparent before the patient has completely recovered from the anesthetic.

In case the injury to the facial nerve is slight, the resultant paralysis is rarely complete; it develops gradually and often it does not appear until some days subsequent to the operation.

It is not an uncommon occurrence for facial paralysis of otitic origin to appear in patients upon whom no operation has been performed, in which event its advent is considered to be of serious import, especially when accompanied by labyrinthine symptoms, or when due to the encroachment of tumors. The extent of the paralysis of the facial muscles is ascertained by requesting the patient to smile, to close the eyes, or to whistle.

Cases have been recorded where facial p a r a l y s i s has disappeared after long periods, even when the nerve trunk has been completely severed, and in a few instances where the nerve has not only been severed, but with more or less destruction to the tissue (Zezold and Pierce). Pierce records one case in which a quarter-section of nerve trunk was destroyed, causing complete facial paralysis, which finally was restored after a period of nine months. The prognosis, therefore, so far as it relates to the restoration of function, depends upon the nature, severity, and extent of the injury which the nerve trunk has received. If due to temporary p r e s s u r e upon the nerve trunk, to traumatism without destruction of tissue, or to inflammatory effusion into its sheath, a cure may be expected. Notwithstanding the experience above recorded facial paralysis, occurring as a result of complete destruction of the nerve trunk at any point, is almost invariably permanent.

Facial paralysis of otitic origin should not be confused with that known as Bell's paralysis, which is not due to pyogenic invasion of the middle-ear spaces.

Some of the methods of treatment seem good for some cases and useless in others. Some of the methods seem too conservative, while, at times, the most radical seems to be the most conservative treatment.

HISTORY

FAURE, in 1898, joined the distal end of the paralyzed seventh nerve to the spinal accessory.

KARTE, in 1903, first did a hypoglossal facial anastomosis, and this has been done many times since then. The objection to this hypoglossal anastomosis is — the associated movements of the face with the tongue.

NEY states that most lesions of the facial nerve in the canal are probably compressive in nature, and that most cases recovering in a few hours or a few days postoperative are of this naure. MARTIN, of

San Francisco, has seen five such cases as a result of a radical, all of which recovered in a few months with no treatment except loosening the packing plus massage and electrical stimulation.

Two English surgeons, LODGE and BROOKE, each report cases of plastic operations with grafts from the fascia lata for facial paralysis, but to me the results are poor consolation.

Without leaving conspicuous scars, three new ligaments are grafted into the face, corresponding in position to the inferior portion of the orbicularis oculi, the levator palpebrae superior nasi and the zygomatic major. These sustain the drooping lower lid and palsied side of the mouth and make them conform to a more pleasing facial expression. The material employed is a continuous strip of fascia lata. Two short incisions are made, exposing the temporal fascia and the internal palpebral ligament respectively. A third, tiny incision is made at the junction of the skin and mucous membrane at the angle of the mouth. Next, a strip of fascia lata five mm. wide from the thigh has been threaded along a triangular course between the three facial incisions, a m o n g the atrophied muscles, with the aid of a packing needle. The two free ends are drawn taut and woven into the fibres of the temporal fascia.

The advantages advanced for this operation are: Its immediate effect; its simplicity; can be done under local anesthesia; needs no s p e c i a l technique or detailed anatomical knowledge, and is less dangerous. The disadvantages are that in time the fascia may stretch, and it does not cure the distressing condition.

ROBERT C. MARTIN, of San Francisco, reports a case of intra-temporal suture of the facial nerve, done in 1930. He states that: 1. Only those with peripheral facial paralysis should be operated. These palsies are complete, whereas the central palsies due to crossed innervation, as well as homolateral innervation of the upper facial division, shows a complete loss of the lower division only. 2. More successful are those showing a complete loss on waking from anesthesia. 3. There should be no nerve d e a f n e s s or labyrinthine symptoms, as

these suggest a lesion proximal to the geniculate ganglion.

J. MORRISSETT SMITH, of New York, reports two cases of decompression of facial nerve for post-operative paralysis. He believes that facial paralysis resulting from a mastoid operation should immediately be followed by a decompression of the facial nerve.

NEY has pointed out that an intact nerve trunk is very resistant to surrounding suppurative processes and that nerves may lie for many months in immediate c o n t a c t with an active suppuration without functional impairment, w h i l e, on the other hand, the facial nerve is extremely susceptible to "compressive" lesions. It completely fills the bony canal which it traverses and its sheath is intimately attached.

In the facial canal the inflammatory exudate and swelling accompanying the i n j u r y are immediately converted into compressive factors by the solid bone surrounding the nerve.

The removal of the bone permits the swelling of the nerve and the reparative processes to occur without compression, and it offers the quickest possible repair and restoration of function. After the bone has been removed it is very important to remember that the sheath of the nerve must be opened at the site of injury.

Report of two cases of decompression done for paralysis—one following a simple and the other following a radical mastoid:

Case No. 1. A girl of 10 years developed facial paralysis immediately following a radical mastoid one year and 10 months ago. Forty per cent return of function had already taken place. A left secondary radical was done and decompression of the tympanic and most of the mastoid segments done. The nerve was found to have been injured but not severed in tympanic portion.

Result: Ear dry. Seventy per cent of function recovered four and a half years later.

Case No. 2. Girl, six and one-half years of age, complete facial paralysis the day after simple mastoidectomy. M a s t o i d wound was immediately reopened. Nerve found injured but not severed in the mastoid segment from horizontal semicircular canal almost to stylo-mastoid foramen. Facial ridge lowered; mastoid segment of the nerve decompressed. The drum and ossicles were left in place—flap out.

Result: Facial p a r a l y s i s completely cleared up four months post-operative.

This next operative procedure done by DR. ARTHUR DUEL, of New York, and SIR CHARLES BALLANCE, who has recently died, of London, seems to me to be one of the most radical yet the m o s t conservative methods yet developed and to offer much more hope which will fit in any case of peripheral paralysis. They w o r k e d together on a series of anastomosis with every possible and s o m e well nigh impossible nerves. Many of these were repeated many times. About 140 experiments were done.

In England when a surgeon desires to do an experiment on an animal, he has to obtain a license from the government to do so. In trying to develop some method of restoring facial function without associated movements they did a series of 24 autoplastic grafts varying from one to 16 mm. in length in the facial nerve. These were in baboons, monkeys, and cats. They tried many different n e r v e s, reversed facial grafts, intercostal grafts, cutaneous grafts and the ext. respiratory (long thoracic) nerve of Bell grafts. They tried this last nerve over many times—different lengths, different technique; different animals—in all 24 trials. There were no failures. The face was restored in three to six months. The usual repair in injury cases would not be more than five or six mm.

The length of time since injury due to loss of function and atrophy of the facial muscles and the length of graft required to bridge the gap are important factors. It may be that the perfect results obtained in animals, who require facial motions rather than expressions of e m o t i o n s, will not prove so perfect in man. Direct repair by an autoplastic graft is obviously a much better method than indirect r e p a i r by anastomosis to another nerve.

In some of the anastomosis on monkeys, as in all on man, there are associated movements. These occur when the hypoglossal, the decendens-noni, or the glossopharyngeal nerves are united to the facial. In a lady in whom hypoglosso-facial anastomosis was done nine years ago, a ripple of muscle contractions occurred over the face during fixation of the tongue and swallowing. What surgeon would enjoy eating opposite a patient in whom he had done this operation?

The new method here recommended gets rid of all associated movements.

They give a brief history of 12 cases. Here is one:

Case No. 1: A girl, age eight and one-half years, showed immediate, complete facial paralysis following operation. Exploratory operation was done two days later. The stump was found in the neck at the posterior border of the parotid gland. A faradic current applied to the stump caused contraction of all the muscles of the face on that side. The proximal end was found at the level of the horizontal semicircular canal. The ossicles and drum were removed and the nerve uncovered to the geniculate ganglion (ganglion formed in the fallopian canal just before chorda tympani is given off). The measured distance of the gap was 27 mm. An autoplastic graft was laid in the gutter from the proximal without suture to the distal end which was sutured by one strand of finest silk attached to a needle without a knot.

These cases were operated from a few days to 13 years after operation. In a few of the cases no division of the nerve was found but a depressed fracture of the fallopian canal.

There can be no associated movements because of the gap of the injured nerve has been replaced by a living autoplastic nerve graft which c o n v e y s impulses from the cortical center in the brain to the peripheral endings of the facial nerve.

In most cases the operator has no accurate knowledge of how, when, or to what extent the nerve was damaged.

It seems that the most careful watching of the face by the anesthetist during operation for sudden spasm of the face muscles is unreliable. It can be totally severed and no muscular twitching of the face be noted. In nine of the 12 cases, the area of destruction varied from 15 to 40 mm. in length.

SIR CHARLES BALLANCE asks the question, "When shall we operate?" and then he supplies the answer, "NOW!" Delay may make all the difference between success and f a i l u r e. When facial palsy immediately follows an operation on the mastoid it is advisable to uncover the nerve at once to determine the extent of damage, because compression or slight injury may be remedied by decompression, where delay, bolstered by vain hope, is often most unsatisfactory.

A graft may be introduced at once when the nerve has been destroyed while there can be only a slight atrophy of the muscles and a quick and more perfect result is assured.

DUEL definitely demonstrated, in his animal experiments, t h a t a n y autoplastic nerve grafts — either motor or sensory — with the nerve direction either maintained or reversed, will successfully bridge the gap and restore the function of a divided facial nerve.

The use of the faradic electrical current in finding the facial trunk is inestimable before the reaction of degeneration has taken place. This reaction probably does not last more than 72 hours.

DUEL reports one case of bilateral facial paralysis, one for 11 years and the other side paralyzed for two weeks. At operation both nerves were uncovered from the stylo-mastoid foramen to the horizontal semicircular canal. In one case the result was amazing. As the sheath was split open the nerve swelled to twice its normal size. Both have now recovered about equally to a marked degree—although not complete.

With human beings, he used the sixth, seventh, or eighth intercostal nerves in all but two cases. It is more easily found than Bell's nerve, especially in fat people, and the length of the nerve required is often too long to enable us to anastomose the ends, and a paralysis of the serratus magnus results, which is more serious than letting the intercostal nerve stay unrepaired.

DUEL and BALLANCE state that no delay in operating is justifiable. We have seen patients treated for six months, a year, or even three years by galvanism, massage, etc. The result is—there is a continuation of the distortion and the facial paralysis. It does not matter to the patient that he has a slight faradic response; what matters to him is that the horrible deformity of facial palsy still persists.

DR. BALLANCE states that he remembers quite well when the first operations for appendicitis were done. They were not performed until the patients were dying. The patients were kept in the m e d i c a l wards. They had to be "protected" from the surgeons.

Slight suppuration is not a risk in doing this operation. Finer nerves effect more rapid and complete r e c o v e r y than the larger nerves. There is less probability of a central necrosis. The divided ends of the nerve should not only be united in the facial canal, but it must be decompressed. The periosteal fibrous sheath must be split up. It lies around the neural sheath of the nerve. This is a fundamental principle and the best results will not be gotten unless this is done.

In man it is justifiable to complete the radical mastoid operation if it has not already been done except in cases in which the operation involved only the lower half of the descending portion of the fallopian canal. We are not in favor of an operation which displaces the nerve from the canal.

Case Report: An eight and one-half year old girl operated at Manhattan Eye and Ear Hospital for a post-auricular-subperiosteal abscess, was operated by a house surgeon. Facial paralysis followed. In the next few days Dr. Duel tried to find the facial nerve as it emerged from the stylo-mastoid foramen, but could not. Searching in the neck wound the stump of the nerve was found just as it entered the parotid gland. The nerve had been severed at its entrance to the sterno-mastoid foramen.

The mastoid had been s c r a p e d away removing the nerve up to the bend; not being able to find the nerve in the bone he did a radical mastoid, locating the nerve in the anterior wall of the tympanum, and followed it down. It had been curetted away from the bone. There was a shortage of 27 mm. Thinking there would be very little chance for recovery of such a long graft in a suppurating wound, he decided to identify the stump by suturing a graft of 27 mm. from Bell's nerve to the end near the parotid gland with black silk, thus locating it for future anastomosis if the graft failed. In three months there was a response to foradic current. All of the muscles of the face move. He believes that in three months more it will be impossible to tell which side was the operated one.

The most careful dissection, the most successful placement of a graft, may easily fail for want of meticulous care in the after treatment. Daily dressings are done, and may be done more often in the midst of suppuration.

Dangers that menace the life of a skin graft are: (1) The use of *any* antiseptic. (2) Bungling the dressing causing disturbance of the graft by ever so slight a manipulation before it is protected by a bed of healthy granulations. (3) Pus. (4) Blood clot.

The nerve should be compressed five to 10 mm. above and below the graft. The graft should be laid in position with great care that no bleeding shall prevent perfect apposition of its ends. A thin layer of dentist's gold should be laid over the whole length of the graft and decompressed facial segments. The wound should be left *wide open* and lightly dressed with small bits of sterile packing gauze wrung out of sterile N.S.S.—nothing else! At the daily dressings curiosity should be curbed to the point of refraining in looking at the graft by lifting the gold foil for several days. If frequent dressings have kept it free from pus, it should be found pink and healthy. On lifting the gold foil in another two weeks the nerve should be found embedded in a velvety layer of healthy granulations. When the whole wound looks h e a l t h y enough to warrant it—a plastic operation to close the wound may be done. Daily, gentle massage of the facial muscles and galvanic m a s s a g e once or twice daily, should be kept up until the muscles begin to respond to faradic stimulation. Let the emphasis be made again that there is no reason for delay should the facial paralysis immediately follow the mastoidectomy.

DR. DUEL—If the nerve is operated at once they can find the exact damage—if a definite injury is found graft will be more likely to succeed and will repair more

quickly—the patient would have a "better deal" and the surgeon would sleep much better.

In the March issue of the Archives of Otolaryngology, DR. STERLING BUNNELL, of San Francisco, who is undoubtedly a plastic surgeon, discusses very thoroughly and extensively his work on surgical repair of the facial nerve. The rest of my discussion shall be from DR. BUNNELL's paper. He states: "Present indications are either to repair the facial nerve directly, by decompression, suture or free nerve graft, or, if the nerve is irreparable or the facial muscles have undergone degeneration, to perform a p l a s t i c reconstruction operation using muscle and fascia. He states the first successful suture of this nerve intratemporally was done by him in 1925.

His operative procedure is as follows: Through an incision excising the old mastoid scar and running well down the neck, paralleling the flexion crease, the facial nerve is first located as it emerges from the stylo-mastoid foramen. It will be found to be one inch deep and directly under the lobule of the ear. The nerve is uncovered from below upward, the mastoid process being chiseled away, and the nerve exposed in the fallopian canal until the lesion is located. Care is taken to preserve the external auditory meatus intact in order to maintain a clean field. The nerve will be found to be 7/8 of an inch deep in the bone. T h e r e f o r e, the bone should be chiseled away widely to afford space in which to work. The nerve is also exposed above the lesion as it lies in the fallopian canal and is uncovered downward to the lesion, where it will be found to terminate in a neuroma if it has been severed as long as three months. Both nerve ends are trimmed back boldly until g o o d a x o n bundles present.

If the gap between the nerve ends is not too great, namely, 16 mm. at the bend, or 23 mm. at the geniculate ganglion, rerouting of the nerve is resorted to instead of free grafting, because direct suturing of the nerve gives a somewhat better end result than does a graft. If the vaginal process and part of the tympanic plate of the temporal bone are removed, the nerve can be made to run straight from the parotid gland to the middle ear. One cm. of length is thus gained. By freeing the nerve well into the parotid gland, two mm. more is gained, and by displacing the p a r o t i d gland another four mm. is gained. Thus, if the lesion is at the bend, 16 mm. can be gained by rerouting.

If the gap is too great to be overcome by rerouting, a free nerve graft is advisable. BUNNELL uses the sural nerve in the back of the calf. The nerve ends are accurately sutured together with four stitches of the first silk using the shortest curved atraumatic eye needles. Sufficient bone must be chiseled away to afford space for this difficult task. By a p l a s t i c maneuver, viable soft tissue should be laid over the nerve suture or graft to obliterate all dead space and to maintain the growing nerves surrounded by clear and vascular tissues, which will aid in the quality or degree of perfection of their union. DR. BUNNELL states he has repaired over one thousand peripheral nerves, and is convinced that the degree of eventful regeneration of the sutured nerve will be exactly in proportion to the accuracy of the union. As a rule, even the most a c c u r a t e l y joined nerves regenerate not 100 per cent, but more nearly 80 per cent in degree of perfection. The sheath should be so accurately sewed that no axon escapes at the suture line and the amount of scar formation at the juncture should be minimal. The presence of hematoma, pus, or acute infection, greatly detracts from the accuracy of healing just as does merely laying the nerve ends together in contrast to accurate suturing. It is only the location of this nerve which makes the repair mechanically difficult. The repair of this nerve should be good for three reasons: (1). The lesion is

well out in the periphery, where regeneration in the nervous system is best. (2) It is a purely motor nerve. (3). The nerve is small, which allows its free ends to maintain sufficient nourishment from lymph without central necrosis until new vasularity is established.

BUNNELL believes it inadvisable to attempt to unite a severed facial nerve at once after an operation for mastoiditis, as good healing cannot take place in an infected field. It is best to repair the nerve during the first year and preferably four months from the completion of healing, but even after four years considerable return of muscle function will occur. After ten years only a trace of movement can be expected.

CONCLUSION: In the treatment of facial palsy emotional expression should be restored by repairing the nerve itself intratemporally or extratemporally, instead of resorting to anastomosis with other nerves. If repair of the nerve is impossible, reconstruction of the face by a plastic operation involving the muscle and fascia is indicated. Decompression of the nerve often restores function. Direct union of severed ends by means of rerouting the nerve is preferable to the use of a free nerve graft when possible, because with it a more perfect degree of regeneration can be expected. Free nerve grafts should be used if the gap is too great for rerouting and will give good results. The degree of regeneration is in direct proportion to the accuracy of the union of the nerve ends. This argues for accurate, aseptic, surgical repair of the nerve in a clean field by suture at some time before more than a year has elapsed since the time of injury.

The Treatment of Carcinoma of the Cervix Uteri*

RALPH E. MYERS, M. D.

OKLAHOMA CITY, OKLAHOMA

More than two decades ago radiation therapy began making its contribution to the treatment of carcinoma of the cervix

*Read before the Section on Dermatology and Radiology, Annual Meeting, Oklahoma State Medical Association, Tulsa, Okla., May 11, 1937.

u t e r i. In the beginning the pioneering work was largely performed on cases that were quite hopeless from a surgical standpoint. It was soon discovered that symptoms were often ameliorated and life prolonged. Occasionally these pioneers experienced the thrill of apparent cures in what were formerly hopeless cases. I recall with much pleasure seeing some of the early cases treated by Bailey and Janeway which showed no evidence of active malignancy three or four years after the treatment had been given.

In those days the gynecologist generally looked with a critical eye on this new form of therapy. When he referred what he sometimes called "border-line" cases for radiation treatment, one could feel sure that they would usually be considerably beyond the "border." However, as a group they proved very open-minded and rapidly changed to enthusiastic advocates of radiation treatment. In fact some[1] of them were among the first to accept it as the treatment of choice, even in the early cases.

Today in this c o u n t r y, and in many places abroad, the surgical treatment of cancer of the cervix, even though it seems to be well localized, is generally looked upon as a rather questionable procedure. Few surgeons have had sufficient experience to warrant their attempting the radical operation, while on the other hand, inadequate surgery is ineffective and often quite disastrous in its results. Even those few with extensive experience in radical hysterectomy have a mortality which most surgeons do not like to contemplate. Recently the great English surgeon, Bonney[2], admitted a percentage of 9.5 in his previous 200 operations. But to reach this point of perfection the surgeon has to pass through a period of much higher mortality, and he, who does the operation only occasionally, always f a c e s such a situation. What the average percentage figure is for all who perform this radical procedure, one can only guess. Suffice it is to say, it is high enough to tip the scales decidedly in favor of radiation therapy with its low mortality, its b e t t e r palliation in those cases which prove incurable, and its fair percentage of cures which is at least as good as those of surgery.

While the treatment of cervical carcinoma at present seems rightfully to be wholly a radiological problem, we are still far from the point where we can be content with our results. We must be open-minded and willing to accept whatever seems to improve the chances of cure. Perhaps in certain types of cases we may yet find that surgery can aid us. Above all we as radiologists must strive to keep our methods of treatment in step with scientific facts.

Early in the history of radiation therapy it was discovered that, following repeated non-lethal doses, epithelial tumors of the skin gradually became more and more resistant until finally no dose could be safely given which had much therapeutic effect. Later the same observation was made in cases of other tumors. The explanation formerly given was that the tumor cells themselves became radioresistant. However, experimental work[3] has not borne out these conclusions. Tumors have been rayed in vitro and in vivo with doses of X-ray just insufficient to destroy them, and then transferred to new hosts and the process repeated. Even though this procedure has been followed many times, these cancer cells showed no d i f f e r e n c e in the amount of the required lethal dose from that of untreated cancer cells of the same tumor strain.

On the other hand, if we turn our attention to the tumor bed, we find changes there after heavy radiation which offer a very logical explanation for the phenomenon. Within a short period after intensive dosage, microscopic examination reveals swelling of the walls of the arteries, especially the intima, and thrombosis of some of the terminal arterioles. In addition, edematous changes take place in the perivascular connective tissue. This is followed later by a devitalization of the connective tissue and permanent changes in the blood vessels so that they are incapable of reproducing the previous response. If radiation is again repeated, necrosis of the connective tissue is likely to result, while the tumor cells continue to live.

Since these observations indicate quite definitely that the effect of the radiation on the tumor bed is more important in the destruction of cancer than its direct action on the tumor cells, we must also question another oft quoted theory. The explanation frequently given, especially by the French school, for the advantages of protracted radiation over m a s s i v e dosage given in a short period, is that by the former more or less continuous treatment the cancer cells are caught during mitosis when they are most susceptible to radiation. It would appear more logical to conclude that the protracted method of treatment owes its advantages to a more favorable reaction in the cancer bed which is accompanied by less damage to normal structures.

Unfortunately the fundamental principles and conceptions just enunciated are frequently i g n o r e d. All too often one hears of the radium treatment being applied in broken doses over a period of a few days and followed some weeks later by a c o u r s e of X-ray treatment. Perhaps after an interval of another few weeks a second course is given. Sometimes these two procedures are handled by two separate physicians, unassociated with each other, as if they produced different results rather than causing one and the same type of reaction. At the best, the fight against cancer is a hard struggle. Practically all of the chances of a cure are locked up in the first effort. If responsibility and treatments are divided, the results are bound to fall short of the attainable goal.

There are, of course, no generally accepted methods of radiation therapy. Leading radiologists do, however, all agree that the treatment should be continuous, somewhat protracted and very intensive. Naturally variations in individual cases call for some changes of procedure. Bearing in mind certain fundamental f a c t s, one should endeavor to follow as l o g i c a l a method as possible.

In the use of radium especially, we must always keep before our minds the inverse square law. If we do, we will realize that no worth while effect by this agent alone will be produced more than three to four cm. from its site of application. Even at this distance the reaction will often need to be enhanced by X-ray therapy, if the cancer is to be destroyed. Beyond this quite local area we must trust to the intensive X-ray therapy to stamp out the disease. That it can be quite effective in accomplishing this is well shown by results reported by Coutard[4] in far advanced cases.

When the cancer seems to be wholly con-fined to the cervix (Group I), should our procedure be fundamentally different than when it has reached the vaginal wall or begun to invade the parametrial tissues (Group II)? In my opinion it should not. Our grouping is necessarily inaccurate. Inspection and palpation reveal to us only those changes produced by large numbers of cancer cells. They tell us nothing about small groups of cells which may have permeated lymph channels and tissue spaces for some distances. If the growth was actually confined to the cervix in all Group I cases, then we should have few failures either by surgery or radiation. The fairly high percentage of such failures shows definitely that the growth had already spread in many of them into the realm of the Group II cases. It seems to me the conclusion is inescapable that all of what appear to be early cases should r e c e i v e thorough combined treatment.

Turning now to the very advanced Group III cases, we are faced with a much different situation. Here a large part of the growth is beyond the point where internal radium therapy can have any appreciable effect on it. If there is to be any chance for a cure (and some of these cases can be cured), or if we are to produce good palliation, our treatment must be applied so as to cause a heavy reaction throughout the whole of what we estimate to be the probable tumor area. This can only be brought about by Roentgen therapy. It is hard to conceive how increasing the reaction in a small localized area by the use of radium could contribute any aid to the final result. In fact, if too severe a local reaction were produced, it might interfere some with the intensive X-ray treatment which should be given.

Since a certain number of cures are obtained in Group III cases, it is quite evident that some of the cervical carcinomas are sufficiently radiosensitive that a reaction intensive enough to destroy them can be produced by the Roentgen rays alone. In a very few early cases I have given my full course of X-ray therapy before applying the radium. In some of these it has been quite interesting to watch the cervical growth shrink rather rapidly and finally change into a whitish slough, while the reaction of the normal part of the cervix was only a moderate hyperemia — a beautiful example of selective action. One could not help but gain the impression that no radium was necessary. Nevertheless we have been afraid that there might be some groups of more resistant cancer cells lurking around the cervix which required that greater intensity of reaction which the radium would give. This suggests my conception of the treatment which may be stated as follows: By means of Roentgen therapy one can safely produce a moderately intensive reaction throughout the greater part of the pelvis. If the growth is sufficiently radiosensitive and is within the field radiated, it will be entirely destroyed. If it is too resistant for the above intensity of reaction, but is within the confines of the cervix or very closely adjacent, the increased intensity of the reaction brought about by the radium may still destroy it.

A moment ago I was speaking of giving the whole course of Roentgen radiation first. The method did not find special favor with me. In the first place it was discovered that in some cases there was a marked tendency of the X-ray therapy to bring about a closure of the uterine canal. If not discovered in time, this would prevent proper application of radium. In the second place with a stenosis of the canal perhaps in the offing, there was a natural tendency to wind up the radium phase of the treatment rather quickly. This is quite contrary to the principle of gradually increasing reaction followed in the Roentgen therapy. Accordingly I shortly returned to my previous method of giving occasional moderate doses of radium interspersed in the X-ray treatment. The time of these treatments is, of course, modified according to the general condition of the patient, her symptoms and the changes noted in the cervix during rather frequent examinations. If there is quite a little infection in the growth, the radium therapy is delayed somewhat in order to give the healing effects of the X-rays time to eradicate it.

As our experience broadens, we may find it also advisable to modify somewhat the method of treatment according to the type of growth found by microscopic examination. Most surely we should try to get a good biopsy specimen from every case treated, not so much for diagnosis as to increase our knowledge in the hope that it may aid the treatment. If one has had a fairly extensive experience in dealing with cervical cancer, he can make the diagnosis with absolute certainty in a large percentage of cases by simple inspection and palpation. This leads me to another rule which I feel advisable to follow. In the majority of cases the taking of a biopsy specimen c e r t a i n l y causes no harm, if treatment is instituted within a reasonable length of time. Occasionally, however, I have seen instances where such a procedure has been followed by l i g h t i n g up of a rather quiescent g r o w t h, which subsequently spread like the proverbial "wild fire." I am not aware of any such instances in cervical cancer. However, I have made it a rule in all cases where I think the diagnosis is sure, to wait ten days to two weeks after treatment is instituted before removing a specimen for microscopic study. At this time the radiation reaction is beginning to develop whereas the cancer cells are still unchanged. Perhaps it is unnecessary to do it this way, but at any rate I feel safer about it. In case the diagnosis is questionable, the biopsy and microscopic study should, of course, be made first.

Speaking of safeguards, I have learned what I believe is another important point from b i t t e r experience. The radiation treatment of cancer of the cervix does have its mortality. There will probably always be the possibility of lighting up some latent infection, but, judging from my observation, the chances of this can be distinctly lessened, if the patient is carefully watched and if the radiation reaction is not built up too rapidly. Some patients can tolerate a rather rapid administration of the treatment and respond as well as other cases where it is administered more slowly, but every now and then a case will appear which will cause one very much regret for having attempted it. This has driven me to the conclusion that there are no circumstances which justify haste in applying the treatment.

As brought out previously, the chances of a cure or of good palliation are almost always sealed in the first series of treatments. I do not make the rule absolute because there are occasional exceptions, even if an intensive protracted treatment has been applied the first time. A well advanced proven case of carcinoma of the lung which was first treated intensively by me nearly five years ago according to the protracted m e t h o d well illustrates this. Because of return of symptoms I gave him another intensive protracted Roentgen treatment about a year later with most gratifying results. He is alive and well today. Judging from this case and others, it seems to me that after a period of many months some of the former reactivity of the tissue to radiation may return.

In case the initial radiation treatment was so inadequate that it did not exhaust the reactivity of the cancer bed, a second but thorough course of treatment has a good chance of some success, especially if the growth was quite radiosensitive at the start. A case like this fell in my hands about three years ago. She had been treated for carcinoma of the cervix in another city by a long series of interrupted X-ray and radium treatments. Because she was gradually getting worse she discontinued them. When she came to me she was losing weight rather rapidly, she had a copious foul-smelling discharge and was suffering much pain. Under a continuous intensive course of radiation therapy she rapidly improved. At her last visit a few months ago she seemed perfectly well and showed no evidence of a return of the trouble. This case well illustrates the contrast in effectiveness b e t w e e n repeated non-sterilizing irradiations and a continuous course of intensive therapy. Furthermore, one can hardly condemn too strongly the practice so commonly seen of physicians gambling with human life under a display of such inadequate knowledge.

Early in my work in radiation therapy I gained the impression that the intensity of the reaction produced was the main factor in determining the chances of a cure. Accordingly this i d e a has a c t u a t e d me throughout my whole period of therapy of cancer of the cervix. My first cases treated more than a decade ago followed in most respects the same general principles as used today. Even then the treatments were continuous and quite intensive and protracted over a period of four or five weeks. As I reviewed these old cases recently, I found I had attained some fairly gratifying r e s u l t s which I believe are worth reporting.

Prior to five years ago I had treated a total of 34 cases. Many of these were so far advanced that there was no hope except of some palliation. Out of this whole group two have since died of intercurrent d i s e a s e unrelated to their malignancy. They should not be considered in this statistical report. Of the remaining 32, 11 are still alive, one has been lost track of and the remainder have died of their malignancy. This figures to slightly over 34 per cent of five year cures for the entire group. I should, however, mention the fact that one of the 11 cases, treated almost ten years ago, has recently developed a carcinoma of the bladder which is thought to be primary there. Peculiarly, two of the cures are cervical stump (Group IV) cases, both of which were treated nearly 11 years ago. Only one Group IV case proved a failure. As might be expected the greater number of the c u r e s came from Group I cases where there were seven successes and one probable failure.

One should not attempt to draw any definite conclusions from this small series. As it stands, it compares favorably with the reports from many of the large cancer centers. In the light of more knowledge and experience one naturally entertains the hope that the future holds in store further progress toward the goal of success.

BIBLIOGRAPHY

1. Ward, George Gray, and Farrar, Lillian, K.P.: Eleven Year's Experience with the Radium Treatment of Carcinoma of the Cervix at the Woman's Hospital, Surg., Gynec. and Obst. 52:556, 1931.

2. Bonney et Al. Lancet 2:1000, 1166-1167, 1936.

3. Editorial, Am. J. Cancer 16:1246-1249, 1932.

4. Coutard, Henri: Roentgen Therapy of the Pelvis in the Treatment of Carcinoma of the Cervix. Am. J. Roentgenol. and Rad. Therapy, 36, 603-609, 1936.

Carcinoma of the Cervix and Breast*
Prognosis and Preferable Therapy

EDWARD D. GREENBERGER, M.D.
MCALESTER, OKLAHOMA

The average practitioner knows little as to what procedures the surgeon or radiologist performs in the treatment of these two types of carcinoma, comprising about 40 per cent of all cancers. The average practitioner usually is unable to give the patient or her family a proper prognosis of her condition either as to a five year cure or palliation of symptoms. The purpose of this paper is to give you a general outline of the preferable therapeutic procedures in the treatment of these two important types of carcinoma, and also to enable you to render a more correct prognosis to the patient and her family.

* * *

CARCINOMA OF THE CERVIX

The chief factor in determining the prognosis of this group of carcinomas is the extent of the local involvement, which is determined chiefly by clinical methods. A good classification of carcinoma of the cervix based on the extent of the lesions is offered by Dr. H. Schmitz of Chicago.

Group 1—Clearly localized carcinoma; beginning nodule.

Group 2—The doubtly localized carcinoma; beginning ulceration.

Group 3—Invading carcinoma; paracervical a n d parametrial involvement.

Group 4—Terminal carcinoma; f i x a t i o n of the uterus, generalized pelvic metastasis, distant metastasis.

	Approximate number of cases in each group	Percentage 5 year cures
Group 1	5-10%	70-95%
Group 2	10-25%	30-50%
Group 3	} 75%	10-20%
Group 4		None

The p a t i e n t who can be classified in group one and two should therefore be given a fairly good prognosis, if correct treatment is instituted. Patients in group three and four should be given a poor prognosis as to a five year cure.

*Presented before the Southeastern Oklahoma Medical Society at McAlester, Oklahoma, December 9, 1937.

The long controversy regarding the relative merits of surgical and radiation treatment in carcinoma of the cervix has been fairly well settled in the last few years. Surgery is excellent for patients who are definitely in group one. Radium accomplishes the same results. Patients falling into groups three and four are, of course, inoperable. It is often impossible to determine by bimanual examination whether a patient is in group two or three. Radiation has therefore supplanted surgery in the treatment of almost all cases of carcinoma of the cervix.

It has been repeatedly shown by statistical studies and post-irradiation pathological studies of the cervix, that large cervical cancers can be completely destroyed by adequate radium therapy applied by any of the several methods. The problem therefore in the treatment of 75 per cent of all patients with cancer of the cervix (groups three and four), is to destroy the cancer cells outside the range of the radium action, i.e., the cancer cells in the parametrium or other pelvic organs. Deep X-ray applied externally to the pelvis combined with radium in and around the cervix is the best approach to this problem today. A patient in group three who has not been treated by the combination of X-ray and radium, has not received sufficient irradiation and therefore has been inadequately treated. The five year cures in the future will increase according to our ability to deliver lethal doses of X-ray to the cancer cells w i t h i n the parametrium and pelvis.

GENERAL METHODS OF IRRADIATION

There are two schools on the preferable sequence of X-ray and radium irradiation:

1. X-ray series is given before the radium therapy and often again about two months after the radium treatment.

2. Radium therapy f i r s t, then X-ray about four to six weeks later.

The first procedure is used if there is some pelvic infection present. It is preferable in group three and four cases. The second procedure is preferable in group one and two and borderline group three cases.

RADIUM

There are two major types of technique of radium therapy to carcinoma of the cervix:

1. Large massive doses of radium given a few to 24 hours in one to several treatments.

2. The F r e n c h or Regaurd technique whereby small doses of radium are given continuously from four to seven days. The principle of this technique is to irradiate the different cells during their mitotic stage.

The Regaurd technique was recommended by the Radium Society this past year, because fistulas, bowel adhesion and obstruction rarely occurred by this protracted irradiation. The Regaurd technique is the one I therefore use. Also, because I have but 50 Mg. of radium. The total dose, with the different techniques, varies from 2,000 to 4,000 mg/hr. around the cervix and 3,000 to 6,000 mg/hr. within the uterus. The dose depends on the extent of the carcinoma, size of the uterus, amount of radium used, type of filter, and whether it is given in massive or protracted doses. The distribution of the radium needles or tubes is likewise very important not only as to correct dosage but as to proper treatment. When radium therapy is given by means of tandem in the uterus for about 3,000 mg/hr., seven to 15 skin doses reach the serosa two cm. away, four to seven skin doses affect the parametrium and paracervical lesion three cm. away, and only one to four skin doses five cm. away. (Approximately 10 skin doses is required to destroy a squamous cell carcinoma.) But, when radium is applied around the cervix for 2,000 mg/hr. by means of a colpostat, combined with the uterine tandem in the above dose, 25 skin doses is given around the cervix, seven to 15 skin doses four cm. distant around lower half of the uterus, and one to five skin doses reaches the lateral pelvic wall[1].

X-RAY

X-ray irradiation in carcinoma of the cervix, and breast, is administered according to the protracted fractional method as advocated by Coutard; i.e., 150-200 r units to a portal every other day over a period of two to four weeks for a total of 1,200 to 2,500 r per portal. Usually, three to six portals are used in irradiating the pelvis. Only 30 to 40 per cent of dose delivered to the skin, actually reaches the tumor 10 cm. within the pelvis. By the use of multiple ports and cross-firing, a large dose can be delivered to the cancer growth within the pelvis.

* * *

II   CARCINOMA OF THE BREAST

The numerous available statistics on the five year cures of cancer of the breast, treated by surgery alone, show a range from 15 to 52 per cent, or an average of 28 per cent cures. Such wide variations of percentage cures indicates that these excellent surgeons operated on patients in different c l i n i c a l stages of the disease. When the operated cases are divided into two main groups: (1) carcinoma localized in the breast, and (2) extension of the cancer into the axilla, then a more correct evaluation of surgical procedures is obtained. The percentage of cures now varies from 50 to 80 per cent in the first group and 15 to 25 per cent in the s e c o n d group. A proper classification of breast cancers is therefore necessary for a more c o r r e c t prognosis and to better evaluate various therapeutic procedures. The classification offered by Doctor Portmann of the Cleveland Clinic, I believe is very practical for this purpose[2].

Group 1—(a) Tumor localized to the breast and movable.
   (b) Skin not involved.
   (c) Metastasis not present in the axillary lymph glands.

Group 2—(a) Tumor localized to the breast and moveable.
   (b) Skin not affected (or only slightly edematous or ulcerated).
   (c) Metastasis p r e s e n t in the axillary lymph glands but only few are involved.

Group 3—(a) Tumor diffusely involving the breast.
   (b) Skin involved (edematous ulcerated), multiple nodules.
   (c) Metastasis to n u m e r o u s axillary glands, supraclavicular glands, distant metastasis.

In more than half of the cases, axillary

metastasis cannot be palpated. Groups one and two in the above classification therefore often cannot be differentiated without a pathological examination of the axillary contents. Only 50 per cent of all cases operated at the Cleveland Clinic were in groups one and two.

The patient that is definitely in group one is almost entirely a surgical problem, and the results, as stated, are very good. Radiation assumes a very minor role in these cases. Most of the deaths in this group are due to spread of the cancer cell to the lungs and abdomen through the back door before the mastectomy was performed.

The patients in group three are essentially a radiological problem. Palliation, cessation of growth and destruction of the glands and tumor, and often an attempt to make an inoperable case an operable one, are the objectives of radiation. Not one patient in this group who was operated at the Cleveland Clinic, survived five years without obvious evidence of the disease. It seems, from their statistics, that surgery actually does harm in these cases and shortens the life of the patient.

The evaluation of the correct therapeutic procedures in group two and borderline group three cases has been the big problem to the surgeon. Does irradiation increase his percentage of five year cures? Is irradiation of more value when given pre- or post-operatively, or when combined? Many of the statistical reports in the past comparing the results of surgery alone and surgery plus irradiation are not of true value, for these authors did not classify their cases in groups two or three. Also, many of these writers were unfamiliar with radiological procedures and could not correctly state how, when, and why irradiation was administered. Many of the patients were inoperable to start with and post-operative irradiation, of course, was given a black eye in these cases.

As mentioned above, the percentage five year cures by surgery alone in group two and borderline group three cases are very melancholy, about one in six surviving. The statistics in this same group when treated with surgery plus adequate post-operative irradiation show: (1) an increase

in the five year cures varying from five to 25 per cent as compared to surgery alone; (2) a drop of local recurrences varying from five to 25 per cent to a minute fraction or no recurrences.

Surgery plus proper post-operative irradiation produces better results in group two than surgery alone, but the results still are poor. An attempt to improve the number of cures in this group has stimulated the surgeon and radiologist to try preoperative irradiation. Small series of cases now being reported throughout the country are very encouraging and indicate that we are on the right track in the treatment of this group of cases.

Dr. F. Adair[3], of Memorial Hospital in New York City, has recently published an excellent paper on the value of pre-operative irradiation, employing doses of 1,800 to 2,400 r to each of three or four portals. The diagnosis in each case was proven by punch biopsy. Radical operation was performed six to eight weeks after irradiation was completed. In 70 per cent of his cases, there was a very definite shrinkage of the tumor mass. In 23 per cent of the cases, no evidence of carcinoma cells could be found on microscopic examination of the resected breast. This and other similar studies prove that irradiation alone can cure completely a certain percentage of breast cancers. This should convince many of the skeptical surgeons that X-ray is of definite value when applied properly.

Pre-operative irradiation has been belittled by many, because histological studies have shown that the majority of breast tumors are adeno-carcinoma, which are resistant to moderate doses of X-ray. But, Ewing, Cutler, and others have repeatedly shown that many sections in such tumors show very anaplastic cells, which are extremely responsive to moderate doses of X-ray. Again, most of these anaplastic cells are at the periphery of the breast tumor, where the blood supply is best, and therefore are readily destroyed by X-ray.

Pre-operative X-ray irradiation is therefore indicated: (1) to destroy the more sensitive cancer cells, (2) to confine the field of the cancer growth, and (3) to prevent surgical transplantation.

Pre-operative irradiation has been used for a long time in other types of cancer, as kidney tumors, cancer of the body of the uterus, cervical metastatic n o d e s, bone tumors, etc. Many surgeons object to pre-operative irradiation because of the delay in operation from four to eight weeks. But as Dr. Bloodgood once said, "The moment the X-ray begins, the moment the danger of spread ends."

GENERAL METHODS OF IRRADIATION

The C o u t a r d technique as described under carcinoma of the cervix is used in the pre- and post-operative techniques.

The pre-operative irradiation is administered: (1) a c c o r d i n g to technique of Adair, as mentioned above, i.e., 1,800 to 2,000 r, operation two months later, (2) according to the technique of Phahler, Merrit, Christie, etc., employing a moderate dose, 900 to 1,200 r to three or four portals, operate two weeks later and further irradiation given three to six weeks after operation.

Radium packs to the chest has been used in larger clinics in place of the X-ray, but the method is impractical and the results are inferior to X-ray.

In patients under 35 years of age, sterilization by irradiation or surgery is recommended.

* * *

CONCLUSION

(1) Classifications of carcinoma of the cervix and breast, based on the clinical extent of these diseases, have been presented. The statistics on the five year cures of these cases in their respective groups were presented in order to emphasize the importance of grouping or classifying a patient, if a proper diagnosis is to be reached and the proper therapeutic procedure evaluated.

(2) Patients in g r o u p two and three with carcinoma of the c e r v i x are best t r e a t e d by the combination of radium therapy in and around the cervix and deep X-ray externally.

(3) In the treatment of carcinoma of the breast, group three cases should be carefully differentiated from group two; operation is to be avoided in the definite group three cases. The percentage five year cures by surgery alone in group two and borderline group three cases has been shown to be poor. Post-operative irradiation increases the percentage somewhat but the results still are unsatisfactory. Pre-operative irradiation in these groups of cases appears today to offer the greatest percentage of cures, which, I feel, will be verified in the next five year statistics.

REFERENCES

1. Distribution of Radiation Within the Average Female Pelvis for Different Methods of Applying Radium to the Cervix. A. N. Arneson, Journal of Radiology, July, 1936.
2. Classification of Mammary Carcinoma. W. V. Portmann, Journal of Radiology, October, 1937.
3. Effect of Pre-operative Irradiation in Primary Operable Cancer of the Breast. Dr. F. Adair. Journal of Roentgenology and Radium Therapy, March, 1936.

Cardio-Vascular Syphilis*

F. REDDING HOOD, M.D.
OKLAHOMA CITY, OKLAHOMA

In the discussion of a d i s e a s e entity there seems to be three questions that need answering. How can the disease be prevented? If it occurs how can it be recognized? And when recognized what can we do about it?

*Read before the Section on Genito-Urinary Diseases and Syphilology, Annual Meeting, Oklahoma State Medical Association, Tulsa, Oklahoma, May, 1937.

Cardio-vascular syphilis is here taken to mean the invasion of the structures of the cardio-vascular system w i t h Treponema Pallida and the physiological-pathological changes that follow such invasion or as a result of an invasion elsewhere in the body with secondary c h a n g e s in the cardio-vascular system. When there is an invasion into the human body with this organism and it becomes generalized it is reasonable to a s s u m e that along with the other organs that the heart and blood vessels are involved. It is then that cardiovascular syphilis begins. For the sake of brevity and clarity let us divide the invasion into that of involvement of the myocardium and the aorta.

It has long been considered that myocardial involvement was quite rare, but the organisms have been found at post mortem examinations in young individuals with acquired syphilis without signs of cardio-vascular disease who died from other causes. Worthen and others contend that this invasion is a more common cause of heart failure than coronary or rheumatic heart disease. He demonstrates Treponema Pallida in almost all of his cases. There is another school who believe that the myocardial damage is due to interference with coronary circulation as a result of the involvement of the ostia of the coronary vessels as part of the pathological changes in the aorta. Both sides base their conclusions on the finding of fibroid and hyline scars on post mortem examinations. To one it means fibroblastic proliferation and scar formation as in any other syphlitic lesion and to the other myocardial infarction with necrosis, and s c a r formation. They are both probably right but the fact remains that myocardial damage does occur, that the process begins early and gradually progresses for many years without clinical manifestation.

There is an acute spyhilitic myocarditis that may occur at any time from one day to 40 years following the initial invasion. It may result in sudden death or it may start out as a severe attack and continue to grow worse. It is manifested clinically by marked dyspnea, cynosis, precardial distress and dilation of the heart and pathologically by yellow to gray areas, which are distinguished from infarcts by the presence of lymphocytes, plasma cells and interstitial edema.

Gummas do occur in the heart and are usually located in the upper posterior part of the intraventricular septum and hence interfere with the conduction apparatus, producing partial or complete a-v block, bundle branch block, Stokes Adams syndrome, or may similate a myocardial infarction of the posterior basal type.

In early syphilis the aorta is probably always involved. This simple aortitis begins at the commencement of the aorta and extends upward. This is influenced by the rich network of the lymphatics, and as they become less marked so does the degree of pathological changes due to spyhilis and so we find our most marked change in the ascending aorta, the arch, and the first part of the descending aorta and in that order. The invasion of the aorta is followed by healing and scar formation as in any other syphilitic lesion and results, in late syphilis, in the a o r t a becoming nodular or ridged, a sort of longitudinal folds, with a dilatation of the aorta. The pathological changes of simple aortitis do not produce symptoms, but the condition is apt to progress into aortic insufficiency or aortic aneurysm or both.

When the valve becomes involved it is the free edge which undergoes a proliferative valvulitis, this in turn is replaced by fibrous tissue which then contracts shortening the cusps and become incompetent. Adhesions do not occur and so the cusps do not adhere together to produce stenosis. However as the aortic ring dilates and the cusp margins being shortened by fibrous tisue are made taut a triangular opening is formed which is relatively stenotic and the blood flow past these taut crisp edges may produce sounds which heretofore were explained on a basis of a roughened aorta or stenotic valve which could not be demonstrated at post mortem.

If the pathological p r o c e s s of simple syphilitic aortitis should involve the media of the vessel with a resultant loss of the elastic tissue then aneurysm will result.

The most important factor in regards to the pathological changes is the time required for these processes to take place. It is one of the unsolved problems of medicine, why an organism remains in a tissue for 20 or more years with gradual progressive changes and produces no symptoms, and then suddenly causes great damage. That is the story of cardio-vascular syphilis. An indiscreet youth today contracts primary syphilis, today begins cardio-vascular syphilis and if he is an average individual, between 20 and 25 years from now his cardio-vascular syphilis will be recognized and then as an average individual he will have two y e a r s to live. Needless to say the prevention of these manifestations is the recognization a n d cure of early syphilis.

Now to the second question. If the disease is not prevented how may it be recognized, and more important still how can it be recognized early in order that the grave consequences may be avoided? If we investigate the text books we find that we can divide the symptoms into three groups. Those that result from aortic valve disease with strain and cardiac failure. Those resulting from narrowing or closure of the mouths of the coronary arteries to cause myocardial infarction or angina pectoris. And those resulting from pressure from an aneurysm. These are all late, so late that when found the battle is almost over, hope almost gone. And even with these symptoms, signs may be entirely absent. One might write a .thesis on these symptoms and their use in the diagnosis and differential diagnosis of these late manifestations of cardio-vascular syphilis but our problem is early diagnosis. Most patients who come to late cardio-vascular syphilis will give a history of having had earlier, maybe years earlier, two outstanding symptoms.

It is on these two symptoms that we base our hopes for early recognition of this serious condition. It is true that these two symptoms occur together, or separately in many other conditions and that a diagnosis of cardio-vascular syphilis cannot be made with them alone but in any patient of any age in which they occur one should investigate the possibility of early syphilis. These two symptoms are disturbances of respiration and substernal distress.

The dyspnea may occur in any form or to most any degree. It may be expressed as a shortness of breath which occurs following ordinary e x e r c i s e. This is the earliest sign of myocardial weakness from any cause and hence may attract attention to the heart and then be dismissed as functional, psychic, neuro-circulatory asthemia because no other evidence can be found to support it. But more often it takes on the form of a paroxysmal nocturnal dyspnea, waking the patient from sound sleep, last-

ing for 20 to 30 minutes, may gradually subside but most often passes away suddenly. It is usually accompanied by fear of death and profuse sweating, and leaves the patient in a state of exhaustion. One patient may complain that only the top of the lungs can be used for breathing, another that it is difficult to e x p a n d the lungs, another of sighing, but almost all patients that come to late syphilis with cardio-vascular pathology will give a history of some disturbance of the respiratory mechanism.

This disturbance i s n o t accompanied with pain as a rule, but about the time that it began the patient began to notice a substernal distress which may be expressed as a tightness in the upper chest, a band like constriction of the chest, a dull ache, or actual pain. It may be anginal in type, occuring in response to effort. It may occur at rest. May be spasmodic or continuous. May or may not r a d i a t e. Probably the most common history is that of a continuous aching pain or distress occuring under the upper half of the sternum, or in the back, radiating to the shoulders and arms and occuring without relationship to effort.

The one important thing is that any disturbance with respiration, associated with any discomfort of the upper chest in which there is any doubt as to the diagnosis should be investigated for early syphilis. The battle against late syphilis with its cardio-vascular manifestations can be won only by d i a g n o s i s and cure of early syphilis.

There are two schools of thought in regards to s p e c i f i c treatment of cardiovascular syphilis. One group believes that arsenicals should never be used and the heavy metals but rarely as they are afraid of the too rapid destruction of the organisms with resolution of the inflammatory tissue with a resultant accident. The other believes in pushing the treatment in hopes of stopping the invasion. The more logical method is that in between as advocated by Stokes and others.

In treating cardio-vascular syphilis we must remember that we are dealing with a patient who has structural damage due to invasion with a foreign organism and that that damage will continue until the invasion is conquered. We must also realize that this damage has brought about certain disturbances of function that will continue because of irreparable structural damage unless treated. We must therefore t r e a t both conditions concurrently and according to indications as they arise.

The effect of the arsenicals on the heart is that of vagus stimulation or interference w i t h the controlling mechanism of the heart and on the heart muscle itself interfering with muscle conduction and resulting in tachycardia or fibrillation, particularly of the ventricles. These reactions can be avoided by pre-courses of heavy metals and by guarded doses. In those cases presenting high grade myocardial damage, anginal attacks, those similating coronary occlusion with infarction and in the very old, arsenicals should not be used. In cases of hypertension or with renal insufficiency the arsenicals will be better

tolerated than the heavy metals and in these the iodides deserve a high and intangible place. In those patients in which the arsphenamine can be used will have a longer life expectancy than those in which the heavy metals are used alone.

One observes in many cardio-vascular patients that p r o p e r response to usual treatment is not reached until anti-leutic treatment is instigated, while syphilitic patients will need rest and digatilis in myocardial failure, nitrites and the theophyllum compounds in anginal attacks, morphine and oxygen in coronary accidents, diuretics and other cardio-vascular drugs when indicated.

I would like to conclude with the warning and statement by Stokes, that "The high points of syphilis of the cardio-vascular system may be touched with three words: ubiquitous, insidious, disastrous."

---o---

Congenital Deformities of the Mouth and Face*

GEORGE H. KIMBALL, M.D., F.A.C.S.
OKLAHOMA CITY, OKLAHOMA

For the past 10 years I have been interested in the examination and treatment of cases presenting various types of congenital deformities of the face and mouth.

As a medical student my curiosity was directed toward this subject by hearing it said that few men cared to operate these cases, and the fact that most men preferred not to do them at all. The hazards encountered apparently discouraged a great many surgeons from attempting this kind of work.

Congenital deformities and mal-formations of the mouth have occurred in the human race since time immemorial. Smith and Dawson in their work entitled "Egyptian Mummies" reported the finding of only one case of cleft palate and one case of club foot. Hippocrates does not mention either hare-lip or cleft palate in his writings. Celsus mentioned operations on

lips, but probably referred to mutilated lips rather than the c o n g e n i t a l type. Antyllos, a pioneer plastic surgeon of an-

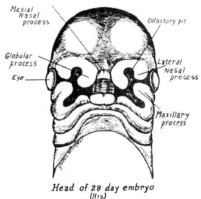

Head of 28 day embryo
(His)

FIGURE I

Shows the potential non-union which occurs in every case about the mouth and face.

*Read before the Section on Surgery, Annual Meeting, Oklahoma State Medical Association, Tulsa, May, 1937.

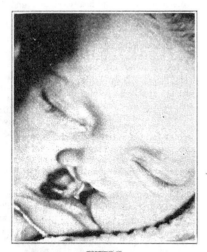

FIGURE II

A rather large angioma of the upper lip associated with a complete cleft of the lip and palate.·· (The angioma was treated by Lain-Eastland clinic.)

cient times described operations for defects a b o u t the nose, ears, eyelids, and cheeks. Galen mentioned cleft lip and a method of repair. In 1500 Pierre Franco, a contemporary of Pare wrote about con- .genital split lip. Pare himself, the cele- brated F r e n c h surgeon, introduced the term (bec-de-lievre) or hare-lip.

Le Monnier in 1776 is said to have suc- cessfully operated and closed a cleft palate. In 1861 von Graefe, the founder of modern plastic surgery introduced to the profes- sion the first comprehensive s u r g i c a l method in closing clefts of the palate. In Europe, Diffenback and Roux, Stevens and Warren in America contributed to the ad- vances in this field of surgery. Ferguson, von Langenback, and Wolff were pioneers in this field and so in this field of surgery as in other fields we find gradual improve- ment in methods so that today the work is fairly well standardized.

ETIOLOGY: In the past we have been con- tent to say that there is no causative fac- tor known. A great many theories have been offered such as the position of the t o n g u e, systemic disease, malnutrition, maternal impression, etc. Recently (1932- 1935) Fred Hale of Texas A.&M. has pro-

duced a great variety of congenital de- formities in pigs by reducing the Vitamin A content in the diet before gestation and ap- proximately a month after gestation. He was able to deplete the Vitamen A element in the diet in 160 to 190 days before the birth of the litter to a very low point, and then to withhold Vitamin A for approxi- mately a month after the birth of the pigs. These litters were found to be born prin- cipally without eyes. Associated anomalies were hare-lips, cleft palates, sub-cutaneous c y s t s, misplaced kidneys, and accessory ears. This work then is the first definite experimental evidence that we have in the production of congenital anomalies from the maternal diet standpoint. (Maternal Vitamen A deficiency.)

EMBRYOLOGY: The embryo at a very ear- ly period does not have fusion of all parts which make up the face and mouth. Hence all embryos have a potential condition for

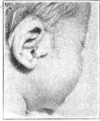

FIGURE III

Enlarged accessory ear in a new born.

development o f non-union. Hence everyone is a po- tential subject.

H E R E D I T Y: In about 50 per cent of the cases we f i n d that other members of the family either on t h e father's or the mother's side have some defect of mouth or face.

RACE: The negro race is particularly free from these congenital deformities of the face.

CLASSIFICATION OF DEFORMITIES

In 1,000 consecutive cases reported by Davis there were 948 which had a harelip or cleft palate or a combination of the two conditions. The other combinations in- cluded in this series are namely:

Rudimentary mandible.
Micro-glossia.
Atresia of nares-anterior.
Atresia of choanae.
Absence of naso-lacrimal ducts.
Colobomas extending into facial clefts.
Mucous pits in lower lips.
Hemangiomas of lip.

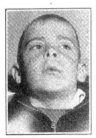

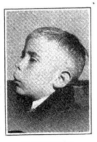

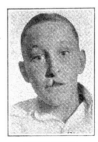

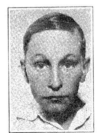

FIGURE IV (A)
AP view of lymphoma in a boy of 6. This had been operated twice. The treatment is radiation sometimes followed up by surgery.

FIGURE IV (B)
Lateral view, same case.

FIGURE VI (A)
Incomplete hare-lip in a boy of 13. Stopped school because of ridicule by associates.

FIGURE VI (B)
Final result following plastic surgery.

Hemangiomas of cheek.

Lymphangiomas of lip.

Dermoid cysts of dorsum nares.

Meningocele.

Microtia and atresia of exterior auditory canal.

Macrotia.

Ethmocephalus and cyclopia.

Ethmocephalus and anophthalmia.

Anophthalmia and atresia of choanae.

Hemi-cephalus, median.

Cleft lip, rudimentary nasal bones.

Temporomandibular fibrous ankylosis with incomplete fusion of mandibular and maxillary gingival margins.

So one can see that the surgical correction of the harelip and palate makes up the major problem in this series.

TIME OF OPERATION

I should like to say first that these cases are not emergency in nature. All of them must be thoroughly studied and adequately prepared before operation is performed. Since the new-born child does not stand surgery well, it is my opinion that it is best to wait until the child is at least three to six months of age before the lip is operated on. Also the child must be on the upgrade. He must be making a daily gain in weight. He must be free of all infections and he must be surgically a good risk.

The cleft palate is best repaired between the age of 18 months or two years on up to four or even six years of age.

CONTRA INDICATIONS TO OPERATION

1. Mal-nutrition.

2. Anemia.

3. Infection, such as in ears, tonsils, or impetigo.

4. Any cardiac condition which will not permit general anesthesia.

5. An associated mal-formation or defect such as hydrocephalus, mental insufficiency, mental retardation.

6. Prolonged coagulation time.

The pediatrician is our best friend in aiding us to thoroughly prepare the child. One cannot appreciate the value of a well-trained man in this work until he has experienced his help.

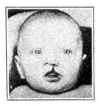

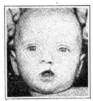

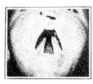

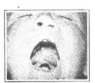

FIGURE V (A)
Incomplete uni-lateral hare-lip.

FIGURE V (B)
Two weeks post-operative.

FIGURE VII (A)
Complete cleft of palate, pre-operative view.

FIGURE VII (B)
Post-operative view. One operation.

TYPES OF OPERATION

A. *Harelip*: Most harelip operations to-day are modifications of various contributions made by pioneers in this work. I believe the modified Mirault plan gives uniformly the best results in harelip operations. This operation allows a result that is functionally perfect; and from an appearance standpoint, the lip has normal contour, normal thickness, and mobility.

B. *Cleft Palate*: Most palates can be successfully c l o s e d by a modified Von Langenbeck operation. Modifications are used as suggested by Blair, Burdick, and Dorrance. In the extremely wide clefts it has been f o u n d advisable to operate in stages. This avoids the excessive sloughs that will be encountered if too much is done at once. The "push back" operation as outlined by Dorrance is quite valuable in the so-called congenital insufficiency c a s e s. B r o w n has recently used the modified "push back" operation for the congenitally short, as well as the short immobile palates which followed surgery. Speech has been improved in these cases.

PRINCIPLES OF OPERATION

Lip

1. C o m p l e t e anesthesia, preferably ether so that the anesthetic may be deepened or lightened and if necessary completely withdrawn.
2. Land marks should be placed before incisions are made.
3. Complete mobilization of lip.
4. Denudation of the margins of the cleft enough to allow the muscles to be united.
5. Reconstruction of the floor of the nose so as to prevent deformity of the nostril.
6. Careful skin closure so as to secure the minimum of scar.
7. Closure of mucous membrane in such a way as to obtain thickness of the lip.
8. Splint (Logan Bow).

Palate

1. C o m p l e t e anesthesia, preferably ether.
2. Mobilization of flaps.
3. Preservation of blood supply.
4. Complete hemostasis.

5. Freshening of the medial borders of the cleft with relaxation.
6. Careful suture of the flaps without tension.

POST-OPERATIVE CARE

Lip: Frequent cleansing adds much to the final result. The arms must be restrained. If infection develops early drainage should be established. Sedatives are indicated for a few days, feedings are continued as soon as tolerated.

Palate: Some sedation is helpful, arms are restrained, packs are removed at the end of 24 hours. Repacking is necessary in case of hemorrhage. The suture line is perhaps best kept clean by peroxide and saline. The child is given liquids for about 10 days.

As a rule the lip is operated first and thus pressure is brought to bear on the cleft palate. Occasionally in adults the palate is done first for the reason that there is more room to work, the lip being done separately.

CONCLUSIONS

These cases present an interesting study, both from the standpoint of etiology and as to their repair. The operative technique is fairly well standardized.

One should remember that *none of these operations are emergency in nature*. They should n e v e r be done until the case is thoroughly studied and carefully prepared.

BIBLIOGRAPHY

1. "Relation of Vitamin 'A' to Anophthalmos in Pigs," by Fred Hale. American Journal of Ophthalmology, Vol. 18, 1935.
2. "Congenital Deformities of Face," by Warren B. Davis, M.D., S. G. & O., August, 1935.
3. "The Operative Story of Cleft Palate." 1933 by George Morris Dorrance.
4. "Elongation of Partially Cleft Palate," by James Barrett Brown, M.D., S. G. & O., December, 1936.
5. "Congenital Deformities of Mouth and Face," by Dr. Curt Von Wedel, Journal of the Oklahoma Medical Association 15:46, 1922.
6. "Mirault's Operation for Single Harelip," by Vilray P. Blair and J. B. Brown, M.D., S. G. & O., 51-81-1930.

* * *

DISCUSSION

Dr. John F. Burton, Oklahoma City: I rather hesitate to discuss this subject because it has been so w e l l presented. I think this type of work is really highly specialized. There are three points I would like to stress. First, this type of operation is not an emergency; it is elective. Second, the patient should be amply prepared before operation. Third, the work should be done by someone who is doing this line of work rather often.

About 50 per cent of the work we are now doing is re-doing cases that have been done elsewhere. I think that fact should be given rather serious thought.

I think that Dr. Kimball has prepared a very interesting paper on a common condition that we see throughout the state. Unfortunately, people are not in a position to pay for the work and for that reason it is quite often neglected.

----------0----------

Common Diseases of the Nails

JOHN HENDERSON LAMB, M.D.
OKLAHOMA CITY, OKLAHOMA

Due to the great frequency of nail disturbances the diseases of the nails have become of interest in all fields of medicine today. White[1] has given a fine summary of various nail conditions seen in dermatological p r a c t i c e. Pardo-Castello[2] has edited a new book on the subject. Still many of us are at a loss when presented with nail conditions as to whether the disease is local or constitutional.

A review of the anatomy of the normal nail must be made before a study of the disease processes is understood. The nails are similar to the epidermis in that they are formed by keratotic cells which retain fragments of their nuclei and are closely adherent. The nail substance is very similar to keratin and serves as a protection to the extremities of the toes and fingers.

The nail proper or nail plate may be divided into a distal portion which is smooth, shiny and pinkish in color, and the lanula or proximal end. The nail rests upon a layer of cuboidal b a s a l cells called the matrix. It is the productive part of the nail and the cells grow distally, becoming cornified. The matrix can be seen through the proximal portion of the nail plate or the white, crescentic lanula. The nail bed lying under the nail plate is composed of an epithelial layer of cells similar to the matrix with which it is continuous. It does not take part in production of the nail plate, but plays a role in the nail nutrition. The nail plate and the nail bed apparently grow together from the matrix outward.

INFECTIONS OF THE NAIL

The first nail diseases to be discussed are those disturbances of the nails which are caused by infectious organisms which include the Staphylococcus and ringworm organisms. The most common of these is that discussed under the title of onychomycosis or ringworm of the nails. Pardo-Castello states that 18 per cent of all nail disturbances belong in this group.

Fungus diseases are becoming more common due to the popularity of the modern age for every kind of sport which has seemed to increase the amount of ringworm of the feet and b o d y, and consequently of the nails. The nail is a common foci of infection and many times although the skin of the fingers and feet may be cleared of the infection the nails still harbor the vegetable parasite.

The ringworm organisms found to cause these infections are usually the dermatophytes, the yeast-like group of fungus or the monilia, sometimes the true yeasts or baker's yeasts, and in a limited number of cases favus has been cultured.

Pencillium and aspergillus h a v e also been found to produce nail lesions.

The disease caused by the dermatophyte is characterized by first a slight scaling of the nail surface and is usually always dry. It is accompanied only rarely by a slight paronychial infection. There is then further development to a worm-eaten malformation and finally presents a peculiar destruction affecting the entire thickness of the nail in striations resembling "split bamboo." The nail becomes brittle, discolored, grooved and pitted, while beneath the partially separated bed there is an accumulation of debris and horny material from which the organism usually can be found by microscopical examination in 15 to 20 per cent s o d i u m hydroxide. This preparation must soak one to two hours to dissolve the nail substances. Contrary to belief, heating the slide does not hasten the process and may destroy the mycelium. The infection in the finger nails starts sometimes without any intercurring cutaneous involvement but with toenail involvement an infection usually can be found on the surrounding skin.

The infection usually involves one nail only at first and then later it seems to spread to the other nails. E x c e p t for monilia there is practically no pain involved in ringworm of the nails. Monilia infections as a rule are accompanied by paronychia and the infection is more of an exudative type. Often the paronychia precedes nail i n v o l v e m e n t. Kingery[3] & Thiennes have reported an epidemic of paronychia (caused by monilia) accompanied by dermatitis of the hands due to handling fresh fruits. Sutherland Campbell[4] also report a similar epidemic among orange workers.

In treatment a valuable preparation is Whitfield's ointment of double strength applied by a stiff brush following curettement and cutting of the nail. Sometimes a valuable agent is chrysarobin powder made into a paste with lysol to be applied to the infected nail only, the skin surface surrounding the nail protected by some bland salve. Tincture of iodine and mercuric tincture (Metaphen and Merthiolate) have been useful as an application in some instances.

Use of the X-ray is e f f i c a c i o u s in all types of onychomycosis but it is of special value in monilia and yeast types of infection. Each nail is windowed off with lead and treated with separate exposures. Frequently surgical removal must be resorted to, although almost invariably there is a reinfection after removal.

Several authors have suggested that X-ray therapy following surgical removal be employed. Artificial nails can now be obtained for the more particular patients with malformed nails. These are sealed on the deformed nail, hiding all deformity.

Syphilis—Syphilitic involvement of the nails with atrophy or deformity has been noted by many observers, but there seems to be some question whether the atrophy is due to local disturbance caused by the spirochete, or whether the disturbances are due to lowered vitality generally, disturbing circulation and nutrition of the nail bed. Of course, chancres of the nail bed and periungual regions have been seen, especially in professional m e n. Stokes[5] states that changes in the nails are not particularly distinctive in syphilis.

Diagnosis of syphilis should be thought of, though, in nail dysfunctions associated with paronychia and dactylitis of the terminal phalanx.

Pardo-Castello describes two c a s e s of secondary lesions on the body with superficial onychia affecting the outer surface of the nails. White of Chicago states that he has yet to see one case of nail disturbance due locally to the spirocheta pallida.

Psoriasis—Although this skin disease is usually on the glaborous skin it can involve the nails. Most cases are associated with skin lesions but there are frequently cases in which the nails alone are infected. Pardo-Castello finds 15 per cent of previous cases presenting nail lesions. Diagnosis is usually made by punctiform depressions, irregular transverse grooves, a brownish discoloration, hypertrophy of the free margins with tendency to erosion and distal nail plate destruction with irregular crustaceous deposits. Some n a i l s with psoriasis may have only simple manifestations as dryness, loss of luster with fine desquamation. The nails should be scraped always and examination made for ringworm organisms. Cases of fungus infections of the nails of several years' duration in many instances have turned out to be psoriasis.

Treatment of the nails for psoriasis is very unsatisfactory and there is a temptation for over-treatment. A f e w X-ray treatments — two or three exposures of fractional doses windowed to each nail —

are worth a trial. Improvement may not take place until three to six weeks from the initial dose; otherwise, the therapy is the same in general as that of psoriasis of the skin. Strong keratolytic agents, chrysarobin in collodion five to 10 per cent have been recommended. Anthralin ointment has helped in one of our cases but it stains the nails a dark purple.

Eczema—In e c z e m a of the nails the m a t r i x and the p e r i u n g a l regions are attacked. C o m m o n l y known are nail changes due to occupational dermatoses and irritation from various irritants. R. Prosser White[6] in his textbook on "Occupational Diseases" gives a list of irritants to the nails and includes lime, plaster, caustic soda, etc. Cleveland White says "Cases have been observed in which there is no question of irritation of the nails due to nail polish and polish remover."

I have lately seen a dentist with squamous eczema of the hands and atrophic nails on the right hand with longitudinal ridges and undermining of the distal end; the cause is probably from medicines or chemicals used in dental work. Nail deformities are also seen in the so-called allergic eczemas. These apparently disappear as the dermatosis is cured. Chronic eczema of the feet of old people usually produces hypertrophied and d i s t o r t e d nails (onychogryphosis).

The clinical picture of eczema of the nails varies greatly. In occupational disturbances they may be s i m p l y stained yellowish-green or gray, or they may be completely destroyed. In most cases the adjacent skin is usually affected, being red and swollen, or dry and cracked with an eczematous paronychia.

The nails become malformed with irregular edges and depressions, the free margins cracked, thickened, everted and discolored. Sometimes longitudinal ridges are noted. Treatment is usually slow but successful. X-ray is the method of choice in the subacute and chronic stages. Change of occupation in many cases is necessary for complete cure.

Atrophy of the nails must a l w a y s be ruled out in diagnosis of nail disturbances. These conditions may be congenital or acquired; the atrophy is more often sym-metrical. Sometimes nail atrophy is associated with cases of alopecia areata. We see various other types such as paronychia, dryness and transverse line sometimes seen in lichen planus; leuconychia with white spots under the nail which is thought to be caused by the presence of air in the interstitial corneal spaces produced by local trauma or by p r e s e n c e of imperfectly cornified cells which causes the cells to l a c k cohesion. Ridging and furrowing with brittleness are noted in endocrine disturbances as myxedema, and where constitutional disorders are present. Tuberculosis has been found to p r o d u c e acute paronychia w i t h lymphangitis. One of the most common types is known as verruca necrogenica and has been contracted by autopsy attendants in careless handling of tuberculous material.

In chronic pulmonary tuberculosis the hippocratic nails are seen with clubbing of the fingers. The nails are enlarged and curve over the end of the finger as a cupulo.

We recently saw a severe arsphenamine dermatitis with high fever which caused a recession in the growth of the nail with transverse furrows across the nails, progresssing to undermining and nail destruction. The nail gradually grew distally as the patient recovered with new, well nail in its place.

Cleveland White has recognized nail disturbances due to lack of Vitamin B and D and improper usage of these vitamins. The n a i l s show transverse depressions with longitúdinal striations; in s e v e r e cases, nail destruction.

We have observed one case which we believed to be due to avitaminosis but were discouraged with the use of v i t a m i n therapy. We have not seen nail disturbances in our cases of pellagra.

Tumors and Trauma — Various tumors can occur around the nails as elsewhere in the body. Malignancies, keloids, angiomas, melanotic Whitlows develop from collections of nevus cells in the nail bed, xanthomas and warts. Warts around the nails should be treated conservatively. Electro-diathermic methods sometimes leave bad scarring. They respond well sometimes to X-ray therapy with bismuth injections and mercurial ointments.

Epithelioma may develop from the nail bed or the matrix. It is usually prickle cell in type and of malignant order. We have recorded no cases in our files.

CONCLUSION

1. Fungus diseases are the most common of nail disturbances.

2. Psoriasis, lichen planus and eczema sometimes attack the nail.

BIBLIOGRAPHY

1. White, Cleveland, Diseases of the Nails, Urologic and Cut. Review, August, 1936, Vol. 40:562-564.

2. Pardo-Castello, V., Diseases of the Nails. Charles C. Thomas, Publisher.

3. Kingery, L. B., and Thiennes, Mycotic Paronychia and Dermatitis, Arch. Dermat. & Syph., February, 1925, p. 186.

4. Sutherland-Campbell, Paronychia, An Attempt to Prove the Etiologic Factor in an Epidemic Among Orange Workers, Arch. Dermat. & Syph., February, 1929, p. 233.

5. Stokes, John H., Modern Clinical Syphilology.

6. White, R. Prosser, Occupational Diseases.

The School-Child's Breakfast

Many a child is scolded for dullness when he should be treated for undernourishment. In hundreds of homes a "continental" breakfast of a roll and coffee is the rule. If, day after day, a child breaks the night's fast of 12 hours on this scant fare, small wonder that he is listless, nervous, or stupid at school. A happy solution to the problem is Pablum, Mead's Cereal cooked and dried. Six times richer than fluid milk in calcium, ten times higher than spinach in iron, and abundant in vitamins B and G, Pablum furnishes protective factors especially needed by the school-child. The ease with which Pablum can be prepared enlists the mother's co-operation in serving a nutritious breakfast. This palatable cereal requires no further cooking and can be prepared simply by adding milk or water of any desired temperature. Its nutritional value is attested in studies by Crimm et al. who found that tuberculous children receiving supplements of Pablum showed greater weight-gain, greater increase in hemoglobin, and higher serum-calcium values than a control group fed farina.

Mead Johnson & Company, Evansville,. Indiana, will supply reprints on request of physicians.

Early Diagnosis Campaign

Next month, April, is the occasion of the nation-wide Early Diagnosis Campaign conducted by the tuberculosis associations of the United States. This is the 11th annual campaign. Wherever possible physicians should join in observance of this educational effort. Any sound program designed to better inform the public about disease is more than worth while; intelligent patients are the most satisfactory to manage.

It would be a good plan to feature a paper, or program, on tuberculosis at the county medical society session; physicians need to know more about its early diagnosis. With a better informed public they must be alert to meet the expectations of their patients.

The Oklahoma Tuberculosis and Health Association, 22 West Sixth street, Oklahoma City, has special literature for this campaign, and other up-to-date pamphlets and publications on tuberculosis; copies of these will be mailed anywhere on request.

Progress Report of Type Incidence of Pneumococcal Infections in Oklahoma.

This survey was started December 1, 1937. One hundred and forty-one registered hospitals, laboratories, sanatoriums and related institutions were contacted with 21 replies to date. Eleven institutions reported that they did no typing. We have records to date of 167 cases of pneumococcal infections, two of which on checking proved to be streptococcal pneumonia. In 74 cases the organisms were not typed. In 91 cases the types have been determined and are distributed as follows: Type I, 25 cases; Type II, 19 cases; Type III, 11 cases; Type IV, three cases; Type V, one case; Type VI, one case; Type VII, 18 cases; Type VIII, one case; Type IX, one case; Type XI, one case; Type XIV, two cases; Type XIX, two cases; Type XXI, two cases; Type XXII, two cases; Type XXXII, one case, and one case of mixed infection of Types I and II.

The Bacteriology Department has determined the type in 31 cases, the others are from sources throughout the state.

We appreciate greatly the cooperation which the various hospitals, laboratories, and individual physicians have given thus far, and trust we will eventually hear from all of them. In our final report the record from each institution will appear separately in order to give due credit to all concerned.

The money for this project has been supplied from the fund for medical research given to the University of Oklahoma School of Medicine by the last legislature. This problem should be of interest to everyone throughout Oklahoma since the State Department of Public Health informs us that pneumonia has ranked second as the cause of death in the state for the past ten years.

Signed: H. D. MOON, Prof. of Bact.

Protamine Zinc Insulin Squibb

Physicians will be interested to know that Protamine Zinc Insulin Squibb is now available in two strengths, 10 cc. vials of 40 units per cc. and 10 cc. vials of 80 units per cc.

Protamine Zinc Insulin has been available in the 40-unit strength since February 1, 1937. It was felt, however, that a higher potency was also needed for the many diabetics who require large amounts of Insulin daily.

While the efficiency of the two strengths of Protamine Zinc Insulin may be identical, the transfer of a patient from one strength to the other should be made only under the careful supervision of a physician until more experience has been accumulated.

Protamine Zinc Insulin Squibb is marketed under license from the Insulin Committee, University of Toronto.

Spring Medico-Military Symposium

March 28th and 29th brings to the doctors of the Southwest another banner program — the Spring Medico-Military Symposium will be presented by the Kansas City Southwest Clinical Society in conjunction with the medical officers of the Seventh Corps Area in Kansas City, Missouri.

Other than the army and navy representatives, guest speakers will include Dr. J. Albert Key, professor of clinical orthopedic surgery, Washington University, and Dr. Ovid O. Meyer, associate professor of medicine, University of Wisconsin.

The medical profession of the southwest is invited to attend this two-day meeting. There will not be a registration fee and complimentary luncheon will be served each day to the registrants.

THE JOURNAL
OF THE
Oklahoma State Medical Association

Issued Monthly at McAlester, Oklahoma, under direction of the Council.

Copyright, 1938, by Oklahoma State Medical Association, McAlester, Oklahoma.

| Vol. XXXI | MARCH, 1938 | Number 3 |

DR. L. S. WILLOUR..Editor-in-Chief
McAlester, Oklahoma

DR. T. H. McCARLEY..Associate Editor
McAlester, Oklahoma

Entered at the Post Office at McAlester, Oklahoma, as second-class matter under the act of March 3rd, 1879.

This is the official Journal of the Oklahoma State Medical Association. All communications should be addressed to The Journal of the Oklahoma State Medical Association, McAlester Clinic, McAlester, Oklahoma. $4.00 per year; 40c per copy.

The editorial department is not responsible for the opinions expressed in the original articles of contributors.

Reprints of original articles will be supplied at actual cost provided request for them is attached to manuscripts or made in sufficient time before publication.

Articles sent this Journal for publication and all those read at the annual meetings of the State Association are the sole property of this Journal. The Journal relies on each individual contributor's strict adherence to this well-known rule of medical journalism. In the event an article sent this Journal for publication is published before appearance in The Journal the manuscript will be returned to the writer.

Failure to receive The Journal should call for immediate notification of the Editor, McAlester Clinic, McAlester, Oklahoma.

Local news of possible interest to the medical profession, notes on removals, changes of addresses, births, deaths and weddings will be gratefully received.

Advertising of articles, drugs or compounds unapproved by the Council on Pharmacy of the A. M. A., will not be accepted.

Advertising rates will be supplied on application.

It is suggested that wherever possible members of the State Association should patronize our advertisers in preference to others as a matter of fair reciprocity.

Printed by News-Capital Company, McAlester.

EDITORIAL

WE MUST ASSIST

The American Medical Association has undertaken, through the State and County Societies, a survey to obtain information as to m e d i c a l needs and to formulate preferable procedures to supply these needs in accordance with established policies and local conditions.

A pamphlet has been distributed by the Bureau of Medical Economics of the American Medical Association and your officers have requested sufficient copies of these in order that one or two may be sent to the officers of each County Medical Society. This is the first time that organized medicine has assumed leadership in undertaking these studies and they must have the complete cooperation of the State and County Medical Societies in determining medical needs.

It will be well if each County Medical Society will have appointed a Committee on Economics and they will, by the means at their command, complete the survey in their respective counties; a report of the survey will be submitted to the Committee on Medical Economics of the State Association and they will compile a report for the American Medical·Association.

Organized Medicine has seen the threat of socialization and this can only be avoided by these matters being adjusted by the doctors themselves. This present plan will place in our hands not only the information required as to medical needs but we can formulate the plan to meet these needs.

Let us do our share to keep the practice of medicine in the hands of the medical profession and avoid bureaucratic control from Washington.

HOSPITALIZATION FOR THE VETERAN

The Veterans Administration hospitalizes Veterans on submission of an application form, of which one page is devoted entirely to the medical findings of the local examining physician. The only exception to this is in case of emergency in which event the Veteran may be admitted by authority over the telephone. Everyone is interested in securing hospitalization for those Veterans who are in need of such hospitalization and who, under the Veterans Administration regulations, are unable to pay for same.

On the Veterans Administration Form P-10 the local physician is asked to state briefly the history of the veteran's physical condition. This history should give, as closely as possible, the approximate time the veteran first became aware of the condition and accurate history of previous, similar attacks.

The second section of the physician's portion of the application p e r t a i n s to symptoms. This would include subjective findings—it being necessary that the veteran's word be taken for these conditions, and in this portion of the application many "gold brickers" can be eliminated.

The third section pertains to physical findings and of course include the active objective symptoms and laboratory findings. In this portion also is given the local physician's d i a g n o s i s and while these would undoubtedly have to be tentative they should be made as accurately as possible.

The Veterans Administration, American Legion, and all good citizens would like to find some means of eliminating hospitalization of veterans actually not in need of such treatment, and this can be accomplished to a greater or lesser degree, in proportion to the completeness of the examination and report made by the local physician.

The physicians of Oklahoma can and will be of the utmost assistance in culling the wheat from the chaff. We should play no favorites in any instance in recommendation for hospitalization as it is the taxpayer's money that is being spent and we, as taxpayers, should try our best to protect our own money.

The Veterans Administration, the American Legion, and the good citizens of Oklahoma feel that they have the cooperation of the medical profession of the State. If the local physicians know and can be made to realize the importance of these examinations, unnecessary hospitalization can be avoided.

"POLITICS"

During the last session of the Legislature Organized Medicine in Oklahoma had some experience with politics and we have been thoroughly convinced that it will be much easier to select officers who will support the program of organized medicine than to convert them to our way of thinking after they have been elected.

The above remark has been the text of many speakers before various meetings of doctors in this State and we hope they have elaborated upon the subject sufficiently so that each doctor believes that the above statement is correct and believes it so thoroughly that he will take an active interest in the selection of our state officers in the coming primary.

Candidates for office, from Governor down, are announcing and starting their campaign and this is the time when County Medical Societies should pay their debts to the Senators and Representatives who supported our program, and see to it that those who place themselves before the coming primary and who opposed our program during the last session of the Legislature are defeated.

We have been in politics, we owe political debts and these debts should receive our earnest consideration, the same as a financial obligation, and if we do not pay off, our credit will be destroyed.

There are candidates who have already announced for governor, who have done everything possible to wreck organized medicine in this state. All doctors are familiar with their attitude toward development of medicine in Oklahoma. There is no reason why we should not have a commitment of the candidates before the primary, in order that we may know how best we can protect the health of the people of our State, as well as elevate the standard of the practice of medicine.

Now is the time for us to think clearly, investigate the candidates thoroughly and after this not only vote intelligently, but use our influence to bring about the nomination and election of officers who can best serve the State, protect the Medical School, all other medical institutions and the health of our people.

IMPORTANT REPORT

Report of Cancer Committee of Oklahoma State Medical Association and S t a t e Executive Committee of Women's Field Army.

The Women's Field Army is an organization of the Federated Women's Clubs and doctors, under medical control, for the dissemination of factual information about cancer. The National Federated Women's Clubs and the American Society for the C o n t r o l of C a n c e r have formed the Women's Field Army, under the control of the latter. In Oklahoma its controlling body is the state executive committee of the Women's Field Army, composed of the state commander, Mrs. W. M. Van Divort of Nowata; the members of the cancer committee of the State Medical Association—Dr. Wendell Long of Oklahoma City, Dr. Paul Champlin of Enid, Dr. Ralph McGill of Tulsa; the state chairman for the American Society for the Control of Cancer, Dr. E. S. Lain of Oklahoma City; and the State Public Health Officer, Dr. C. M. Pearce.

The control of all lay medical educational efforts must rest in a medical majority in order to avoid the pitfalls incident to faulty lay interpretation of medical speakers and information. There is such control in this organization both nationally and in the state.

In Oklahoma this control rests not only with doctors but principally in the appointed representatives of the State Medical Association, rather than in the government agencies (public health departments) or a small group of doctors. It is a direct challenge to the doctors of this state to demonstrate that they are able to carry out a program of medical education for the public with satisfaction to both public and themselves.

The success of this movement in Oklahoma depends on following certain fundamental principles and the cooperation of every doctor of the State Medical Association.

ORGANIZATION

It is the general policy of your committee (State Executive Committee of Women's Field Army and Cancer Committee of State Medical Association) that each county medical society have control through its county cancer committee of all medical activities within its county. This holds even to support the withdrawal of the Women's Field Army from a county should the county medical society reject it.

A dual organization of State Federated Clubs and the State and County Medical Societies is a necessity to proper function.

There is an organization of the women under the able state commander, with a chairman for each of the nine districts and a county lieutenant for each county.

A cancer committee of three members must be appointed by each county medical society. In counties where this committee is not appointed, the secretary of the county society is now considered the chairman of that committee.

The COUNTY EXECUTIVE COMMITTEE is composed of four members, the county lieutenant of the Women's Field Army and three members of the county cancer committee. This committee will have the responsibility for all medical activities in its county.

A working plan for organization of county executive committees will be sent each county before the publication of this report.

SPEAKERS

All medical speeches *must* be by doctors.

Each county cancer committee will carefully form its own county speakers bureau from its own members.

The State Executive Committee has a tentative State Speakers Bureau of doctors selected by the Cancer Committee of the State Medical Association and the state chairman for the American Society for the Control of Cancer. Its members have reviewed the medical material to be used and the endorsed speakers policies.

Assignment of a speaker for each request from the women's organization *must* be made by the chairman of the county cancer committee. The only restriction upon the county in this assignment is that any speaker from outside the county *must* be chosen from the approved list of speakers of the State Executive Committee. A speaker outside the county can be obtained through the Oklahoma City office, Medical Arts Building, Oklahoma City, in charge of your committee's chairman.

There should be reasonable uniformity of medical information. The basis for every speech should rest on the approved material produced and furnished by the American Society for the Control of Cancer. It should be carefully reviewed by each speaker in order to obtain facts rather than opinions.

This material includes three film strips and projector, available to county cancer committees and members of the State Speakers Bureau by writing the Oklahoma City office. Each speaker on county and state speakers bureau will be supplied a "Speakers Compend" (general information). This medical material will be supplied *doctors only.*

Pamphlets for the public, also produced and supplied by the American Society for the Control of Cancer, will be given each person in each audience.

SPEAKERS' POLICIES

The success of the Women's Field Army in Oklahoma depends upon the highest ethical conduct of those who speak. They must remember that they represent the entire profession by their speech and conduct.

(1) The *family doctor* must be protected and considered basic in all such situations as requests for consultation, examination, and information about cancer specialists. The family doctor is best able to supply this information to his patients and if he does not feel he has sufficient information, he can easily obtain it.

(2) Information about treatment should be very general, emphasizing that only surgery, radium and X-ray are recognized, importance of avoiding all quacks, uninvestigated lay persons who advertise, etc.

(3) Giving only known facts and admitting when facts unknown.

(4) No discussion of theories.

(5) Use of as few technical terms as possible.

(6) Avoidance of expressing individual opinion, sticking to supplied film strips and facts in compend as closely as possible.

(7) Maintainance of high ethical conduct by all speakers.

WHY DOCTORS SHOULD SUPPORT WOMEN'S FIELD ARMY

(1) This organization is medically controlled and in Oklahoma control rests in representatives of the State Medical Association.

(2) Lay fear and cancerphobia is largely based on ignorance of facts and articles published by laymen. It can be best counteracted by factual medical information.

(3) The State Executive Committee of the Women's Field Army is making every e f f o r t to establish and maintain sound fundamental policies, which are essential.

(4) The women's organization will have an enlistment campaign in April or May

when each member enrolled will pay one dollar or more. Therefore, the women will pay for the supplies and organization and all we doctors will supply is the effort. (Incidentally, no member of the Women's Field Army in Oklahoma receives any salary for his or her work.)

(5) It is an opportunity to prove to the public that organized medicine can ably supply the necessary medical information they desire.

State Executive Committee of Women's Field Army	State Medical Association Cancer Committee	Wendell Long, Chm. Paul Champlin Ralph McGill Mrs. W. M. Van Divort E. S. Lain C. M. Pearce

---

THE GENERAL PLAN OF POST-GRADUATE INSTRUCTION
SPONSORED BY THE
OKLAHOMA STATE MEDICAL ASSOCIATION

THE INSTRUCTOR

Your state committee on post-graduate medical teaching of the Oklahoma State Medical Association was fortunate in securing the services of Dr. Edward N. Smith as instructor of our obstetrical program. The general outline of Dr. Smith's ten lectures and clinics is attached for your information.

This course of modern methods in obstetrics is being offered by giving one lecture of approximately one hour in length, followed by a clinic of one hour, making a total of two hours of instruction once a week for ten weeks (ordinarily, lectures will not be given on Saturdays or Sundays). It will require, as will be seen, two and a half months for the complete course in each of the centers. The course will be offered in county-seat towns or centers where physicians customarily m e e t for county medical meetings. This, however, is not always a necessary rule.

It is proposed to open the course in the cities in northeastern Oklahoma, and our field representative will, in the near future, be in your community to discuss the most logical centers with you. Between lectures, as far as his time for travel will permit, Dr. Smith will be available for free consultation with doctors registered in the course. He will also be available for talks before local civic clubs, P.T.A., and Women's Federation Clubs. You can readily see from this that physicians will have the advantage of discussing the theories advanced in the lectures over their cases in actual practice.

Many doctors appreciate this post-graduate instruction offered under this plan, and receive more direct benefit than if the course were presented on a larger plan. National meetings with national clinics do not give individual instruction afforded under the plan sponsored by our State Medical Association. This does not minimize the value of our national medical meetings, but we raise this point to emphasize the individual instruction to be received on a circuit plan of this type.

Some years ago, the Oklahoma medical profession was privileged to have many valuable courses presented on a circuit plan. That plan, of course, was abolished as most of you remember. In the past, when we sponsored this circuit medical and surgical post-graduate instruction, you recall that you were asked to pay a fee of from $30 to $35 for each course of some nine lectures, and no consultation privileges included. Under the present plan, the State Medical Association, with the financial assistance of the Commonwealth Fund and the State Health Department, is offering ten lectures giving the doctors consultation privileges with the instructor for the small fee of $5. As stated above, this is made possible by reason of funds your committee has assembled from endowment resources. We wish we could offer this course to you without even the minimum $5 fee, but the fee will be needed to assist in financing the general plans of this ten weeks' circuit in your local community.

QUALIFICATIONS OF MEDICAL INSTRUCTOR AND OUTLINE OF COURSE

Dr. Edward N. Smith has been selected by your committee as the medical instructor in the obstetrical program. Dr. Smith is highly qualified to handle this work. He is a graduate of Washington State College, and of the University of Pennsylvania School of Medicine. He has had an excellent background of experience including rotating internship, Camden, New Jersey, several residences in obstetrics and gynecology including Cornell Medical Center, New York City; Margaret Hague Maternity Hospital, Jersey City, New Jersey; Columbia Medical Center, Sloane Hospital; New York Post-Graduate Hospital, and is a diplomate of the American Board of Obstetrics and Gynecology. He is also the recipient of the Degree of Med. D. Sc. in Obstetrics and Gynecology, Columbia University.

In addition to Dr. Smith's very thorough post-graduate training in obstetrics, he did general practice in Livingston County, New York, for four years following his graduation, serving also as County Health Officer and secretary of the local medical society.

In view of his broad experience as a general practitioner and teacher, he is cognizant of their problems and particularly adapted for his present position.

Dr. Smith is very pleasing of personality, and has the ability of conveying his world of information to others in a manner easily understood.

The following is the tentative outline of the course which Dr. Smith will present:

1. Sterility and Fertility.
   Contraceptive and conceptive advice.
2. History and Examination.
   Pelvic measurement. Practical office, laboratory and instrumental aids.
3. Normal and abnormal pregnancy, by trimesters.
4. Normal labor and delivery.
5. Operative obstetrics.
6. Obstetrical emergencies and danger signs.
7. Dystocias. Breech, transverse and compound presentations. Elderly primigravida.
8. Normal and abnormal puerperium.
   Retroversion and pessaries. Lacerations.
9. Care of infant.
   Prematurity. Follow-up.
10. Medical and surgical complications.

Editorial Notes—Personal and General

· We recently received an announcement to the effect that the Medical Arts Laboratory of Oklahoma City had sold its assets to Dr. W. F. Keller, director and principal stock-holder. This change was made to conform to the requirements of the Oklahoma Basic Science Law.

The Profession has always considered this laboratory and Dr. Keller as synonymous, and we are glad to hear that he is now sole owner.

DR. and MRS. E. T. ROBINSON, Cleveland, vacationed in Texas and Mexico City for three weeks in January and February.

DR. JOE C. RUDE, formerly located at 525 E. 68th St., New York City, The New York Hospital, announces his change of address to the Collis P. Huntington Memorial Hospital, Harvard Medical School at Boston.

DR. CHARLES K. MILLS, McAlester Clinic, McAlester, Oklahoma, is visiting Clinics in California.

DR. L. C. KUYRKENDALL, Councilor, McAlester, was guest speaker of LeFlore County Medical Society at their meeting in Poteau in February.

DR. L. S. WILLOUR, McAlester, spent a week in March at the Willis C. Campbell Clinic in Memphis.

The medical staff of the Menninger Clinic will conduct its fourth annual Postgraduate Course on "Neuropsychiatry in General Practice," April 25 to 30, inclusive, at the Menninger Clinic, Topeka, Kansas. The course this year will include a brief introduction to the fields of neurology and psychiatry and a specific application of this knowledge to the large group of cases of psychoneuroses, psychoses and psychogenic and neurological disorders which every physician meets in his daily practice. Suggestions made by those who took the course last year have been embodied in this year's program in order to make it applicable to the most common practical problems of the physician.

As in previous years, several guest speakers, prominent in the fields of neurology and psychiatry, will appear at the evening sessions of the course.

---o---

News of the County Medical Societies

CARTER County Medical Society reports the following program of the joint meeting with the Oklahoma Regional Fracture Committee, at Ardmore January 14th:

An afternoon session at 2:30 p.m., "Pneumonia," Dr. G. E. Johnson, Ardmore, Okla.; "Smith Peterson Fixation of Fracture of the Neck of the Femur, with Moving Pictures," Dr. Earl D. McBride, Oklahoma City; "Reconstruction Operation of the Hip, with Moving Pictures," Dr. Paul C. Colonna, Oklahoma City; "Fractures of the Spine, with Moving Pictures," Dr. E. Payne Palmer, Board of Regents of American College of Surgeons, Phoenix, Arizona; "Demonstration of Airplane Ambulance," Mr. Sidney Maxfield, Oklahoma City.

Dinner at 6:00 p.m. at Hotel Ardmore.

The night program, open to the public, at 7:30

p.m., Convention Hall. "Invocation," Rev. George H. Quarterman; "American College of Surgeons Program for the Treatment of Fractures," Dr. Earl D. McBride; "The First Aid Care of the Injured Child," Dr. Paul Colonna; "First Aid in Fracture Work," Dr. E. Payne Palmer; "Presentation of Emergency Arm and Leg Splints to Ambulance Drivers of Carter County," by Dr. Walter Hardy.

PITTSBURG County Medical Society met February 18th at the Aldridge Hotel, McAlester, and heard papers on "Diagnosis of Cancer" and "Ectopic Pregnancy," by Drs. Hugh Jeter and Joseph W. Kelso, respectively, both of Oklahoma City.

OKMULGEE-OKFUSKEE County Medical Societies met February 28, 1938, for a joint meeting and dinner. The speakers were: Dr. O. L. Magruder, Superintendent of the Veterans Hospital, Muskogee, who spoke on the relationships between the veteran, the general practitioner and the Facility service. Dr. I. W. Bollinger, Henryetta, read a paper on "Compression Fractures of the Back" and showed X-ray pictures of an interesting series of cases.

WOODWARD County Medical Society met February 8th, as guests of the physicians of Woodward. Following dinner at 7:30 papers were read by Drs. Basil Hayes, Oklahoma City, on "Phases of Nephritis"; and C. J. Fishman, Oklahoma City, on "Socialized Medicine." The next meeting will be held at Laverne, Oklahoma.

POTTAWATOMIE County Medical Society elected the following officers for 1938 at their meeting in February: President, Dr. E. Eugene Rice; vice-president, Dr. Horton E. Hughes; secretary-treasurer, Dr. Clinton Gallaher, all of Shawnee.

RESOLUTIONS

Report of Committee on Resolutions

Cleveland County Medical Society., February 10, 1938

Dr. G. W. Wiley

WHEREAS our friend and esteemed co-worker, Dr. G. W. Wiley has been called by the Great Physician, and

WHEREAS for many years he was a prominent and active member of our Society, and our profession, and

WHEREAS his professional attainments, and sterling qualities were known and admired both within and without the profession,

Therefore, Be It Resolved, by the Cleveland County Medical Society, that we record our sadness in his untimely passing, holding in memory his splendid skill and personality as a professional man, a loving and generous husband and father, an active leader, a citizen above reproach, and withal, kindly and generous, and

Be It Further Resolved, That a copy of these resolutions be spread upon the Minutes of the Cleveland County Medical Society, and that a copy be sent to the members of the family, and that official copies be sent to the Journal of the Oklahoma Medical Association, and the Journal of the American Medical Association.

Respectfully submitted,
        Dr. E. F. Stephens,
        Dr. D. G. Willard,
        Dr. M. M. Wickham,
            Committee on Resolutions.

ABSTRACTS : REVIEWS : COMMENTS
and CORRESPONDENCE

SURGERY AND GYNECOLOGY
Abstracts, Reviews and Comments from
LeRoy Long Clinic
714 Medical Arts Building, Oklahoma City

Results of Radiation Therapy for Carcinoma of the Uterus. Ward and Sackett. The Journal of the American Medical Association, January 29, 1938, Page 323.

This is an excellent review of the work done at the Woman's Hospital. The following quoted summary contains the important results and the opinions of the authors.

"During the 18 years that we have been treating carcinoma of the cervix with radium at the Woman's Hospital as part of a regular gynecologic service, we have salvaged for five years 27.4 per cent of the 595 patients seen and 28.5 per cent of the patients treated. In the cases of early carcinoma, in which the disease was limited to the cervix, we saved 56.2 per cent, showing the importance of treating the disease in the beginning stages.

"For the 359 patients seen over a period of ten years the absolute cure rate was 17.3 per cent and the relative rate was 18 per cent. In spite of lowered life expectancy, 73 per cent of those who survived five years lived ten years or longer.

"We believe that the extent of the disease is of greater importance than the type of cell in determining the probability of cure. In our series early carcinoma had twice the curability of advanced carcinoma, irrespective of the maturity of the cells and of whether they were of the squamous or adenocarcinomatous type.

"The highest incidence of carcinoma of the stump after supravaginal hysterectomy points to the desirability of doing a panhysterectomy whenever possible if no added risk is involved.

"In 108 cases of carcinoma of the fundus an absolute five year cure rate of 42.6 per cent was obtained and a relative rate of 45.5 per cent. We believe that a panhysterectomy is the most essential part of the treatment of carcinoma of the corpus and should be employed whenever possible. Combined radiotherapy and hysterectomy seems to us the most promising method. However, surgical intervention is contraindicated in nearly 50 per cent of the cases, and radiotherapy is our only resource for this group.

"There is a great need for comparative studies of the improvement obtained in combining high voltage roentgen therapy with radium therapy, and the conclusions should be based on the absolute survival rates over five and ten year periods and not on generalized clinical impressions. With the adoption of the Coutard fractional technic definite improvement may be hoped for.

"Finally, a survey of the six statistical reports of our results shows an improvement in the relative five year cure rates we have obtained as follows: 1925, 23.6 per cent; 1928, 23.1 per cent; 1930, 25.5 per cent; 1932, 24.8 per cent; 1934, 25.28 per cent, and 1937, 28.5 per cent."

There are excellent tables from which the statistical summary was obtained.

Comment: The results given in this article are very good. They emphasize the tremendous advantage of patients with carcinoma of the cervix receiving treatment while the disease is still limited to the cervix. They also show a gradual but steady improvement in the succeeding years in which the treatment has been employed.

The opinions of the authors relative to the importance of the extent of the disease and the type of cell in determining the probability of cure are entirely sound and generally accepted.

Because of the high incidence of carcinoma of the stump after supravaginal hysterectomy in their series, they have raised the question as to the advantage of complete hysterectomy with the removal of the cervix also as against supravaginal hysterectomy. It is generally agreed, in patients where the cervix is sound, that complete hysterectomy is desirable only if the operative mortality risk is less than the possible incidence of malignancy. Judging from statistical reports, the average incidence of carcinoma of the stump after supravaginal hysterectomy is about two per cent. It, therefore, becomes an individual problem for the surgeon to determine whether or not the mortality risk in each individual patient will be increased greater than two per cent by doing the complete hysterectomy rather than the supravaginal hysterectomy.

Wendell Long, M.D.

Notes on Cutaneous Healing in Wounds. J. Herbert Conway. Surgery, Gynecology and Obstetrics, February, 1938, Page 140.

In focusing its attention on the more serious problems of morbidity, mortality, and functional results, the surgical world has somewhat neglected the subject of the healing of the skin in clean incised wounds.

The author of this paper has observed a great variation in the degrees of fibroblastic response in healing by first intention while making post-operative examinations at the New York hospital.

He points out that the purpose of his paper is to show that certain details in the technique of surgical incision and suture have a direct effect upon the degree of fibroblastic response in a clean incised wound and also upon the ultimate cosmetic result. This observation is based on the appearance of scars, photographed one to three years after operation, and consideration of the ultimate result in relation to the variations in the surgical technique employed.

Numerous investigators have shown that a healing wound undergoes a latent or quiescent period which ends abruptly and is followed by a period of contraction. It has been demonstrated that the tensile strength of a healing wound depends upon the firmness of fibroblastic response. The maximal strength of the wound, according to experimental work on animals, is attained in from 10 to 14 days. It is well known that the rate of cicatrization as well as the extent of fibroblastic response varies in different individuals. Furthermore, these variations may be influenced by alteration of certain external factors which are under the control of the surgeon during the incision, suture, and subsequent care of the wound.

He is convinced of the following: "In order to promote ideal cutaneous healing of wounds and minimal cicatrization the following points in the technique and suture of clean surgical wounds are emphasized: the importance of placing the long axis of an incision parallel to Langer's lines of elasticity of the skin whenever possible; attention to the technique of incision so that the incision into the skin is not beveled; adequate undercutting of the skin and subcutaneous tissue flaps so that tension on the cutaneous line of suture is minimized; the use of silk legatures and sutures; and the use of fine arterial silk for approximation of the edges of the skin in the suture of wounds of the face."

LeRoy D. Long, M.D.

An Inexhausible Source of Blood for Transfusion and Its Preservation. Goodall, Anderson, Altimas and MacPhail. Surgery, Gynecology and Obstetrics, February, 1938, Page 176.

The authors believe they have found a safe, constant, efficient and lucrative source of blood for transfusion.

They became convinced that it was unnecessary to waste fetal blood from the placenta. They have established means to preserve this lost blood.

After experimentation they determined that the preservative proposed by the Moscow Institute of Haematology was the best available. The formula for this preparation is given.

A simple means of collecting the blood without contamination was established and considerable study was given to determining best atmosphere for conserving the blood in its freshness. Blood grouping and Wasserman reactions received due consideration.

They believe that the result of their work has been to provide an inexhaustible source of blood for transfusion and to preserve the blood at a minimum of cost and in a condition suitable for a transfusion medium for at least 60 days.

The technique used collecting the blood is extremely simple and blood is always available when it is needed for transfusion. An average of about 125 cubic centimeters of fetal blood is collected from each obstetrical patient.

The details of technique for preservation of the blood in an ice box at a temperature between 33 and 38 degrees Fahrenheit are given.

There are certain conditions which become axiomatic as regards mother, child, and accidents of labor. Blood of the placenta will, of course, not be taken in cases of obvious transmissible disease in either mother or child. Eclampsia is not a contra-indication, however. Blood will not be taken in cases in which the membranes have ruptured for more than 48 hours before delivery, nor in cases of definite prematurity. In cases of marked asphyxia pallida, the amount of blood in the placenta is so small as to make it worthless.

Babies at full term have a fixed blood group. Consequently, the groups of donors of placental blood are relatively numerically the same as in the recipients. Major reactions are all that are necessary in cross-matching. Cultures of the preserved blood are unnecessary because, at the low temperature for preservation, contamination, if present, could not propagate, and consequently would be so attenuated as to be innocuous. There occasionally occurs hemolysis which does not seem to cause any difficulty. It would seem that the hemolysin is in infinitesimally small quantity and is inoperative in the recipient. This subject is under further study.

Fetal blood, as regards cellular content, contains quantitatively approximately 7,000,000 red blood cells to 4,500,000 of the adult. Its cellular strength, therefore, is about 150 per cent that of the adult. Less fetal blood is therefore required. Every normal child at birth has therefore a well marked polycythemia. After birth, when the lungs become operative, the excess of red blood cells becomes unnecessary. This explanation is advanced to meet the argument that in taking the blood from the placenta, one is depriving the newborn of its rightful due, and that one should wait until the contractions of the uterus have squeezed some of the placental blood into the fetal circulation.

Fetal blood contains from 20 to 35 per cent more coagulation power than that of adult blood. From the point of view of transfusion, this is an advantage in hemorrhagic cases, and it does not appear a contra-indication of septic thrombophlebitis.

Preserved blood has many advantages over fresh blood. In the first place, food and other extraneous allergic reactions are eliminated. It is now a standing rule that, when possible, donors should not be used for some hours after ingestion of food. This is to obviate food allergic reactions. In preserved blood, autodigestion occurs and allergic reactions do not occur after 48 hours of preservation.

The author states that they have done many transfusions with fetal blood without a single untoward reaction, nor a single rise of temperature, even to a fraction of a degree, attributable to the transfusion. Before transfusion the fetal blood is heated and strained through gauze. Two or more fetal bloods may be given simultaneously, if necessary, after separate matching.

LeRoy D. Long, M.D.

PREGNANCY TESTS

The Aschheim-Zondek pregnancy test, using mice, later modified by Friedmann, using rabbits, has proven itself a reliable test for pregnancy with an established accuracy of about 95 per cent. However, it is time consuming, relatively expensive, and requires meticulous care of the animals employed.

The following four articles deal with the application of two pregnancy tests which were devised to provide simpler, quicker, and more economical tests for pregnancy.

Visscher-Bowman Pregnancy Tests (Chemical).

This is a chemical test devised by Visscher and Bowman, based upon presence of gonadotropic hormones in the urine of pregnant women. In the test 1 c.c. of urine is employed and to it are added reagents listed in the next two articles. The reading for the test depends upon the color and the precipitate produced.

The Chemical Pregnancy Test of Visscher and Bowman. By Messinger, Presberg, Fellows. American Journal of Obstetrics & Gynecology, February, 1938.

These authors examined 187 urines by the technic of Visscher & Bowman for the determination of pregnancy, finding 69.5 per cent agreeing with the clinical diagnosis.

The chemical test agreed with the Friedmann modification of the Aschheim-Zondek test in 72.5 per cent of 69 cases.

"A russet color and flocculent precipitate could not be obtained with histidine, creatine, glucose, lactose, or galactose, which indicates that these substances are not responsible for the reaction.

"A russet color and a flocculent precipitate should be present before a test be considered positive.

"The titration method described by Visscher and Bowman in their original article could not be confirmed."

Results with the Visscher-Bowman Pregnancy Test. By Dunn and Northway. American Journal of Obstetrics & Gynecology, February, 1938, Page 298.

The conclusions drawn by these authors and their summary concisely state their experience and are therefore quoted.

"Our results show a higher percentage of error than that recorded by other workers. Elimination of urines of low specific gravity and those containing undesirable catabolic products might better our results. In the suspected pregnancies, where these elements do not come into play, our findings were 87.6 per cent correct, the highest percentage of accuracy we found in any group. Contrasted with this, the fewest number of correct results (54.8 per cent) occurred in urines of nonpregnant febrile patients.

"We must conclude from our results, as well as from the results of other investigators, that the Visscher-Bowman test for pregnancy is, as yet, not sufficiently reliable to supplant the biologic methods now in use. A modification of the technique, aiming at the elimination of the sources of error, may ultimately yield a very useful diagnostic method.

SUMMARY

"1. Three hundred ninety-five urines were tested by the Visscher-Bowman method for the determination of pregnancy. Correct reactions were obtained in 84.8 per cent of 250 known pregnancies, 87.6 per cent of 65 suspected pregnancies, and 54.8 per cent of 62 nonpregnancies.

"2. Urines of low specific gravity or containing unusual amounts of catabolic reducing agents tend to give false reactions.

"3. The test in its present form is subject to too high a percentage of error to replace the Friedman and Aschheim-Zondek tests."

Skin Tests For Pregnancy

These tests are intro-dermal in character. They are based upon the hypothesis that since there is an anterior pituitary-like substance in the urine of pregnant women, pregnant women should not be sensitive to its intradermal application, while nonpregnant women should be sensitive and give a dermal reaction after injection. In other words, a skin reaction indicates the absence of pregnancy.

Antuitrin-S Cutaneous Test for the Diagnosis of Pregnancy. By Isadore Gersh, American Journal of Obstetrics & Gynecology, February, 1938, Page 301.

His study was based upon 113 individuals, 50 normal men and non-pregnant women, 48 known cases of pregnancy of two or more months duration, and 15 one to nine days post-partum.

"Using antuitrin-S, 20.8 per cent false negative results were obtained in our pregnant patients and 6.6 per cent in the postpartum cases, while 81.6 per cent of the men and 66.6 per cent of the non-pregnant women showed false positive tests for pregnancy (based on skin reactions one hour after the injection)."

Their conclusions are:

"In our hands the anterior pituitary-like hormone (antuitrin-S) cutaneous test for pregnancy was found to be entirely unreliable."

Skin Tests for Pregnancy. By Frank and Wahrsinger. American Journal of Obstetrics & Gynecology, February, 1938, Page 303.

Antuitrin-S was employed in 112 definitely pregnant women with 28 positive skin reactions, falsely indicating that there was no pregnancy present. Eight patients gave doubtful reactions and 76 no reactions at all. In their pregnancy cases, therefore, the accuracy was 68 per cent.

They also employed the antuitrin-S test on 22 medical non-pregnant, 21 postpartum and eight pediatric patients with a high percentage of positives.

They also ran a series of six patients using another anterior pituitary-like hormone but derived from the placenta. The results were only 50 per cent accurate and the work was discontinued.

Another short series was conducted, using progestin (Upjohn) which is a corpus luteum extract. Ninety-eight per cent of all these patients, including pregnant women, produced positive skin reactions, rendering the test definitely inaccurate.

"We must conclude, therefore, that the use of anterior pituitary-like . hormone injected intradermally in the manner suggested by Gilfillen and Gregg, and scientifically controlled, in a series of 198 cases, did not provide an accurate or reliable skin test for pregnancy."

COMMENT

This is an interesting series of four articles, demonstrating the present status of pregnancy tests. While there are certain objections to the Friedmann modification of the Aschheim-Zondek test, it still remains the most accurate and reliable. It is hoped that certain sources of error may be eliminated from the urine chemical test and that such modification will ultimately yield a satisfactory diagnostic method which is quicker, more economical, and simpler.

Wendell Long, M.D.

EYE, EAR, NOSE AND THROAT
Edited by Marvin D. Henley, M.D.
911 Medical Arts Building, Tulsa

Treatment of Herpetic Keratitis With Vitamin B. J. Nitzulescu and Ecaterina Triandaf, Jassy, Roumania. The British Journal of Ophthalmology, December, 1937.

From the role that vitamin B1 played in the cure of beriberic polyneuritis, Minot, Strauss and Cobb, were lead to try its action in other nerve diseases. Betaxin is the trade name of the product used.

It was found effective in a case of bilateral trigeminal neuralgia. Corneal Herpes following gonorrhoeal conjunctivitis, in a patient age 16 years did not yield to the usual treatment of anti-neuralgic powders and urotropin, the pain becoming intolerable. Injections of Betaxin daily immediately reduced pain and brought about progressive healing of the lesions. In another patient age 33, with a diagnosis of Keratitis herpetica, a similar result was obtained after the routine treatment had proved futile. A history and detailed treatment is given on both cases. Where, before both patients had not been able to rest at all, after the first injection of Betaxin, a peaceful night was spent.

There is quite a discussion of the theoretical action of the vitamin B1 by the author. He does not consider the manifestations of herpes as a process of hylovitaminasis. He is "inclined to attribute to the vitamin the action of a real medicament, exerting a specific influence, functional and trophic on the nerves, which can be injured by very different aeteological agents."

While two cases furnish no data for a definite conclusion, the author is of the opinion that the results derived are more than a coincidence.

New Technique in the Surgical Treatment of Severe and Progressive Deafness From Otosclerosis. Dr. Maurice Sourdille, Nantes, France. The Laryngoscope, December, 1937.

Barany, Jenkins and Holmgreen pioneered the surgical treatment of otosclerosis.

There are two groups: One which presumes the pathogenesis of otosclerosis and attacks the disease at its root; the operation is performed outside the ear as the "elevation of the supra tympani dura mater" or even far from the ear as the removal of one parathyroid or suppressing its function by ligature of its principal vessels. These operations are designed to arrest the progress of the disease. They are indicated early in the disease. The second group attacks the local functional troubles. The operation is a fenestration of the labyrinth. The technique presents both an acoustic and surgical problem. The author's operation is called a "tympanolabyrinthopexy." It associates "the opening of the external semi-circular canal to the new tympanic system derived from the normal system."

When the semi-circular canal is opened the perilymph in turn flows out which in the opinion of the author causes a formation in the labyrinth of a free surface of perilymph. He likens this to the mechanism of the half-filled flask which is discussed. Hearing acuity was immediately noticeably increased under the above conditions, but the problem was to prevent the closing of the aperture, for when this occurred, hearing acuity was gradually decreased.

In order to prevent this the author joins the covering membranes of the labyrinthine fistula with the superior border of the membrana tympani after a resection of the head of the malleus has been done to increase the membrana's excursions.

This is a three stage operation with intervals of four or five months between. The first two stages transforms the tympanic system and modifies the mastoid region. The third stage establishes the labyrinthine fistula at the level of the new tympanic system. This is one of the disadvantages of the procedure, the length of time, and repeated operation. The other disadvantage is the putting of the interior of the mastoid cavity in direct communication with the cavity of the external auditory canal so making the hazard of an external otitis greater.

Some of the advantages of the procedure are:

1. The definite assurance of function if the operative work is successfully done.
2. It is possible to test the tympanic system and the labyrinthine fistula with a manometer because they are constantly in sight.
3. Only the horizontal canal is opened.
4. No foreign material is added.
5. It is not a one step operation.
6. If it becomes necessary the operation may be touched up without difficulty.

In considering the operative indications one must consider the nature and degree of the deafness, the state of health and indications of primary otospongiosis. The author says the external auditory meatus should be wide and straight and the middle ear of large dimensions, well vascularized and resistant. The contra-indications are mentioned and discussed. A sterioscopic radiogram is a necessity as well as a correct interpretation of same before any operative work is started.

The operative technique of the three stages is given in detail as is also a table recapitulating the results obtained. The author claims 80 per cent positive results. The results according to him are comparable to those obtained in ophthalmology, in cataract and glaucoma.

Clinical Evaluation of Short Wave Diathermy in Otolaryngology. A. R. Hollender, M.D., F.A.C.S. The Eye, Ear, Nose and Throat Monthly, January, 1938.

Conventional and short wave diathermy are discussed. Short wave diathermy creates heat at much greater depth than conventional diathermy. Short waves pass easily through bony structures, while with the longer waves use, this bony structure was an insurmountable obstacle. Therefore this particular therapeutic measure is particularly applicable in the field of otolaryngology.

Heat induces hyperemia and stimulates circulation of lymph. Infection is controlled through increase of the inflammatory process. This form of treatment should be indicated in all conditions accompanied by inflammation and infection.

Some precautions to be observed are: removal of metals from the field of treatment, the proper spacing of electrodes and the special attention to dosage in case of patients suffering from diminished or abolished sensation of heat.

The author's summary follows:

1. Heat has for a long time been used empirically in otolaryngology for the alleviation of pain, but its influence on underlying inflammatory processes is now recognized.
2. The limitations and disadvantages of conventional diathermy, especially in otolaryngology, have largely been overcome by short wave diathermy.
3. The results of several workers on the relation of clinical effects to experimental temperature determinations, especially in the sinuses, are reviewed.
4. For otolaryngological purposes special electrodes are required but any apparatus of adequate wattage utilized in general medicine is suitable.
5. Clinically short wave diathermy is a valuable adjunct in the treatment of nasal sinusitis but insufficiently effective in itself to replace classic therapeutic procedures.
6. Short wave diathermy is of value in promptly relieving the pain of acute tonsilitis, pharyngitis and laryngitis and in shortening their course when combined with indicated constitutional measures.
7. In otology short wave diathermy is an effective remedy for auricular infections, otalgia, acute myringitis and eustachian catarrh, but is of doubtful value in chronic pathological processes.
8. Every practitioner should be thoroughly familiar with dosage and method of application, and avoidance of undesirable reactions.

Some Practical Considerations Relative to Complications of Mastoiditis. J. Hallock Moore, M.D., Huntington, West Virginia. Southern Medical Journal, February, 1938.

Simple sinusitis is listed as the most common and most neglected complication of acute purulent otitis media and early mastoiditis. Over 90 per cent of the author's otitis medias have an additional sinusitis. The antra are the most frequent offenders; pan-sinusitis is not uncommon. He recommends for treatment, irrigation through the natural orifice.

The simplest complication is a cortical perforation. Here must be differentiated either skin or scalp infections with a secondary lymphadenitis, an external otitis and the reaction resulting from the improper use of X-ray therapy.

The external otitis may result from the patient using some blunt object in the canal, irritation from the discharge of an acute otitis media or an actual furunculosis.

Impetigo or eczema are two frequent skin or scalp infections at this site. Lymphadenitis usually accompanies these adding more confusion to the picture.

Overdosage of an X-ray treatment may produce all the signs and symptoms of a cortical perforation.

The author's outline of differential diagnosis is as follows: First be reasonably sure of the diagnosis before operation, a wait of a day or two probably will have no more ill effect than the discomfort suffered by the patient during that time.

The X-ray helps little in the differentiation. It will be cloudy in both cortical perforation and cellulitis with secondary broken-down lymphadenitis.

A careful history and treatment of the local condition will aid most in the making of an accurate diagnosis. The author recommends an alum acetate pack for treatment of a furunculosis or an external otitis. Two or three days thus should reduce the swelling or bring the furuncle to the point where it can successfully be incised. Likewise scalp and skin infections properly treated for the same period of time will clear the diagnostic atmosphere. Amelioration of the X-ray reaction will have taken place also in this space of time.

An exploratory incision is made after two or three days if the symptoms have not subsided with the proper treatment. The surgeon should be prepared at this time to continue with the incision and do a complete mastoidectomy, if indicated.

Sinus thrombophlebitis is treated with a complete ligation of the jugular and anterior facial vein, securing free bleeding from the central end of the lateral sinus. The elapse of more time between the myringotomy and the mastoid operation will cause a less number of blood stream infections. Two or three weeks is the suggested interval.

Too much reliance should not be placed on the Tobey-Ayres test. It is of value only in the normal individual.

The aid that sulfanilimide offers is still problematical.

In case of otitic meningitis an immediate complete radical mastoidectomy is advised; an exception is micrococcus meningitis. Extension occurs from the middle ear by simple erosion of the internal cortex, a rupture of a petrosal cell, through the diploic veins or by the way of the internal meatus through the labyrinth.

Petrositis should be operated early and drained. Either the burr method (Kopetsky & Almour) or the subdural route to the apex, depending upon the operator, may be used.

Extra or intradural brain abscess, according to the author, many times is the result of an improperly performed mastoidectomy. Early operation is necessary.

Concerning labyrinth involvement the author feels that "the average case of acute purulent labyrinthitis is safer in the hands of an internist than in the hands of the otologist."

Discussion by McHenry, Boebinger and Daily.

INTERNAL MEDICINE

Edited by C. E. Bradley, M.D., Medical Arts Building, Tulsa; Hugh Jeter, M.D., 1200 North Walker, Oklahoma City

HUGH, JETER, M.D., F.A.C.P., A.S.C.P.

The Present Status of Rheumatism and Arthritis: Review of American and English Literature for 1936. By Philip S. Hench, M.D., F.A.C.P., Rochester, Minn.; Walter Bauer, M.D., F.A.C.P., Boston; David Ghrist, M.D., Los Angeles; Francis Hall, M.D., Boston; W. Paul Holbrook, M.D., Tucson; J. Albert Key, M.D., St. Louis, and Charles H. Slocumb, M.D., Rochester, Minn. Annals of Internal Medicine, Vol. 11, No. 7, January, 1938.

This is the fourth annual review which abstracts material from 593 magazine articles and 15 books, the latter published in 1936.

The references alone are of very great value.

The following is an abstract of only one portion of the review:

The authors state that gout was called a "forgotten disease." Statistics, the authors believe, do not give an accurate index of the disease, because the requirements of different physicians for a diagnosis of gout differs so materially. Hench stated that only one of four or five cases of gout is correctly diagnosed in its early stages. However, he adds, that in some quarters where physicians are loose with the diagnosis of gout, only one of two or three patients who receive such a diagnosis actually have the disease. Hench reviewed the features of classical gout and divided the course of gouty arthritis into two stages, each consisting of two phases: Stage I is that of acute recurrent gouty arthritis with complete remissions and stage II is that of chronic gouty arthritis with acute exacerbations but incomplete remissions. Hench further lists 20 points as the criteria for the diagnosis of gout. Hench believes that in a case presenting a number of the features listed in the criteria for diagnosis, one must not hesitate to entertain a diagnosis of gout in the absence of the four most characteristic features, namely: Podagra, hyperuricemia, tophi and punched-out areas in roentgenograms.

In a review of the laboratory data it was generally agreed that hyperuricemia is usually, but not always, present in classical gout. Furthermore, they conclude that roentgenograms are generally negative in early cases and are of no help in diagnosis until late in the disease. Roentgenograms of the hand may show characteristic changes not seen elsewhere. The etiology, pathogenesis and treatment are reviewed. The reports of cinchophen toxicity are also reviewed. Comfort believed its use was justified since there is no pharmacologic substitute for it in gout, but it should not be used otherwise. He adds that its dangers can be reduced by discontinuing its use permanently, not temporarily, at the first sign of toxicity and by strictly avoiding surgical procedures on those so affected.

The uric acid problem is reviewed and mention is made of insulin's affect upon purine metabolism; with the conclusion that insulin's action is not direct, but indirect, through an increased secretion of epinephrine (adrenal secretion) brought about by insulin hypoglycemia.

Our Arthritis. By Logan Clendening, M.D. The Saturday Evening Post, February 12, 1938.

The author has herein written a lay article which speaks for itself and is well worth every doctor's attention.

PLASTIC SURGERY
Edited by
GEO. H. KIMBALL, M.D., F.A.C.S.
404 Medical Arts Building, Oklahoma City

A Three-Stage Operation For The Repair of Hypospadias. Report of cases, Oswald Swinney Lowsley, M.D., and Colin Luke Begg, M.D., New York. A. M. A. Journal, February 12, 1938.

The authors describe the types of hypospadias in detail. They also give a resume of different methods that have been tried personally. The authors follow a three-stage operation, utilizing scrotal skin for making the urethral canal. They report 10 cases which they have done since 1932. The results have been good in seven cases. One case died the third day post-operative; one case incomplete.

The paper was discussed by Dr. J. Eastman Sheehan, New York, who points out that we must use skin on its own terms. In order to do that we must know the demands of skin.

In 1933 Dr. Vilray P. Blair reported a plan which utilized scrotal tissue to cover the newly-made urethra which was constructed from the ventral surface of the penis.

Comment: The authors are to be congratulated on what apparently is a very sensible plan for the repair of hypospadias. In utilization of any plan that has been put forth, one will meet with some difficulty, as far as healing is concerned, occasional fistula, breaking down of skin and delay from various causes. The principal delay often is infection. I think the preliminary diversion of the urinary stream by super-pubic drainage is sensible.

The technique of Drs. Lowsley and Begg differ in several respects from that of Blair. Each one seems to have succeeded in his efforts. The high percentage of good results obtained by the more recent method is certainly commendable.

Complete Avulsion of the Scalp and Loss of the Right Ear. James A. Cahill, Jr., M.D., F.A.C.S., and Philip A. Caulfield, M.D., Washington, D.C. S. G. & O., February 15, 1938.

The authors describe in detail a case of avulsion of the scalp with the loss of the right ear which was subsequently repaired by pedicle grafts and costal cartilage. The authors relate the historical phases of this type of work and report altogether 96 cases found in the literature of complete industrial scalping.

A case reported by the authors sustained a complete avulsion of the scalp and the right ear secondary to catching her hair in a fly-wheel. The authors describe in detail the manner of repair.

Comment: It is interesting to note the result in this case following rather extensive tube pedicle grafts taken from the back. Personally I have had one case that sustained a rather extensive avulsion of part of the scalp which was sutured and later developed infection with destruction of considerable portion of the skull.

Another case in a male of 72 years of age, lost one-half of his scalp, right ear and skin of back of neck following a burn. This case was repaired by cleansing the area and supplying split grafts to the neck, removing the sequestra from the skull which was from the outer table, later stimulating granulation by boring small holes down to the diploe and after granulations were well established, covering the area with small grafts.

I say this for the reason that some of these cases are not suitable for transplanting pedicle grafts to the scalp. Each case, of course, is a problem in itself.

ORTHOPAEDIC SURGERY
Edited by Earl D. McBride, M.D., F.A.C.S.
717 North Robinson Street, Oklahoma City

Trauma as a Factor in Pott's Disease. Max H. Skolnick. Amer. Review of Tuberculosis, XXXVI, 429, September, 1937.

The author points out that trauma has a definite relationship to later development of Pott's disease. Considerable time may elapse between the trauma and the development of active disease, and the slighter forms of t r a u m a seem to be a greater causative factor than severe injury. Symptomatology plays the most important part in the early diagnosis. Considerable time is required for such lesions to become clinically and objectively manifest, but if roentgenograms were taken in every case where symptomatology indicates possible activity, many cases would be discovered before irreparable damage had resulted.

The Regeneration of Bone Transplants. Hans May. Annals of Surg. CVI, 441, September, 1937.

A review of the literature on this subject is presented and the author describes his own research as follows:

An investigation directed to the process of vascularization of a bone graft was carried out by subperiosteally removing the radius (including its two articular ends), placing the removed bone in salt solution and then replanting it in its original bed, and suturing the periosteum and closing the joint capsules. Twenty-five such experiments were performed on dogs, but aseptic healing occurred in only four animals. X-rays were made every eight days. The dogs were killed after five weeks, ten weeks, four months, and ten months, followed immediately in each case by injection of the axillary artery with a turpentine-mercury solution. The radii were removed, X-rayed, and studied histologically with the following findings:

The graft a l w a y s dies after transplantation; many nuclei disappear, others degenerate, but in from two and a half to four months regeneration occurs by creeping substitution of dead bone by new bone. Small and large vessels grow from the periosteum into the graft; the former early regress as the large vessels progress until the entire graft is supplied by a well-arranged vascular system. That part of the graft not covered by periosteum becomes destroyed by ingrowing fibrous tissue and only small portions are saved by surviving osteoblasts. The periosteum, therefore, is the reliable factor in regeneration when an entire bone, with its closed medullary cavity, is transplanted.

Lambrinudi's Operation for Drop-Foot. F. P. Fitzgerald and H. J. Seddon. The Brit. Jr. of Surg. XXV, 283, October, 1937.

Twenty-four cases in which the Lambrinudi operation has been used are cited. The operation may be used for drop-foot or flail-foot. There have been five failures in the series due to lateral instability at the ankle. Previous to the operation, the procedure is planned from tracings of lateral roentgenograms with the idea that in certain cases the patient will wear a tapering cork to build up the back of the foot. Segments of the astragalus, oscalcis, cuboid, and scaphoid are removed and the calcaneocuboid joint is cleaned out. The cartilage on the posterior surface of the scaphoid left after removal of a notch is not removed. The cuboid is brought up to the anterior surface of the astragalus and arthrodesed. Likewise the scaphoid is brought upward and forward which brings the forward part of the foot partially or completely up in line. The foot is fixed in a short leg plaster.

Earl D. McBride, M.D., F.A.C.S.

UROLOGY

Edited by D. W. Branham, M. D.
514 Medical Arts Building, Oklahoma City

Local Use of Arsphenamines in Acute Gonorrheal Urethritis. John E. Heslin and William A. Milner, Albany, New York. Journal of Urology, February, 1938.

Sulpharsphenamine in aqueous solution was used as a local installation in 42 patients in an attempt to determine whether there is any therapeutic value to this drug in the treatment of gonorrhea.

Such treatment was suggested by the definite therapeutic results obtained in the treatment of cocci infection of the upper urinary tract when the drug was administered intravenously as also the specific local action of neosalvarsan in cases of Vincent's Angina.

In a comparison of 42 patients treated by a daily injection of sulpharsphenamine 0.1 gram to the dram of water, as compared to a similar number of patients treated with other more accepted modes, it was found that less time was required to obtain a cure. Complications in the form of posterior urethritis were of less frequent incidence with this form of treatment.

The authors summarize their experience, that in their hands this drug, while not specific, has proven more efficacious than any other in the local treatment of gonorrhea.

Comment: One hardly knows how to comment on such investigations than to say that gonorrhea is a disease of such clinical variability that small series of cases are practically useless in order to form any definite conclusions as to the therapeutic worth of any particular drug or preparation. While such investigation is praise worthy in its aim the average practitioner had better wait further corroberative evidence before discarding more acceptable and better known methods of treatment.

Primary Syphilis in the Female. Paul F. Stookey and Morris Polsky, Kansas City, Missouri. Urologic and Cutaneous Review, February, 1938.

This article details the physical characteristics of the chancre as it occurs in the female. Unlike the lesion that ordinarily presents, primary syphilitic infections involving the cervix produces a large swollen boggy diffuse inflammatory reaction, the so-called "cold edema." This appearance is due to the rich lymphatic network of the cervix. Dark field examination from such lesions will usually show the typical spirochete. Because the lymphatics of the cervix drain into the deep iliac and para-rectal glands regional adenopathy is not apparent. As statistics show the primary lesion in women more often involves the cervix the authors stress the importance of thoroughly examining the cervix in suspected instances of syphilitic infection.

Comment: Because syphilis in its early stages is infrequently found in the female as compared to that observed in the male this article is extremely practical and timely. The authors' observation of the characteristic appearance of cervical infection should be of value to each practicing physician. More dark field examination should be made in cases of cervical infections and erosions. Only by detecting syphilis in the "dark field positive and Wassermann negative stage" can we improve our therapeutic results in the treatment of this disease.

Lively Interest In Physicians' Tour of America By De Luxe Special Trains En Route to the A.M.A. Convention in San Francisco

According to latest reports reaching us, physicians and their families are evincing a very keen interest in the arrangements made by the American Express Travel Service with the cooperation of your society to see America en route to and returning from the San Francisco Convention. This early interest indicates the assured success of this important Convention.

The "See America" movement by De Luxe Special Trains is endorsed by approximately 25 State Medical Societies. It presents an unprecedented opportunity for our members and their families to join with their colleagues from other states, and enjoy the facilities and service of De Luxe Special Trains, and at the same time visit the many scenic attractions of our western states.

Many physicians, completely immersed in their practices, have hesitated to take such an extended vacation heretofore but now the fact of the A.M.A. Convention and the attractiveness and economical features of this travel program has brought such a trip within the realm of desirable possibilities.

Picture the beauty and relaxation of such scenes as the Indian Detour in New Mexico, the Grand Canyon of Arizona, Los Angeles and the beauties of southern California, Santa Catalina Island, the famous Columbia River Highway in Oregon, Seattle, Washington, Victoria, Vancouver, Lake Louise and Banff in the Canadian Rockies, Yellowstone National Park, Colorado Springs and many others.

The all-inclusive price is unusually low because of the cooperation of so many important medical societies. It is, therefore, recommended that our members avail themselves of this most attractive and unusual program which may not again present itself for some time. An attractive folder, describing these travel arrangements, may be obtained through the Secretary's office or the Transportation Agents, The American Express Travel Service, 1010 Locust Street, St. Louis, Missouri.

Correlation of Positive Reaction to Tuberculin and Shape of the Chest

S. A. Weisman, Minneapolis, (Journal A. M. A., Oct. 30, 1937), believes that his study, which shows that there is a definite correlation between the deep chest and the positive reaction to tuberculin, adds one more link to the chain of evidence supporting the contention that the deep chest is more or less associated with tuberculosis. It also helps to explain why there is such a high incidence of tuberculosis among the poor in the slum districts. The children in the slums are physically underdeveloped. They are not only shorter and lighter but they have on the average a deep, primitive, infantile type of chest, one that has not gone through the normal process of development. Even the newborn and infants are shorter and lighter and have a deeper chest than the average infant from a better environment. In many large cities the government is wiping out the slum districts and replacing them with modern, well built and well ventilated homes.

OFFICERS OKLAHOMA STATE MEDICAL ASSOCIATION

President, Dr. Sam A. McKeel, Ada.
President-Elect, Dr. H. K. Speed, Sayre.
Secretary-Treasurer-Editor, Dr. L. S. Willour, McAlester.
Speaker, House of Delegates, Dr. J. D. Osborn, Jr., Frederick.
Vice Speaker, House of Delegates, Dr. P. P. Nesbitt, Medical Arts Building, Tulsa.
Delegates to the A. M. A., Dr. W. Albert Cook, Medical Arts Building, Tulsa, 1937-1938; Dr. Horace Reed, 1200 North Walker, Oklahoma City, 1937-1938; Dr. McLain Rogers, Clinton, 1938-1939.
Meeting Place, Muskogee, May 9-10-11, 1938.

SPECIAL COMMITTEES

Annual Meeting: Dr. Sam A. McKeel, Ada; Dr. H. K. Speed, Sayre; Dr. L. S. Willour, McAlester.

Conservation of Hearing: Dr. J. A. Morrow, Chairman, Sallisaw; Dr. Howard Brown, Ponca City; Dr. E. A. Hale, Alva.

Conservation of Vision: Dr. Milton K. Thompson, Chairman, Muskogee; Dr. William F. Klotz, McAlester; Dr. O. H. Miller, Ada.

Crippled Children: Dr. D. H. O'Donoghue, Chairman, Oklahoma City; Dr. George S. Baxter, Shawnee; Dr. Ray Lindsey, Pauls Valley.

Industrial Service and Traumatic Surgery: Dr. Earl McBride, Chairman, Oklahoma City; Dr. J. F. Park, McAlester; Dr. G. H. Stagner, Erick.

Maternity and Infancy: Dr. John A. Haynie, Chairman, Durant; Dr. Edward P. Allen, Oklahoma City; Dr. Marvin B. Glismann, Okmulgee.

Necrology: Dr. C. E. Williams, Chairman, Woodward; Dr. James L. Shuler, Durant; Dr. E. P. Green, Westville.

Post Graduate Medical Teaching: Dr. Henry H. Turner, Chairman, Oklahoma City; Dr. H. C. Weber, Bartlesville; Dr. T. H. McCarley, McAlester.

Study and Control of Cancer: Dr. Wendell Long, Chairman, Oklahoma City; Dr. Paul B. Champlin, Enid; Dr. Ralph McGill, Tulsa.

Study and Control of Tuberculosis: Dr. Carl Puckett, Chairman, Oklahoma City; Dr. Will C. Wait, Clinton; Dr. L. J. Moorman, Oklahoma City.

STANDING COMMITTEES

Medical Defense: Dr. L. C. Kuyrkendall, Chairman, McAlester; Dr. O. E. Templin, Alva; Dr. W. A. Howard, Chelsea.

Medical Economics: Dr. Rex Bolend, Chairman, Oklahoma City; Dr. E. M. Gullatt, Ada; Dr. R. B. Gibson, Ponca City.

Medical Education and Hospitals: Dr. Robert U. Patterson, Chairman, Oklahoma City; Dr. W. P. Longmire, Sapulpa; Dr. LeRoy Long, Oklahoma City.

Public Policy and Legislation: Dr. J. M. Byrum, Shawnee; Dr. Sam A. McKeel, Ada; Dr. H. K. Speed, Sayre; Dr. W. P. Neilson, Enid; Dr. R. C. Pigford, Tulsa.

Scientific Exhibits: Dr. W. N. Weaver, Chairman, Muskogee; Dr. Curt Von Wedel, Oklahoma City; Dr. E. Rankin Denny, Tulsa.

Scientific Work: Dr. W. G. Husband, Chairman, Hollis; Dr. C. Stevens, Seminole; Dr. W. N. Johns, Hugo.

SCIENTIFIC SECTIONS

General Surgery: Dr. Stratton E. Kernodle, Chairman, 635 First National Building, Oklahoma City; Dr. H. G. Crawford, Vice-Chairman, Bartlesville; Dr. E. P. Nesbitt, Secretary, Medical Arts Building, Tulsa.

General Medicine: Dr. Minard F. Jacobs, Chairman, Medical Arts Building, Oklahoma City; Dr. Frank Nelson, Vice-Chairman, Medical Arts Building, Tulsa; Dr. Milam F. McKinney, Secretary, Oklahoma City.

Eye, Ear, Nose and Throat: Dr. Chester McHenry, Chairman, Medical Arts Building, Oklahoma City; Dr. A. H. Davis, Vice-Chairman, Medical Arts Building, Tulsa; Dr. Edwin H. Coachman, Secretary, Manhattan Building, Muskogee.

Obstetrics and Pediatrics: Dr. M. B. Glismann, Chairman, Okmulgee; Dr. C. W. Arndell, Vice-Chairman, Ponca City; Dr. C. E. White, Secretary, Muskogee.

Genito-Urinary Diseases and Syphilology: Dr. Chas. B. Taylor, Chairman, Medical Arts Building, Oklahoma City; Dr. D. W. Branham, Vice-Chairman, Medical Arts Building, Oklahoma City; Dr. Shade Neely, Secretary, Commercial National Building, Muskogee.

Dermatology and Radiology: Dr. L. S. McAlister, Chairman, Barnes Building, Muskogee; Dr. M. M. Wickham, Vice-Chairman, Norman; Dr. John H. Lamb, Secretary, Medical Arts Building, Oklahoma City.

STATE BOARD OF MEDICAL EXAMINERS

Dr. Thos. McElroy, Ponca City, President; Dr. C. E. Bradley, Tulsa, Vice-President; Dr. J. D. Osborn, Jr., Frederick, Secretary; Dr. L. E. Emanuel, Chickasha; Dr. W. T. Ray, Gould; Dr. G. L. Johnson, Pauls Valley; Dr. W. W. Osgood, Muskogee.

STATE COMMISSIONER OF HEALTH

Dr. Chas. M. Pearce, Oklahoma City.

COUNCILORS AND THEIR COUNTIES

District No. 1: Texas, Beaver, Cimarron, Harper, Ellis, Woods, Woodward, Alfalfa, Major, Dewey—Dr. O. E. Templin, Alva. (Term expires 1937.)

District No. 2: Roger Mills, Beckham, Greer, Harmon, Washita, Kiowa, Custer, Jackson, Tillman—Dr. V. C. Tisdal, Elk City. (Term expires 1939.)

District No. 3: Grant, Kay, Garfield, Noble, Payne, Pawnee—Dr. A. S. Risser, Blackwell. (Term expires 1938.)

District No. 4: Blaine, Kingfisher, Canadian, Logan, Oklahoma, Cleveland—Dr. Philip M. McNeill, Oklahoma City. (Term expires 1938.)

District No. 5: Caddo, Comanche, Cotton, Grady, Love, Stephens, Jefferson, Carter, Murray—Dr. W. H. Livermore, Chickasha. (Term expires 1938.)

District No. 6: Osage, Creek, Washington, Nowata, Rogers, Tulsa—Dr. W. A. Howard, Chelsea. (Term expires 1938.)

District No. 7: Lincoln, Pontotoc, Pottawatomie, Okfuskee, Seminole, McClain, Garvin, Hughes—Dr. J. A. Walker, Shawnee. (Term expires 1939.)

District No. 8: Craig, Ottawa, Mayes, Delaware, Wagoner, Adair, Cherokee, Sequoyah, Okmulgee, Muskogee—Dr. E. A. Aisenstadt, Picher. (Term expires 1938.)

District No. 9: Pittsburg, Haskell, Latimer, LeFlore, McIntosh—Dr. L. C. Kuyrkendall, McAlester. (Term expires 1939.)

District No. 10: Johnson, Marshall, Coal, Atoka, Bryan, Choctaw, Pushmataha, McCurtain—Dr. J. S. Fulton, Atoka. (Term expires 1939.)

CLASSIFIED ADVERTISEMENTS

THE JOURNAL
OF THE
OKLAHOMA STATE MEDICAL ASSOCIATION

| VOLUME XXXI | McALESTER, OKLAHOMA, APRIL, 1938 | Number 4 |

Congenital Visceral Anomalies As Exemplified By The Developing Vascular System*

CHARLES F. DE GARIS, M.D., PH.D.
Department of Anatomy,
University of Oklahoma School of Medicine

In attempting to discuss congenital visceral anomalies, there are one of two ways to approach the subject. Either I can discuss in a purely descriptive fashion some of the anomalies I have seen myself, or I can seek to arrive at certain conclusions regarding anomalies in general and their causes in particular. I t h i n k you will agree with me that this latter approach is distinctly more appropriate for the present occasion.

My own interest in anomalies has centered largely about those of the vascular system. Regarding vascular anomalies, I believe I am able to say this: that even gross deviations from the normal are due to small early irregularities or arrests in development, whereby the blood stream is diverted from a so-called normal channel into one which is just as good but which is not usually selected. Let me give you an example of how this works.

Take the developing limb, for instance. In early stages, the limb-bud is filled with an equi-potential c a p i l l a r y net, out of which are to develop the definitive arteries and veins, as we find them in the finished product. As growth continues, c e r t a i n channels of the capillary net become larger than others, and acquire thicker walls, because these are the channels through which a greater volume of blood is passing. In other words, the blood flows more rapidly through some channels than others and

*Read as part of a Symposium on Congenital Visceral Anomalies conducted at the University of Oklahoma Hospital Staff Meeting, December 10, 1937.

develops a greater head of pressure. In response to this increased rate and increased pressure the capillary channel enlarges in lumen and develops muscular and elastic coats, in brief, is converted into an artery or vein, as a result of the growth stimulus provided by the increased volume of blood.

Regions of the capillary bed which are transmitting less volume of blood are converted into smaller a r t e r i e s and veins, arterioles and venules, those which transmit still less r e m a i n as capillaries, and those through which the blood has ceased to flow degenerate and finally disappear. Thus by a process of selection on the basis of blood volume a definitive or final pattern of blood vessels is condensed out of the original capillary net.

I have called this original capillary net equi-potential, b e c a u s e, theoretically at least, any one channel has an equal potentiality with any other for becoming the path of the main artery or vein. Then what is the factor which decides the path to be selected? There is one all-pervading factor governing the operation of the developing vascular system. This is the factor of *minimum work* (see Murray, 1926, and Weyrauch and De Garis, 1937). Blood, like any other liquid, flows most rapidly and under a greater head of p r e s s u r e through those channels which offer it the least work to do in overcoming friction.

Then the question arises: Since we start w i t h an equi-potential capillary system,

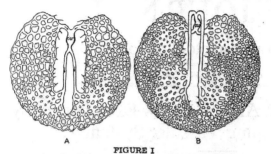

FIGURE I

This figure shows two early stages in development of the area vasculosa in the chick. It is seen that parts of the capillary net receiving blood from the heart and delivering it back to the heart are becoming enlarged by reason of the direction of flow (increased rate and pressure) imparted by the heart itself.

how does it happen that the blood does not flow with equal velocity and equal pressure through the whole system? We assume that in very early stages it does. But we must remember that in the case of the limb-bud, for instance, growth is going on very rapidly. The undifferentiated mesenchyme soon begins to lay down muscles, skeletal elements, fascias; and the nerves find their way from the neural tube into the various fields of muscles and integument. In brief, the bud is becoming a limb, with all the complexity of structure which characterizes a limb.

Let us also remember that this complexity of structure is being laid down right in the midst of our original capillary net, in fact is being laid down as a result of the metabolic exchanges provided by the blood in that capillary net. Then what happens to the capillaries?

I have already indicated the answer to this question, but am now able to answer it more fully. The environment of those capillaries has ceased to be undifferentiated mesenchyme, and has now become muscles, cartilages, fascias. And the large nerve trunks have found their way to these various differentiated parts. To this rapidly growing and changing environment the capillary net must adjust itself, and this it does very early by the enlargement of those of its channels through which the blood is passing most rapidly, and by the disappearance of those other channels through which blood has ceased to flow. The developing vascular system, then must be regarded as very labile and adjustable

to the other contents of the limb, or of any other part we may be considering. In fact, we may say that just what arteries and veins we find in a given part, such as the limb, are determined by a process of selection, or in truth by several processes of selection, wherein the vascular system always conforms to its surroundings, i.e., the muscles, nerves, etc., which form its environment. And the guiding f a c t o r in all t h e s e selections or adjustments is the factor of minimum work.

At this point I could go into much detail on the various stages of development of the forelimb arteries, since many investigations have been carried out on this subject. Rather than burden you with these details, I shall confine my illustrations and comments to a few stages in development of the area vasculosa, which exemplifies the capillary net, and to but three stages in development of the early limb arteries. The first four figures are from the work of Thoma 1893) on the histogenesis and histomechanics of the vascular system.

The question may be asked: Since we start with an equi-potential s y s t e m of capillaries, meaning a system out of which

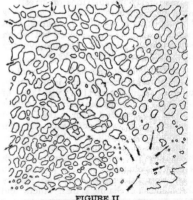

FIGURE II

This is a much enlarged view at a slightly later stage. The arrows indicate the direction of blood away from and to the heart. Some distinctly enlarged channels are apparent throughout this sample of the area vasculosa.

any sort of vascular pattern may develop, then why do we have, for instance, in the dissecting room, very much the same arteries in one arm after another? There are, of course, variations of arterial branches, great numbers of them, some quite large and conspicuous. But in general it is fair to say that the human arm has the axillary, brachial, radial, ulnar and other large arteries in rather surprising

(The following three figures are from the work of Woollard (1922) on the forelimb arteries of the pig.)

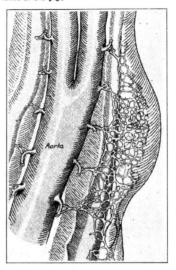

FIGURE V

A very early limb-bud stage, where the invading capillary net is shown with five segmental supplies from the dorsal aorta.

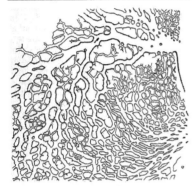

FIGURE III

A vascular tree is here clearly demonstrated as leading away from the heart through the area vasculosa. Much of the area is, and will continue to be, occupied by the capillary net.

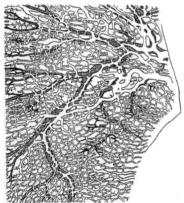

FIGURE IV

Between this and the previous figure many stages have been omitted. This figure shows well differentiated arteries (in black) and veins (in white), with an extensive capillary plexus filling the space between the larger vessels.

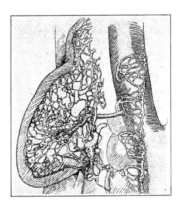

FIGURE VI

An older limb-bud stage, showing a wide-meshed capillary net and an axial artery beginning to condense in the central substance of the bud. All segmental supplies from the dorsal aorta have been lost except one, which is to become the definitive subclavian artery.

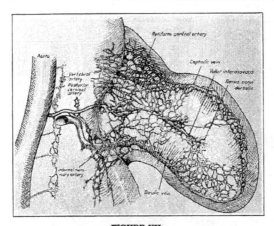

FIGURE VII

A still more advanced limb-bud, where the retiform central artery foreshadows the axillary-brachial channel. Also some elements of the subclavian artery, e.g., the vertebral, superior intercostal and internal mammary branches, are present in retiform extensions. The marginal veins, namely the cephalic and basilic, are here fairly definite structures.

regularity. In other words the text-book picture of arm arteries, at least of the larger ones, is usually not far from what one finds in the cadaver.

Then in the light of what we have already said about the development of these arteries, how do we account for this regularity? Paradoxically we are now asking, not how do we account for anomalies, but how do we account for the absence of them? The answer is not far to seek. If we go from arm to arm in the laboratory, we find the same muscles, nerves, bones. These are the inherited equipment of the arm, and this equipment does not show a wide range of variation in the human arm. Now since these structures are the ones to which the vascular system has had to adjust itself during development, we therefore have much the same arteries in one arm after another.

In some cases it is true that certain developmental stages of the arm arteries are carried over to the definitive or final pattern. Persistence of the median artery as a large trunk in the forearm is one such instance; persistence of both superficial and deep channels in the upper arm is a much more frequent instance. Such gross deviations from the normal we call anom-

alies. That they serve the arm just as well as the normal pattern, and therefore have remained, must be attributed to the fact that from the time of their early selection they have served as the paths of minimum work, to such an extent, in fact, that the normal pattern, which would usually follow such developmental stages, has either not developed at all, or has failed to compete as a path of minimum work, and therefore has not attained its customary size and distribution. This is directly analogous to the situation arising where two competing railroad systems serve the same territory. If there is a time or tariff differential in favor of one of the roads, the less favored road can not for long compete, and must eventually go out of business or restrict its service to such part of the territory as it can serve economically. In the case of arteries the tariff differential is simply a matter of work required to overcome friction.

Now if you push the question beyond this point and ask why in any given case an embryonic pattern, i.e., an anomaly, has persisted, then I am obliged to become rather general. In some few cases the presence of an unusual muscle or an aberrant arrangement of nerves, especially in the brachial plexus, may be found to explain the arterial anomaly. But in most cases one is merely confronted with an anomalous artery and nothing else. Then in such a case the best and most that anyone can say is that at some critical stage in development such an artery became and remained the path of minimum work, because of some arrest or irregularity in the development of its environment, that is, its related muscles, nerves, etc. Such an arrest or irregularity was obviously transient, and was fully compensated as development went on, since no trace of it is left, except as reflected in the anomalous artery itself.

I have discussed this question of arterial anomalies at some length, first because it is a field with which I am familiar; second because it illustrates as c l e a r l y as any other one of the fundamental categories of anomalies. Anomalies of the kind I have been discussing are the ones due to early transient arrests, which as a rule do not affect at all the economy of development or of post-natal life. A very large number of the anomalies found in the dissecting room are of this type.

Another type of anomaly which I can only mention briefly in closing, does as a rule affect the economy of development, and may even cut it short. This is the type due, not to some small local arrest or irregularity, but to an arrest of the whole embryo at an early critical stage. The first and most critical of these stages is that of gastrulation, or what corresponds to it in the mammalian embryo. If gastrulation is in any way delayed or suppressed, then the consequences are far reaching and profound. Anencephaly, cyclopia, doubling of the head or doubling farther down the axis, or complete doubling with production of single ovum twins are a few of the many things that may happen, depending on just when, to what extent and for how long the delay occurs. My time is much too short to permit a discussion of this dramatic category of anomalies.

But I do wish to leave with you the one generalization which I will allow myself on this occasion, namely that anomalies of whatever type are due to an altering of the developmental sequence, are due to a delay at some critical stage in development, either of the whole organism, or of one of its various parts. This, I believe, is the verdict of experimental morphology and by implication, of nature's own experiments which comprise the body of science called teratology.

LITERATURE CITED

Murray, C. D. 1926. The physiological principle of minimum work. I. The vascular system and the cost of blood volume. Proc. Nat. Acad. Sci., vol. 12, pp. 207-214.

Thoma, R. 1893. Untersuchungen ueber die Histogenese und Histomechanik des Gefaesssystems. 91 pp. Stuttgart.

Weyrauch, H. B. and C. F. De Garis, 1937. Normal and interrupted vascular patterns in the intestinal mesentery of the rat. An experimental study on collateral circulation. Am. Jour. Anat., vol. 61, pp. 343-372.

Woollard, H. H. 1922. The development of the principal arterial stems in the forelimb of the pig. Contributions to Embryology, No. 70, vol. 14, Carnegie Inst. Washington, pp. 141-154.

* * *

EXPLANATION OF FIGURES

Figure 1. (1 to 4 are from R. Thoma, 1893). A. Schematic representation of the area vasculosa in chick prior to torsion of the heart. B. The same after torsion of the heart.

Figure 2. A much enlarged sample of the area vasculosa in the region receiving blood from the heart. Some capillary channels are enlarged as a result of the direction of blood (increased rate and pressure).

Figure 3. A later stage of the same area; the enlargement and thickening of certain channels are clearly indicated.

Figure 4. A much advanced stage of the area vasculosa; arteries (in black) and veins (in white) are fully differentiated.

Figure 5. (5 to 7 are from H. H. Woollard, 1922). An early limb-bud stage in the pig; a capillary plexus has invaded the limb-bud and is fed by channels from the dorsal aorta.

Figure 6. A more advanced stage of the limb-bud, now showing but one channel of supply from the dorsal aorta; within the capillary plexus a central artery has begun to form.

Figure 7. A further limb-bud stage, now showing differentiation of branches from the subclavian artery, an extension of the retiform central artery and condensation of the marginal veins.

Chronic Arthritis and Undulant Fever
Their Interrelationship

E. GOLDFAIN, M.D.
OKLAHOMA CITY, OKLAHOMA

He who would treat arthritis in an informed and intelligent manner needs to approach the p r o b l e m from the broad standpoint of the internist. Arthritis is a symptom and the causes of same are many and quite varied. The joints, after all, are much like the fundus of the eye. They may r e f l e c t locally general diseased states such as tuberculosis, trauma, specific infections such as staphylococcus, gonococcus, pneumococcus, syphilis, rheumatic fever, neurologic states such as syringomyelia, constitutional states such as gout, hemophilia, intermittent hydrarthrosis, as well as atrophic arthritis and hypertrophic arthritis.

Over the entire country, as well as in Oklahoma, an intensive campaign to eradicate brucellosis or what is also known as Bang's disease in cattle, is being waged. We, as physicians, are awakening to the fact that brucellosis in man is a not at all uncommon disease state. It will often explain many cases of chronic illness otherwise unexplainable.

That being the case, a careful study of the relation of undulant fever to chronic arthritis is not only timely but important.

Six types of undulant fever now are being listed. In the order of their importance they are:

1. Chronic or subclinical.
2. Ambulatory.
3. Latent infections.
4. Undulating fever.
5. Continuous fever.
6. Rare acute malignant type.

It is the ambulatory and especially the chronic or subclinical cases of brucellosis in man that are of interest to him who would study carefully any case giving a history of rheumatic or arthritic symptoms.

The following symptoms are often found in the subclinical or chronic type of brucellosis: arthralgia, arthritis, headache, backache, malaise, weakness, neuritis or neuralgia, myositis, leukopenia, secondary anemia, spondylitis, persistent joint stiffness.

These symptoms, in toto or in part, may well lead to a diagnosis of chronic rheumatic disease or chronic arthritis without ever suspecting brucellosis unless tested for properly.

It has been quite definitely proven that the agglutination test may be negative in at least five per cent of the cases. In our experience the per cent of negative agglutination tests will run higher, in the chronic cases at least.

Other diagnostic m e a s u r e s therefore must be used to determine definitely its presence. Those other means are the opsonocytophagic test and the skin test. These two tests may well give information as to whether a patient is actively infected, immune or simply susceptible. K e l l e r,

Pharris and Gaub, in their J. A. M. A. article October 24, 1936, bring out this diagnostic procedure v e r y nicely. Utilizing their procedure 50 cases of apparent rheumatic and arthritic disease were tested. Fourteen cases gave positive agglutination tests; 26 gave opsonic index tests of slight to marked phagocytosis to a degree of 0 to 20 per cent; 16 cases yielded 20 to 60 per cent mild, moderate or marked phagocytosis, and eight cases gave 60 to 100 per cent phagocytosis of moderate to marked degree. Of the 50 cases skin tested, 36 gave positive skin tests of mild to severe degree.

The results are best shown in Tables I, II and III.

TABLE I

Determination of phagocytosis activity as reported by Keller, Pharris and Gaub, and adapted from Huddleson, J o h n s o n and Hamann. The opsonocytophagic activity of the blood.

Classification	Number of bacteria per polymorphuclear cell
1. Negative	None
2. Slight	1 to 20
3. Moderate	21 to 40
4. Marked	41 or more

TABLE II

The diagnosis of undulant fever according to results of the skin, agglutination and opsonocytophagic tests as reported by Keller, Pharris and Gaub, and adapted from Huddleson, Johnson and Hamann.

Agglutina-tion Test	Skin Test	Opsonocytophagic Power of Blood	Status Toward Brucella
Negative	Negative	Cells negative to 20% slight phagocytosis	Susceptible
Negative	Positive	Cells negative to 40% marked phagocytosis	Infected
Positive	Positive	Cells negative to 40% marked phagocytosis	Infected
Negative	Positive	Cells 60% to 100% marked phagocytosis	Immune
Positive	Positive	Cells 60% to 100% marked phagocytosis	Immune

In other words, 31 cases of apparent rheumatic or arthritic disease were diagnosed as cases of active brucellosis, in addition to other diagnoses. Five c a s e s were diagnosed as having a c q u i r e d immunity to brucellosis.

Of the 31 cases diagnosed as actively infected with brucellosis only 11 cases, or 35.5 per cent, yielded partial or complete agglutination. These 31 cases yielded opsonocytophagic tests and skin tests indicating active infection with brucellosis.

TABLE III

Fifty cases of apparent rheumatic or arthritic disease studied as shown below.

Agglutina-tion Test	Skin Test	Opsonocytophagic Power of Blood	Status Toward Brucella
14 cases positive or complete agglutination		26 cases 0% to 20% mild to marked phago-cytosis	14 cases suscept-ible; 15 actively infected
		16 cases 20% to 60% moderate to marked phago-cytosis	16 cases actively infected
36 cases mild to severe allergic skin reaction		8 cases 60% to 100% moderate to marked phago-cytosis	31 cases actively infected; 5 cases immune

A list of symptoms most commonly present in those cases diagnosed as actively infected with brucellosis and the percentage of cases in which these symptoms were noted are:

		Approximate per cent
1.	Arthralgia	100.0
2.	Backache	90.0
3.	Neuritis and neuralgia	48.4
4.	Myositis	32.0
5.	Malaise	38.7
6.	Spondylitis	6.4
7.	Neurasthenia	26.0
8.	Anorexia	38.7
9.	Constipation	77.0
10.	Slight pyrexia	29.0
11.	Headache	61.0
12.	Persistent joint stiffness	26.0
13.	Psychasthenia	3.0
14.	Secondary anemia	93.0

TABLE IV. Detailed report on the fifty cases studied as shown in Table III.

	Skin Test	Opsonic Index	Agglutination	Brucella Status	Other Diagnosis
EH	Negative	16% slight phagocytosis	Negative	Susceptible	Atrophic arthritis
WBH	Negative	16% slight	Negative	Susceptible	Fibrositis
JCH	Negative	24% marked	Negative	Susceptible	Atrophic arthritis
WBP	Negative	8% marked	Negative	Susceptible	Hypertrophic arthritis
WHM	Negative	2% moderate	Negative	Susceptible	Atrophic arthritis
WES	Negative	None	Negative	Susceptible	Atrophic arthritis
CKM	Negative	64% marked	Negative	Susceptible	Atrophic arthritis
MH	Negative	1% slight	Negative	Susceptible	Fibrositis
LBC	Negative	4% slight	Negative	Susceptible	Psychoneurosis; fibrositis
BR	Negative	16% slight	Negative	Susceptible	Hypertrophic arthritis
LR	Negative	Negative	Negative	Susceptible	Atrophic arthritis
NH	Negative	Negative	Negative	Susceptible	Hypertrophic arthritis
PC	Negative	20% slight	Negative	Susceptible	Chr. fibrositis
BDJ	Negative	20% slight	Negative	Susceptible	Psychasthenia
AJB	Positive	16% slight	Negative	Active	Chr. fibrositis
RFC	Positive	16% slight	Negative	Active	Hypertrophic arthritis
GE	Positive	20% marked	Negative	Active	Neurasthenia; chr. fibrositis
EWH	Positive	20% marked	Complete	Active	Chr. choroiditis
CNH	Positive	8% moderate	Negative	Active	Hypertrophic arthritis
JBT	Positive		Partial	Active	Chr. fibrositis
JT	Positive	12% slight	Negative	Active	Hypertrophic arthritis
JGS	Positive	4% marked	Partial	Active	Chr. fibrositis
MD	Positive	8% moderate	Negative	Active	Hypertrophic arthritis
CHH	Positive	12% slight	Partial	Active	Atrophic arthritis
LEM	Positive	None	Complete	Active	Atrophic arthritis
CWI	Positive	20% slight	Negative	Active	Psychasthenia; chr. fibrositis
FEC	Positive	24% slight	Negative	Active	Sciatica
CE	Positive	32% marked	Negative	Active	Atrophic arthritis
MI	Positive	40% marked	Complete	Active	Chr. fibrositis
JH	Positive	40% slight	Negative	Active	Chr. fibrositis
CDM	Positive	28% moderate	Complete	Active	Ankylosing spondylitis
AMM	Positive	20% to 60%	Complete	Active	Hypertrophic arthritis
ELL	Positive	36% slight	Negative	Active	Atrophic arthritis
RAL	Positive	24% slight	Negative	Active	Atrophic arthritis
GT	Positive	32% moderate	Negative	Active	Atrophic arthritis
BF	Positive	27% slight	Negative	Active	Atrophic arthritis
AAL	Positive	28% moderate	Negative	Active	Psychoneurosis
CAW	Positive	40% moderate	Complete	Active	Atrophic arthritis
GWB	Positive	60% marked	Partial	Active	Asthenia; psychoneurosis
WJC	Positive	64% slight	Negative	Active	Atrophic arthritis
HLD	Positive	80% slight	Negative	Active	Hypertrophic arthritis
GJP	Positive	20% to 60%	Complete	Active	Psychasthenia
MO	Positive	45% slight	Negative	Active	Psychoneurosis
POW	Positive	96% slight	Negative	Active	Sciatica
WHS	Positive	52% moderate	Negative	Active	Neurasthenia; salpingitis
BB	Positive	72% marked	Negative	Immune	Atrophic arthritis
GG	Positive	82% marked	Complete	Immune	Atrophic arthritis
AP	Positive	76% marked	Negative	Immune	Atrophic arthritis
CAF	Positive	98% marked	Complete	Immune	Hypertrophic arthritis
RS	Positive	100% marked	Partial	Immune	Atrophic arthritis

Before a case of active brucella infection was so diagnosed, the skin test had to be definitely positive. In addition, the presence of an active opsonocytophagic test in which up to 60 per cent of the neutrophiles were revealing mild, moderate or marked phagocytosis, was required. The presence of a positive agglutination test was desirable. However, a diagnosis of active brucellosis was made even though the agglutination test was not positive in the presence of the above skin and opsonic index tests.

Treatment has been that of v a c c i n e therapy with the brucella bacterine, and general medical measures.

A report on the results of treatment in these cases with the specific bacterine and the effects of such treatment on the opsonic index and skin test as well as agglutination test will be made at a later date.

I desire at this time to give credit to Miss Rita Robinson of the State Health Laboratory, who cooperated with me in compiling statistics for this s u r v e y, she doing the agglutination tests and opsonic index tests on all of the cases. I also wish to thank Dr. M. R. Beyer of the State Health Department for his suggestions in respect to paying more attention to this disease as having etiologic significance in many c a s e s of apparent rheumatic and arthritic disease.

LITERATURE REFERENCES

1. Huddleson, I. F.; Johnson, H. W., and Hamann, E. E.: A Study of the Opsono-Cytophagic Power of the Blood and Allergic Skin Reaction in Brucella Infection and Immunity in Man, Am. J. Pub. Health 23:917-929 (Sept.) 1933.

2. Huddleson, I. F.: Brucella Infections in Animals and Man, Commonwealth Fund, 1934.

3. Glynn, E. E. and Cox, G. L.: Variations in the Inherent Phagocytic Power of Leukocytes, J. Path. & Bact. 14:90-131, 1910.

4. Angle, Fred E.: Treatment of Acute and Chronic Brucellosis (Undulant Fever), Personal Observation of One Hundred Cases Over a Period of Seven Years, J. A. M. A. 105:12, 939-941, Sept., 1935.

5. Bruce, David: Notes on the Discovery of a Micro-Organism in Malta Fever, Practitioner 39:161, 1887.

6. Bang, Bernhard: The Etiology of Contagious Abortion, Ztschr. f. Tiermedizin 1:241, 1897.

7. Evans, Alice C.: Further Studies on Bacterium Abortus and Related Bacteria, J. Infect. Dis. 22:580 (June) 1918.

8. Evans, Alice C.: Chronic Brucellosis, J. A. M. A. 103:665 (Sept. 1) 1934.

9. Simpson, W. M.: Undulant Fever (Brucellosis), J. Indiana M. A. 27:564-570 (Dec.) 1934.

10. Cumston, C. G.: The Treatment of Malta Fever, M. J. & Rec. 121:219-220 (Feb. 18) 1925.

11. DeFinis, G.: L'immunoterapia dii tifo, dei paratifi a della febbre mediterranea con i vaccini lisizzati di Christina e Caronia, Pediatria 31:11-23 (Jan.) 1923.

12. Schilling, G. S.; Magee, C. F., and Leitch, F. M.: Treatment of Undulant Fever, with an Autogenous Antigen, J. A. M. A. 96:1945-1948 (June 6) 1931.

13. Harris, H. J.: Undulant Fever: Difficulties in Diagnosis and Treatment, New York State J. Med. 34:1017-1021 (Dec. 1) 1934.

14. Angle, F. E.: The Treatment of Undulant Fever with Vaccine, J. Kansas M. Soc. 30:323 (Oct.) 1929.

15. Janbon: Diagnosis, Arch. Med. Chir. de Normandie, pp. 3803-3844, Aug., 1936.

16. Winans, H. M.: Internat. Clin. 3:131-142 (Sept.) 1936.

17. Fillipovich, A. N.: Abortin in Allergic Diagnosis in Man, Sovit. vrach. zhur. pp. 34-36, Jan. 15, 1936.

18. Kemp, H. A.: Applications of Bacteriology of Brucella Group to Clinical Problems of Brucellosis, Texas St. J. of Med. 32:279-284 (Aug.) 1936.

19. Engel, C., and Vigilain, M. R.: Bacterial Allergy, Experimental Studies, Klin. Wchnschr. 15:638-640, May 2, 1936.

20. Baserga, A.: Clinical Diff. Diagnosis of Various Forms of Brucellosis, Riv. san siciliana 24:357-363, April 1, 1936.

21. Denham, C. R., and Fitch, C. P.: Modified Technic for Agglutination, J. Inf. Dis. 59:287-295, Nov.-Dec., 1936.

22. Higginbotham, M., and Heathman, L. S.: Precipitin and Complement Fixation Reactions of Polysaccharide Extracts of Brucella, J. Inf. Dis. 59:30-34, July-Aug., 1936.

---o---

Consideration of the Varied Symptomatology* of the Prostate and Verumontanum

ALLEN R. RUSSELL, M.D.
McALESTER CLINIC

It is well to consider in the beginning that the symptomatology associated with a prostatitis or prostatic condition cannot be complete without including also the verumontanum and the posterior urethra, because in practically all cases there is an associated involvement of the latter two, just as there is in the kidney tissue with pyelitis. The purpose of this paper is for the consideration and we might say review, of the more common symptoms, and some s p e c i a l attention to the unusual symptoms that arise from the above named tissues. Prostatic hypertrophy w i l l be omitted except where it is referred to as a

*Read before the Section on Genito-Urinary Diseases and Syphilology, Annual Meeting, Oklahoma State Medical Association, Tulsa, May, 1937.

direct association of an inflammatory process.

. With the anatomy of the prostate in mind, it can readily be understood why the urethra, seminal vesicles ,and the verumontanum, are so closely related in their pathological conditions. Regardless of which may be primarily involved, the infection will extend through the ducts, posterior urethra, and the minute openings, to result also in an infection of the rest of the group. Also further extension may involve the vas deferens and epididymis, as is commonly the case. With an inflammatory condition in the small ducts and minute openings of these different structures, it may be entirely closed temporarily or permanently, and as a result, absorption of pus takes place in the same manner as it would from an abscessed tonsil.

Locally, c h r o n i c infections of these structures are common causes of a persistent urethral discharge, or secretion, especially in the morning, which persists for an indefinite period of time to re-occur, and with acute exacerbations of the chronic process, even after long periods of absence from any subjective or objective symptoms.

Here it is well to consider the rich nerve supply of the prostate and it's associated tissues, which accounts to a large extent for the great variety of symptoms. The principal nerve supply is from the hypogastric plexus, which also supplies to some extent, all the viscera of the pelvic cavity, and is formed by the union of numerous filaments, which descend on each side from the abdominal aortic plexus, and from the lumbar ganglia, being continuous by dividing below into two lateral portions which form the pelvic plexus, often termed the i n f e r i o r hypogastric plexus. This also enervates the viscera of the pelvic cavity, and is situated along the side of the rectum, giving off many filaments to the rectum. There is a separate plexus which is called the prostatic plexus, which enervates directly, the prostate gland, seminal vesiculae, portion of the posterior urethra, and the erectile t i s s u e s. From the above plexuses there are many trunks and filaments, continuous with the nerve supply to practically all of the tisues from the level of the umbilicus to the knees.

Therefore, it is readily seen that generally the symptomatology may be almost unlimited, and from these poorly drained foci of inflammation, s e p t i c material, either in the form of infectious emboli or toxins may at any. time escape into the circulation, and lodge in the various parts of the body, producing most any systemic manifestation, but especially in the form of disturbances in the synovial membranes, the myocardium, meninges, or eye, or may result in a group of symptoms dependent upon a toxemia which produces mental derangement in the form of neurasthenia in it's broadest sense. The train of symptoms dependent upon prostatic inflammations, and it's associated conditions, varies enough to make up definte groups which may be considered separately.

First: Inflammatory group. This may be characterized by a febrile state, obstinate or intermittent urethral discharge, associated with a varied degree of tenderness, swelling, and distention of the pelvic organs, with one or many of the various systemic conditions resulting from a toxic absorption.

Secondly: The rheumatic or metastatic group, which includes joints, tendons, muscles, bones, and eye lesions, as a secondary inflammatory process.

Third: The pain group. Under this may be included those with persistent perineum pain, sometimes accentuated by defecation and often referred to the rectum, and extremely disturbing to the individual. There may also be associated neurasthenic symptoms, painful erections without s e x u a l stimulus, frequent nocturnal emissions, and associated bloody semen. The great percentage of disturbance of sexual function is the alleged sequence of an inflammatory condition of the prostate and it's associated pelvic organs in practically every case, but is allied rather definitely to the verumontanum. In this group there is usually a history of previous urethritis, obscure pain under the glans penis, along the shaft, in the perineum, over the pubes, in the region of the sacro-iliac joint, down the thighs, or along the sciatic nerve, practically assimilating a sciatica. In short, the pain may be anywhere in the pelvis or the adjacent regions. On the other hand it may amount only to a discomfort or sensation which the patient will not refer to as an actual pain, then again he may classify it merely as an itching. There may be any degree of pain or discomfort in the form of burning urination, tenesmus, frequency, etc. It may be well to mention here that often times patients who have had their prostate massaged over a long period of time, and the secretions be practically free of pus and these symptoms not having been relieved, until endoscopic treatment with dilatation and direct application to the veru alone, will the distressing symptoms be relieved. There is no doubt that some of the patients who have been termed sexual neurasthenias have been the result of just such conditions, which could have been relieved by thorough examination of these structures for the various conditions above mentioned, because a thorough, systematic, treatment of these will often secure surprisingly good results.

Frequently symptoms of urinary obstruction and irritability find their cause a l m o s t entirely in the verumontanum, which is found enlarged, swollen, tender, and at times irregular and cystic. The so-called urethritis cystica chronica. These types of cases are as a rule, only relieved

by endoscopic treatments with local applications, puncture, removal, and treatment of the cysts. It is also well to mention that in some patients, with the above conditions, the healing process leaves the patient with a vesicle contracture, which is chiefly the result of the bladder having emptied itself so frequently that it has not been subjected to normal distention, and if this does not take care of itself, after clearing up the condition of the veru, it may be necessary to gradually dilate the bladder by hydraulic distention until it is remedied.

In closing, I would like to say, that rectal palpation, massage, and microscopic examination of the prostatic fluid, are not in themselves sufficient and complete when the patient continues to have symptoms, and these tests show no evidence of pathology, because this is a very sensitive area, and a little pus can go a long ways in causing trouble in such a highly sensitive locality; and in many cases, unless you go further, with endoscopic examination of posterior urethra and verumontanum, to find the cause, treat it, and eliminate it, these symptoms cannot be completely relieved.

————o————

Endocrinology; Its Practical Application in Gynecology*

P. N. Charbonnet, M.D.
E. O. Johnson, M. D.
TULSA, OKLAHOMA

INTRODUCTION

To the average clinician the implication in the title of this paper, "Practical Endocrinilogy," is a paradoxical one. For some time endocrinology has been regarded as a fertile field for research workers, but inasmuch as there is a lag between academic discoveries and clinical application, most practicing physicians have been reluctant to accept or try endocrinological

*Read before the Tulsa County Medical Society on April 12, 1937.

therapy on their patients. This has been a j u s t conservatism f r o m the clinicians' standpoint, especially since the early preparations of whole glandular extracts, dessications, etc., contained so little of the active hormone principle that they were practically inert pharmacalogically. However, since the methods of extraction have improved, the active principles not only identified but also synthesized chemically with their structural formulae becoming known, an added impetus has been brought about so that all branches of medicine are necessarily interested. Practically every speciality has a hormonal aspect. The pediatrician explains the brown vaginal discharge of the newborn babe on a hormonal basis. The orthopedist must always keep in mind calcium intake and parathyroid function; the general surgeon has to remove certain glands which produce hormones, as the thyroid; the brain surgeon deals with abnormalities of the pituitary, and so it goes with each speciality. Any one who does not have a working knowledge of the physiology of the endocrine system in their particular speciality will miss the proper interpretation of many maladies therein.

There are several f a c t o r s which have necessarily impeded the dissemination of knowledge in endocrinology. One is the great confusion in the nomenclature of the hormones and active chemical principles, with the many synonyms for the same hormone. The original discoverer attaches a name as a rule, then others who are first to verify his experiment give a different name. These added to the various drug manufacturers' trade names for the same principle have placed the nomenclature in a furious state of chaos. Recently, however, in regard to the ovarian hormones, Allen, C a r v e r, Butenandt, and Slatta[88] agreed to use the term *"Progesterone"* for progestin, the corpus luteum hormone. Also the A.M.A. council on pharmacy[89] recently took the following action in regard to the estrogenic substances, and the follicular hormone of the ovary, or the so-called female sex hormone. "Accordingly, the council, on the recommendation of the advisory committee, decided (a) to adopt the system of nomenclature based on the root estr-; (b) To retain *Theelin, Theelol,* and *Dihydrotheelin* as synonyms for the compounds known in the aforementioned system as *Estrone*†, *Estriol*, and *Estradiol*, respectively, and (c) To adopt the term *Estrogenic* to describe those compounds or extracts which, in addition to their other physiologic properties, produce estrus, and to adopt the noun Estrogen as the collective term for all the substances having those properties." These rules were made with the courteous withdrawal of trademark rights of some of the drug com-

†Estrone is used as a synonym for Theelin, estrin, etc., in this paper and does not refer to a trade name, or product of any particular drug company.

panies. Further active regulatory participation in the naming of hormones by the A.M.A. council should aid the clinician materially in grasping the essentials and keeping up with the progress in endocrinology.

Another factor which causes great confusion is that of the dosage. This was adequately and impressively brought out by Dr. C. D. Leake[24] of San Francisco, who in his discussion of Mazer and Israel's paper said: "—it might be b e t t e r to express dosage of that agent (estrone) in terms of milligrams than in terms of rat units. The situation is quite comparable to such a proposition as prescribing m o r p h i n e in terms of pain-relieving units; no one does that. One should remember, of course, that bio-assay is merely a method of estimating chemical concentration by means of a biologic end-point." Not only is this biologic dosage confusing, but the dosage for each individual patient is based on a clinical estimation (refer to General Principle—B) which requires much clinical experience. Laboratory tests to determine the lack or excess of hormones are still too elaborate and expensive for the general practicing clinician.

The third factor contributory to confusion is that which is brought about by the various drug houses in their descriptive catalogues of their endocrine products. In their haste to be the first to produce and distribute glandular preparations for hormonal therapy, they have included many of such products which have no established value clinically as yet. We have one such catalogue which lists preparations from 22 separate structures of animals, including s u c h structures as tonsils, parotid, and prostate tissue. While this particular company states in the first of their booklets that many of the preparations are not of established value, the busy practitioner who rarely reads it but glances over those preparations which are for sale, gets a very misleading conception of the status of therapy in endocrinology.

While much of the foregoing discussion has been directed toward endocrinology in general, we intend to take up only that part of endocrinology which pertains to gynecology, keeping in mind that this is a necessity for discussion only and that one must be familiar with all the general principles of endocrinology as well as those pertaining to gynecology.

Novak and others have pointed out that outside of pain the most frequent symptom encountered in gynecology is that of a disturbance in menstruation. When one considers that practically all that is known about menstruation is based on an endocrine interpretation, then one can conceive of the importance of a c l e a r working knowledge of endocrinology to the gynecologist. And the gynecologist who fails to see this will soon fall behind in this rapidly developing, fascinating subject, the therapy in which applies to a great many of his patients in d a i l y practice. The gynecologist interested in menstruation, is concerned with the gonad stimulating hormones of the anterior pituitary gland, prolan A which stimulates the follicular development of the ovary and prolan B which stimulates lutenization; also, the ovarian hormones estrone (theelin, progynon, estrin) which is derived from the follicle, and the progesterone (progestin) which is the hormone of the corpus luteum. Our discussion will then be limited entirely to these hormones, and oftimes they will be spoken of collectively as the sex hormones. A detailed discussion of the physiology and hormonal relationship between the ovaries, pituitary and endometrial development will not be taken up.

While there are many interesting speculative fields being opened up by the chemist with his fascinating structural formulae[112] showing the relationship between the sterols of plants, vitamin D, various coal tar carcinogenic compounds, and the sex hormones; and by the far reaching clinicians in their attempts to produce simple methods of contraception[90-91-92-93-95] and sterilization[94-98] by using hormones, no attempt will be made to d i s c u s s them. Rather we will adhere to those conditions in gynecology in which definite results have been obtained clinically on the human. Every attempt will be made to leave out, even in the discussion, therapy which has been used on animals only, or therapy of conditions which are still disputed, such as ovarian cysts[100] and Involutional Melancholia[96-97].

ENDOCRINOLOGICAL PRINCIPLES

Just as with other forms of therapy, there are certain principles which must be followed. The principles of treatment of general endocrinological disorders also apply to those in gynecology. Thus, we may divide the principles of treatment into general and those pertaining to gynecology. It is assumed that one has a knowledge of the potency and cost of the various commercial products, if economical and effective results are to be obtained. Some of the principles of treatment are:

General[1-2]

A. Glandular function is not restricted to a single gland, but an interrelationship exists between the many glands of internal secretion.

B. Glandular dysfunctions are based on the gland being hyper, or hypoactive, or absent. Therefore, one should try to determine w h e t h e r the therapy desired s h o u l d be substitutional, inhibitive, or stimulative.

C. No hormone, when administered, has any direct effect on its parent gland.

D. Adequate vitamins and other necessary food factors are essential to gland function, as iodine, calcium, etc. Vitamin E deficiency interferes with gonadal function, just as lack of vitamin D does with parathyroid, vitamin B with thyroid, vitamin C with adrenal cortex, and vitamin A with anterior pituitary hormone.

E. Methods used elsewhere in medicine are of value, such as good hygiene, adequate rest, treatment of secondary factors, as anemia, etc.

Gynecological[4-5-6-7]

A. Mode of administration: The effectiveness of many of the sex hormones depends on the mode of administration. The most common routes are: hypodermic, percutaneous[8], oral, rectal (enema), and vaginal[9-10] methods of administration. Tachezy[11] treated oligomenorrhea, and amenorrhea, with good results by giving urine of pregnant women as e n e m a s in 100 c.c. d o s e s. Mazer and Israel[12] showed that Theelin given by hypodermic injection is t w i c e as effective as by oral injection when judged by the rate of excretion and absorption. Zondek[8] obtained good results by percutaneous route in treating acne and suggested its use over joints in arthritis in cases of menopause.

B. The sexual glands are characterized by their periodicity of function in the female as manifested by menstruation, pregnancy, and lactation.

C. The third principle is that of the threshold of effectiveness. Hormone storage apparently does not occur in the body, so that the response of an organ depends upon a minimum hormone level over a period sufficient for such a response to occur.

D. The gonads do not have the power of self-regulation. Zondek has referred to the pituitary as the "motor" of the gonads.

E. Hypophyseal activity is modified by the gonad hormones; there is a reciprocal interaction between the gonads and the pituitary.

F. Frequent pelvic examination with inspection of the vagina and cervix in order to watch for untoward results is also necessary. Inasmuch as the dosage of these sex hormones is a matter of clinical judgement, subject to error, and because adverse reports of side actions are being reported (see contraindications) frequent examination should be made, watching the size and consistency of the ovaries, uterus and cervix. No doctor who does not have his patients willing to submit to periodic pelvic examinations should treat them for any length of time with large doses of gonadotropic or estrogenic hormones. This should be axiomatic until further d a t a proves them to be entirely harmless.

ORGANOTHERAPY IN GYNECOLOGY

Of the many gynecological disorders in which hormonal therapy has been tried, there are only comparatively a few conditions in which definite results of value have been attained. These are: gonorrheal vulvo-vaginitis in prepubertal girls, senile v a g i n i t i s, the vasomotor symptoms of menopause, pruritus vulvae, functional uterine hemorrhage, primary dysmenorrhea, habitual abortion, and some cases of amenorrhea and sterility. These will be taken up in order, listing the dosage used by various authors.

Gonorrheal v u l v o-vaginitis in girls: Lewis[13] in 1933 advocated the use of daily injections of 50 rat units (150 IU) of es-

trone for a period of as long as two months. He showed that by the use of estrone the epithelial lining of the vagina of the prepubital girl which is very susceptible to the gonococcus could be built up[14] to a close simulation of the postpubertal vagina which is known to be very resistant to the gonococcal infection. Also the reaction of the vaginal secretion is changed from neutral or alkaline to acid[104] which helped. Many were afraid of the harmful effects on the breasts from the occasional swellings that were noted. Also, some felt that the hyperemia of the internal pelvic structures which was produced might favor the ascent of the infection or later on cause some disorder in the menstruation. With the exception of Witherspoon[15] all investigators[16-17-18-19-20-24] have been getting good results with no ill effects. Te Linde[21] and others [19] have obtained better results from the use of vaginal suppositories containing estrone (Amniotin suppositories, 1,000 I.U.) which remove the necessity of so many hypodermic injections, and can be inserted by the mother. The dosage as suggested by some authors are:

A. [20]Estrone 10,000 units intramuscularly the first day, 4,000 units daily by mouth thereafter until the smears are negative (14-18 days). Then give 3,000 units daily for 14 days.

B. [19]Daily use of vaginal suppositories containing estrone 1,000 units for 14-18 days supplemented with oral or hypodermic thereafter.

C. [24]Estrone, 1,000 rat units by hypodermic three times a week for six-eight weeks.

Senile Vaginitis: Davis showed in 1935 that the use of estrogenic substances (amniotin) relieved the ill effects of the atrophic vaginal epithelium with its concomitant, discharge, and burning which is found in postmenopausal life and cases of artificial menopause produced by X-ray, radium, or surgery. Jacoby et al.[23] did not get as good results, but felt that its use was justified. The justification of the treatment with estrogenic substance is b a s e d on building up the atrophic epithelium of the vagina. The treatment may have to be repeated from time to time if symptoms recur.

Dosage: [22]500 IU estrone, three times a week for six weeks.

Vasomotor Symptoms of Menopause: While there is no unanimity of opinion on the etiology of menopausal symptoms, it is considered that either the withdrawal of estrin or the hyperfunctional state of the anterior pituitary lobe[24-25-26-27] is the chief factor. Several investigators[25-26-27-31-38] have shown that the amelioration of the symptoms is concomitant with a definite decrease of the gonadatropic factor of the hypophysis. The good results obtained by estrone therapy is explained by Albright[26] in that estrone stops the over production or decreases the production of prolan A.

The menopausal symptoms are many, varied and include besides hot flashes and sweats, headaches, nervousness, insomnia, and fluctuant hypertension. In no condition has the use of estrogenic substances been so valuable and effective. Several early investigators[28-29-30] used folliculin with excellent results. Pratt[34] has been skeptical of his results, however, and tried injections of saline instead of estrogenic preparations without noticing any difference. Not infrequently a low grade fluctuating hypertension has been noted in the menopause. Liebhart reported excellent results in controlling this by the use of estrogenic substances. However, others [25-36] reported poor results and were unable to duplicate Liebhart's work. Shaefer[37] reports that with the use of two c.c. of aqueous Theelin three times a week the hypertention was held in abeyance. In spite of a few controversial reports in regard to the results with particular symptoms, the use of estrogenic substances has been a very valuable form of therapy in menopause. The treatment need only be used periodically when the symptoms are worst, so that continuous treatment is not necessary. The dosages as used by several investigators are:

A. [24]Estradiol benzoate 10,000 rat units hypodermically every fourth day until the major symptoms subside. Then gradual withdrawal of the medication.

B. Novak[6] gives estrone (Theelin) 1,000 IU hypodermically every day, or every other day until symptoms are relieved, then gradual withdrawal of the hypodermic medication and changing to oral tablets.

C. [38]Frank finds that estrone in hypodermic doses of 4,000 R. U. on alternate days until a total of 24,000 R. U. has been taken is satisfactory. He finds that the relief is not permanent.

Migraine[39-40]. Glass[39] finds that a total dosage of 8,000 to 32,000 IU of estrone gives relief of headaches for a period of six to 36 months.

The use of vaginal smears[57] has been suggested as a clinical laboratory test of the results of the use of estrone in these cases of menopause.

Pruritis Vulvae[106-110]: Kaufman[41] used injections of estrogenic substances in a case of pruritis vulvae which had menopausal symptoms, also with excellent results.

Functional Uterine Hemorrhage: The endocrinological disorders of uterine bleeding have been known to be due to the ovarian dysfunction of a failure of ovulation[52-6], with abnormal persistence of estrin stimulation and absence of progesterone effect since corpora lutea are not formed. This is associated with a hyperplastic endometrium[58-59]. Progesterone is employed along with Antuitrin "S." Wilson and Kurzrok[42] attribute the effectiveness of these substances to their action on the anterior pituitary causing an inhibition of the bleeding hormone. Therapy is directed toward stimulating the formation of corpora lutea by giving the luteinizing factor of the anterior pituitary (prolan B) and substitution therapy of progesterone.

A. Progesterone[6] 1 R. U. is given by hypodermic for one to six doses if the bleeding is menorrhagic in type. These injections are started as soon as the menstrual flow starts. If the bleeding is of metrorrhagic type, Antuitrin "S" is given in doses of 200 R. U. for several injections before the progesterone is started.

B. We use the combination of Antuitrin "S" and progesterone in the menorrhagic type of bleeding.

Primary Dysmenorrhea: Reynolds has shown that in general, with an increase in estrone, there is an increase in rhythmic activity of the uterus while progesterone is the normal inhibitant. Based on this conception the endocrine therapy has been directed towards the administration of prolan B (Follutein, Antophysin, Antuitrin "S") and progesterone. The results have been very unsatisfactory previous to the chemical synthesis of progestin by Butenandt in 1934. However, clinicians using the newer preparations since show that this is a valuable form of treatment in selected cases. Israel[43] made a careful study and along with Campbell[44] who used corporin, and Browne[45] and Witherspoon[85] who used follutein obtained good results but only for a short duration. They found that there was no assurance of permanent r e l i e f. Elden[46] using progesterone, obtained good results and observed no delay in the menstruation or change in the character of the succeeding periods. T h e s e authors use the following dosage:

A. [6]Progesterone one rat unit, or pregnancy urine preparations (Follutein, Antuitrin "S," Antophysin) 100-200 units as daily intramuscular injections beginning three-four days before the period and continuing until the flow is well established.

B. [30]Progesterone 2/25 to o n e R. U. three-six days before the period in a single or divided doses.

C. [24]Estrone with poor results.

Habitual Abortion: Whereas previous results with c o r p u s luteum extracts, and residue have been of questionable value, the newer preparations which have been marketed since the chemical synthesis of progestin (progesterone) are encouraging. Kane[47] reported unusual success in 36 out of 40 cases with progesterone.

Dosage: [1-6]Progesterone 1/5 to 1 rabbit unit two-three times a week as soon as pregnancy is definitely established and continued past the period when the previous miscarriages occurred.

Amenorrhea: Several investigators[33-34-35-24-0-107-48-50-51-32] have been able to produce menstruation in cases of amenorrhea and even in castrated women after Kaufman[49] was first able to show that it could be done. However, it requires massive doses of estrin and progesterone to accomplish this and there is no assurance that it will be permanent, but a repetition of the treatment may be necessary for each menstruation. Amenorrhea may be classified[60-51-53] into several groups b a s e d upon lack of proper function of the ovarian hormones

and, or the gondatropic hormones which stimulate the ovary to their production. Several c l i n i c i a n s use the following dosage:

A. [6]Estrone 10,000-20,000 IU, intramuscularly daily or every other day for 6-10 doses. Thyroid therapy can be used in addition.

B. [24]300,000 rat units of estrone in three divided doses and repeated monthly yielded 20 per cent results.

C. [51]Dosages of estrone 100,000 R. U. are usually required to bring about the first menstruation in primary Amenorrhea and about 50,000 R. U. in secondary Amenorrhea.

D. [83]In a castrated woman: E s t r o n e 50,000 rat units and 12 to 14 rabbit units of progestin produced bleeding.

With doses of this magnitude it is a q u e s t i o n whether the unmarried girl should take them if she feels well, since her sexual glands have had only a partial test of their function.

Sterility: Very little of the endocrine factors involved in certain cases of sterility is known, especially since Novak has discovered that many of these girls have an anovulatory menstruation. We do n o t know yet just exactly which endocrine factors cause ovulation. However, there are three glands[56] the hypofunction of which are responsible for most sterilities; anterior pituitary, ovaries, a n d thyroid. They are listed in descending order of frequency, the pituitary being the most frequent offender.

Endometrial biopsies according to Novak's suction curette technique[71] aids materially in diagnosing the ovarian sterilities. If the endometrium[109] s h o w s evidence of proliferation without a secretory stage then one can conclude that there is an absence of progesterone which in turn shows the absence of a corpus luteum and therefore ovulation has not occurred.

The treatment is directed toward the correction of the under-functioning gland at fault. Thyroid seems to be of value in small doses in all types of sterility based on a hormonal disturbance.

Some investigators[61-62] h a v e reported good results from the use of estrogenic substances (Progynon B) in doses of 100,-

000 to 500,000 IU given intramuscularly on the ninth to eleventh day of the cycle. Others[56] feel that ovarian hormones are contraindicated inasmuch as these hormones cannot stimulate (rule in endocrinology) their parent gland (the ovary) into activity, and inasmuch as some reports have been made on the harmful effects in animals on the parent gland there is no hope in this therapy. These same observers feel that the use of the gonadotropic hormones (Prolan A and B) may aid in stimulating the ovary and be of some benefit in the treatment of sterility. The treatment as suggested by several authors is:

A. [6]Thyroid in small doses. Gonadotropic hormones of the anterior pituitary (Prolan A and B).

B. [56]Progesterone and Estrone are contraindicated. Anterior pituitary hormones are of value.

C. [24]Mazer used 30,000 to 430,000 R. U. of Estradiol Benzoate on each of four cases over a period of one-two months as treatment for amenorrhea with subsequent conception following withdrawal of treatment.

There are several additional conditions in gynecology in which good results from sex hormonal therapy are being obtained, and are worthy of mention: Hypoplasias of the uterus[63-64], "Mazoplasis" or adenosis of the breasts[65-66-67-68-24-6-79-101-102-103] excessive lactation post-partum (24 - Discussion[105]) and more recently Schneider[69] has described a syndrome indicative of estrogenic deficiency. No attempt has been made to discuss other conditions outside of gynecology in which estrogenic therapy as well as the gonadotropic hormones have been used efficaciously, such as acne, cryptorchism, and David's disease.

In closing there are some points worthy of reiteration, namely that while no stress has been made on the use of other glandular therapy in conjunction with the sex hormones one should remember that it is often necessary. Of all glandular therapy, thyroid extract has been the most reliable and beneficial as stressed by Novak[6] and Hoskins[70]. Thus, the possibility of other glandular disorders must be kept in mind when treating gynecological patients.

A word in regard to the contraindica-

tion to the use of the sex hormones might not be inapropos before closing. It is known that thyroid and the estrogenic hormones have an antagonistic reaction (Year Book of Obstetrics and Gynecology, 1936). Aside from this, side reactions[72] such as urticaria, parotitis, anaphylactic shock, and generalized dermatitis have been reported. Witherspoon[73-74] points out that an excess follicular hormone may be a common etiological factor in hyperplasias of the endometrium, uterine fibroids, and endometriosis. This theory is supported by the fact that fibroids do often increase rapidly in size during pregnancy[75]. Bauer[76] disagrees with this belief, however. Loeb[77] and Novak[78] discuss the estrogenic hormones in relation to the carcinogenic hydrocarbons. Hofbauer[80] demonstrated changes in the cervical epithelium in the form of hyperplasia, and metaplasia by injection of female sex hormones. This was confirmed by Philip Smith and Engle. Watson[81] cautions the use of all sex hormones during the reproductive period. Some authors[87-90] state that women who have been treated for carcinoma of the breast, and carcinoma elsewhere in the body should never be given ovarian hormones.

Damm[82] advises that all large doses of estrin should be followed by progestin. In animals (rabbits) Zondek[83] found a glandular cystic hyperplasis of the endometrium and atrophy of the uterus by prolonged use of estrin. Mazer[84] found no effects from doses of 100,000 to 200,000 units of estrogenic principle given to women over a period of two-three months on the weight, B. M. R., blood pressure, blood count, coagulation time, bleeding time, urine and blood chemistry. The only conclusions that one can draw from the foregoing reports is that while the sex hormones are proving to be of definite clinical value, care should be taken in their use. A definite indication should be present, and they should not be regarded as just something else to try if other things do not work. A very appropriate word of caution was made recently in an editorial in the J. A. M. A.[86] "Rather are they (the editorial comments) intended (a) To emphasize that there is a great discrepancy between laboratory knowledge of the hormones and their clinical application, (b)

To suggest that for the present only those clinicians with facilities for critical study be encouraged to administer the new endocrine preparations to patients and that these clinicians be urged to publish their negative results as well as their positive results, and (c) To suggest that a large group of physicians not represented in either of the groups mentioned cease their undiscriminating injection of u n k n o w n substances into unsuspecting patients."

In spite of this warning, one should not have a futile aspect towards endocrinology. Dr. Novak has made the comparison between the present status of endocrinology and that of the cancer problem. He points out that even though we know little about the etiology of cancer, still the most cynical clinician does not feel that a careful familial history for cancer, a biopsy and pathological examination of the tissues along with the best known methods of therapy X-rays, and radium is not worthy of trial. The same enthusiasm and diligence should be applied to gynecological endocrinology, bearing in mind the safeguards which have been mentioned previously.

BIBLIOGRAPHY

1. Wolf, "Endocrinology in Modern Practice," Saunders Pub. 1936.
2. Engelbach, "Endocrinology," C. C. Thomas Pub. 1932.
3. Zondek, Acta obst. et gynec., Scandinav 15:1-10, 1935.
4. Payne, J. M. Soc. New Jersey, 31:629, Nov., 1934.
5. Novak, J. A. M. A. 105:562, Aug. 3, 1935.
6. Novak, Am. J. Obst. and Gyn. 32:887, Nov. 1936.
7. Moore, Am. J. Obst. and Gyn. 29, 1, Jan. 1935.
8. Zondek, Schweiz Med. Wehnschr 65:1168, Dec. 7, 1935.
9. Berger, Klin. Wehnschr, 14:1601, Nov. 9, 1935. Abstract: J. A. M. A. 105:2191, Dec. 28, 1935.
10. Te Linde, A. J. Obst. and Gyn. 30:512, Oct. 1935.
11. Tachezy, Zentralbl f. Gynak 59:972, April 27, 1935.
12. Mazer and Israel, J. A. M. A. 108:163, Jan. 16, 1937.
13. Lewis, Am. J. Obst. and Gyn. 26:593, Oct. 1933.
14. Lewis, Am. J. Obst. and Gyn. 29:806, June, 1935.
15. Witherspoon, Am. J. Obst. and Gyn. 29:906, June, 1935.
16. Archivos Argentinos de Ped, Buenos Aires 7:460, July, 1936.
17. Miller, Am. J. Obst. and Gyn. 29:553, April, 1935.
18. Phillips, N. Eng. J. Med. 213:1026, Nov. 21, 1935.
19. Lewis et al., J. A. M. A. 106:2054, June 13, 1936.
20. Hobarst, Med. Klin. 32:179, Feb. 7, 1936.
21. Te Linde, Am. J. Obst. and Gyn. 30-512, Oct. 1936.
22. Davis, Surg. Gyn. and Obst. 61:680, Nov. 1935.
23. Jacoby, Am. J. Obst. and Gyn. 31:654, April, 1936.
24. Mazer, J. A. M. A. 108:168, Jan. 16, 1937.
25. Mazer and Israel M. Clin. North America 19:205, July, 1935.
26. Albright, "Endocrinology" 20, 24 Jan.-Feb. 1936.
27. Frank, Proc Soc Exp. Biol and Med. 33, 311, Nov. 1935.
28. Sevringhaus, Am. J. Obst. and Gyn. 25:361, March, 1933.
29. Sebringhaus, Am. J. Med. Sc. 178:638, 1931.
30. Hamblen, Endocrinology, 15, 184, 1931.
31. Fluhmann, Endocrinology, 15, 177, 1931.
32. Macfarlane, Am. J. Obst. and Gyn. 31:663, April, 1936.
33. Goldberg, Endocrinology 19:649, Nov.-Dec. 1935.
34. Pratt, Am. J. Obst. and Gyn. 31, 789, May 1936.
35. Wallis, Zentralbl. f. Gynak 60:2839, Nov. 28, 1936.
36. Gisen, Zentralbl. f. Gynak 60, 370, Feb. 15, 1936.
37. Shaefer, Endocrinology 19, 705, Nov.-Dec. 1935.
38. Frank et al. N. Y. State J. Med. 36:1363. Oct. 1936.
39. Glass, Endocrinology, 20:333, May, 1936.
40. Dunn, Am. J. Obst. and Gyn. 30, 186, Aug., 1935.
41. Kaufman, Zentralbl. f. Gynak 60:850, April 11, 1936.
42. Wilson, Am J. Obst. and Gyn, 31, 911, June, 1936.
43. Israel, J. A. M. A. 106, 1698, May 16, 1936.
44. Campbell, Am. J. Obst. and Gyn. 31:508, March, 1936.
45. Browne, Am. J. Obst. and Gyn. 29:113, June, 1935.
46. Elden Am. J. Obst. and Gyn. 32:91, July, 1936.
47. Kane, Am. J. Obst. and Gyn. 32:110, May, 1935.
48. Neustaedter, Am. J. Obst. and Gyn. 29:68, May, 1935.
49. Kaufman, J. Obst. and Gynec. Brit. Emp. 42:431, June, 1935.
50. Watson, Canad. M. A. J. 34:898, March, 1936.
51. Kurzrok, Am. J. Obst. and Gyn. 29:771, June, 1935.
52. Crossen, Am. J. Surg. 33, 345, Sept., 1936.
53. Elden, Endocrinology 20:47, Jan., 1936.
54. Monatschr f. Geburtsh u. Gynak 102, 203, June, 1936.
55. Tschertak, Gynec et obst. 30:423, Nov. 1934 (See page 544 yearbook, 1935).
56. Chute, J. A. M. A. 107:1857, Dec. 5, 1936.
57. Papanicolaou, Am. J. Obst. and Gyn. 31:806, May, 1936.
58. Witherspoon, New Orleans M. and S. J. 88:205, Oct., 1935.
59. Burch, J. Indiana M. A. 27:560, Dec., 1934.
60. Tchertok, Monatschr. f. Geburtsh, U Gynak, 102:202, June, 1936 (Year Book Obst. and Gyn. 1936, page 499).
61. Breschbeck, Muncheon Med. Wehnschr 82:1677, Oct. 18, 1935.
62. Keene, J. M. Soc. New Jersey, 31, 629, Nov., 1934.
63. Clouberg, Zeitscher. f. Geburt u. Gynak, 107:331, March, 1934.
64. Iko and Nagai, Zentralbe f. Gynak, 59, 1336, June 8, 1935.
65. Lewis and Geschickter, Am. J. Surg., 24, 280, May, 1934.
66. Leriche, Lyon Chir. 30, 54, Jan.-Feb., 1933.
67. Whitehouse, S. G. and O. 58, 278, Feb. 2A, 1934.
68. Mazer, M. Rc., 140, 417, Oct. 17, 1934.
69. Schneider, Am. J. Obst. and Gyn. 31, 782, May, 1936.
70. Haskin, J. A. M. A., 105:948, Sept., 1935.
71. Novak, J. A. M. A. 104, 1497, April 27, 1935.
72. Zieman, Illinois M. J. 70, 198, Aug. 1936.
73. Witherspoon, Surg. Gyn. and Ob. 61:743, Dec., 1935.
74. Witherspoon, Am. J. Cancer, 24, 402, June, 1935.
75. Enge, Am. J. Obst. and Gyn. 28, 682, 1934.
76. Bauer, Am. J. Obst. and Gyn. 32, 183, Aug., 1936.
77. Loeb, J. A. M. A. 104, 1597, May 4, 1935.
78. Novak, Am. J. Ob. and Gyn. 32, 674, Oct., 1936.
79. Cutler, J. A. M. A., April 11, 1931.
80. Hofbauer, Zentralbe f. Gynak 59:2534, Oct. 26, 1935.
81. Watson, Canad. M. A. J., 34, 293, March, 1936.
82. Damm, Octa Obst, et Gynec. Scandinav. 15, 58, 1935.
83. Zondek, J. Exp. Med., 63, 787, June, 1936.
84. Mazer, et al, J. A. M. A., 105, 257, July 21, 1935.
85. Endocrinology, 19:408, July-August, 1935.
86. Editorial, J. A. M. A., 107, 1390, Oct. 24, 1936.
87. Yearbook of Obstetrics and Gynecology, 1936, page 556.
88. Science 2, 153, Aug. 16, 1935.
89. J. A. M. A. 107, 1221, Oct. 10, 1936.
90. Zuckerman, Lancet 2,9, July 4, 1936.
91. Okomoto et al., Jap. J. Obst. and Gynec. 18, 105, April, 1935.
92. Zondek, J. Exp. Med. 63, 789, June 1, 1936.
93. Zondek, Wien. Klin., Wehnochr. 49, 455, April 10, 1936.
94. Kurzrok, J. of Contraception, 2,27. Feb., 1937.
95. Taylor, The Practice of Contraception, Williams and Wilkins, Co., 1931.
96. J. A. M. A. 103, 13, July 7, 1934.
97. Carlson, Northwest Medicine, 36, 55, Feb., 1937.
98. Haberlandt, Monatschr. f. Geburtsh u. Gynak, 87:320, 1931.
99. Schockaert, Bruxelles-Med., 15-1010, July 14, 1935.
100. Taylor, Am. J. Surg. 33, 558, Sept., 1936.
101. Geschickter, Arch. Surg. 32, 598, April, 1936.
102. Taylor, Surg., Gynec. and Obst., 62, 129, Feb., 1936.
103. Taylor, Surg., Gynec. and Obst., 62, 562, March, 1936.
104. Lewis, Surg. Gyn. and Obst., 63, 640, 1936.
105. Mayor, Zentralb, f. Gynak, 60, 2379, 1936.
106. Schockaert, Bruxelles-Med., 16, 1667, 1936.
107. Foss, J. Obst. and Gynec. Brit. Emp., 43, 1091, 1936.
108. Novak, Surg. Gynec. and Obst., 60, 330, Feb., 1935.
109. Rock et al., J. A. M. A., June 12, 1937, 108,24, page 2022.
110. Klaften, Medizinische Klinik, 33:566, April 23, 1937.
111. Grey, James et al., J. A. M. A., Sept. 15, 1937, 109:13, 1032.
112. Koch, F. C., Physiological Reviews, 17:153, April, 1937.

The Relative Value of the Various Methods of Diphtheria Immunization

DR. C. E. BRADLEY

TULSA, OKLAHOMA

The value of diphtheria immunization is unquestioned by the medical minds of to-day, but there is still some question and uncertainty about the best method of producing this immunity; i.e., the method which will result regularly in the maximum percentage of permanent immune patients with a minimum of injections and unpleasant reactions. The high incidence of susceptibility in children, especially those of pre-school age, has led to the general acceptance of the view that preliminary Schick testing in pre-school children is unnecessary, and that all pre-school children, excepting those showing decided allergic tendences, should be given the benefit of active immunization against diphtheria routinely. This immunization should not be given before the sixth month of life as the infant possesses a natural immunity acquired from its mother up until this time. This immunity is gradually lost after the fifth-sixth month, and in view of the fact that about 80 per cent of the cases of diphtheria occur in the pre-school group (six months to six years) the sooner this immunity can be given after the sixth month, the better it is, as only in this way can a child be given the protection during this hazardous period, and in addition unfavorable reactions, especially with toxoid, are rarely if ever seen in children at this age.

At the present time there are three accepted methods of actively immunizing a child against diphtheria.

TOXOID

By giving two to three, 1 c.c. d o s e s of diphtheria toxoid (Ramon's anatoxin) with interval between injections of three weeks. This method may be used routinely in all children under six years, since they seldom if ever manifest other than slight local reactions. Older children and adults show more local and general reactions.

Therefore, if this method is used in the older group it is advisable to test them by injecting 0.1 c.c. of the anatoxin intradermally. If no urticarial wheal appears at the site of injection within a period of 15 minutes, then the 1 c.c. immunizing dose may be given. If an urticarial wheal appears at the site of injection, no further injection should be made until three days have elapsed, and then the doses should be modified as follows: the first dose on the third days should be 0.1 c.c., then 0.25, 0.5, 1 and 1 c.c. should be given at intervals of one week.

ALUM PRECIPITATED TOXOID

The desirability of minimizing the number of injections necessary for the immunization of young children prompted a number of investigators to undertake the development of material capable of producing active immunity after a single dose.

The manner in which immunization is accomplished with alum precipitated toxoid is dependent upon its slow absorption, and some investigators believe the one dose toxoid is able to maintain a more or less continuous antigenic stimulus, extending over a period corresponding to that of two doses of the Ramon toxoid. On the other hand, there is a dissenting minority who, while admitting the desirability and advantages of a single injection, have presented conclusive evidence that the protection effected by a single dose of 1 c.c. of alum precipitated toxoid is not of sufficient permanency to justify the continued use of a single dose as the method of choice.

Pansing and Shaffer[1] made an accurate and reliable study on a group of school children in Ohio. An analysis of the data on this group indicated that a very high immunity results from one dose of 1 c.c. of alum precipitated toxoid by the 28th to the

60th day after innoculation as evidenced by a negative S c h i c k test. A further analysis of data on these same children indicated that 57.8 per cent of them had lost protection at the end of two years as evidenced by a positive Schick reaction. They also found that a second injection of alum precipitated toxoid offered protection to the 57.8 per cent of children who had lost their immunity at the end of two years.

More recently Jean V. Cooke[2], of Washington University, St. Louis, in a study of 1,000 adult student nurses immunized by T.A.T., toxoid and alum precipitated toxoid over a period of 18 years, found that the most effective procedures were two injections of alum precipitated toxoid with an interval of several months between, or three injections of plain toxoid with intervals of several weeks between the doses.

This tends to confirm the well known experimental observations that the immunity following the first or "primary" response to diphtheria is feeble and transient, but the "secondary" response following a later antigen stimulus results in rapid, pronounced and persistent antitoxin formation. It would appear, therefore, that those who become immune following a single injection or series of injections have already responded previously to the diphtheria antigenic stimulus, such as occurs in the development of "natural immunity," and develop the permanent immunity characteristic of secondary stimulus. On the other hand, those who have not reacted previously to the diphtheric antigen, and consequently do not become immune following a single injection or series of injections, will require a second immunization.

It should be emphasized that there are certain individuals who are absolutely incapable of responding to any antigenic substance. They are referred to as being immunologically inert. Fortunately, however, the percentage of persons incapable of developing immunity is very small.

TOXIN ANTITOXIN

Many continue to favor the use of toxin antitoxin in the immunization of o l d e r children and adults, because of the fact that it is said to give fewer reactions. The procedure is to administer three successive injections of toxin antitoxin in doses of 1 c.c. each, given at intervals of from one to three weeks. It should be remembered, however, that toxin antitoxin contains some horse serum to which the patient may be sensitive, or develop a sensitivity following this administration of the toxin antitoxin mixture.

SCHICK TEST

Material for the Schick test consists of diphtheria toxin diluted in peptone, and can be purchased commercially, and is stable for a period of months. Experience indicates it is as reliable as freshly diluted toxin and its use is recommended for general use. To perform a Schick test 0.1 c.c. of the diluted toxin (representing 1/50th of M.L.D. of toxin) injected intracutaneously in the flexor surface of the forearm at the junction of the upper and middle third. The Schick test should be read at the end of 72 hours. A positive reaction consists of redness, edema, and possibly induration, 1 cm in diameter or larger. This signifies lack of immunity. If the test is negative it should be read again on the seventh day. A control test may be performed on the opposite arm if desired. Similarly diluted toxin heated to 176° F. for 10 minutes is used for this purpose. Practically a control test is unnecessary in the younger age groups, where pseudo-reactions seldom occur.

This following report summarizes the r e s u l t s of 3,203 immunizations against diphtheria in pre-school children over a 12 year period with the use of the different antigens.

Year	Serum	Number Doses	Number Given	Number Schicked	Number Positive
1925-26	T.A.T.	3	193	43	0
1927	T.A.T.	3	272	229	8
1928	T.A.T.	3	286	146	8
1929	T.A.T.	3	147	68	6
1929	Toxoid	2	64	37	0
1930	T.A.T.	3	78	27	1
1930	Toxoid	3	83	41	3
1930	Toxoid	2	23	4	0
1931	T.A.T.	3	123	42	0
1931	Toxoid	3	744	283	9
1932	Toxoid	3	298	104	7
1933	Toxoid	1	6	4	0
1933	Toxoid	3	341	87	9
1934	Toxoid	3	179	97	2
1935	Alum Toxoid	1	12	10	5
1935	Toxoid	3	205	142	2
1936	Alum Toxoid	1	139	49	0
TOTALS			3,203	1,413	60

Approximately 4½ per cent positive.

CONCLUSIONS

1. No immunization program is complete without the follow-up Shick test, as

many lay people have a false security in thinking their children are 100% protected after the immunization is completed, when in reality we know a definite percentage is still susceptible to diphtheria.

2. It would seem that efforts to simplify the technique of diphtheria immunization to a single dose of antigen has led to a sacrifice of reasonable permanency of immunity for greater convenience of administration.

3. Past experience indicates that the use of the two or preferably three doses of plain toxoid given at intervals of several weeks, or the administration of two doses of 1 c.c. each of alum precipitated toxoid given with a 60-day interval between them is better than running the risk of a child losing its protection too soon after the administration of the single dose of the alum precipitated toxoid, and are the methods of choice at the present time.

BIBLIOGRAPHY

1. Pansing, H.H., Shaffer, E. R. American Journal of Public Health, 26 :786-788, August, 1936.

2. Cooke, Journal of Pediatrics, 9 :641-646, November, 1936.

Further Experience With Prostatic Resection*

HENRY S. BROWNE, M.D.
TULSA, OKLAHOMA

The trouble in prostatic obstruction is caused by those portions of the gland which project into the bladder and urethra. By prostatectomy the whole gland is removed in order to relieve this obstruction. By resection it is possible to remove the obstructing portions only. This is possible in all cases except those in which the resectoscope cannot be introduced and in the occasional huge glands, which amount to less than 10 per cent. Following a properly done resection the patient voids a full, free stream and empties his bladder so that the results are excellent and permanent in the vast majority of cases. By fulfilling the above requirements the operation can be called anatomically and physiologically correct.

Preliminary preparation has proven its worth over many years in prostatic surgery and I deplore the tendency in some quarters to get away from this proven safety factor. In the last 100 cases under my care two deaths followed immediate operation and one other after insufficient preparation. So in all but the hale and hearty I practice preliminary preparation. Catheter drainage has been used entirely and in no case has cystotomy been necessary.

*Read before the Genito-Urinary Section, Annual Meeting, Oklahoma State Medical Association, Tulsa, May, 1937.

At first I did vasectomy routinely, then in 75 cases I did not. While only four developed epididymitis, one had a severe disability lasting three months with loss of the testicle from abscess formation. Another developed huge abscesses of both testicles which contributed materially to his death one month after resection. I am, therefore, again doing vasectomy in all cases except the younger men. This is done at the same time as the resection. No case of epididymitis has developed from an indwelling catheter.

As to the operation itself, much has been written but points which to me seem important have not been emphasized. After the sheath is introduced, the bladder neck is carefully examined with a retrograde telescope to determine the amount and location of intravesical protrusion of the prostate. The operating unit is then introduced. This is equipped with the latest foroblique telescope (No. 68A) which gives much greater magnification and a wider field of vision than the original telescope. Resection is then carried out layer by layer, for it is then easier to tell when the level of the floor of the bladder is reached. The intraurethral portions are then removed to just below the level of the verumontanum, which of course is kept inviolate. In making all cuts the sheath is pressed firmly against the tissue, so that a deep bite is obtained; otherwise, the loop will ride up and out and a thin shaving will be the result. Cutting tissue near the veru is delicate work and it is usually necessary to cut away from it toward the bladder. The next point I consider very important: the sheath is withdrawn to the veru, carefully centered and then turned first clockwise then counter-clockwise, and as long as tissue falls into the sheath it is removed, for otherwise it would later on fall into the u r e t h r a and cause further obstruction. This, of course, r e q u i r e s cutting clear around the clock, but when it has been done one can be fairly certain that all of the obstructing tissue and usually much more has been removed. A finger is then inserted into the rectum and the prostate massaged against the sheath. This will sometimes express more tissue out where it can be removed. Bleeding points are systematically sought out and coagulated with a strong, hot spark. The new telescope is a great aid in finding these quickly. It is very important that at the finish the irrigating fluid return clear, for I am firmly convinced that the time to stop hemorrhage is at the time of operation. The area is then inspected with the retrograde telescope, and any remaining tissue projecting into the bladder is located and then removed. There is now a wide, cone-shaped opening where the prostatic urethra was, with its apex at the veru, and base at the neck of the bladder, and one is fairly certain that there is no longer any obstruction present. A 22F retention catheter is then placed in the bladder. Following the advice of Alcock and others, no case is kept on the operating table more than one hour. If there is more tissue to be removed, this is done a week later. This has been necessary in five per cent of my cases.

In the post-operative care f l u i d s are forced by mouth, or by needle if necessary. The catheter must be kept open by frequent irrigations, the solution being injected and withdrawn each time by suction with a piston syringe, for a bulb syringe has not the power to withdraw clots which may form, and the bladder must be kept empty. If it overdistends hemorrhage may result, or severe chills and high fever. As soon as the urine becomes clear, irrigations are discontinued.

At the end of a resection, there is a wide area of raw s u r f a c e in a closed sac bathed in urine which is usually infected. Even with continuous drainage there is bound to be a slight absorption, which I believe is the cause of the post-operative rise in temperature which nearly always occurs. This raw surface quickly seals over so that the temperature returns to n o r m a l usually within 72 hours. The catheter is removed in 96 hours, or 24 hours after the temperature returns to normal, if it should be elevated for a longer time.

There has been no post-operative hemorrhage, immediate or late, in more than 100 consecutive cases under my care. I attribute that partly to luck but more to the fact that complete hemostasis in each case was obtained at the time of operation, and that the catheter was kept open afterward.

When the catheter is removed the patient should void a full, free stream at once and be proud of it. On checking the residual urine it should be less than 50 c.c. The two go together, and if this is not the case the resection is incomplete and the result will not be satisfactory. So instead of waiting and hoping for several months and then having to reoperate eventually, I now reoperate within a week and in each instance have removed considerable more tissue, usually from overhanging lateral lobes. A second resection has been necessary in eight per cent of the cases. Rotation of the sheath at the level of the veru in the first operation has largely obviated the need for a second one by revealing the overhanging laterals at that time. There has been only one definite recurrence, occuring four years after the first operation. In all other cases reoperated on later, the trouble was due to not removing enough tissue the first time.

If the temperature is normal for two days after the catheter is removed the patient is allowed to leave the hospital. Occasionally after that there is a rise in temperature, poor appetite and signs of septic absorption. The prompt reinsertion of a retention catheter and bladder irrigations has corrected this in less than a week in all cases.

What is the appearance of the operated

area later on? An autopsy was obtained in one case in which death had occurred 60 hours after resection. The patient, age 79, general health good, NPN 42 with 120 c.c. of residual urine, was operated on without preliminary preparation. Thirty-nine grams of tissue was removed in one hour. Bleeding was more than usual but controlled readily. Complete suppression of urine developed with death in 60 hours. In removing the ureters, bladder and prostate, the surrounding tissues were found normal; the ureteral orifices, base of the trigone and verumontanum were intact; the prostate was found to have been completely removed down to the capsule, except for a small amount of tissue just behind the veru. The operated area had a healthy pink color and no area of coagulation was visible. One case had cystotomy for stone 15 months after resection. There was a visible cavity present at the bladder neck into which the index finger was easily inserted. The majority of patients have been cystoscoped one or more times from two months to several years afterward and the cone-shaped opening appears to be permanent. In other words, instead of a prostatic urethra, there is a prostatic cavity which is continuous with, and to all intents and purposes a part of, the bladder.

There has been an almost complete absence of burning and frequency afterward. They get up not at all or not more than three times at night and void promptly, quickly and completely.

In the last 100 cases under my care there have been five deaths. Sixty-five grams of tissue was the most removed in one case—44 grams in one hour and 21 grams a week later. In 28 cases more than 25 grams was removed. During the same period I performed two prostatectomies.

Prostatic resection is a difficult, delicate and technical procedure, but when done properly the results are uniformly satisfactory and lasting in the vast majority of cases. Like many others I have had my troubles and worries, but nothing has given me more satisfaction than, time after time, to see a grave surgical risk of advanced age come through the operation without shock or discomfort, and be alive and enjoying life two or three years later.

Many Physicians and Their Families Will "See America" En Route to the Convention in San Francisco

Officials of this Society were pleased to learn from the American Express Company, Official Transportation Agents for the Convention tours, that they have already received a very excellent response from physicians and their families, which indicates that the San Francisco Convention will be a great success. It is recommended that members of this Society who intend to participate in the Convention apply at an early date to the American Express for their tour reservations, as this will assure them of receiving the type of pullman accommodations they desire.

This is the first time that the physicians have been offered the facilities of de-luxe special trains visiting the scenic attractions of the west, at a very nominal all-expense cost from your home city. Traversing a route that contains many wonders, one's particular preferences are bound to be among them. For instance, the Indian Pueblo District with its remnants of an ancient civilization long vanished from this continent. The Grand Canyon offers its grandeur of scenic attractions. Southern California, its glowing, sun-filled cities and orange empires, Spanish Missions, Catalina Island and the Pacific rolling up to the edge of white sands. That is the route to San Francisco and the Convention.

Returning, there is a choice of two routes. One includes the charming cities of America's Northwest: Portland, Seattle, Victoria, Vancouver and the majestic Canadian Rockies and its resorts. Route Two winds through Yellowstone National Park and its world-famous geyser region, through Salt Lake City, and the scenic beauties of the Royal Gorge, Colorado Springs and the mile-high city, Denver.

That is but a rough outline of the itineraries offered to physicians planning to attend the Convention this June. These special train tours are restricted to physicians, their friends and families, and have been made possible through the united interest and support of 25 state medical societies which makes it possible to offer the tours on an economical, all-expense basis. This is an ideal opportunity to enjoy a wonderful vacation with your family and in the company of friends and colleagues in the Society and in other state Societies.

---o---

Recent Statement by the Judges of the Mead Johnson Vitamin A Award

"The Vitamin A Award offered by Mead Johnson & Company was supposed to be made on the basis of papers published or accepted for publication by December 31, 1936. The judges of this award, meeting in New York, June 4, 1937, feel that its presentation at this time is not warranted since no clinical investigation on vitamin A has yet been published which completely answers any of the objectives of the original proposal. The judges, therefore, agreed to defer further consideration of the granting of this award until December 31, 1939. This action was taken because of the existence of pronounced differences of opinion among investigators as to the reliability of any method yet proposed for determining the actual vitamin A requirements."

Statement by Mead Johnson & Company

In view of this action by the judges of the Mead Johnson Vitamin A Award, and as an earnest of our good faith in the matter, we have segregated from our corporate funds on deposit with the Continental Illinois National Bank & Trust Company of Chicago, the sum of $15,000. This cash deposit has been placed in escrow and will be paid promptly when the board of judges decides on the recipient of the Main or Clinical Award. The Laboratory Award of $5,000 was made on April 10th, 1935.

THE JOURNAL
OF THE
Oklahoma State Medical Association

Issued Monthly at McAlester, Oklahoma, under direction of the Council.

Copyright, 1938, by Oklahoma State Medical Association, McAlester, Oklahoma.

Vol. XXXI	APRIL, 1938	Number 4

DR. L. S. WILLOUR................................Editor-in-Chief
McAlester, Oklahoma

DR. T. H. McCARLEY................................Associate Editor
McAlester, Oklahoma

Entered at the Post Office at McAlester, Oklahoma, as second-class matter under the act of March 3rd, 1879.

This is the official Journal of the Oklahoma State Medical Association. All communications should be addressed to The Journal of the Oklahoma State Medical Association, McAlester Clinic, McAlester, Oklahoma. $4.00 per year; 40c per copy.

The editorial department is not responsible for the opinions expressed in the original articles of contributors.

Reprints of original articles will be supplied at actual cost provided request for them is attached to manuscripts or made in sufficient time before publication.

Articles sent this Journal for publication and all those read at the annual meetings of the State Association are the sole property of this Journal. The Journal relies on each individual contributor's strict adherence to this well-known rule of medical journalism. In the event an article sent this Journal for publication is published before appearance in The Journal the manuscript will be returned to the writer.

Failure to receive The Journal should call for immediate notification of the Editor, McAlester Clinic, McAlester, Oklahoma.

Local news of possible interest to the medical profession, notes on removals, changes of addresses, births, deaths and weddings will be gratefully received.

Advertising of articles, drugs or compounds unapproved by the Council on Pharmacy of the A. M. A., will not be accepted.

Advertising rates will be supplied on application.

It is suggested that wherever possible members of the State Association should patronize our advertisers in preference to others as a matter of fair reciprocity.

Printed by News-Capital Company, McAlester.

EDITORIAL

FORTY-SIXTH ANNUAL MEETING

Since the organization of the Oklahoma State Medical Association there has never been a more attractive program presented than the one published in this issue of the Journal. Our Guest Speakers, Doctors Frank C. Neff, Kansas City; William S. Middleton, Madison, Wisconsin; and Edward H. Ochsner, Chicago, are international authorities on the particular subjects they present and their special ability to present these subjects will make their presentations not only instructive but interesting.

The Scientific Programs of the various Sections have been prepared with careful attention as to their timeliness and acceptability of the subjects, and many of the leading physicians of the state have allowed their names to go on the program and will be prepared to give to the Sections material well worth while.

The officers of the Association will have many things of importance to consider. The Council and House of Delegates will have many important decisions to make, consequently each delegate should make it a point to familiarize himself with the various questions that will be presented and see to it that he is in his place on time at the meetings of these important bodies.

The Medical Profession of Muskogee County has put forth every effort to make this meeting enjoyable. There will be ample hotel facilities to care for the crowd. The Golf Tournament, Tour of Inspection of the Veterans Hospital and Fort Gibson, together with the President's Reception and dance will contribute to enjoyment of the time spent in Muskogee.

No matter how far you may live from the meeting place you can ill afford to miss this very important meeting and participate in the programs and discussions.

———o———

Editorial Notes—Personal and General

DR. WANN LANGSTON, Oklahoma City, attended the College of Physicians Postgraduate Course in Cardio-Vascular Diseases in Philadelphia, in March, and the meeting of the College in New York in April.

———

DR. JOSEPH FULCHER, Tulsa, announces the opening of his office at 210 Medical Arts Building.

———

DR. E. P. HATHAWAY, Lawton, has been appointed County Health Superintendent of Comanche County.

———

DR. GEORGE A. KILPATRICK, McAlester, recently made an extensive tour of the medical centers of the Pacific Coast.

———

DR. E. K. WITCHER, Tulsa, announces the opening of his office for the practice of Internal Medicine, 511 Medical Arts Building.

———

DRS. PHIL McNEILL and R. Q. GOODMAN, Oklahoma City, were guests of the Pittsburg County Medical Society, Friday, March 18th, at their monthly meeting, in McAlester.

———

DR. J. C. REYNOLDS, Frederick, is reported ill in Rochester, Minn.

———

DR. E. S. CROWE, Olustee, attended the Dallas Clinical Society in Dallas, in March.

———

DR. HARRY R. CUSHMAN, Clinton, has been appointed County Health Superintendent of Custer County.

Oklahoma Pediatric Society

The Board of Directors of the Oklahoma Pediatric Society have decided to have the annual meeting of the Society in the fall instead of with the state meeting. There will be a short business meeting after the program of the section on Pediatrics.

Alpha Epsilon Delta Convention

The Fifth Biennial Convention of the Alpha Epsilon Delta Honorary Premedical Fraternity was held at Chapel Hill, North Carolina, March 24-26. The North Carolina Beta Chapter, at the University of North Carolina, acted as host to 85 visiting members and delegates from 21 chapters in 14 states.

One of the most important reports to the convention was the success reported by the various chapters for their social hygiene programs among the college students. Many of the chapters have well conducted programs on mental and social hygiene for the students. Two of the high points of the convention were the illustrated lecture by Dr. Addison G. Brenizer of Charlotte, N. C., on "Surgical Anatomy of the Thyroid Gland and Thyroidectomy," and the address by Dean Wm. deB. MacNider, of the University of North Carolina Medical School, on "The Biologically-Minded Physician," at the convention banquet Saturday evening.

The Oklahoma Alpha Chapter of Alpha Epsilon Delta is located at the University of Oklahoma.

Officers elected to the Grand Staff were: Grand President, Dr. Charles F. Poe, Professor of Chemistry, University of Colorado; Grand Vice-President, Dr. K. P. Stevens, Professor of Biology, Central College; Grand Secretary-Historian, Dr. Maurice L. Moore, Drexel Hill, Pa.; Grand Treasurer, Dr. Warren H. Steinbach, Professor of Chemistry, University of Arkansas. Members elected to the Executive Council were: Dr. Emmett B. Carmichael, School of Medicine, University of Alabama; Dr. H. R. Henze, Professor of Chemistry, University of Texas; and Dr. R. W. Bost, Professor of Chemistry, University of North Carolina.

News of the County Medical Societies

MUSKOGEE County Medical Society had as their guest of honor Dr. Robert U. Patterson, Dean of the Oklahoma University School of Medicine, on March 21st, at their monthly meeting held in Muskogee.

OKMULGEE-OKFUSKEE County Medical Societies held their monthly meeting in Okmulgee March 21st with the following program: "Toxic Goiter," illustrated with lantern slides, Dr. J. C. Brogden, Oklahoma City. "Diaphragmatic Hernia," (X-ray Findings) by Dr. E. G. Hyatt, Oklahoma City.

News Notes of Woman's Auxiliary

Women's Auxiliary to Woodward County Medical Society Elects Officers

The Women's Auxiliary to the Woodward County Medical Society at its annual meeting held at the Baker Hotel in Woodward elected the following officers for the ensuing year: Mrs. D. W. Darwin, president; Mrs. T. C. Leashman, vice-president; Mrs. C. W. Tedrowe, recording secretary; Mrs. O. C. Newman, treasurer; Mrs. H. K. Hill, corresponding secretary. Dues were paid. Other business was shortened that the invitation to meet with the Medical Society might be accepted.

A seven o'clock turkey dinner was enjoyed by all.

An interesting and instructive paper on, "Socialized Medicine" was read by Dr. C. J. Fishman of Oklahoma City. Dr. Basil Hays of Oklahoma City gave an illustrated lecture on "Urology." This lecture received comment from several of the doctors present.

It may be of interest to some who read this report to know that the organization known as "Woodward County Medical Society" is composed of members from Beaver, Ellis, Harper and Dewey Counties as well as from Woodward County. Wives of members of the medical society are eligible to membership in the women's auxiliary.

So far as we know, this society and auxiliary embrace the largest area in the state, organized under one unit.

Mrs. J. C. Duncan, Publicity Chairman.

OBITUARIES

JOSEPH ALEXANDER MILROY

Dr. Milroy passed away at his home in Okmulgee the evening of February 7, at the age of 67. His wife, children and a few close friends were at his bedside when the end came.

The doctor had been suffering with heart disease for a number of years, but did not give up active practice until the two or three years passed. The last county medical meeting he attended, a year ago now, he said would no doubt be his last meeting with his doctor friends.

Dr. Milroy was born in Northwood, Ohio, April 15, 1870, where he attended public school, grew up and went to Geneva College, after this graduating from the old Starling Medical College now the Medical College of the State University. His first two years' practice was at Lakeview, Ohio, after which time he came to Oklahoma, stopping for awhile at El Reno hoping to draw some of that land thrown open to settlers. Failing in this quest he rode horseback to Okmulgee in 1901, settled down and remained in the practice of his chosen profession there until the time of his death—36 years. He married an Okmulgee girl, Miss Florence Weirick, in 1906. From this union came six children, five boys and one girl, all grown but one.

The deceased was a useful citizen and successful doctor, a member of the Presbyterian church, a church he helped to organize in the early days of Okmulgee. He assisted very materially in the erection of the present magnificent church now standing at the corner of Ninth and Seminole streets. From this church his funeral was held. Dr. A. E. Bleck, the pastor, officiating, assisted by the Rev. E. L. Watson, pastor of the First Baptist church of Okmulgee.

Mr. President, your committee feels very keenly the loss of a good citizen and close associate in medicine, we being among the oldest physicians left in Okmulgee. We suggest this simple resolution be placed in the records of the Okmulgee County Medical Society, a copy sent to the Journal of the Oklahoma Medical Society for publication, and one sent to the family:

First, That the doctor's cheerful and happy disposition in administering to the needs of the sick and afflicted of Okmulgee County, often without compensation, has been an inspiration to the profession and a benediction to all the people. This we feel is worthy of emulation.

Second, That our sympathy is hereby extended to the family and all who mourn his loss.

Committee: L. B. Farmer,
W. C. Milchener,
S. B. Leslie.

PROGRAM

Forty-Sixth Annual Session of the Oklahoma State Medical Association at Muskogee, May 9, 10, 11, 1938

GENERAL INFORMATION

Headquarters—Severs Hotel, Telephone 4900.

Registration, Scientific and Commercial Exhibits—Basement, S e v e r s Hotel. All physicians, except those outside the state and visiting guests, must hold membership receipt for the year 1938, before registering. Please attend to this, if you are not in good standing, by s e e i n g your County Secretary at once.

Woman's Auxiliary—Registration, Severs Hotel, Mezzanine floor. Meeting place, First Presbyterian Church, 5th and Broadway.

Guests of Honor—Dr. Wm. S. Middleton, Madison, Wisconsin; Dr. Frank C. Neff, Kansas City; Dr. E d w a r d H. Ochsner, Chicago.

Council—The Council will meet at 3:00 p.m., Monday, May 9th, in Parlor A, Mezzanine floor, Severs Hotel, for the transaction of business affairs and thereafter on call of the President.

House of Delegates—The House of Delegates will meet at 8:00 p.m., Monday, May 9th, in the Ball Room, Mezzanine floor, Severs Hotel, and at 8:00 a.m., Tuesday, May 10th, same place.

Resolutions—Any resolutions that you may desire to submit to the H o u s e of Delegates should be forwarded to the State Secretary at least one week before the Annual Meeting.

General Sessions—Will be held, beginning 10:00 a.m., Tuesday, May 10th, and 9:30 a.m., Wednesday, May 11th, in the Ritz Theater, 3rd and Court Streets.

Golf Tournament—The Oklahoma State Medical Association golf tournament will be held at Muskogee Country Club on Monday, May 9th. You may tee off for play any time after 1:00 p.m.; the course being open to any member of the State Medical Association, all day Monday. Please have your credentials with you. G r e e n fees paid. Each player will take care of his own caddy. There will be several prizes, so please help the committee in correctly posting your s c o r e s after play Monday evening. It is necessary to furnish us with your handicap, signed by either Pro or Secretary of your club. Arrange your own foursomes if possible, otherwise these will be arranged by the committee. No twosomes allowed, unless necessary in the afternoon play, nor more than foursomes. All arrangements of and participation in trophies will be under the personal supervision of Mr. Gordon Jones, the Club's Professional.

The Annual Golf Tournament Banquet will be held immediately following play, 7:00 p.m., M o n d a y evening. Price per plate $1.50. Please see that your reservation is in the hands of the committee, Shade D. Neely, Commercial N a t i o n a l Bank Building, Muskogee, not later than Sunday, May 8th.

Muskogee business firms donating prizes.

Oklahoma Internists' Association — A luncheon for the members and guests of this Association will be held on the balcony of the Arrow Cafeteria, Tuesday, May 10th, at 12:30 p.m. Please notify Dr. Fred C. Dorwart, Barnes Building, Muskogee, one week before the meeting if you plan to attend.

The Chairman of the Committee on Hotels, Dr. C. E. DeGroot, anounces the following hotels will be available: Severs, Muskogee, Baltimore, Milner, Huber and Jefferson. Correspond with Dr. DeGroot, Surety Bldg., Muskogee, if you wish reservations made.

COMMITTEES IN CHARGE

H. T. BALLANTINE, General Chairman

Advisory Committee: J. H. White, J. S. Fryer, C. M. Fullenwider, W. R. Joblin, James G. Rafter, L. S. McAlister.

Finance—I. B. Oldham, W. P. Fite, W. D. Berry.

Entertainment— I. B. Oldham, R. N. Holcombe, E. H. Coachman.

Registration—H. A. Scott.

Meeting Places—Finis W. Ewing.

Hotels—C. E. DeGroot.

Golf—Shade D. Neely.

Memorial Ceremony—Floyd E. Warterfield.

Medical Reserve Corps Dinner — I. C. Wolfe.

Reception—M. K. Thompson.

Scientific Exhibits—George L. Kaiser.

WOMAN'S AUXILIARY
MONDAY, MAY 9, 1938
Registration on Mezzanine Floor, Severs Hotel

7:30 P. M.—Meeting of State Executive Board, First Presbyterian Church, Social Hall, 5th and Broadway.

TUESDAY, MAY 10, 1938

9:30 A. M.—Annual Meeting of State Auxiliary, First Presbyterian Church. Visiting Doctors' wives invited.

1:00 P. M.—Luncheon, Muskogee Town and Country Club.

4:30 P. M.—Board Meeting for new and retiring State Officers, First Presbyterian Church, Social Hall.

WEDNESDAY, MAY 11, 1938

10:00 A. M.—Motorcade. Leave from Severs Hotel.

SECTIONS

All Sections will meet at 1:30 p.m., Tuesday, May 10th, and at the same hour on Wednesday, May 11th. Meeting places will be as follows:

Surgery—Ball Room, Mezzanine Floor, Severs Hotel.

Medicine—District Court Room "A," 3rd Floor, County Court House.

Eye, Ear, Nose & Throat—District Court Room "B," 3rd Floor, County Court House.

Obstetrics & Pediatrics — County Court Room "B," 3rd Floor, County Court House.

Genito-Urinary Diseases & Syphilology —North Parlor, Mezzanine Floor, Severs Hotel.

Dermatology & Radiology—East Parlor, Mezzanine Floor, Severs Hotel.

(Court House across the street east from Severs Hotel.)

TUESDAY, MAY 10, 1938

8:30 to 10:00 A. M.—Tour of Inspection of Veterans Hospital.

(Transportation furnished from Severs Hotel.)

GENERAL SCIENTIFIC SECTION

Ritz Theater, Third and Court Streets.

10:00 to 10:40 A. M.—"The Surgery of Pulmonary Tuberculosis from a Medical Standpoint," Wm. S. Middleton, Madison, Wisconsin.

10:40 to 11:20 A. M.—"The Management of the Hypertonic Period of Early Infancy," Frank C. Neff, Kansas City.

11:20 to 12:00 Noon.—"The Middle Way," Edward H. Ochsner, Chicago.

SECTION ON GENERAL SURGERY

Ball Room, Mezzanine Floor, Severs Hotel

Chairman—Stratton E. Kernodle, Oklahoma City.

Vice-Chairman—H. G. Crawford, Bartlesville.

Secretary—P. P. Nesbitt, Tulsa, Okla.

TUESDAY, MAY 10, 1938
1:30 P. M.

"*Inguinal Hernia*"—W. P. Fite, Muskogee. Discussed by H. C. Weber, Bartlesville.

"*Acute Appendicitis*"—LeRoy Long, Sr., Oklahoma City. Discussed by M. M. DeArman, Miami.

"*Surgery of the Gall Bladder*"—David L. Garrett, Tulsa. Discussed by Roscoe Walker, Pawhuska.

"*Treatment of Acute Intestinal Obstruction*" — Geo. A. Kilpatrick, McAlester.

Discussed by LeRoy D. Long, Oklahoma City.

"Acute Pelvic Infections"—P. N. Charbonnett, Tulsa. Discussed by W. C. Vernon, Okmulgee.

"Treatment of Acute Empyema"—H. Dale Collins, Oklahoma City. Discussed by R. B. Gibson, Ponca City.

SECTION ON GENERAL MEDICINE

District Court Room "A," 3rd Floor
County Court House

Chairman—Minard F. Jacobs, Oklahoma City.

Vice-Chairman—Frank Nelson, Tulsa.

Secretary—M i l a m F. McKinney, Oklahoma City.

TUESDAY, MAY 10, 1938
2:00 P. M.

(Tuesday's program is sponsored by the Oklahoma Internists' Association.)

"Diabetes Mellitus—Recent Advances in its Treatment"—Alexander Marble, Boston, Mass.

Chairman's Address — "Constipation" — Minard F. Jacobs, Oklahoma City.

"The Indication of Thoracoplasty as an Adjunct in the Treatment of Tuberculosis"—R. M. Shepard, Tulsa.

"Lobar Pneumonia" — Samuel Goodman, Tulsa.

SECTION ON EYE, EAR, NOSE AND THROAT

District Court Room "B," 3rd Floor
County Court House

Chairman—Chester McHenry, Oklahoma City.

Vice-Chairman—A. H. Davis, Tulsa.

Secretary—E. H. Coachman, Muskogee.

TUESDAY, MAY 10, 1938
1:30 P. M.

"Bronchoscopy in Oklahoma"—L. Chester McHenry, Oklahoma City. Discussed by Ruric N. Smith, Tulsa.

"Ocular Therapeutics"—Tullos O. Coston, Oklahoma City. Discussed by D. L. Edwards, Tulsa.

"The Sinus Problem"—Wm. L. Bonham, Oklahoma City. Discussion by Hugh Evans, Tulsa.

"Iritis Occurring in Undulant Fever"—Illustrated with Slides—James R. Reed and E. Goldfain, Oklahoma City. Discussed by F. M. Cooper, Oklahoma City.

"The Use and Abuse of Cautery and Escharotics in the Nose"—O. Alton Watson, Oklahoma City. Discussed by Weldon Sanger, Ponca City.

"Cavernous Sinus Thrombosis"—Theodore G. Wails, Oklahoma City. Discussed by C. M. Fullenwider, Muskogee.

SECTION ON OBSTETRICS AND PEDIATRICS

County Court Room "B," 3rd Floor,
County Court House

Chairman—M. B. Glismann, Okmulgee.

Vice-Chairman—C. W. Arrendell, P o n c a City.

Secretary—Carl F. Simpson, Tulsa.

TUESDAY, MAY 10, 1938
1:30 P. M.

"Chairman's Address"—M. B. Glismann, Okmulgee.

"Birth Control"—George R. Osborn, Tulsa.

"Prenatal Care"—George L. Kaiser, Muskogee.

"Relief of Pain"—E. P. Allen, Oklahoma City.

"Placenta Accreta—Case Report"—J. M. Byrum, Shawnee.

"Still Births"—E. O. Johnson, Tulsa.

"Syphilis in Pregnancy"—F. A. Demand, Oklahoma City.

SECTION ON GENITO-URINARY DISEASES AND SYPHILOLOGY

North Parlor, Mezzanine Floor, Severs Hotel

Chairman—Charles B. Taylor, Oklahoma City.

Vice-Chairman — D. W. Branham, Oklahoma City.

Secretary—Shade D. Neely, Muskogee.

TUESDAY, MAY 10, 1938
1:30 P. M.

"Chairman's Address"—Charles B. Taylor, Oklahoma City.

"Symposium on Gonorrhea"—
   "Acute Gonorrhea"—R. H. Atkin, Oklahoma City.

"Chronic Gonorrhea" — J. H. Howe, Ponca City.

"Complications of Gonorrhea"—Allen R. Russell, McAlester.

"Twenty-Five Years' Progress in Urology" —Floyd E. Warterfield, Muskogee.

"Treatment of Infections of the Prostate"— Basil Hayes, Oklahoma City.

SECTION ON DERMATOLOGY AND RADIOLOGY

East Parlor, Mezzanine Floor, Severs Hotel

Chairman—L. S. McAlister, Muskogee.

Vice-Chairman—M. M. Wickham, Norman.

Secretary—John H. Lamb, Oklahoma City.

TUESDAY, MAY 10, 1938
1:30 P. M.

"Chairman's Address" — L. S. McAlister, Muskogee.

"Treatment of Poison Ivy" — Hervey A. Foerster, Oklahoma City.

"New Aspects of Fever Therapy and Its Relationship to the Treatment of Syphilis"—Onis G. Hazel, Oklahoma City.

Election of Officers.

GENERAL MEETING

TUESDAY, MAY 10, 1938
8:00 P. M.

Ball Room, Mezzanine Floor, Severs Hotel

H. T. Ballantine, General Chairman, Presiding

Invocation—Rev. H. J. Lloyd.

Music—Quartette.

Introduction of Guests—H. T. Ballantine, Muskogee.

Address of Welcome — Finis W. Ewing, President, Muskogee County Medical Society.

Response—J. D. Osborn, Jr., Frederick.

Music—Violin Solo.

Introduction of President-Elect—Sam A. McKeel, Ada, Retiring President.

President's Address—H. K. Speed, Sayre.

9:30 P. M.

President's Reception and Dance — Ball Room, Mezzanine Floor, Severs Hotel.

WEDNESDAY, MAY 11, 1938

8:00 to 9:30 A. M.—Tour of Fort Gibson. (Transportation furnished from Severs Hotel.)

MEMORIAL SERVICE

9:30 to 10:00 A. M.—Ritz Theater, Third and Court streets.

Presiding Officer—Dr. F. E. Warterfield.

Invocation—Rev. W. G. Letham, Muskogee.

Music—Quartette.

Report of the Necrology Committee—Dr. C. E. Williams, Woodward, Chairman.

Memorial Address—Dr. LeRoy Long, Sr., Oklahoma City.

Music—Quartette.

Benediction—Rev. W. G. Letham, Muskogee.

GENERAL SCIENTIFIC SECTION

Ritz Theater, Third and Court Streets

10:00 to 10:40 A. M.—*"Observations from the Current Year's Experience with Medical Cases in a Children's Hospital"*—Frank C. Neff, Kansas City.

10:40 to 11:20 A. M. — *"Acute Coronary Occlusion"* — Wm. S. Middleton, Madison, Wisconsin.

11:20 to 12:00 Noon—*"The Socialization of Medicine"* — Edward H. Ochsner, Chicago.

SECTION ON GENERAL SURGERY

Ball Room, Mezzanine Floor, Severs Hotel

WEDNESDAY, MAY 11, 1938
1:30 P. M.

"Chairman's Address"— Stratton E. Kernodle, Oklahoma City.

Election of Officers.

"Management of Burns"—Patrick Nagle, Oklahoma City. Discussed by F. L. Flack, Tulsa.

"Diagnosis and Treatment of Trigeminal Neuralgia" — Roland M. Klemme, St. Louis, Mo. Discussed by Harry Wilkins, Oklahoma City.

"Factors of Safety in Thyroid Surgery"— R. M. Howard, Oklahoma City. Discussed by A. S. Risser, Blackwell.

"Colles Fracture" — John E. McDonald, Tulsa.

SECTION ON GENERAL MEDICINE

District Court Room "A," 3rd Floor
County Court House

WEDNESDAY, MAY 11, 1938
1:30 P. M.

"Gastro Intestinal Allergy" — George J.
Seibold, Oklahoma City.

Election of Officers.

"Masked Intermittent Malaria, A Study"—
David W. Gillick, Shawnee.

"Coronary Artery Disease" — Harry C.
. Daniels, Oklahoma City.

"Interesting Aspects of Nephritis"—Elmer
Musick, Oklahoma City.

SECTION ON EYE, EAR, NOSE
AND THROAT

District Court Room "B," 3rd Floor
County Court House

WEDNESDAY, MAY 11, 1938
1:30 P. M.

"Surgical Treatment of Pyogenic Infection
of the Paranasal Sinuses" — F. Clinton
Gallaher, Shawnee. Discussed by H. F.
Vandever, Enid.

Election of Officers.

"Syphilis of the Eye" — F. T. Gastineau,
Vinita. Discussed by Gordon Ferguson,
Oklahoma City.

"Lateral Sinus Thrombosis"—Donald Mishler, Tulsa. Discussed by J. C. Matheney,
Okmulgee.

"Intra-Capsular Cataract Extraction"—A.
J. Metscher, Enid. Discussed by Chas.
H. Haralson, Tulsa.

"Functional Hearing Tests"—C. A. Pavy,
Tulsa. Discussed by W. R. Mote, Ardmore,

"Necessity of Accurate Eye Examinations"
—Milton K. Thompson, Muskogee. Discussed by Dr. A. H. Davis, Tulsa.

SECTION ON OBSTETRICS AND
PEDIATRICS

County Court Room "B," 3rd Floor
County Court House

WEDNESDAY, MAY 11, 1938
1:30 P. M.

"Treatment of Gonorrheal Vulvo-Vaginitis"—Ben H. Nicholson, Oklahoma City.

Election of Officers.

"Nephritis"—C. E. Bradley, Tulsa.

"Pyloric Stenosis and Pyloro Spasm in
Infants"—John H. Walker, Muskogee.

"Presentation of Congenital Bone Deformities"—Luvern Hays, Tulsa.

"Acute Infective Laryngotracheobronchitis" — Carroll M. Pounders, Oklahoma
City.

SECTION ON GENITO-URINARY
DISEASES AND SYPHILOLOGY

North Parlor, Mezzanine Floor, Severs
Hotel

WEDNESDAY, MAY 11, 1938
1:30 P. M.

"Symposium on Syphilis"

"Acute Syphilis"—David Hudson, Tulsa.

"Somatic and Latent Syphilis"—James
Stevenson, Tulsa.

"Cerebro-Spinal Syphilis"—C. R. Rayburn, Norman.

"Public Health Aspect of Syphilis" —
Charles M. Pearce, Oklahoma City.

Election of Officers.

"Carcinoma of the Prostate" — Henry S.
Browne, Tulsa.

---o---

COMMITTEE REPORTS

These reports are made in compliance with provisions
of the Constitution and By-Laws which call for publication of such matter in the issue of The Journal
preceding the Annual Session.

1938 Report of Committee on Post-Graduate
Medical Teaching

Your Committee met February 5, 1937, and unanimously voted to submit a request to the Commonwealth Fund for financial aid in re-establishing
post-graduate medical teaching in Oklahoma. This
request was unanimously authorized by the House
of Delegates at the annual State Meeting held in
Tulsa last year (1937). Your Chairman was then
requested to communicate with the Commonwealth
Fund, and a personal interview was arranged with
the Director and Aassociate Director of the Fund,
which was held in New York June 9, 1937. We were
advised that the Commonwealth Fund would consider our application but desired the active cooperation of all agencies in the state interested in
post-graduate medical instruction. At a later
meeting of the Committee, Dr. Chas. M. Pearce,
State Commissioner of Health, offered the cooperation and financial assistance of the Oklahoma
State Department of Health. Dr. Robert U. Patterson, Dean of the Medical School of the University
of Oklahoma, advised that the school would be
unable to participate financially but was in sympathy with the program and would aid in an advisory capacity. The Committee suggested that the
President of the State Association apoint an advisory committee, and Dr. McKeel named the following: Dr. Chas. M. Pearce, Dr. Robert U. Patterson, Dr. Otis G. Bacon, Dr. J. B. Eskridge, Dr. M.

J. Searle, and Dr. C. W. Tedrowe. It was decided to present a two-year course in obstetrics.

A budget was prepared and submitted to the Commonwealth Fund, which called for a total yearly expenditure of $19,500.00, distribution to be as follows:

Clinical Instructor, salary and traveling
  expense $10,000.00
Field Director, salary and traveling expense   6,000.00
Office Secretary 1,500.00
Miscellaneous account, for stationery, postage and other office supplies, motion pictures, lantern slides, projectors, manikin, etc., for teaching purposes, etc., for first year only............................ 2,000.00

The Council of the State Medical Association voted to provide $2,000; State Health Department $5,000; and the Commonwealth Fund was asked to supply the balance, in the amount of $11,500. An additional $1,000 is anticipated from registration fees.

We were advised by Miss Quin, the Associate Director, October 29, 1937, that our application had been approved at the October meeting of the Board. Your Chairman was then requested to communicate with prospective instructors. Knowing that Tennessee State Medical Association had recently begun a similar program and had interviewed a number of prospective instructors, we communicated with Dr. James R. Reinberger, Chairman of the Tennessee Committee. Your Chairman met with Dr. Reinberger in New Orleans in December, and discussed a number of applicants with him. After much correspondence and after carefully going over the credentials of a number of applicants, it was decided to invite Dr. Edward N. Smith, of Spokane and New York, to come to Oklahoma City for a personal interview with the Committee.

Much valuable time was lost in selecting a Field Director in waiting for a decision of the Tennessee Committee on whether or not they would permit Mr. L. W. Kibler to act in a dual capacity as organizer for both states, and a final negative decision was not reached until January 18. Immediately, we wired Dr. Smith to report to our Committee, which he did on February 4. After interviewing Dr. Smith, the Committee unanimously chose him as our Instructor. Because of his experience and knowledge of post-graduate teaching in this state, Mr. Kibler was asked to meet with us and aid us in outlining our first program and in selecting a field organizer. It was finally voted that your Committee go forward with the work of securing temporary field assistance in the organization of our first course and in training some one for the permanent position. Miss Mary Frances Carpenter was selected as office secretary. The treasurer of the State Medical Association was named to disburse the funds upon approval of vouchers by the Committee Chairman.

The state has been temporarily divided into 12 teaching circuits. Five cities in each circuit are to be selected as the teaching centers. It was decided to begin the first course April 4, 1938, in northeastern Oklahoma, including the counties of Cherokee, Craig, Delaware, Mayes, Osage, Ottawa, Rogers, and Washington, at the centers of Claremore, Pawhuska, Bartlesville, Vinita, and Miami.

The response of the physicians in this circuit has been most gratifying. Registrations totaling 85 per cent have already been received, as this is written two weeks before the scheduled opening of the course. Other circuits now are being organized, and a minimum of 15 registrations in each center is required. The registration fee of $5.00 is added to the general Post-Graduate Fund.

Dr. Edward N. Smith has been selected by your Committee as the medical instructor in the obstetrical program. Dr. Smith is highly qualified to handle this work. He is a graduate of Washington

State College, and of the University of Pennsylvania School of Medicine. He has had an excellent background of experience including rotating internship, Camden, New Jersey, several residencies in obstetrics and gynecology including Cornell Medical Center, New York City; Margaret Hague Maternity Hospital, Jersey City, New Jersey; Columbia Medical Center, Sloane Hospital; New York Post-Graduate Hospital, and is a diplomate of the American Board of Obstetrics and Gynecology. He is the recipient of the Degree of Med. D. Sc. in Obstetrics and Gynecology, Columbia University.

In addition to Dr. Smith's very thorough postgraduate training in obstetrics, he did general practice in Livingston County, New York, for four years following his graduation, serving also as County Health Officer and secretary of the local medical society.

In view of his broad experience as a general practitioner and teacher, he is cognizant of their problems and particularly adapted for his present position. Dr. Smith is very pleasing of personality, and has the ability of conveying his world of information in a manner easily understood.

Between lectures, as far as his time for travel will permit, Dr. Smith will be available for free consultation with doctors registered in the course. You can readily see from this that physicians will have the advantage of discussing the theories advanced in the lectures over their cases in actual practice.

There will be ten lectures given in each circuit consisting of five teaching centers. The instructor will give one lecture each week in each center. The sessions include approximately one hour of didactic lecture followed by demonstrations on clinical patients, manikin, female pelvic skeleton, etc. The lecture, itself, will be supplemented by the answer and discussion of questions submitted the previous week, and in addition, any clinical material available will be utilized for study. The accessory equipment will consist of actual demonstrations of the instruments, chemicals, and procedures advocated, supplemented by charts, graphs, lantern slides and 16-millimeter moving picture projection.

The supply of patients for these clinical lectures will be assured through the cooperation of the local committee chairman. Any physician enrolled in the course may submit a patient for examination or group discussion when time permits by notifying the local committee chairman.

Your Committee expresses its appreciation to Dr. James R. Reinberger, Chairman, and Mr. L. W. Kibler of the Tennessee Committee on Post-Graduate Medical Instruction for their cooperation and suggestions.

A supplemental verbal report will be given to the House of Delegates at the annual meeting of our State Association.

Respectfully submitted,
Committee on Post-Graduate Medical Teaching,
    Henry H. Turner, Chairman,
    H. C. Weber,
    T. H. McCarley.

Report of Committee on Control of Cancer of Oklahoma State Medical Association

Your Committee has actively joined with the State Federated Women's Clubs in organizing the Women's Field Army in Oklahoma with the majority control resting in this committee as laid down in our special report appearing in the March issue of the Journal, page 94.

We have communicated with every county medical society in the state and they now have full information and instructions as to the fundamental principles and the actual operation of this public educational effort.

To the date of this writing 18 county medical

societies have appointed active cancer committees. Most of these have formed county speakers' bureaus and are supplying speakers for small and large public meetings arranged by the women's organization. The reports coming to us give ample evidence that both the profession and the members of the federated clubs are taking this work seriously and are pleased with the results.

Appointments of additional county cancer committees are being received daily and they are satisfactorily coordinating their educational activities with the women's organization.

Several large meetings have been held in the state where the county cancer committees have requested speakers from outside their county and these have been supplied through this committee from the State Speakers' Bureau which is under the direction of this committee.

Every county which has not completed its organization is urged to do so at once and in the event of misunderstanding or desiring more information they should write a member of this committee.

The American Society for the Control of Cancer is liberally furnishing materials for all educational efforts. This assistance in supplying uniform sound factual information for both speakers and public is of tremendous value and should be appreciated by the members of the State Medical Association.

RECOMMENDATIONS

1. Continued active cooperation with the American Society for the Control of Cancer.

2. Encouragement of frequent programs and discussions about cancer in all county medical societies.

3. Avoidance of abrupt changes in personnel of this committee in order to maintain a continuity of purpose and activity.

4. Assignment of funds for secretarial assistance and other necessary expense to this committee for the success of this work.

5. Rigid adherence to the ethical principles outlined and followed by this committee in recent years.

Wendell Long, Chairman.
E. S. Lain.
Paul Champlin.
Ralph McGill.

Report of the Committee on Public Policy and Legislation

The Committee soon after appointment was faced by a protest on Initiative Petition No. 166, which was filed with the Secretary of State.

During this time the Committee has held four meetings in Oklahoma City, one in Tulsa, one in Enid and one in Shawnee. In addition to this each member of the Committee has visited various groups and County Medical meetings in the various parts of the state.

The Committee has also sent out three different letters to each member of the State Medical Association and a number of letters to the officers of the County Societies.

All this effort was made to raise money to cover expense of protesting the Initiative Petition above mentioned.

In protesting the Initiative Petition 166 a lawyer, handwriting experts and clerical help were employed to handle the hearing before the Secretary of State. These expenses, with all other expenses such as printing, postage, stenographic hire, have been paid.

The printing above referred to includes 5,000 copies of the Initiative Bill, one of which was mailed to each Doctor in the state, and a sufficient supply retained to supply the attendance at the meeting of the State Association in Muskogee and for any other Doctor desiring additional copies of the same.

This, itself, has not been without considerable expense.

The protest on the bill at this time is before the Supreme Court. Whether we will have sufficient funds to carry on through the Court remains yet to be seen.

The Committee desires to make a detailed report on all its activities before the House of Delegates in the meeting of the State Association and a copy of the Auditor's report on the funds collected and expended will be presented at that time in detail.

Respectfully submitted.

S. A. McKeel, President,
H. K. Speed, President Elect,
W. P. Neilson,
R. C. Pigford,
J. M. Byrum.
By: J.M.B., March 15, 1938.

Report of the Committee on Industrial Service and Traumatic Surgery

The function of the Industrial Service and Traumatic Surgery Committee should be a very important one, but the present committee, as well as committees of other years, has faced a situation in which there has seemed to be very little general interest on the part of the members of the State Medical Association.

Thus far this year, no definite problems have arisen which would require the investigation or consideration of this Committee. A few years ago a state law was enacted, setting up a State Insurance Fund, which to a very great extent has taken over the greater portion of the compensation insurance business. Most of the private casualty insurance companies have ceased writing this kind of business, except companies where the compensation policy must be written in order to secure and render satisfactory service to the employer on his many other insurance necessities. As a result of this alteration in the status of compensation insurance, a greater proportion of all injury cases of a compensable nature, occurring throughout the state are handled through the State Insurance Fund, who has its own claim adjusters and attorneys. These adjusters and attorneys must settle for disability through the action and judgment of the State Industrial Commission, under exactly the same rules as a private insurance company. However, the State Insurance Fund, as well as the State Industrial Commission is at the State Capitol building, so that many details and daily difficulties may be ironed out between members of the two organizations, without formal procedure. In many instances this is of advantage to the doctor who is treating an injured employee, especially if the doctor takes the trouble to make his reports clear and understandable so that the adjusters of the State Fund can properly consider the problems. The adjusters of the State Fund have made an especial effort to cooperate with the profession throughout the state in the care of injured employees who come under their jurisdiction. They make no special appointments to doctors for the care of their cases, and try not to discriminate or interfere with the professional rules or methods, in any way. However, the adjusters of the State Insurance Fund have become experienced to the extent that they quickly recognize inefficient medical service, and in many instances give notification that certain cases must be sent to recognized specialists for treatment. The expression from these adjusters is that the medical profession is cooperating in an extremely satisfactory manner. As far as this Committee is able to determine, the profession of the State seems very well satisfied with the present status of compensation industrial practice, as compared with some of the difficulties which arose a few years ago when many of the insurance companies continuously complained about exorbitant hospital and professional fees and instructed their claim adjusters to secure reduction of fees in all cases possible. The Fund has not established any definite fee schedule but has an average fee schedule in their office, which as a whole has seemed fair to all concerned. Many items on a fee schedule cannot be adhered to strictly, and when an unusual situation arises the doctor should correspond with the adjusters of the State Fund before going too far with the case, in order to give them a chance to record complications and difficulties in the case, and make an investigation if necessary.

Your Committee welcomes any discussion or criticisms or difficulties which may arise, and will be willing to present formally any reasonable resolutions or requests for investigation to the State Insurance Fund or the State Industrial Commission for consideration.

Earl D. McBride, Chairman.
J. F. Park.
G. H. Stagner.

Report of Crippled Childrens Committee

The Crippled Childrens Committee of the Oklahoma State Medical Association has had a fairly active year, particularly in cooperation, and consultation in regard to the recent epidemic of infantile paralysis. In cooperation with the Oklahoma State Health Department, a pamphlet was prepared and published by the Oklahoma Commission for Crippled Children, recapitulating our present knowledge on infantile paralysis. This pamphlet was distributed by the Commission and we are informed that it had a very good reception among the doctors of the state.

We have consulted on various occasions with the Oklahoma Commission for Crippled Children and will attempt to cooperate with them in augmenting their program.

Yours very truly,
D. H. O'Donoghue, Chairman.
George S. Baxter.
Ray Lindsey.

Report of the Committee on Medical Education and Hospitals

During the past year, this Committee has been ready to cooperate with all medical agencies in the state looking to the advancement of educational standards, and to increase the opportunities for post-graduate education within the reach of physicians practicing in the state. The Committee took an active part in the work of the Oklahoma Clinical Society during its conference held in Oklahoma City during November, 1937. While this presented interesting and valuable lectures and conferences available to physicians residing in other states, its greatest benefit was for physicians practicing in our own state.

While the University of Oklahoma School of Medicine (the only one in the state) more than two years ago presented comprehensive plans calculated to increase the teaching facilities of the medical school, and also to amplify the teaching facilities and the capacity of the University and Crippled Children's Hospitals, the Legislature made no appropriations for the indicated new additions and construction. The Legislature did, however, appropriate more funds for the medical school for salaries and maintenance, and for the two teaching hospitals than ever before in the history of the school. There are now a sufficient number of full-time teachers in the first two years (preclinical years) of the medical school to carry on the teaching on a very high plane for the number of students for which the school now has accommodations. It is hoped that the next Legislature (meeting in January, 1939) will grant additional funds in order to build up a nucleus of full-time teachers in the important clinical departments of the last two, or clinical years of the medical school. A few full-time and part-time teachers in the clinical departments to work with the larger fine staff of clinical teachers who are also engaged in private practice, will go far to place our medical school in the forefront of like institutions in the United States. It is hoped that the next Legislature will also furnish some of the funds which are needed to begin the construction program which will expand the facilities of the two teaching hospitals, so that in addition to providing more clinical material for teaching medical students, the state will also be able to care for a greater number of its underprivileged citizens who look to it for help when they need it.

One of the most unfortunate situations which the authorities of the two teaching hospitals have to face from time to time is their inability to take in patients who need hospital treatment, because the present limited bed capacity of these two institutions makes it impossible.

The Committee is deeply interested in plans which will supply the needs of the other fine state hospitals which care for those afflicted with mental diseases and tuberculosis.

Members of this Committee of the medical school are co-operating in the conduct of postgraduate courses of instruction in Obstetrics which are to be given throughout the state of Oklahoma for one year. This work is being given under the auspices of the Oklahoma State Medical Association from funds provided by the State Health Department and the Commonwealth Fund of New York.

Robert U. Patterson, Chairman.

ANNUAL REPORT
of the Secretary-Treasurer-Editor
March 31, 1937, to March 31, 1938

TO THE MEMBERSHIP OF THE OKLAHOMA STATE MEDICAL ASSOCIATION:

The Constitution and By-Laws provide that the Secretary-Treasurer-Editor shall s u b m i t to the Council and through it to the House of Delegates a report of the various activities of his office during the previous year

Detailed statements of all financial transactions, duplicate deposit certificates and other business matters I hereby submit for audit to the Council.

MEMBERSHIP: On March 31, 1937, we had 1,350 members; on March 31, 1938, we find our membership to be 1,313. We, of course, expected some decrease in membership when the dues were increased to $8.00 per year. However, we are greatly surprised to find the decrease to be as small as is apparent. It is unfortunate that our membership is not sufficient so that we can retain three Delegates to the American Medical Association, but as the quota has been increased for each state we will only be represented by two Delegates for the next three years.

DEATHS OF PHYSICIANS: We, of course, regret to have to mention the names of our members who have died during the past year. A list of these members will be _____ with the report of the Necrology Committee _____ they will be properly honored at the Mem____ Service which will be held during the Musk____ Meeting.

MEDICAL DEFENSE: The following cases have either been settled, dropped or disposed of in the following manner:

Settled: Cleveland County, No. 13226.
Pottawatomie County, No. 6064.
Roger Mills County, No. 5875.

Pending: Caddo County, No. 9407.
Carter County, No. 16262.
Choctaw County, No. 8644.
Logan County, No. 1693.
Mayes County, No. ——
Pontotoc County, No. ——

In addition to the above the following cases are now pending, the progress and status of which is unknown as they are pending or dormant in the courts:

Blaine County, No. ——
Carter County, No. ——
Craig County, No. ——
Hughes County, No. ——
Payne County, No. ——
Pottawatomie County, No. ——

I want to mention in particular our very intimate relationship with the Cooperative Medical Advertising Bureau, whose offices are in the American Medical Association building. We have received from the Bureau every consideration and we have been very careful to accept no advertising which has not been approved by this Bureau. Our advertising material is kept clean and strictly ethical even though we are offered, every month, advertising that is not of the type which we would care to use. You may be sure that any products that you see advertised in your Journal have received the approval of the Council on Pharmacy and Chemistry of the American Medical Association. It would be a great advantage to the Journal if every doctor would ask the "detail men" who visit them whether or not his product is Council Approved, as there have been several accidents during the past year from the use of products submitted by detail men that were not Council Approved and by their use many deaths resulted. It would be to the advantage of the members of the State Association to patronize the pharmaceutical houses that carry Council Approved products, that use the Journal for advertising, and exhibit at our annual meetings.

The Journal, during the past year, has maintained its usual size and there have been some issues that have been quite voluminous. We have been glad to accept the high type papers that have been presented by the members and there has been sufficient material so that our scientific section has been well filled with worth while material.

Again we want to thank the physicians who give so graciously of their time in the preparation of our abstract department. There is much favorable comment from the subscribers as to the scope, detail and excellent manner in which these abstracts appear in the Journal. The men who prepare these abstracts are the busiest physicians and surgeons in the state and the time consumed means much to them, and their contributions add greatly to the value of our Journal.

As usual we are not in position to list our Bills Receivable, however, a schedule of same is hereby submitted to the Council.

From the reports which you will find published in the Journal you will note that there have been decided activities by the various Committees, and of special importance is the work by the Post Graduate Medical Teaching Committee, who have been able to bring to the state post graduate work on Obstetrics, with a full time instruc? r ,who is assisted by a director and stenograp ??s work has been made possible by fin· ??istance from the Commonwealth Fund ?8? ? ??al money obtained through the State H ?·lth _ ?· nent.

The Legislative (n.mittee has a job on their

hands which no doubt will receive the attention of both the Council and House of Delegates.

The Committee on Study and Control of Cancer has been very active and is organizing throughout the state a campaign which, if carried on over a period of years, will without question reduce cancer mortality. This Committee deserves the cooperation of every county medical society.

At the beginning of 1938 we had an indebtedness with the First National Bank of McAlester of $9,000.00. Since payment of 1938 dues, $2,000.00 of this indebtedness has been paid, showing our indebtedness to the Bank, at this time, to be $7,000.00. The expense has been carefully budgeted for the next few years, and it would appear that about $2,000.00 each year, together with the $2,000.00 which has been allocated by the Council for Post Graduate Medical Teaching in Obstetrics is all that can be paid, and satisfactory arrangements have been made so that our indebtedness can be liquidated in this manner.

AUDIT REPORT

Oklahoma State Medical Association
Dr. L. S. Willour, Secretary-Treasurer
McAlester, Oklahoma
For Period From April 1, 1937, to March 31, 1938
By J. K. Pemberton, McAlester, Oklahoma

April 4th, 1938.

Dr. Sam A. McKeel, President,
Oklahoma State Medical Association,
Ada, Oklahoma.

Dear Dr. McKeel:

Upon request, I have audited the books of account, records and investments of

Dr. L. S. Willour, Secretary- Treasurer
Oklahoma State Medical Association,
McAlester, Oklahoma,

for the period beginning April 1st, 1937, and ending March 31st, 1938, and submit the following schedules, together with comments and supporting exhibits.

Cash receipts were traced into the bank through a detailed check of the items received, against deposit tickets as shown by the files of the bank. Cash expenditures and disbursements were c h e c k e d against bank records, all vouchers and checks were examined and compared with original entries; endorsements scrutinized and found to be in order.

In company with Dr. L. S. Willour, Secretary-Treasurer, I have examined the following investments which are kept in a safety deposit box in the First National Bank, McAlester, Oklahoma, which box is registered in the name of the Oklahoma Medical Association; except at this date the bonds are held by the bank as collateral to a loan totaling $5,000.00 executed by the Oklahoma Medical Association:

GENERAL FUND:

3¼ % U. S. Treasury Bonds of 1944-46—

Bond No.	Par Value	
94180L	$ 500.00	
94181A	500.00	
95099K	1,000.00	$2,000.00

MEDICAL DEFENSE FUND:

3¼ % U. S. Treasury Bonds of 1943-45—

Bond No.	Par Value	
878J	$1,000.00	
879K	1,000.00	
880L	1,000.00	$3,000.00

April 15, 1937, and October 15, 1937, coupons were attached to the bonds and had not been clipped and deposited, however on April 4th, 1938, these coupons were clipped and deposited to their respective accounts. April 15th, 1938, and subsequent coupons are attached to the bonds.

The books of the Association are kept on an actual cash receipts and disbursements basis, and for that reason accrued items are not included in the audit, however upon investigation I find no unpaid or accrued accounts payable, all bills having been paid prior to the date of the audit; there are certain accounts receivable owing to the Association and a list or schedule in detail has been prepared showing these accounts and the amounts due, and is attached hereto and made a part of this audit report.

I find upon examination the following Notes and Accounts payable made and owing by the Association:

ACCOUNTS PAYABLE:

To the General Fund O. S. M. A.............$3,824.00

NOTES PAYABLE:

To the General Fund O. S. M. A................ 3,800.00

To the First National Bank, McAlester, Okla. (Secured by the above described U. S. Treasury Bonds of the par value of $5,000.00) 5,000.00

To the First National Bank, McAlester, Oklahoma (Unsecured) 2,000.00

I further find that proper resolutions were passed authorizing the execution of said borrowings which are therefore in order, and constitute valid and binding obligations of the Oklahoma State Medical Association.

I respectfully submit the following Audit and Report for your information.

J. K. PEMBERTON, Auditor.

* * *

The above and foregoing statement and following Audit is submitted as my report for the period from April 1st, 1937, to March 31st, 1938.

L. S. WILLOUR, Secretary-Treasurer, Oklahoma State Medical Association.

THE FIRST NATIONAL BANK
McAlester, Oklahoma
April 2nd, 1938

Dr. L. S. Willour, Secretary-Treasurer,
Oklahoma State Medical Association,
McAlester, Oklahoma.

Dear Dr. Willour:

This is to certify that according to our records the following accounts reflected a credit balance, subject to check, at the close of business March 31st, 1938, as follows:

Oklahoma State Medical Association:

General Fund $6,014.37
Medical Defense Fund 1,185.00
Post Graduate Fund 4,125.84
Legislative Fund 1,195.27

It is further certified that the following direct obligations of the Oklahoma State Medical Association were owing to the First National Bank, McAlester, Oklahoma, at the close of business on March 31st, 1938, as follows:

Date of Note	Description of Collateral	Date Due	Amount
Feb. 23, 1937	Unsecured	May 23, 1938	$2,000.00
Feb. 12, 1937	3¼% U. S. Treasury Bond of 1944-46 No. 95099K	April 10, 1938	1,000.00
Feb. 18, 1937	3¼% U. S. Treasury Bonds of 1944-46 Nos. 94180L, 94-181A, 2 at $500.00; and 3¼% U. S. Treasury Bonds of 1943-45 Nos. 878J, 879K, 880L, being 3 at $1,000.00	April 10, 1938	4,000.00

TOTAL Indebtedness $7,000.00

Yours very truly,

J. K. PEMBERTON,
Vice-President and Cashier.

Oklahoma State Medical Association
Dr. L. S. Willour, Secretary-Treasurer
McAlester, Oklahoma
March 31, 1938

BALANCE SHEET

ASSETS

CURRENT ASSETS:
First National Bank, McAlester, Oklahoma:

General Fund $5,764.22
Medical Defense Fund 1,198.00
Post Graduate Fund 2,630.08
Legislative Fund 1,144.07 $10,736.37

INVESTMENTS—U. S. GOVERNMENT BONDS:
General Fund (Par Value).... 2,000.00
Defense Fund (Par Value)— 3,000.00   5,000.00

NOTES AND ACCOUNTS RECEIVABLE:
Due to General Fund............. 7,624.00   7,624.00

TOTAL $23,360.37

LIABILITIES

EXCESS OF ASSETS OVER LIABILITIES:
Balance March 31, 1937.........$4,518.87
Add:
Excess of Income over Expenditures:
General Fund 466.52
Medical Defense Fund............ 1,151.00
Post Graduate Fund.............. 2,630.08
Legislative Fund 902.94   8,736.37

NOTES AND ACCOUNTS PAYABLE:
To General Fund 7,624.00
To Bank (Secured U. S.
Gov't. Bonds) 5,000.00
To Bank—Unsecured 2,000.00   14,624.00

TOTAL $23,360.37

CASH RECEIPTS AND DISBURSEMENTS
Oklahoma State Medical Association
Dr. L. S. Willour, Secretary-Treasurer
McAlester, Oklahoma
April 1, 1937, to March 31, 1938

GENERAL FUND:
Balance .... $ 4,282.99
RECEIPTS:
Advertising $7,556.54
Memberships 9,135.10
Transfer from Medical De-
fense Fund 1,447.75
Repayment from Legislative
Fund 500.00
Proceeds Loan from First Na-
tional Bank 2,000.00

Total Receipts 20,639.29

Total Cash to Account for....................$24,922.38
DISBURSEMENTS:
Dr. L. S. Willour:
Salary to 4-1-38 at $200.00
per month $2,400.00
Oltha Shelton:
Salary to 4-1-38 at $125.00
per month 1,500.00
Oltha Shelton; Salary advance 14.36
Other Office Salaries 30.00
Social Security Tax 35.75
Rent 313.80
Telephone and Telegraph 73.55
Postage 266.22
Stationary and Printing 170.78
Treasurer's Bond and Audit 75.00
Printing Journal 6,065.54
Press Clipping Service 36.00
Expense Annual Meeting 606.24
Expense Council and Delegates 804.04
Expense Post Graduate Work.. 341.85
Expense Medical Defense 100.00
Expense—Legislature 201.03
Purchase Typewriter 84.00
Interest Paid Borrowed Money 165.00
Sundry Expense 51.00
Payment of Loan First National
Bank 2,000.00
Loan to Public Policy and
Public Relations Committee 3,824.00

Total Disbursements 19,158.16

Balance on Hand March 31, 1938............$ 5,764.22
MEDICAL DEFENSE FUND:
Balance March 31, 1937 ....$ 1,494.75
RECEIPTS:
Fees Collected $1,301.00   1,301.00

Total Cash to Account for...................$ 2,795.75
DISBURSEMENTS:
Transfer to General Fund $1,447.75
Medical Defense of Members.. 150.00

Total Disbursements 1,597.75

Balance on Hand March 31, 1938............$ 1,198.00
POST GRADUATE FUND:
Balance March 31, 1937 0
RECEIPTS:
Received from Commonwealth
Fund March 3, 1938 .... $ 4,175.00
Dues Collected 240.00   240.00

Total Cash to Account for...................$ 4,415.00
DISBURSEMENTS:
Salaries, Executive $1,333.32
Salaries, Clerical 187.50
Stationary and Printing 50.19
Postage 17.68
Sundry 47.61
Office Furniture and Fixtures 148.62

Total Disbursements 1,784.92

Balance on Hand March 31, 1938..........$ 2,630.08

CASH ON DEPOSIT
Oklahoma State Medical Association
Dr. L. S. Willour, Secretary-Treasurer
McAlester, Oklahoma
March 31, 1938
FIRST NATIONAL BANK,
McALESTER, OKLAHOMA.
GENERAL FUND:
Balance as per Records ....$ 5,764.22
ADD:
Outstanding Checks: No.   Amt.
3617   4.00
3574   1.00
4115   4.00
4663   6.50
4677   6.50
4683   6.24
4688   486.50
4689   1.61
4690   26.15   542.50

6,306.72
DEDUCT:
Deposits, Shown on Records
3-39-38   194.35
Shown Banks Records 4-4-38   98.00   292.35

Balance as per Bank Statement
and Verification Letter.....................$ 6,014.37
MEDICAL DEFENSE FUND:
Balance as per Records ....$ 1,198.00
DEDUCT:
Deposit, Shown on Records
3-29-38; Shown Bank Rec-
ords 4-4-38 .... 13.00   13.00

Balance as per Bank Statement
and Verification Letter ....$ 1,185.00
POST GRADUATE FUND:
Balance as per Records ....$ 2,630.08
ADD:
Outstanding Checks: No.   Amt.
2   350.00
4   47.61
5   21.52
6   18.92
7   95.43
8   53.19
9   132.69
10   9.75
11   416.66
12   350.00   1,495.76

Balance as per Bank Statement
and Verification Letter ....$ 4,125.84

INCOME AND EXPENDITURES
Oklahoma State Medical Association
Dr. L. S. Willour, Secretary-Treasurer
McAlester, Oklahoma
For Period from April 1, 1937, to March 31, 1938
GENERAL FUND:
INCOME:
Advertising $7,556.54
Memberships 9,135.10

Total Income $16,691.64
EXPENDITURES:
Salaries: Secretary-Treasurer 2,400.00
Salaries: Assistant Secretary.. 1,500.00
Salary Advance: Assistant Sec-
retary 14.36
Other Office Salaries 30.00
Social Security Tax 35.75
Rent 313.80
Telephone and Telegraph 73.55
Postage 266.22
Stationary and Printing 170.78

Treasurer's Bond and Audit.... 75.00
Printing Journal 6,065.54
Press Clipping Service 36.00
Expense, Annual Meeting 606.24
Expense, Council and Delegates 804.04
Expense, Post Graduate Work.. 341.85
Expense, Medical Defense 100.00
Expense, Legislature 201.03
Purchase Typewriter 84.00
Interest Paid Money Borrowed 165.00
Sundry Expense 51.00

Total Expenditures $13,334.16

Excess of Income Over Expenditures........$ 3,357.48
DEDUCT: Loan to Public Policy
and Public Relations Committee........... 3,824.00
Balance Net—Excess of Income over
Expenditures ....$ 466.52

MEDICAL DEFENSE FUND:
INCOME:
Fees Collected ....$1,301.00 $ 1,301.00

Total Income·...................$ 1,301.00
EXPENDITURES:
Medical Defense of Members.$ 150.00

Total Expenditures ....$ 150.00

Excess of Income over Expenditures........$ 1,151.00

POST GRADUATE FUND:
INCOME:
Received from Commonwealth
Fund $4,175.00
Fees Collected 240.00

Total Income ....$ 4,415.00
EXPENDITURES:
Salaries, Executive $1,333.32
Salaries, Clerical 187.50
Stationery and Printing 50.19
Postage 17.68
Sundry Expenses 47.61
Office Furniture and Fixtures 148.62

Total Expenditures 1,784.92

Excess of Income over Expenditures........$ 2,630.08

————o————

Books Received and Reviewed

HERNIA, Anatomy, Etiology, Symptoms, Diagnosis, Differential Diagnosis, Prognosis and the Operative and Injection Treatment, by Leigh F. Watson, M.D. Member of Attending Staff of California Lutheran Hospital and Methodist Hospital of Southern California, Los Angeles. Second Edition. The C. V. Mosby Company, St. Louis, 1938.

This work, by a surgeon who for some years was an honored member of the Oklahoma profession, is the most complete treatise on the subject of hernia to be presented. The book is beautifully illustrated and well edited.

The various operative procedures for every sort of hernia are considered in detail, diagnosis, preoperative and post-operative care are considered. The anatomy of all types of hernia is thoroughly described and illustrated.

Several chapters give in the most minute detail the treatment of hernia by injection. Indications and contra indications for this sort of treatment, formulae of injection materials, dosage, truss fitting and all other phases of the procedures receive the most careful attention of the author.

Medico-legal and compensation f e a t u r e s with many pertinent suggestions are presented.

In all this is a most interesting presentation of the subject of hernia and when carefully read will add much to the surgeon's knowledge of this subject.

———

SHADOW ON THE LAND — SYPHILIS, by Thomas Parran, M.D., Surgeon General of the United States Public Health Service, Washington, D. C.

This is well presented in a story like form of syphilis and its dangers to the people of this nation.

It presents all the dangers of its contagiousness and complications as well as end results in form of delinquents, deformities and various other effects on economic status of the people as a whole. It is equally well written for medical men and for laity and is a challenge to both.

———

A TEXTBOOK OF SURGICAL NURSING, by Henry H. Brookes, Jr., M.D., Instructor in Clinical Surgery, Washington University School of Medicine; Surgeon to the Out-Patients, Washington University Dispensary; Assistant Surgeon to Barnes Hospital. Illustrated. The C. V. Mosby Company, 1937.

This very complete textbook covers not only the nursing problems but many of the surgeon's problems. The preoperative care, essential preoperative laboratory examination; preparation of the patient in all respects, including the operative field, are thoroughly covered, as well as the post operative care, including diagnosis of nursing treatment fully described.

Not only does this serve as a most complete text for nurses but might well be read by physicians and surgeons interested in surgical subjects. I would say that any nurse, who would conscientiously read and digest this treatise, would very satisfactorily specialize in the nursing of surgical patients. It is a most complete text and I heartily recommend it.

———

MENTAL THERAPY, Studies in Fifty Cases, by Louis S. London, M.D., formerly passed Assistant Surgeon (R) United States Public Health Service; Medical Officer United States Veterans Bureau; Assistant Physician Central Islip State Hospital, Central Islip, New York, and Manhattan State Hospital, Wards Island, New York. Two volumes, price $12.50. Covici-Friede Publishers, New York.

This is no doubt one of the best works on abnormal psychology published in a long time. Dr. London has been interested in Freudian theories since 1913. Through his long and distinguished career in state hospitals for the insane and his boundless opportunity for taking the working measure of the genius of Freud, he has been one of those instrumental in bringing about the acceptance of psychoanalysis as a vital method of research into the enigma of the psychosis. Hence, this book is a work of unquestionable authority.

This book is a presentation of 50 cases and is divided into six parts. Part one is entitled "Meta-psychology" and describes the historical evolution of psychotheropeutics. Part two takes us into the case histories. Here we see the minor psychoses clearly dramatized and detailed. Part three takes us into the graver paraphilias (sexual perversions). Part four concerns cases that are borderline between nemoses and major psychoses. Part five deals with schizophrenia and with paranola. The last part deals with the manic depressive psychoses.

There is an extremely valuable glossary at the end of the second volume.

This book should become an extremely valuable reference volume for psychologists, neurologists, psychiatrists and general practitioners.

ABSTRACTS : REVIEWS : COMMENTS
and CORRESPONDENCE

SURGERY AND GYNECOLOGY
Abstracts, Reviews and Comments from
LeRoy Long Clinic
714 Medical Arts Building, Oklahoma City

The Injection Treatment of Hernia; Kansas City Medical Journal, January, 1938; A. S. Jackson.

In 1933 Bratrud and McKinney of the University of Minnesota brought forth their views in regard to the injection treatment of hernia. The idea of injecting a hernia by a solution was not new since various investigators during the past century have written and talked of the subject. Few if any of these, however, served to awaken the interest of the medical profession by reliable scientific investigation based upon animal experimentation and pathological studies. That the latter was conducted under the guidance of Drs. Wangensteen and Bell of the Surgical and Pathological Departments of the University of Minnesota is sufficient to attract attention to the subject.

In attempting to ascertain the facts for himself, the author began a study of the problem in 1934 and with his associate, Dr. Holmgren, injected approximately 280 hernias in 230 patients. He is not yet prepared to give any opinion as to the efficacy of the method in his hands, feeling that three years is not sufficient time to form definite conclusions regarding any method of treating hernias.

There are reports in the literature regarding the injection treatment of hernia based on short periods of observation with high percentages of cures. Their value is questionable. What is wanted are the facts. Can a hernia be cured by the injection of a solution? As a surgeon the author tried to look upon this subject with an open mind to determine whether or not this method was successful.

He says that after a study of nearly 300 cases he is not as enthusiastic as many who claim over 90 per cent cures, nor can he accept a report claiming less than three per cent cures.

It seems that there is no generally accepted successful method of curing hernia. It is apparent that surgery has not alone entirely settled the hernia problem. Even the promising Gallie fascial suture operation appears to be ineffective according to a report from the Hospital for Ruptured and Crippled at New York City, which shows 284 or 29 per cent recurrences in 975 operations. It is significant that 63 per cent of the recurrent cases developed after one year so that the longer the study is continued the higher is the percentage of recurrence. This excellent fact finding study covered a period of 11 years. As a consequence of these disappointing results, the fascial suture method of Gallie has been largely abandoned at the New York Hospital for Ruptured and Crippled and silk is now used routinely. Many other surgeons have returned to the use of silk and the technique advocated by Halstead.

The author now believes that the incidence of recurrence of hernia following herniotomy in this country is about 15 per cent. His former idea was that this figure would be about 10 per cent.

In this article he merely summarizes the findings of his own study and does not attempt to review the historical aspect of the injection method for the treatment of hernia nor does he attempt to give the technique for the method.

He concludes that the injection treatment of hernia has already shown sufficient results in the hands of capable scientific investigators to warrant a careful study by all who are interested in the problem of hernia. Until more time has elapsed and the end results of large series of cases have been carefully tabulated, final judgment concerning the success or failure of this method of treatment must be withheld. With increasing knowledge and the development of more effective sclerosing solutions (he used Proliferol, the solution developed by Bratrud and his associates at the University of Minnesota) undoubtedly better results may be expected than are now apparent.

LeRoy D. Long.

Distribution of Ureteral Pain; An Editorial appearing in Wisconsin Medical Journal, December, 1937; Dr. George H. Ewell.

The difficulties sometimes encountered in a differential diagnosis between lesions of the urinary tract and lesions of adjacent abdominal viscera has long been recognized by most clinicians. Particularly is this true when the lesions involve the right side of the urinary tract.

The frequency with which symptoms ordinarily attributed to diseases of the gastro-intestinal tract occur with lesions of the urinary tract is also well known. Brooks in a discussion of this subject stated that nausea and vomiting were in many instances the outstanding symptoms of renal disease. Braasch, in a discussion of this subject in 1920, stated that in his clinic approximately half of the patients with lesions in the right kidney and ureter had had previous operations on the adjacent abdominal organs and in most instances the pathology of the ureter and kidney was not recognized.

Bumpus and Thompson found in the study of 1,001 cases of ureteral stone, that nausea and vomiting occurred in 30 per cent; that in 22 per cent of their patients the symptoms were of such nature that appendectomy had been performed; that in 16 per cent a diagnosis of cholecystic disease had been made. Others have reported similar findings. Ockerblad and Carlson studied the distribution of renal and ureteral pain following stimulation of various portions of the ureter with a faradic current by means of a specially constructed electrode introduced through cystoscope. This excellent piece of work was awarded a certificate of merit in the Scientific Exhibit of the American Medical Association at the last meeting at Atlantic City. Ockerblad's and Carlson's study was done on normal subjects and pyeloureterograms were made to rule out the possibility of any pathologic change in the urinary tract.

The stimulations were applied at intervals of 5 cm. along the course of the ureter and from these studies was noted that stimulation of the interior of the kidney produced pain which was referred to the back. Stimulation at 25 cm. from the ureteral orifice produced pain which was felt over the anterior portion of the iliac crest and anterior iliac spine. Stimulation at 26 and 27 cm. produced pain in the region of the anterior iliac spine. Stimulation at a point 10 to 20 cm. from the ureteral opening produced pain which was felt at the same abdominal levels.

This corroborates the clinical reports of many series of cases of ureteral calculi where pain was entirely abdominal in as high as 30 per cent in some series. Stimulation at points between 10 and 20 cm. produced pain on the inside of the leg also, in some instances radiating to the toes.

Stimulation of the ureter at a point 5 cm. above the ureteral orifice, which is within the area where calculi are often found, produced pain slightly lateral to the midline, below the iliac crest and mesial to McBurney's point. In some instances, pain on the inner or outer side of the thigh was obtained from stimulation at this area.

Stimulation of the lower 2 cm. of the ureter produced pain most always in the midline and in the suprapubic region.

This work of Ockerblad and Carlson provides us with experimental information which should be an aid in the differential diagnosis of intra-abdominal lesions and lesions involving the urinary tract, particularly urinary tract calculi.

LeRoy D. Long.

The Effect of Iodine in Adenomatous Goiter; Arnold S. Jackson and H. E Freeman; Journal of the American Medical Association, April, 1936.

There is still some misunderstanding among certain of the profession with regard to the action of iodine in the various types of goiter.

It is generally recognized that iodine in any form (Lugol's solution is usually used) causes a very beneficial response when used in exophthalmic goiter. This occurs practically without exception, but the iodine is especially useful in the preoperative treatment of exophthalmic goiter.

There are, undoubtedly, certain cases of "iodine fast" exophthalmic goiter patients who have been overtreated with iodine. These patients, with the long-continued administration of iodine, finally reach a stage at which their toxic symptoms fail to r e c e d e with iodine medication and may even progress. We do not know just how or why this occurs, but it does occur. To be entirely on the safe side, one should not persist too long in iodine medication, even in exophthalmic goiter.

It has been known for over a century that iodine administered in adenomatous goiter often resulted in injurious effects. These "injurious effects," of course, are the development of symptoms of thyrotoxicosis brought on by the iodine. These patients have nontoxic adenomatous goiter which is made toxic by the administration of iodine. The term "iodine hyperthyroidism" has been suggested for this condition. The condition occurs only in the presence of an adenomatous goiter, and since it does not result from the use of iodine in a normal thyroid gland, the term "iodine hyperthyroidism" in an adenomatous goiter was suggested as best describing this entity. There are very few men, notably Means and Lerman, who do not accept this fact that hyperthyroidism is often induced in adenomatous goiter by the use of iodine. Many men, on the other hand, have issued the warning against the danger of the administration of iodine in nontoxic adenomatous goiter. Unfortunately, this warning is often not heeded and, as a result, many patients are rendered hyperthyroid.

The authors hold to the opinion that iodine, injudiciously administered, may be and often is the precipitating f a c t o r in producing thyrotoxicosis from a previously nontoxic thyroid adenoma.

It has been shown that adenomatous goiter does not become toxic in patients less than 30 years of

age unless this is brought on by the injudicious use of iodine.

However, a simple adenoma, even in a young individual, is a definite contraindication for iodine.

It is felt that when the profession generally is cognizant of the danger of the prolonged use of iodine in exophthalmic goiter, and also cognizant of the danger of producing a toxic adenoma from a nontoxic adenoma by the administration of iodine, that there will be a general lowering of the death rate in goiter throughout the country.

The authors desire to call especial attention to the effect of iodine (they use the aqueous solution) in toxic adenomas. Scant mention has been made of the effect of iodine in toxic adenomas, although since 1923 the literature has been voluminous on the use of iodine in exophthalmic goiter.

Since the response to iodine in exophthalmic goiter and in toxic adenoma is so essentially different, it is difficult to conceive the idea of those men who maintain that these two clinical entities are but variations of the same disease.

Their toxic adenoma cases show many instances in which not only was the basal metabolic rate increased after aqueous solution of iodine, but the various symptoms of hyperthyroidism were aggravated noticeably.

There was noticeable improvement in toxic symptoms, including the basal metabolic rate, in many of their cases (the majority) following aqueous solution of iodine, but it is impossible to estimate just how much of this was due to rest, quiet, sedation and symptomatic treatment and how much was due to iodine.

Their study reveals that approximately 62 per cent (of the toxic adenoma cases) were benefited or were not affected and approximately 38 per cent of the cases the basal metabolic rate, tremor, tachycardia and the like were definitely made worse by iodine.

The authors summarize their conclusions as follows:

1. There may be produced iodine fast cases of exophthalmic goiter.

2. Iodine not only does no good but is definitely contraindicated in nontoxic a d e n o m a s of the thyroid.

3. There is danger, in administering iodine in cases of adenomatous goiter, of producing "iodine hyperthyroidism."

4. Adenomatous goiter does not become toxic before the patient has reached the age of 30 unless the toxicity is brought on by the injudicious use of iodine.

5. We have shown that iodine may and does produce thyrotoxicosis in adenomatous goiter as opposed to the contention of Means and Lerman.

6. The effect of aqueous solution of iodine in toxic adenoma is not constant or specific and is not the same as that produced in exophthalmic goiter.

7. Approximately 62 per cent of all cases of toxic adenoma are benefited by iodine or are not affected, while 38 per cent are made worse.

8. In a series of cases of toxic adenomas, toxic symptoms and the basal metabolic rate were aggravated by aqueous solution of iodine.

9. Owing to its variability of action, we believe that iodine should be given as a routine in all cases of toxic adenoma before and after operation, because two-thirds of the cases will be improved, and the harmful effect on the other third is negligible over a short time.

Their final conclusions are as follows:

1. Iodine should not be given to patients with nontoxic thyroid adenomas.

2. The condition termed iodine hyperthyroidism is a definite clinical entity.

3. Aqueous solution of iodine has an inconstant effect in toxic adenomas.

Diabetic or Mycotic Vulvovaginitis. Supplementary Report. H. Close Hesseltine and L. K. Campbell, Chicago, Ill. American Journal of Obstetrics and Gynecology, Vol. 35, No. 2, February, 1938, Page 272.

These authors have studied 58 diabetic patients with vulvitis and pruritis. They have also studied 53 diabetic women without vulvitis or pruritis and 38 control individuals. They have convincing results that the etiological agent of "diabetic vulvitis" is usually, if not always, a fungus.

Of the 58 diabetic patients with vulvitis all but three had a positive fungus culture. There were unusual circumstances about these three patients including fungicides used immediately before culture and menstruation at time of culture which may have vitiated the result.

Of the 53 diabetic women without vulvitis five had positive fungus cultures and have been considered by the authors as probable "carriers" of yeast organisms.

Large quantities of glucose solution were poured over the vulva of patients without fungi five times daily without the appearance of symptoms. However, when glucose was similarly poured over the vulva of patients with fungi present, symptoms and findings typical of mycotic vulvitis appeared in one to five days. This demonstrated the direct relationship of fungi to the vulvitis in diabetic individuals.

In addition, in several instances, all vulva irritation was relieved where fungicidal therapy was employed before patient was placed under diabetic management. There were others who did not improve under diabetic management and the vulvitis was promptly cured by fungicidal therapy.

The following conclusions are justifiably drawn by the authors:

1. In the presence of monilia or cryptococci the application of glucose in powder or aqueous solution will be associated usually, if not always, with the development of a vulvovaginal mycosis or will cause exacerbations of mycosis.

2. In the absence of yeastlike fungi the application of glucose in powder or aqueous solution has produced no symptoms or tissue changes.

3. The incidence of fungi in diabetes mellitus patients with vulvitis, and the similarity of the clinical appearance of mycotic vulvitis and of "diabetic vulvitis" justifies the previous statement that "diabetic vulvo-vaginitis is an infection, usually a mycosis, and rarely, if ever, an irritation from products in the urine."

4. Glucose available in the urine or the tissues favors the development of a vulva mycosis, just as its topical application may do.

5. Fungicidal therapy will cure "diabetic vulvitis."

6. Vulval mycosis occurred in diabetic patients from 12 to 73 years of age.

7. Whenever mycotic vulvitis is found in a nonpregnant patient one should exclude the possibility of diabetes mellitus.

8. Either "mycotic vulvitis" or "fungous vulvitis" is correct and accurate and should replace the incorrect, misleading and obsolete term "diabetic vulvitis."

9. Even such terms as "a p h t h o u s vulvitis," "thrush vulvitis," or "yeast vulvitis," do not conform to the modern taxonomy."

Comment: This is a very excellent piece of work demonstrating the etiological agent of vulvitis and pruritis in diabetic women.

Wendell Long.

EYE, EAR, NOSE AND THROAT
Edited by Marvin D. Henley, M.D.
911 Medical Arts Building, Tulsa

Retained Intra-Ocular Foreign Bodies. William H. Stokes, M.D., Omaha. Archives of Ophthalmology, February, 1938.

This is an analysis of 300 cases of retained foreign bodies in the globe. The review of available literature on this subject shows much confusion as to procedure; it finally depended, apparently, on the preference of the individual. It seems that the older the oculist is in experience, the more conservative is his method of handling these cases.

In 12 of these patients there was absolutely no history of an accident, the foreign body having made a painless entrance into the eyeball.

Roentgenograms were made in all the 300 cases. Demonstration and localization was possible in 97.5 per cent of them. Other routine aids to diagnosis were the ophthalmoscope and corneal microscope. There were 101 cases of this series that had a retained foreign body in the globe.

There are two tables given stating type of foreign body, period retained and end results. The first table has 26 cases in which the foreign body has retained in the vitreous for a period of from one month to 35 years. The second table has 49 cases in which the foreign body was retained either in the retina or in the sclera for a period of one month to 25 years.

Of the nonmagnetic foreign bodies copper was present in 13, brass in 5, lead in 5, glass in 2 and stone in 1. Analysis showed preservation of perfect vision even when the foreign body was present for years in the anterior chamber of the iris. If present in the vitreous, uveitis or panophthalmitis caused loss of the eye. In all cases of the foreign body being brass, enucleation became necessary. Lead, glass and stone in the vitreous had the same end result.

The author's conclusions are:

This study has brought my attention to the following points:

While an inquiry into the history of an accident should always be made of all patients coming to the oculist for examination, a negative subjective history is no criterion that none occurred.

It is of paramount importance to have accurate localization before extraction is attempted, and this can be obtained in all but a few exceptional cases by roentgenographic studies.

Rarely should the magnet be used for the mere detection of a foreign body.

A foreign body located in the anterior segment is best removed by the anterior route, and one in the posterior segment, through the scleral route. Electrocoagulating pins should be used in all cases in which extraction is done by the posterior route. It is best to remove a foreign body from the interior of the eye in cases of recent injury.

The view that the retention of a foreign body in one eye will cause a sympathetic inflammation in the other eye is not sustained by my observations.

On the contrary, I have found that sympathetic irritation developed only in cases in which ill advised efforts at removal were utilized.

Preservation of useful vision or of the eyeball is possible perhaps for the entire lifetime of the patient in spite of the retention of a foreign body in the posterior segment of the globe. One may assume that such a patient could not have fared better had intervention been adopted.

The knowledge that a foreign body within the eye may be tolerated for prolonged periods of time is worthy of consideration when one is deciding on the management of such cases, and conservative treatment is more often indicated than recommended by the majority of writers on the subject. However, the patient must be under the observation and care of a competent oculist for a period of years.

Treatment of Lateral Sinus Infections Without Operation on the Jugular Vein. E. Miles Atkinson, M.D., F.R.C.S., New York. Archives of Otolaryngology, February, 1938.

Zaufal in 1880, first suggested ligature of the internal jugular vein in thrombosis of the lateral sinus. Since that time the argument has gone on— to tie or not to tie. The orthodox procedure is to tie the internal jugular if a thrombosed lateral sinus is found.

The author maintains that ligature of the vein does not stop the spread of the infection. Collateral channels in the inferior petrosal sinus and the venal condyloidae afford additional channels along which the infection may travel. Also when the internal jugular is tied off, the point of the ligature may well become another focus even aiding an additional thrombosis rather than inhibiting the formation. Length and severity is added to the operation by tying the vein. There is a resulting neck scar.

A review of the literature shows: Korner in his 1925 book shows 60 per cent recovery, either with or without ligation; G r u n b e r g shows 21 cases ligated of which only 15 per cent recovered—40 cases were not ligated with 60 per cent recovered; Undritz from his experiment concluded:

1. That ligature of the vein exercises no noticeable influence on the course of the disease.

2. That experimental sinus thrombosis shows a tendency to spontaneous recovery and,

3. That the thrombus is to be regarded as a protective mechanism not lightly to be interfered with.

The 15 cases reported are divided into three groups.

1. Cases in which there were granulations on the sinus wall without demonstrable thrombosis—8.

2. Cases in which there were inflammatory changes in the sinus wall with gross thrombus formation—5.

3. Cases in which there was necrosis of the sinus wall without thrombosis—2.

Five of the 15 cases showed thrombosis. Ligature of the internal jugular was done on two cases. Positive blood culture was found in two cases. Nine cases of perisinus abscess or pathologic exposure of the sinus were treated by full exposure of the sinus. One case was complicated by a cerebellar abscess. All cases recovered.

The author as the above shows does not abandon the ligature of the internal jugular altogether. He has three indications for ligature.

1. Tenderness along the internal jugular vein.

2. Unexplained lymphadenitis (palpable) m a y signify phlebitis and thrombosis.

3. If the patient has as many as three rigors postoperative, the jugular vein is explored.

The External Operation on the Maxillary Sinus. Arthur M. Alden, A.M., M.D., F.A.C.S., St. Louis, Mo. The Southern Medical Journal, March, 1938.

Lamorier first did the external operation in 1743. Luc and Caldwell, in 1897, working independently, improved the original operation by making a permanent opening into the inferior meatus from the antrum. This has remained a fundamental principle although different operators have variations.

Indications for the operation: Continued suppuration from the antrum even after adequate intranasal drainage, antral disease of dental origin (fistula through the alveolus or tooth fragment in the cavity), degeneration of the mucosa (shown by lipiodol X-rays or antroscopy), presence of a cyst or new growth.

Before operation: If lues is present, p a t i e n t should be well medicated before operated; X-ray of all teeth under the floor of the sinus—if dental disease is present then remove before operation to p r e v e n t reinfection; cytologic and bacteriologic study of pus lavaged from the antrum (if Vincent's is present, give neoarsphenamine intravenously—if streptococcus, give sulfanilamide—if staphylococcus, then there is possibility of a later osteomyelitis).

Two factors are to be considered at operation, the comfort and safety of the patient and the method that will insure the greatest ease and efficiency to the operator. The author thinks general anaesthesia makes the operation more difficult for the surgeon in addition to the added hazard of a later lung complication. He prefers local anaesthesia. Avertin has been discarded. A grain and a half of pentobarbital is given an hour before operation; a half hour before operation a quarter of a grain of morphine (H) is given and the same dose of pentobarbital is repeated. This leaves the patient cooperative and relaxed but not unconscious.

Blair's method with a Barnhill needle is used to block the maxillary division of the nerves trigeminus on the affected side. Three c.c.'s of two per cent procaine with 10 drops of epinephrine are used. The author states that in over 200 injections he has had no following complications.

Three or four minutes after the injection the operation is started. Intra-nasal medication is not used. The gum and lower part of the canine fossa are injected with the same solution for ischemia only. A new approach is used to prevent severing of the nerve endings and the subsequent postoperative anaesthesia.

A horizontal incision extends from the canine tooth backward including the second molar; a vertical incision next extends from the gum margin between the lateral incisor and canine teeth upward one inch (including the periostium); the periostium is elevated and the whole triangular flap is retracted upward. The operation then proceeds in the routine manner. Time consumed is usually about 30 minutes.

Two or three black silk sutures are used to close which are removed on the fourth or fifth day. No packing is left in. Iced compresses are used on the operated side for 24 hours. The sinus is irrigated with a curved cannula with warm saline solution the fifth day. Inspection is made with an antroscope or a nasopharyngoscope from time to time.

The Development of Modern Methods of Estimating Refraction. W. B. E. McCrea, M.B., B.Ch., D.O.M.S., Dublin. The British Journal of Ophthalmology, March, 1937.

This is an interesting historical account of spectacles and methods of fitting them. An enormous amount of time and energy must have been expended during the compilation.

The first account of a glass being used as an aid to reading was by Marco Polo, while traveling in China in 1270. The invention of spectacles is credited to Alessandro Spina, a Dominican friar of Florence, who died in 1313. Salvino D'Armato also claims this honor.

The first reference to glasses in medical literature is made by Bernard de Gordon, a teacher of medicine at Montpellier. They are mentioned casually so evidently had been in use some time. The cost of a pair of glasses at this time was the equivalent of what is now fifty pounds.

During the fifteenth and sixteenth centuries the medical profession was strongly opposed to the use of spectacles. Literature was written on how to protect oneself from wearing glasses as well as how to rid oneself of the habit.

Tourmaline, beryl, quartz and later glass were used in making the lenses. In Germany the first frames were made of leather and reinforced with fish bones. The first side pieces were of string.

James Ware early in the nineteenth century made some very accurate observations and may truly be termed the discoverer of hypermetropia.

Thomas Young in 1793 and Airy in 1827 introduced cylindrical lenses for the correction of astigmatism.

Benjamin Franklin invented bifocals about the end of the eighteenth century.

Among the earlier works on ophthalmology, as "Synopsis of Diseases of the Eye," there was no mention made of any refraction problems.

Sir William Lawrence, 1833, regarded farsightedness and presbyopia as synonymous. Students were generally thought to be myopic. In management of myopia strange procedures prevailed such as avoiding anything that tended to promote the flow of blood to the head. Abstinence of heating drinks, attention to diet, washing eyes with cold fresh spring water, stimulating foot baths, etc.

If anisometropia existed and the one eye was myopic, the good eye was to be occluded and the other eye exercised.

In 1840, William McKenzie of Glasgow published a treatise on diseases of the eye which was widely read on the British Isles, Continent and in the United States. In it he makes the statement that after cataract extraction no glasses should be given as long as the vision is improving.

There were two theories of asthenopia: First that it was a peculiar disposition of the retina to become congested; the second explained it as a painful compression of the eye, caused by contraction of the ocular muscles.

John Whitaker Hulke, 1830, said that in his student days the ophthalmoscope was unknown and a half-dozen convex and concave spherical lens constituted sufficient stock for fitting glasses.

In 1864, Cornelius Donders, Professor of Physiology and Ophthalmology in the University of Utrecht, revolutionized the attitude of the Medical Profession towards problems of refraction with his book, "On the Accommodation and Refraction of the Eye."

The writer continues the tracing of the development and growth of refraction quoting various authors and relating numerous theories and beliefs of that day. The history is carried up to 1870. J. Soelberg Wells is given credit for the beginning of modern refraction as we know it. He deplores the haphazard plan of the opticians in fitting glasses. He advocates the medical man selecting the proper lens, writing this on a piece of paper, which is taken to the optician, who then furnishes the correct lens to the patient.

---o---

UROLOGY

Edited by D. W. Branham, M. D.
514 Medical Arts Building, Oklahoma City

Calculous Disease in the Urinary Tract. Linwood D. Keyser. Bulletin of the New York Academy of Medicine. February, 1938. Roanoke, Virginia.

A comprehensive article in which the author discusses some of the causes for the formation of stone together with an outline of treatment based on modern day concepts of this disease.

He states that stone formation tend to develop when colloids and crystalline material are simultaneously precipitated in the free urinary stream. The colloidal jel enmeshes agglutination crystals and forms the organic framework which around and within these crystals are laid down as building elements. This process may be stimulated both by hyperexcretion of crystalline material through the kidneys beyond the power of the urine to maintain solubility and entrance of foreign colloid into the urinary stream.

The second etiologic factor responsible for the formation of stone is the impregnation or encrustation of cells, bacteria, tissues or foreign bodies with urinary salts.

Other factors that he discusses is the relation of vitamine deficiency, urinary reaction, urostasis, fractures and disease of bone as also parathyroid disease. He is not enthusiastic in support of vitamine deficiency as a cause for stones as he feels that patients with stones for the most part have a dietary adequacy of vitamin A; however, urinary acidity or alkalinity does play a large part in speeding up or retarding the formation of stones.

The relation of urostasis as a primary cause for the formation of stones is entirely lacking. However, in maintaining infection and stagnation it is a matter of great moment. He epitomizes the treatment of stones in a detailed chart and the following procedure is suggested:

1. Remove all stones and fragments as far as possible, by surgery or cystoscopy.

2. A qualitative chemical analysis of the stone removed should be carried out immediately.

3. X-rays should be made immediately and at intervals of six months to one year for several years after the operation.

4. Seek and correct possibly related metabolic errors.

5. The diet should be carefully regulated with regard to the composition of the stone; low oxalate dietary in oxalatic stones and low purin diet in uratic calculi.

6. Vitamin administration as a tonic to the epithelial structures.

7. Elimination of urinary and focal infections.

8. Establish satisfactory renal and ureteral drainage.

9. Shift the urinary reaction to the range which will best keep the stone-forming crystals in solution.

10. Patients with fractures, infections of the bones, or patients long bed-ridden should have their urine kept acid by diet and drugs and furnished ample vitamines as a prophylaxis against stones.

Newer Physiology of Prostate Gland. James L Farrell. Chicago, Illinois. Journal of Urology. February, 1938.

A detailed study of the prostatic secretion in dogs from a pharmacologic standpoint.

By injecting various drugs and noting their effect on the quantity and rate of secretion it was concluded that the innervation of the prostate is chiefly parasympathetic in nature. Pilocorpine markedly stimulates secretion, atropine antagonizes pilocorpine stimulation and renders hypogastric stimulation inactive; Ephedrine stimulates the gland to a slight extent; histamine and yohinbine do not affect secretion from the gland.

The prostate definitely excretes the majority of drugs commonly used for antiseptic purposes in detectable quantities. It was found that prostatic secretion in itself has a difinite bactericidal action, however, this effect was not particularly enhanced by the excreted drugs.

An interesting phase of this study was the observation made on the elimination of alcohol by the gland. The concentration of alcohol found in the secretion nearly approached that found in the urine following administration in standardized amounts. It was also found that a definite deleterious action was exhibited on the viability of the sperm which suggested that alcohol may be a factor in sterility. Also this may explain the bad effects noted clinically from excessive alcoholic ingestion in cases of prostatitis.

--- o ---

PLASTIC SURGERY

Edited by

GEO. H. KIMBALL, M.D., F.A.C.S.
404 Medical Arts Building, Oklahoma City

Vitamin Oils in the Treatment of Burns, an Experimental Study. Charles B. Puestow, M.D., F.A.C.S., Henry G. Poncher, M.D., and Harold Hammatt, B.M., Chicago, Ill. S. G. & O., March, 1938.

The authors have carried out an experimental study to determine the value of several oils and other commonly used agents in the healing of burns.

In 1905 Wuttig produced endothelial proliferations in the liver by injecting cod liver oil into the mesenteric veins of rabbits, whereas olive oil was inert. Bond used irradiated ergosterol in liquid petrolatum as a dressing for ulcers and granulating wounds. He believed that the ointment reduced infection, promoted healthy granulations and stimulated epitheliazation. Loehr has used cod liver oil dressings extensively in the treatment of burns and other wounds. He became quite enthusiastic about this treatment which was used in the form of a paste and when on the extremity was encased by a plaster cast, the dressings were changed infrequently as possible. He further believed that skin grafting was unnecessary in many of these cases due to the fact that the wounds rapidly healed under his form of treatment. He thought the number of late fatalities was reduced, more so than with tannic acid treatment.

Various other workers have indicated that ointments containing vitamin A and D are effective in the treatment of ulcers and burns.

The authors point out the method of producing burns in pigs and rabbits by using an electro-

cautery locally. They attempted to produce a burn of small size and depth for a comparative study. They then used five different preparations in order to study the effect of each on the healing of burns.

The oils employed and their identification numbers are as follows:

1. Olive oil free of vitamins.

2. Cod liver oil containing 1,800 units of vitamin A and 175 units of vitamin D per gram.

3. Irradiated ergosterol in oil containing one million units of vitamin D per gram.

4. Fish liver oil containing 45,000 units of vitamin A and 75,000 units of vitamin D per gram.

5. Fish liver oil containing 380,000 units of vitamin A and 2,000 units of vitamin D per gram.

Five per cent tannic acid solution was applied to other lesions and control lesions were left untreated.

Summary: Controlled burns were produced upon pigs and rabbits and were treated with ointments containing varying amounts of vitamin A and vitamin D content. The time and character of local wound healing was determined and compared with untreated controls and burns treated with tannic acid.

Burns treated with five per cent fresh tannic acid solution healed in the same length of time as untreated controls of similar average size. The application of vitamin free olive oil ointment to slightly larger burns was followed by complete healing in the same length of time as the controls. Cod liver oil ointment shortened by 25 per cent the healing period of burns equal in size to the controls. Burns which averaged 50 per cent larger than the controls were treated with three high vitamin ointments, No. 3 containing no vitamin A but very high vitamin D, No. 4 having a low vitamin A to vitamin D ratio, and No. 5 with a high vitamin A to vitamin D ratio. The time of healing was approximately 25 per cent shorter than in the smaller control lesions and those treated with tannic acid. It was no longer than in the smaller lesions treated with cod liver oil ointment of low vitamin content. The response to the various high vitamin ointments employed was approximately the same. Histological studies of the scars of all healed burns revealed no characteristic difference for the various therapeutic agents employed.

Comment: In the treatment of burns it is often necessary to change the type of treatment. Especially is this true in cases which for some reason or other fail to continue the regeneration of epithelium. These cases might be compared to cases that have non-union of bones especially where fractures are multiple. In other words the power or the ability to continue to heal is lost. In such cases scarlet red ointment sometimes will give the necessary stimulus to the epithelium. In other cases one of the oils containing vitamins will be more successful. In addition to the ointments the general condition of the patient must be improved by adequate care, diet, blood transfusions and any other measure that will improve the vital process. Exposure of burned areas to ultra violet light is of benefit. Recently the so-called bruised yeast cells have been employed and this ointment seems to stimulate the epithelium. Also granulations remain healthy and the periphery of the burned area remains soft and pliable whereby some of the area otherwise treated becomes thick and friable.

The authors in this case have, I believe, shown some evidence of the stimulating value of ointments containing vitamins. Since there are so many varied applications recommended it is difficult to follow each one in detail. Personally I like to cleanse burned areas daily even when using any kind of ointment, then reapply whatever medication is being used. In this way one can follow more accurately the progress of healing.

The ointment containing bruised yeast cells can be readily removed by wet dressings in preparation for a skin graft. Also scarlet red ointment can be readily removed the same way. However personally I like to keep the burned surfaces cleansed by frequent wet dressings if there is a skin graft contemplated.

INTERNAL MEDICINE

Edited by Hugh Jeter, M.D., 1200 North Walker. Oklahoma City

HUGH, JETER, M.D., F.A.C.P., A.S.C.P.

Diseases of Metabolism and Nutrition, Review of Certain Recent Contributions. Russell, M. Wilder, M.D., Ph.D., Rochester, Minn., and Dwight L. Wilbur, M.D., San Francisco. Archives of Internal Medicine, Vol. 61, No. 2, February, 1938.

In this the authors have again reviewed the literature for one year including 224 separate articles covering a great variety of subjects involving metabolism and nutrition such as follows:

1. Disorders of fat metabolism.
2. Obesity.
3. Experimental diabetes.
4. Protamine Zinc Insulin.
5. Other insulins with prolonged action.
6. Nutrition.
7. Reports abstracted separately on the various vitamins.

Diabetes: Many reports concerning protamine zinc insulin have been made. The opinion that it is a definite improvement in treatment continues to prevail. Whitehill and Harrop believe that patients who are not cooperative and who are lax in the management of their diet do badly with protamine zinc insulin and that such patients will find the use of unmodified insulin safer and on the whole more satisfactory. They also point out that in cases with diarrhea as a complication in which absorption of food from the bowel is uncertain, protamine zinc insulin is unsafe to use. Sherrill and Cope question whether any particular advantage is to be gained from protamine zinc insulin in cases in which formerly a normal balance could be maintained with unmodified insulin. Warvel and Shafer emphasize that the use of protamine zinc insulin requires more effort on the part of the physician. Severe diabetes requires more than one dose of protamine zinc insulin and makes it necessary frequently to add unmodified insulin. Experience at the Mayo Clinic and also of Joslin indicates that protamine zinc insulin and unmodified insulin are not satisfactorily given mixed together in a syringe. Protamine zinc insulin of 80 units strength has been recently distributed but reports show its use seems very rarely indicated.

Most American and Canadian physicians continue to administer protamine zinc insulin in one dose daily before breakfast but a few have found other periods during the day satisfactory. One author gives it two hours before breakfast and another reports good results with the administration at 11 p.m. Wilder says "If one insists on having continuously sugar-free urine when only protamine zinc insulin is used, chronic hypoglycemia is unavoidable at least in many cases." There appears from the literature to be a number of observers who believe a trace of sugar in the urine is desirable for the well being and comfort of the patient.

Reports indicate most satisfactory results with a

diet of 150 gm. of carbohydrate or less most satisfactory for protamine zinc insulin therapy. However, some have been able to use higher diets. Four meals or more per day are used by most authorities.

Protamine zince insulin is being used more in emergency than previously, such as acidosis, acute infections and surgery.

Peck reports six cases of allergy to protamine but Wilder has encountered none.

Its Quick Action Prevents Deformities

No antiricketic substance will completely straighten bones that have become grossly misshaped as the result of rickets. But Oleum Percomorphum can be depended upon to prevent ricketic deformities if given early and in adequate dosage. This is not true of all antiricketic agents, many of which are so limited by tolerance or bulk that they cannot be given in quantities sufficient to arrest the ricketic process promptly, with the result that the bones are not sufficiently calcified to bear weight or musclepull and hence become deformed.

Mental Effects of "Benzedrine Sulfate"

Molitch and Sullivan (Am. J. Orthopsych., 7:519, Oct., 1937) report on the mental effects of "Benzedrine Sulfate" (benzyl methyl carbinamine sulfate, S.K.F.).

The New Standard Achievement Test was given to a group of 96 boys aged 10 to 17. A week later the same boys took the test again about 1½ hours after 50 of them had received a 10 mk. "Benzedrine Sulfate" tablet and the remaining 46 a placebo.

The 46 boys on placebos scored a net loss of 29 points, while the 50 boys on "Benzedrine Sulfate" scored a net gain of 63 points, although 26 of the 50 did not show noticeable improvement. Some weeks later these 26 received 20 mg. (or double the previous dose) for a third test. Twenty-four of these boys, or 92 per cent, improved their scores with a net gain of 117 points.

The greatest responses were noted in language usage, geography, physiology and hygiene, and arithmetic. Normals of average intelligence and feeble-minded boys responded better than normals of inferior intelligence. Grouped according to academic age, it was found that the boys in junior high school showed greater improvement on "Benzedrine Sulfate" than those in lower grades.

Reactions were mild and transitory, although hypersensitivity to "Benzedrine Sulfate" induced nausea in the cases of two boys who failed to respond even to the double dose of "Benzedrine Sulfate."

Care Of The Feet In Chronic Arthritis

John G. Kuhns, Boston (Journal A. M. A., Oct. 2, 1937), contends that chronic arthritis in its early stages usually presents the same pedal symptoms which are caused by chronic strain. Differentiation can usually be made from the history of progressive impairment of the general health, involvement of other joints and stiffness of the feet after rest, which lessens with continued use. The swelling is variable in degree but more widespread and not limited to a special location. Limitation of motion in the midtarsal joints is one of the most common early symptoms. The blood sedimentation index is elevated in most instances. Roentgenograms, which usually show nothing abnormal at the onset of the disease except swelling of the soft tissues, show progressive bony atrophy, clouding of the joint spaces and increasing narrowing and irregularity of the articular surfaces. These symptoms and these changes in the feet will be observed in about three fourths of all patients with early chronic arthritis. The only certain method of preventing future disability is to avoid weight bearing until the pain and swelling in the feet subside. Before the patient again becomes ambulatory, proper shoes and adequate support should be given to prevent strain. If inadequate or no treatment is given and the arthritis remains, increasing deformity usually occurs. The deformity most commonly seen is one with the foot stiff in valgus. Because weight bearing is faulty and because normal use of the intrinsic musculature of the foot is prevented, the muscles atrophy and a widening of the anterior part of the foot is seen, a flattening of the so-called anterior arch. This is followed by undue pressure on the heads of the metatarsal bones, and the symptoms are usually pain and tenderness. When this degree of deformity has come, disability is severe, and the patient usually walks with great difficulty. The severe strains, which come chiefly on the foot and the knee, aggravate the arthritis, and no subsidence of the inflammatory processes in the joints can be expected unless the deformity is corrected. When weakening of the intrinsic muscles of the feet and spreading of the forepart of the foot persist, two other deformities develop, hallux valgus and contracted toe deformity. Operative correction is not always necessary in the early stages of these deformities. Temporary cessation of weight bearing and exercise to develop the flexors of the toes and the intrinsic muscles of the forefoot will help greatly. The chief concern is adequate support to the anterior part of the foot. When rigid deformity is present and the arthritis is inactive, a manipulation of the toes into flexion with the patient under anesthesia may be required. After the manipulation, the toes can be held in plantar flexion by adhesive strapping for several days. Repeated manipulations will at times result in normal function of the toes. When subluxation of the proximal phalanx persists and there is marked deformity of the joints, the most rapid and usually the most satisfactory result is obtained by the operative removal of the distal half of the proximal phalanx. If the hallux valgus is severe, operative correction by removing the proximal portion of the first phalanx of the great toe usually gives the best functional result. Extensive reshaping of deformed bones has not proved a desirable procedure. After operation marked changes take place in the atrophied bones as the result of function. The simplest and least traumatic surgical procedure gives the best end result. Operative procedures are undertaken only when the arthritis is quiescent. Ankylosis of the phalanges is not commonly seen. When it has occurred, removal of the entire proximal phalanx has given painless function without the subsequent development of calluses under the toes. Tallux rigidus can frequently be relieved by a long plate or by greater rigidity in the sole of the shoe. Occasionally the ankylosis of the tarsal-metarsal joints can be broken by manipulation, but usually an operation is required. The simplest procedure is removal of the proximal half inch of the metatarsal bone. Ankylosis in the tarsal joints rarely yields to manipulation. If a fair weight bearing position of the foot cannot be secured with proper shoes and foot plates, an operative correction of the deformity is indicated. The most useful procedure is a wedge osteotomy through the subastragalar joint or through the dorsum of the foot, with the foot held subsequently in a good weight bearing position while the site of the osteotomy heals. Spurs are frequently found in feet troubled by arthritis. When a proper weight bearing position of the foot has been obtained and the foot strain has been relieved, the symptoms have disappeared in all but a few cases. A disability constantly associated with arthritic involve-

ment of the feet is epidermomycosis. The infection yields readily to the usual remedies, but reinfection often occurs until the arthritis becomes quiescent and the circulation in the foot improves.

---o---

Malunited Colles' Fractures

Willis C. Campbell, Memphis, Tenn. (Journal A. M. A., Oct. 2, 1937), points out that two entirely different surgical principles may be employed in malunited fractures: one restoring function by a compensatory procedure, the other by reconstructing normal anatomic relationships. The most efficient procedure is a plastic operation of the bone whereby the normal angle of the articular surface is restored, the radial shortening corrected and the prominence of the distal end of the ulna removed, thus reproducing normal external and bony contour. The technic of the operation is as follows: A lateral incision is made over the lower extremity of the radius about two inches in length through the skin and superficial fascia between the brachioradialis and the abductor pollicis longus and the extensor pollicis brevis. The line of fracture is exposed. A transverse osteotomy is made through the radius about three-fourths inch to an inch above the distal articular surface, after which correction of the posterior angulation of the lower fragment can be made by acute flexion of the wrist so that the lower fragment is angulated slightly downward and forward. In this position a hemostat can be inserted between the fragments and opened with moderate force, thus, separating the fracture surfaces and demonstrating the amount of increase that can be obtained in the length of this bone. A skin clip is now placed so as to close this wound temporarily. An incision is then made for about 2 inches over the medial aspect of the lower extremity of the ulna through the periosteum, which is stripped off of the inner half from above downward, exposing the articular surface and the styloid process. With a small osteotomy the inner half or third of the head and inner portion of the shaft is severed from below upward, thus securing a free graft of bone about one inch in length and about one-half inch in thickness at one extremity and tapered at the other. The free graft of bone is trimmed to make a pyramidal wedge with a base on the dorsal as well as the lateral aspect, which is inserted into the space between the fragments. The dorsal wedge maintains the normal angle: the lateral wedge prevents recurrence of radial shortening. Care must be taken that there is slight overreduction of the lower fragment; that is, slight anterior angulation. Both wounds are then closed and dressed with small gauze pads. On inspection the external contour should be approximately normal except that the head of the ulna may not be prominent. The lateral dimension or width of the wrist should be normal, and on palpation the lower extremity of the styloid process of the radius should be distal to that of the lower extremity of the ulna. A sterile flannel bandage is placed from the metacarpophalangeal joints below to just above the elbow, and the sugar tong cast or molded plaster anterior and posterior splints are applied. While this is consolidating, the forearm is held in midposition, the wrist in slight flexion, with pressure over the dorsum of the wrist so as to make the posterior capsule of the wrist joint tense, thus maintaining the lower fragment of the radius. A roentgenogram is then made which should demonstrate practically normal anatomic alinement. Surgical procedures have been carried out in forty-one cases of malunited Colles' fractures; twenty-two were simple osteotomies of the radius; nineteen were plastic procedures on the bone as described. A reasonably high percentage of function was restored by osteotomy alone, but the radial shortening and prominence of the ulna were not corrected: The results from the plastic procedure on the bone have been uniformly excellent, meaning that contour is approximately normal and function restored to a material degree. .

Testing of Activity of Childhood Tuberculosis: Relative Value of the Schilling Differential Count, Sedimentation Rate and Lympho-cyte-Monocyte Ratio

Through the cooperation of Brown, Stafford and Cole of Blue Ridge Sanatorium, Charlottesville, Va., W.Ambrose McGee, Richmond, Va. (Journal A. M. A., March 5, 1938), made a study of the relative value of the Schilling differential blood count, the sedimentation rate and the lymphocyte-monocyte ration on 40 tuberculosis children over a period of approximately six months. A study of the cells in the circulation at regular intervals and under similar conditions by the same person gives a mental picture of the pathologic changes occurring. The laboratory data alone do not in any way suggest the kind of infectious agent, for red and white cells respond only to the type of damage done to the tissues. Total white cell counts by themselves are of relatively little or no prognostic value but when considered from the standpoint of total neutrophils, lymphocytes and monocytes are of value. Through a consideration of the maturity of the neptrophils or the sedimentation rate, the best prognostic information is obtained. Any dfeinite lymphocyte-monocyte ratio was unobtainable because of the great fluctuation in the monocytic percentages. However, a normal monocyte count with an elevated lymphocyte count indicates healing, whereas, the reverse ratio suggests extension of the tuberculous infection. When clinical courses do not parallel laboratory data, especially the shifts and the sedimentation rates, it is advisable to pay more attention to those two tests. Evidence of relapse or rotrogression is first noted in the Schilling shift days or weeks prior to X-ray or physical evidence. A continuous septic type of blood picture is more suggestive of extension of the pathologic process, and there is danger of hemorrhage. The blood picture indicates the status of the infection only at the time the blood is obtained for study.

The Chemistry of Thiamin (Vitamin B₁)

In an endeavor to promote the adoption of a universally acceptable term for vitamin B₁, based on the chemistry of the substance, Robert R. Williams, New York (Journal A. M. A., March 5, 1938), has proposed "thiamin" (chloride, bromide, sulfate and so on) pending action of the Conference on Vitamin Standardization. The greater part of the labor which has been expended on the chemistry of this substance had to do with its isolation. Once a few grams of the vitamin became available, its structure was fully established in three years and its synthesis followed almost immediately. The biochemistry of thiamin, biochemical lesion in thiamin deficiency and the methods of its assay an ddistribution in foods are discussed. The therapeutic response to thiamin remains the most trustworthy diagnostic test. The diagnostic value of thiamin therapy is largely lost if crude natural preparations are used both because of the uncertainty of their standardization and of the presence of other vitamins which may be responsible for the observed effects. After demonstrating a B₁ deficiency and rectifying the immediate shortage, the physician should endeavor to direct the diet of the patient toward a more adequate supply of the vitamin. In the long run one should look to the grocery store rather than the drug store for a normal intake.

Audiometers and Hearing Aids

In order to determine their comparative performances for air conduction tests and the need for pure wave form in clinical practice Austin A. Hayden, Chicago (Journal A. M. A., March 5, 1938), investigated four audiometers of different make. Audiometers, despite their variations, furnish the best means of testing hearing acuity. Any one of the four tested will be more useful in clinical practice than any other means now available for testing and recording hearing acuity. The lack of purity of sound wave apparently did not introduce any serious errors that were not largely explainable by other causes. A quiet room is essential. The need for a soundproof room increases as the loss of hearing to be tested decreases. An audiometer should be part of the office equipment of every otologist.

Index to Advertisers

OFFICERS OF COUNTY SOCIETIES, 1938

COUNTY	PRESIDENT	SECRETARY
Adair		
Alfalfa	F. K. Slaton, Helena	L. T. Lancaster, Cherokee
Atoka-Coal	J. S. Fulton, Atoka	J. B. Clark, Coalgate
Beckham	R. C. McCreery, Erick	P. J. DeVanney, Sayre
Blaine	J. S. Barnett, Hitchcock	W. F. Griffin, Watonga
Bryan	P. L. Cain, Albany	Jas. L. Shuler, Durant
Caddo	J. Worrell Henry, Anadarko	P. H. Anderson, Anadarko
Canadian		G. D. Funk, El Reno
Carter	T. J. Jackson, Ardmore	Emma Jean Cantrell, Wilson
Cherokee	P. H. Medearis, Tahlequah	H. A. Masters, Tahlequah
Choctaw	G. E. Harris, Hugo	F. L. Waters, Hugo
Cleveland	O. E. Howell, Norman	J. L. Haddock, Jr., Norman
Coal	(See Atoka)	
Comanche	E. B. Dunlap, Lawton	Reber M. Van Matre, Lawton
Cotton		G. W. Cotton, Walters
Craig		F. T. Gastineau, Vinita
Creek	C. R. McDonald, Mannford	J. F. Curry, Sapulpa
Custer	Ross Deputy, Clinton	Harry Cushman, Clinton
Garfield		John R. Walker, Enid
Garvin	G. L. Johnson, Pauls Valley	John R. Callaway, Pauls Valley
Grady	L. E. Wood, Chickasha	R. E. Baze, Chickasha
Grant	I. V. Hardy, Medford	E. E. Lawson, Medford
Greer		
Harmon	W. G. Husband, Hollis	R. H. Lynch, Hollis
Haskell		
Hughes	W. L. Taylor, Holdenville	Imogene Mayfield, Holdenville
Jackson	Jas. E. Ensey, Altus	J. M. Allgood, Altus
Jefferson	C. S. Maupin, Waurika	C. M. Maupin, Waurika
Kay		R. G. Obermiller, Ponca City
Kingfisher		
Kiowa	J. M. Bonham, Hobart	J. Wm. Finch, Hobart
Latimer		
LeFlore	E. M. Woodson, Poteau	W. L. Shippey, Poteau
Lincoln	E. F. Hurlbut, Meeker	Ned Burleson, Prague
Logan	F. R. First, Crescent	E. O. Barker, Guthrie
Marshall	J. H. Logan, Lebanon	J. F. York, Madill
Mayes	S. C. Rutherford, Locust Grove	E. H. Werling, Pryor
McClain	J. E. Cochran, Byars	R. L. Royster, Purcell
McCurtain	R. D. Williams, Idabel	R. H. Sherrill, Broken Bow
McIntosh	D. E. Little, Eufaula	Wm. A. Tolleson, Eufaula
Murray		Richard M. Burke, Sulphur
Muskogee	Finis W. Ewing, Muskogee	S. D. Neely, Muskogee
Noble	J. W. Francis, Perry	T. F. Renfrow, Billings
Nowata		
Okfuskee	L. J. Spickard, Okemah	C. M. Bloss, Okemah
Oklahoma	C. J. Fishman, Oklahoma City	John F. Burton, Oklahoma City
Okmulgee	V. M. Wallace, Morris	M. B. Glismann, Okmulgee
Osage	R. O. Smith, Hominy	Geo. Hemphill, Pawhuska
Ottawa	Benj. W. Ralston, Commerce	W. Jackson Sayles, Miami
Pawnee		
Payne	E. M. Harris, Cushing	John W. Martin, Cushing
Pittsburg	A. R. Russell, McAlester	Ed. D. Greenberger, McAlester
Pontotoc	W. F. Dean, Ada	June Yates, Ada
Pottawatomie	E. Eugene Rice, Shawnee	F. Clinton Gallaher, Shawnee
Pushmataha	E. S. Patterson, Antlers	D. W. Connally, Antlers
Rogers	F. A. Anderson, Claremore	W. A. Howard, Chelsea
Seminole	A. N. Deaton, Wewoka	Claude B. Knight, Wewoka
Stephens	W. T. Salmon, Duncan	Fred T. Hargrove, Duncan
Texas		R. B. Hayes, Guymon
Tillman	J. E. Childers, Frederick	O. G. Bacon, Frederick
Tulsa	M. J. Searle, Tulsa	Roy L. Smith, Tulsa
Wagoner	S. R. Bates, Wagoner	Francis S. Crane, Wagoner
Washington	J. E. Crawford, Bartlesville	J. V. Athey, Bartlesville
Washita	J. Paul Jones, Dill	Gordon Livingston, Cordell
Woods	Arthur E. Hale, Alva	Oscar E. Templin, Alva
Woodward	C. W. Tedrowe, Woodward	V. M. Rutherford, Woodward

NOTE—Corrections and additions to the above list will be cheerfully accepted.

THE JOURNAL

OF THE

OKLAHOMA STATE MEDICAL ASSOCIATION

| VOLUME XXXI | McALESTER, OKLAHOMA, MAY, 1938 | Number 5 |

PRESIDENT'S ADDRESS*

H. K. SPEED, M.D.
SAYRE, OKLA.

The 30 years I have been attending Medical Associations it has been almost unanimously the custom of the incoming President to inaugurate in his address a somewhat detailed history of medicine, but if that is what you expect from me, I am going to disappoint you, for I am going to talk about some of the things that are and that I hope will be.

Please be informed that my remarks are not necessarily the ideas or the wishes of Organized Medicine in Oklahoma, for I am sure that many will disagree with me, because they are essentially my own ideas, which I think is improper, because I believe that we should at this meeting appoint a Censure Committee to see that each incoming president says the right thing or things that seem right to the profession in general, as passed upon by this representative group of co-workers.

1. I believe that we should through some central head promote in so far as possible a harmony of purpose of all the members of the Association. Doctors being natural leaders have many individual ideas and will not be easily lead, but by an all time active well balanced man the general views of the entire profession, if approached correctly, can be carried out.

2. It is my very sincere desire that we clean our own house, not by wide spread punishment, of any person or group of people, but many of us know people in the profession that are a discredit to our profession. Why should these not be eliminated?

3. Promote Post-Graduate extension work enthusiastically, and in the future, perhaps at the next legislature make it the duty of the Examining Board to qualify each man's license in so far as the applicant will be required to take so much Clinical or Post-Graduate work every so many years, to be designated by a wise and well selected committee, composed of members of Organized Medicine.

4. That our members be encouraged to use, and our druggist be directed to buy only council accepted pharmaceuticals and appliances, and each doctor or druggist have on his desk a list of these things. If this were done there would not be a repetition of the calamitous misfortune some months back, when more than 100 lives were lost, also the Florida incident of late March of this year, wherein ten lives were lost, which should and did discredit every doctor and pharmaceutical house in America. Why should we set up a Council on Pharmacy and Chemistry and maintain it at an enormous cost and at the same time buy from some fly-by-night company that can sell cheaper products, because they do not go to the expense of maintaining an expensive research laboratory.

5. Some manner of compensating the average doctor for services rendered the indigent, namely, city, county, state or federal government, for I believe they are the charges of all the people, as they have so increased in numbers that it is no longer possible for the individual physician to

*President's Address before Oklahoma State Medical Association, Annual Meeting, Muskogee, May 9, 10, 11, 1938.

give adequate care to all of them, as it has been in the past.

6. Unlimited birth control information to be disseminated by the doctor individually at his discretion and not through a Birth Control Clinic, which usually drifts into the hands of an incompetent Social Service worker.

The health and lives of 700,000 women is jeopardized each y e a r, and 41% of the puerperal deaths each year are caused by criminal abortions.

7. Compulsory pre-employment physical examination for all employees of labor, with subsequent periodical physical examinations.

8. Sponsor a law whereby all Life Insurance companies must have all applicants medically examined and discourage all people from buying non-medical policies.

9. Require physical examinations, including test for gonorrhea, syphilis and tuberculosis for all dispensers of food and food handlers, semi-annually or annually as now incorporated in the Barber Practice Act.

10. A health certificate for both man and woman before entering marriage, and this certificate to be issued by some disinterested medical authority, not the family physician.

11. The sponsoring of a law to be enacted, whereby all owners of cars or trucks driven within the state must carry enough insurance to pay all just doctor bills or hospitalization for any person or persons injured by such car.

12. Some form of Hospital Pre-Payment insurance, to be worked out between the Medical Profession and the hospital authorities, which must not include anesthetics, X-rays, laboratory work or any other medical or surgical service, but hospitalization alone.

13. I request that each County Medical Society co-operate to the fullest extent with the state and county health boards in their most excellent and worth while undertakings, but that any all time or part time health unit be discouraged or barred from practicing m e d i c i n e, in so far as treatment of disease is concerned, but confine their activities to educational infor-

mation regarding sanitation and hygiene, prenatal and postpartum v i s i t s by the public health nurse. Administration of the tuberculin test and the Schick test, but at all time direct the reactors in these cases to report to their family physician for treatment. I am especially opposed to the setting up of free venereal clinics, but that these diseases too be taken care of by the various doctors individually as has been done in the past.

14. I recommend the enactment of a law authorizing a State Health B o a r d, composed of nine members, one retiring each year. The majority of whom must at all times be physicians and that this health board employ and supervise the activities of the state health officer. They to serve without pay, except their per-diem expenses.

15. *Politics.* I am pleased to encourage all men in Organized Medicine to become politically minded, if they have not already done so, for we are in politics from now on whether we like it or not.

I especially would like to encourage doctors and their sons, when convenient to present themselves as candidates for the house and senate, for from personal experience, I can assure you that it is a lot of comfort to the legislative committee to have a doctor or a doctor's son in either of these law making bodies.

I think it is our duty to demand of the legislature a place in the Legislative Sun and see that they give us laws to protect the general public and our own profession as well.

One of which I recommend, known as the Registration Law, passed in the last senate and killed in the house, by a shrewd and designing politician, with no reason at all, except selfish political purposes, as it affected no one except our profession.

Also I w o u l d recommend some few changes in the Basic Science Law, passed in the last legislature, I think it is a good law, but can be i m p r o v e d by minor changes. Also some two or three sections of the Medical Practice Act should have changes, which will work for the benefit of all the people, including the Medical Profession. Especially should it be amended to bar the advertising quack and unscrupulous qualified members of our profession.

16. That we pass a resolution asking congress through both of our senators and various representatives, that the president's cabinet be given a doctor member to supervise and control by co-ordination all of the 12 or more departments of our government that are handling medical matters.

These things, ladies and gentlemen, with others that will present themselves from time to time during my tenure of office will be given attention as whole heartedly as my mental and physical capacity will permit.

SHOCK*

STRATTON E. KERNODLE, M.D.
OKLAHOMA CITY, OKLA.

I. *Definition* — Samuel Gross defined shock as "a rude unhinging of the machinery of life." Dorland defines shock as "a sudden vital depression due to an injury or emotion which makes an untoward impression on the nervous system." Wright describes shock as "a condition in which the sensory and motor parts of the reflex arc are paralyzed to a greater or less degree together with a profound disturbance of the capillary circulation." Cutler states that "shock is a symptom complex resulting from a rapid dimunition of the circulating blood volume below the point of circulatory efficiency." Shock is a syndrome, a group of symptoms and not a disease. It is seen in a wide variety of clinical conditions including extensive surgery or trauma, extensive burns, poisoning with various substances, metabolic intoxications, abdominal emergencies, and severe acute infections. It may occur in association with cardiac disease.

II. *Mechanism* — The mechanism of shock is not very well understood and is still debated in the literature. On account of the length of time alloted me, I can only be dogmatic and state what to me seems to be the most logical explanation of shock. There is first a vaso-motor constriction which maintains the arterial pressure for a time, then there follows a decrease in the return of blood to the heart causing an accompanying decrease in the cardiac output; as a result of this the blood pressure then declines, and vaso dilatation occurs. When there is dilatation of the capillary bed there follows a course of events which consists of increased permeability of the capillaries. There is insufficient supply of oxygen to the tissues, decrease of heat production and increase in viscosity of the blood. The escape of blood plasma into the tissues spaces is associated with stagnation of the blood within the capillaries, diminution of the alkali reserve and accumulation of toxic products. It is well agreed that in shock there is a decrease of blood volume, stagnation within the capillaries and increased permeability of the capillary wall. Hence, shock is due solely to loss of fluids into the tissues outside of the vascular system. The explanation of what causes the above syndromes is still a question. Of the various t h e o r i e s advanced as to the cause of shock, there are none that have been universally accepted and many of the theories that were popular a few years ago have been disproven or at least questioned by other authorities.

III. *Causes*—There are many causes of shock, among them being:

1. Trauma with marked damage to tissues.

2. Prolonged anesthesia.

3. Prolonged operative procedures with rough handling of tissue.

4. Shock that occurs from ruptured abdominal viscera.

*Chairman's Address, Section of General Surgery, Annual Meeting, Oklahoma State Medical Association, Muskogee, May 11, 1938.

5. So-called pleural shock. Shock may be produced by a sudden blow on the abdomen.

6. Obstetrical shock.

7. Shock from freezing or burns.

8. Mental or physic shock, which is generally associated with one of the previous mentioned types.

9. Shock that occurs in cardiac disease, poisonings, and infectious diseases.

Shock is divided into p r i m a r y shock which occurs immediately following an injury and is probably neurogenic. Secondary shock occurs later and post-operative shock is of this type. Primary shock may merge into secondary shock, or so-called secondary shock may occur without evidence of primary shock.

IV. *Symptoms*—Patients in shock may p r e s e n t several or all of the following characteristics:

1. Low venous pressure.

2. Low arterial pressure.

3. Rapid thready pulse.

4. Diminished blood volume.

5. Increased concentration of RBC and Hgb.

6. Leukocytosis.

7. Increased blood nitrogen.

8. Reduced blood alkali.

9. Lowered metabolism.

10. Subnormal temperature.

11. Cold moist skin.

12. Pallid, grayish or cyanotic appearance.

13. Thirst.

14. Shallow rapid respiration.

15. Vomiting.

16. Restlessness.

17. Anxiety progressing to mental dullness.

18. Patient reacts slightly to stimuli.

19. Limbs are toneless, sense of deadness in the limbs, listless, flacidity of muscular system.

20. Decreased or loss of reflexes.

V. *Diagnosis* — The patient following a severe injury may be seen by the physician or surgeon and his general condition appear quite good and the surgeon may be mislead as to the impending shock that will later develop. All physicians have seen patients admitted in apparently good condition and that are not "yet shocked" and then go into profound shock. It is very important for the s u r g e o n to recognize shock in its earliest stages to prevent severe shock developing.

The difference between shock and hemorrhage in a case that has lost a great deal of blood, if seen prior to the onset of shock, may present certain symptoms that are helpful in differentiation. In a case of hemorrhage the capillary bed remains normal and if fluid is introduced into the circulatory system will remain there much better than in a patient with shock where the capillary bed presents marked permeability allowing escape of fluids into the tissues. However, most patients that have had severe hemorrhage will show symptoms of shock. Cannon states that "shock is hemorrhage and hemorrhage is shock." It is a g r e e d by all that hemorrhage in shock is always serious.

At this point I wish to state that there is no difference between medical and surgical shock and shock that occurs in cardiac disease, pneumonia, t y p h o i d fever, and other diseases has the same basis as post-operative shock and the mechanism is the same. In shock there is a concentration of blood in the capillaries and the blood count will show an increase in the RBC and Hgb. This is helpful in diagnosing shock from hemorrhage, as in hemorrhage without shock the reverse is true.

VI. *Treatment* — Assuming t h a t the causes or condition present in shock is due to a decreased blood volume the rational treatment is to restore this lost blood volume. However, this is not as simple as it appears on account of the fact that leaking capillaries allow the escape of fluid through the walls. Shock is not a single entity and no single remedy is sure to give results. However, there are c e r t a i n procedures that can be used that do much in preventing shock deepening and allowing the patient to recover. It is trite to state that the best treatment of shock is to prevent it. This is one of the most important factors in the treatment of shock. As my subject is post-operative shock, I will confine my remarks to that field.

Hasty elective s u r g e r y in a patient whose vitality is lowered by disease or age is to be condemned and every e f f o r t should be made to get these patients in as good condition as possible. In the surgical emergencies and those who have been injured all effort should be made to prevent shock occuring or if shock is present the shock should be treated and surgery delayed if possible until the patient is in b e t t e r condition. Operations should be performed with the greatest of speed and gentleness and care taken to obtain hemostasis. The choice of an anesthetic in a poor risk patient is important as a factor in the prevention of shock. Some surgeons believe s p i n a l anesthesia increases the shock, others oppose this view. Crile advocated "Noci—association" by infiltration of a local anesthetic about the wound combined with nitrous oxide inhalation anesthesia. Ethylene and cyclo-propane probably are as unlikely to enhance shock as any of the anesthetics. Ether especially over a considerable time has a bad effect in a patient susceptible to shock.

Restoration of blood volume is best obtained through blood transfusions, particularly if shock is associated with hemorrhage. Intravenous gum a c a c i a stands next to blood transfusion and should be used in all cases of beginning or advanced shock while waiting for a donor. Next in

order is the intravenous administration of glucose. It is probably true that normal saline is of little value in treatment of shock, as its effects are too transient. However, if there is an associated dehydration and fluid is needed, saline subcutaneously in certain cases may be helpful. The application of heat is very important and every effort should be made to keep the patient warm. Morphine should be given particularly in the early stage of shock. Wallace states that "warmth and rest are the most important factors in the treatment of shock." Cutler and Scott state that "other than transfusions, h e a t and morphine will do m o r e to restore vasomotor tone than all other procedures advocated." The use of other drugs in shock is generally of very little use, except in special instances, as the use of ephedrine in the shock of spinal anesthesia. The use of oxygen and carbon dioxide inhalations has been advocated and is probably of some benefit especially if there is marked anoxemia. Reassurance of the patient is of the utmost importance in the treatment of shock, as fear and other emotions are important in the production of and the deepening of shock.

There is no satisfactory treatment of shock that has persisted for several hours and it is important to reduce the incidence of shock and give adequate treatment of the condition during the early stage of its development. In s p i t e of the fact that shock is very common, our information concerning it is still very incomplete.

——————O——————

CONSTIPATION*

MINARD F. JACOBS, M.D.
OKLAHOMA CITY, OKLA.

Constipation has plagued both the medical profession and the layman since the early history of man when he banded together to live in communities. Hippocrates, Celsius and others in their writings discussed the c o n d i t i o n and suggested sound and reasonable treatment. Even in

*Chairman's Address, Section on General Medicine, Annual Meeting, Oklahoma State Medical Association, Muskogee, May, 9, 10, 11, 1938.

that day a great deal of stress was laid by them on the abuse and harm of cathartics.

As we all know constipation is still today a prominent complaint of many individuals who consult us.

It is my belief that intelligent treatment properly carried out can and will relieve these individuals and as physicians I feel it is our duty to educate them to this fact by proof. Too often the doctor inadvertently suggests to the patient to "take a physic" which leads him to believe that this is quite the thing to do when such I'm sure is not the case. It is also a duty of ours to counteract the misinformation the layman has gained through the commercial exploitation of pseudo-scientific and fraudulent remedies. Today one can not read the advertisements in a magazine or newspaper or listen for any length of time to a radio without seeing or hearing of the dangers of constipation and how this or that particular r e m e d y will harmlessly cure the condition.

GENERAL CONSIDERATIONS

What is constipation? Almost e v e r y person has a different conception. If the stool is large and firm it is called constipation; if there is a feeling as though the rectum did not completely e m p t y it is called c o n s t i p a t i o n; if the passage is thought to be too small in amount it is constipation; or if the bowels do not move regularly it is constipation. Yet with all of the varying ideas there is a common denominator which includes the elements of consistency, volume, and rate of passage. It must be remembered, however, that the colonic function of individuals varies and yet may be within n o r m a l limits. The great majority of individuals h a v e one evacuation daily. A certain percentage have habitually two or three evacuations per day, while occasionally an individual is seen who habitually has an evacuation every second or third day. In all other respects t h e s e individuals are perfectly normal and so we must conclude that this variability is physiological.

ANATOMICAL CONSIDERATIONS

Embryologically the c o l o n is derived from the hind gut. In its formation it goes through a lengthening process, then loops upon itself and undergoes rotation. At this time the cecum normally descends into the right iliac fossa. Any of these transformations may be incomplete or fail to occur or the opposite may take place so that the colon lengthens to such a degree as to favor constipation. In 85 to 90 per cent of individuals the cecum is in the right iliac fossa. The transverse colon varies a good deal in position and is frequently below the interiliac line. The hepatic and splenic flexures vary markedly in position

and in their relation to each other. It is not infrequent to see pelvic positions of the colon without any associated constipation. Conversely, many colons lying in what we consider a normal position are subject to constipation. It is the habitus of the individual that determines the position of the colon. As Spencer has stated the functional efficiency of the colon is more important than the anatomical.

PHYSIOLOGICAL CONSIDERATIONS

The food and liquids arrive at the cecum in a soft mixed fluid state in about two to four hours. The ileum is p r a c t i c a l l y emptied in seven hours. It was formerly thought that a gastro-colic reflex caused a discharge of the i l e a l contents into the cecum. Recently Welch has shown that there is no true gastro-colic reflex as putting food directly into the stomach through a gastric fistula does not result in emptying of the ileum, but feeding by mouth does initiate the reflex. Thus there is an appetite or taste reflex, but not a gastro-colic one. The residue in the cecum and ascending colon remains there the greater part of the time prior to defecation. Alvarez has shown that 15 per cent goes through quickly, 50 per cent passes on the second day, and that approximately four days are required to pass 75 per cent of the mass. The type of food, however, and the number of stimuli arising in adjacent organs have a definite bearing on the muscular activity of the normal colon. In addition and more important as a regulatory mechanism are certain m o t o r phenomena consisting of pendulum movements that mix the cecal contents, and peristaltic and anti-peristaltic waves that cause the material to be retained in the cecum and ascending colon. The purpose of this is to allow the absorption of fluid and salts, which is the chief function of the colon, other than acting as a reservoir. There are also mass movements which occur in the transverse colon about five to six times daily and force the mass into the descending colon and rectum. Bacterial digestion also occurs in the colon and probably should be considered a physiological process.

When food reaches the rectum a reflex is initiated which results in a desire for defecation. With defecation the fecal mass may empty out as far back as the transverse colon or only the rectal contents may e m p t y. It has been demonstrated that after the colon has been at rest a slight stimulus results in extremely active peristalsis which accounts for the frequency of a bowel movement after breakfast. With constipation there is a delay in the passage associated frequently w i t h an excessive absorption of water.

ETIOLOGY

Before discussing the etiology of constipation it should be understood that organic causes both within and without the gastrointestinal tract are not under consideration.

The greatest single cause today is probably poor habits. First, the normal urge to defecate has been ignored so frequently and over such a long period of time that either the reflex is weakened temporarily or the sensorium has become dulled and unresponsive to the m e s s a g e. Second, faulty dietary habits have become prominent. With the supposed progress in our civilization we have become eaters of highly refined foods that o f f e r insufficient stimulation for peristalsis. Many individuals have the habit of eating little or nothing for breakfast and perhaps only a sandwich for lunch. To this there is added insufficient water intake.

Emotional upsets and the constant tension of today's high-pressure living is often an important f a c t o r as they can cause c o l o n i c stasis. Some psychoanalysts as mentioned by Menninger feel that constipation at times is due to repressed tendencies and unconscious desires which serve as a constant stimulation and thus cause chronic dysfunction.

The use and abuse of cathartics, laxatives, and purgatives results many times in constipation. The average layman believes that the retention of waste matter in his bowel longer than a day will materially affect his health and so he takes a physic. He further believes that if the bowels fail to move the day after a physic he is constipated, not realizing that time must be given for the bowel to fill sufficiently to effect normal stimulation. Another misconception is that such symptoms as "biliousness," headache, vertigo and fatigue respond to cathartics. It seems easier and less expensive to reach for a pill rather than consult a physician. But this fault

does not lie entirely with the layman, as physicians have failed to educate the public and have allowed unethical commercial firms to broadcast misinformation. This constant taking of laxatives causes irritation and inflammation of the mucosa of the colon and by abstracting water and reducing the residue causes spasms and alters the normal secretions resulting in a diminished or absent defecation reflex.

In an interesting article by Kraemer he statistically studied a large group of patients to determine the cause of their purgative addiction and found it to be first, advertisers; second, the medical profession; third, parents; and fourth, friends, which included husband and wife. The a d v e r t i s e r s, however, were equal to the other three combined. He also stated that 70 per cent of the populace is addicted.

DIAGNOSIS

The diagnosis of constipation must be established from the patient's history and by a careful painstaking examination. This should include a digital rectal examination and often a sigmoidoscopic examination. Roentgenoscopic observation after giving barium by mouth so as to observe its progress through the colon and a barium enema may be necessary in order to definitely exclude organic causes. The reassurance that this enables the physician to give the patient is often extremely helpful. The presence of vague indigestion, headache, and constipation does not mean that these symptoms may not be secondary to an old peptic ulcer, gall bladder disease, or chronic appendicitis. Occasionally, one sees a patient with a low basal metabolic rate which when elevated to normal corrects the constipation.

TREATMENT

General Hygiene — The treatment of constipation m u s t be approached from many angles. First of all the patient must be reassured that there is no organic pathology. This is extremely important as the nervous woman and the high tension business man are both fearful lest it be something serious. It should be explained to the patient that the normal number of evacuations per day varies in different individuals and that no harm will come if the bowels fail to act for several days. Unfortunately the bugaboo of auto-intoxication is a difficult phobia to separate from the patient. He should be told that experimental proof of such a condition is lacking and that even if bacteria or toxins should get through the walls of the bowel, nature has adequate outposts in the lymph nodes and liver to stop the organisms from getting into the g e n e r a l circulation or change the toxins to harmless products. It is a fact that in Hirshprung's disease the commonly attributed symptoms of autointoxication are not present and yet there are tremendous amounts of retained fecal material.

A regular habit time must be established and physiologically this s h o u l d be after breakfast. However, a "call" should never be ignored. Arising early enough so that time can be given without rush is important. It is probably not a good idea to read at this time.

Rest, relaxation, regular vacations, and if necessary the elimination or reduction of responsibilities are helpful. Sedatives may prove of some benefit but I doubt that I have ever seen any results from the use of antispasmodics such as belladonna.

Exercise is often a worthwhile adjunct for the sedentary worker or housewife as it not only tones up the muscular system, but has relaxing qualities if carried out intelligently. It should not be indulged in to the point of fatigue as this can cause or aggravate the condition. Light massage may at times prove beneficial.

Diet—The diet of the patient must be suited to the individual and it is preferable to give the patient a written or typewritten copy rather than a standard mimeographed one. Frequently one sees diets for atonic constipation and for spastic constipation, yet true atony of the colon without an organic basis is undoubtedly very rare. In the presence of marked redundancies one sometimes does see generalized a t o n y. During roentgenoscopic examinations one may see dilated areas, but they are usually associated with spasticity or the two may sometimes occur in the same individual at different times. H e n c e, in general, the diet usually tends toward a smooth one with the elimination of excessive roughage such as foods with large amounts of fiber or skin. For some individuals raw fruits and raw vegetables must be omitted and temporarily only the pureed ones used.

This does not mean that extra bulk in the form of raw fruits and green vegetables is never indicated.

Occasionally in the thin, undernourished individual a diet high in fats of the type in cream, butter and olive or vegetable oils is helpful as they have a laxative effect. The diet, however, must be balanced. In other words it must c o n t a i n the "protective" foods which include one pint of milk, four servings of vegetables, t w o servings of fruit, one serving of meat, one egg and a tablespoon of b u t t e r each day. Meals should be eaten slowly enough to be properly masticated and this presupposes an adequate set of teeth. Business, worry and arguments should be a v o i d e d at meal times.

Fluid — The amount of f l u i d intake should be at least eight glasses daily. There is no o b j e c t i o n to drinking water with meals as long as it is not used to flush the food in the mouth unchewed into the stomach. Occasionally a glass or two of water in the morning on arising is helpful.

Mechanical Aids—In addition to the general hygienic measures and dietotherapy it is often necessary especially at the onset of treatment to obtain the help of mechanical aids. The most useful of these are probably the mild and non-irritating bulk producers such as plain granular agar and the vegetable mucins. Agar can be taken dry and washed down with water or it may be added to cereals and soups. The average d o s e is from one to three teaspoonsful with each meal. The vegetable mucins are equally as efficient but have the drawback of expense. One to two teaspoonsful with plenty of water at bedtime and occasionally also on arising is the usual dosage.

With some of these products vitamin B has been incorporated. There is no doubt that vitamin B has some effect, but I have not been convinced of its clinical value in constipation. Because of the extensive advertising by the yeast manufacturers many of us have seen patients who on their own initiative have tried yeast and thought it was beneficial, but discontinued its use b e c a u s e of distress from excessive gas formation.

Bran and various seeds are extensively used, but as they are probably irritating to some colons it seems better to use the blander bulk producers. It should be kept in mind, however, that any of them may occasionally form masses in the rectum, especially in older individuals and this may occur even though there is some bowel movement daily. Therefore, an occasional rectal examination should be made.

Oils of various types have been used for many centuries. At the present mineral oil seems to be the one of choice. It is unquestionably a definite aid. How it works is not understood although we glibly speak of it as a lubricant, though it has been shown that it does not act in this manner. Olive oil is equally efficacious. Of course, where o b e s i t y is present its use would naturally be inadvisable.

Physics and laxatives generally speaking have no place in the treatment of constipation e x c e p t possibly temporarily or when the other methods have failed, or in the aged edentulous patient. Fluid extract of cascara and milk of magnesia seem to be the least harmful. If an individual has taken cathartics for 40 or 50 years without apparent harm there is no reason to discontinue them. The fact is the attempt will usually be unsuccessful anyhow.

The use of enemas is still a bone of contention among physicians. As with laxatives they have been used since the time of the early Egyptians. They are only temporary aids and should be considered as such. It is often helpful both mentally and rectally to have the patient use a small enema of physiologic salt solution occasionally at the onset of treatment providing the bowels are not moving otherwise Olive oil retention enemas are also helpful at times in the e a r l y weeks of treatment. High colonic irrigations can be dismissed quickly. They are unphysiologic, o f t e n harmful, and have no place in the treatment of constipation.

CONCLUSION

Constipation is a condition almost as old as man himself. Its marked prevalence is a reflection on us as physicians. Proper treatment which includes attention to the individual's general hygiene as well as his dietary habits can correct the condition.

ROENTGEN THERAPY*

L. S. McALISTER, M.D.
MUSKOGEE, OKLA.

The status of roentgen therapy is well established in the realm of malignancies. For example, in malignancy of the skin, excellent results are obtained in over 90 per cent of the cases, regardless of the quality of the rays we use. The only requirement is that the total dose be administered preferably within two weeks. In my experience, 63 kilovolt X-rays unfiltered are just as effective in malignancy of the skin as 200 kilovolt X-rays through a half millimeter of copper. I have delivered the unfiltered rays at 550 roentgens per sitting every other day for five or six times as suggested by Dr. Martin and his father.

I have protracted and fractionated the 63 kilovolt rays with two milliamperes and one millimeter of aluminum down to a minute "r" afflux of 13. At this rate, 150 or 200 roentgens per day for two weeks has cured several lesions. This reaction never progressed beyond an erythema.

I have also followed the rate of administration advised by Dr. H. G. F. Edwards of Shreveport, in the October, 1937, issue of the Southern Medical Journal. Using five milliamperes and 63,000 volts at eight · inch distance, my equipment delivers 1,200 roentgens in ten minutes. This may be repeated, as he states, at seven day intervals for three or four times, depending on the induration of the growth. The tissues recuperating 70 per cent each week. This method and Dr. Martin's method produce

*Chairman's Address, Dermatology and Radiology Section, Annual Meeting, Oklahoma State Medical Association, Muskogee, May 9, 10, 11, 1938.

severe skin reactions, but not quite so severe as those of Dr. R. L. Sargent of Oakland, California, who advises 2,500 roentgens in air unfiltered in one sitting "just to brush off the surface" and repeats in three days two or three times, depending on the size of the growth.

I recently administered 4,000 roentgens in air through five-tenths millimeter copper to an excavating carcinoma behind the ear. The reaction required four months to heal. To use the farmer's own words, it acted as though some one were in there ploughing and turning up large furrows for that length of time. All of these methods have produced excellent results, but I wish to state that Dr. Sargent's technique keeps the operator awake too much at night. The reactions finally do heal, however.

I have mentioned all of this to s h o w that the treatment of skin carcinoma is almost standardized, providing the operator's equipment is calibrated in roentgens and he follows the technique of some older and more experienced man. The only skin malignancies which the above techniques failed to cure were those which either I or s o m e o n e else had undertreated by the old skin unit dosage system. As you all know, the trend now is to treat these failures with two to five millimeters of copper at short target skin distance. I have had no experience with Chaoul's method of contact therapy, but it seems very promising.

In deep therapy, the techniques are not nearly so well standardized for internal cancer. Every one is riding his own hobby. The filters are thickening and the voltages are rising in an effort to duplicate the gamma ray effect of radium. If this trend continues, the filters will be so thick that the tumor will be receiving more and more of less and less. If one permits his imagination full play, some of the more heavily endowed institutions will finally have such powerful machines and such thick filters that the treatment will be entirely psychic because no X-rays will be getting through.

Seriously, gentlemen, there must be a middle ground. Or, as Dr. Erskine suggests, it might be more b e n e f i c i a l in crowded institutions to d e v e l o p a good quality of X-radiation at a rapid rate, say 200 kilovolts and 100 milliamperes. Then,

as he states, multiple ports could be used to deliver a depth dose of sufficient intensity in a short period of time. This, of course, w o u l d be following the massive dose technique advocated by Seitz and Wintz rather than the protracted fractionated method of Coutard. Parenthetically, we should remember that the slow method of irradiation was advised primarily for carcinoma of the larynx of the intrinsic type and that the work of Seitz and Wintz on carcinoma of the cervix cannot be conscientiously discarded as yet.

I do not wish to create the impression that a million volts against cancer, with thicker filters, is fantastic. It is, however, very uneconomical. I would like to emphasize the fact that it is not the machine, but the man behind it that cures cancer. I also wish to state that the techniques for treating internal malignancy are in a constant state of u n r e s t and that this wholesome state of "rugged individualism" will finally lead to better techniques than we are using at present.

On the other hand, we must admit that irradiation is probably not the final answer to the p r o b l e m of malignancy. I would like to reiterate that we are limited in our attack on the tumor by the amount of irradiation the host of the tumor can "take" and still live and function normally, or nearly normally.

Roentgen therapy is also invading the realm of benignancy to an unprecedented extent. Aside from about 80 skin diseases, various acute and chronic infections are now being treated. Here again rugged individualism plus time will develop definite indications and contra-indications and useful and accepted techniques will be developed.

Erisypelas responds well to 75 roentgens unfiltered, or lightly filtered, daily for two or three days, but according to Dr. Rigler of Minnesota massive doses of ultra violet will produce good results with no possibility of p r o d u c i n g unreversible skin changes. It can also be handled well with sulfanilamide.

Cantaloup sized fibrotic metropathies respond well to a "deep therapy" castration dose. I think roentgen therapy is the method of choice in women near the end of the child bearing age. A few surgeons in my community feel the same way and they also think the same about climacteric hemorrhage. The age limit may be disregarded if for some reason surgery is contraindicated. In these younger women X-ray is to be preferred to radium because of its slow effect in producing the menopause (Kaplan).

Hyperthyroidism, preferably bilaterally symmetrical hyperplastic elastic g l a n d s (Grave's disease), have responded well to multiple doses of roentgen therapy over several months time. Personally I feel that in hyperthyroidism a quality produced by two to four millimeters of aluminum at moderate voltage is more sedative and stabilizing than the quality produced by copper filtration and higher voltages. I have never used Lugol's solution or digitalis except in one post-operative recurrence managed by copper filtration. I would like to remind you that Dr. Alden H. Williams in a large series of hyperthyroidism used only three millimeters of aluminum over a 10 by 15 centimeter port over the thyroid and thymus at seven to ten day intervals, depending on the exigencies of the case.

I have one female patient who has remained stabilized for eight years. She was treated through six millimeters of aluminum through multiple three-quarter inch ports over each lobe and isthmus. In roentgens each port was receiving about 250 in air every ten days. This case was examined by Dr. Hertzler two years or so ago. He reported a fibrotic condition of the thyroid with no evidence of hyperthyroidism. He stated that in his experience she would finally come to surgery. At the present time she is still stabilized and has had no surgery. I feel that I am too young in the game to dispute him.

I have treated two cases of phlegmonous inflammation of large size extending from the mastoid process to the acromion with resolution in seven to ten days. Both had been incised without striking pus. The dose on each case was 250 r o e n t g e n s through six millimeters of aluminum at moderate voltage. They might have resolved anyway? Who can say.

I have t r e a t e d only one case of gas gangrene. He had sacrificed his arm and received anti-tetanic and gas g a n g r e n e serum as well as intra-muscular injections of oxygen. His temperature curve had already started down, but from Kelly's technique he seemed to receive an extra kick which did him a world of good. He is living.

My eye, ear, nose and throat colleagues support me royally. Diphtheria carriers, whether tonsillar or post-nasal, have responded well to nasal syphons and 75 to 200 roentgens at moderate or high voltage.

Chronic adenitis, cervical or otherwise, responds well to 150 roentgens through aluminum or copper. I feel that we need no controls on these cases because of several weeks duration and immediate response to roentgen therapy within a week or ten days. Tubercular adenitis requires several doses and a longer time for resolution. I have treated one case of tuberculous fistula following a biopsy on a supraclavicular gland with excellent results.

I feel that acute adenitis s h o u l d be studied more closely by control series in large institutions. They seem to respond well to 75 roentgens d a i l y at moderate voltage through either aluminum or copper. They either suppurate immediately and require surgical incision or they resolve shortly without suppuration.

I have one eye, ear, nose and throat man who refers his otitis media cases for 75 to 100 roentgens at moderate voltage, through four millimeters of aluminum. He claims that it helps and they dry up more rapidly.

A case of lymphangiitis of the tongue and floor of the mouth was recently treated through four millimeters of aluminum in addition to prontylin, with recovery in 36 hours.

Before I close, I would like to report the treatment of a case of a neoplasm of the cornea in a woman of 84 obscuring vision and the iris and protruding one centimeter anterior to the cornea and of such bulk as to separate the palpebral f i s s u r e quite widely. The ophthalmologist thought it too massive to dissect. She was treated daily with 130 roentgens generated at two milliamperes and 63,000 volts through one millimeter of aluminum at a minute "r" afflux of 13; in other words, ten minutes daily for 14 days. The lesion melted away in three months. The patient could see. In another month a small "striffin," to use the patient's term, still remained across the pupil. At present, the "striffin" has regrown until it is about one-fourth the size of the original lesion. The ophthalmologist still does not feel justified in dissecting it off the cornea. She recently received 700 roentgens through one-quarter millimeter of aluminum, in addition to t w o desiccations with the short wave unit and she can see again. All of these treatments required two per cent butyn and a lid re-

tractor. I know now that pontocaine causes less congestion of sclera. The lashes are still in situ, the cornea is not inflamed and, barring ill-luck, I believe this elderly lady will be able to see throughout the remainder of her normal expectancy.

I wish to take this opportunity to thank my various colleagues for their faith in the new science of modern radiology.

----------o----------

Epidemic Encephalitis, St. Louis Type
Survey of the Outbreak, Summer and Fall of 1937

GEORGE S. BOZALIS, A.B., B.S., M.D.
ANDREW B. JONES, M.D.
ST. LOUIS, MO.

This report is based upon 134 cases of epidemic encephalitis, St. L o u i s Type, treated in the St. Louis City Isolation Hospital, St. Louis, Mo., occurring in the late summer and early fall of 1937.

During this period, a total of 987 cases of epidemic encephalitis were reported to the Health Department of the City of St. Louis and St. Louis County; in the former 431 cases; in the latter 556 cases. A total of 1,097 cases were r e p o r t e d during the 1933 epidemic; 557 from the city and 520 from the county[1].

All cases admitted to the hospital with the diagnosis of epidemic encephalitis that proved to be other conditions have been eliminated. Among the conditions sent to the hospital with this diagnosis were acute poliomyelitis, epidemic meningitis, streptococcus meningitis, tuberculous meningitis, luetic meningitis, brain abscess and acute arthritis.

The problem of differential diagnosis for the referring physicians, as well as for us in the hospital, was made doubly difficult by the presence of acute anterior poliomyelitis in near epidemic proportions within the metropolitan area, and a sizable epidemic just across the river in Illinois.

The summer of 1937 was relatively cool until August. From August on until early

winter it was very dry. There was some hot weather in July, August and September.

The epidemic of St. Louis Type encephalitis of 1933 was preceded by an extremely dry and hot summer. The rainfall in the metropolitan area was the lowest in the history of the weather bureau[2].

Encephalitis is not a new disease. According to medical historians (Jonothan Wright) clinical descriptions of illnesses that correspond closely with the picture of lethargic encephalitis as it is known today occurred as early as the time of Galen. At subsequent periods infrequent references are found to illnesses occurring in epidemic proportions, whose clinical descriptions are much the same as lethargic encephalitis.

In 1890, during an epidemic of influenza that occurred in northern Italy and southern Hungary lasting from 1889-91, Von Economo described a mysterious illness under the title of "Nona." Longuett reviewed this illness and published a complete review of "Nona" in 1892[3]. Their descriptions cover the picture of lethargic encephalitis.

In the winter of 1916-17, an illness characterized by lethargy, stupor, cranial nerve palsies, etc., broke out in Vienna. It was painstakingly described by Von Economo and christened by him "Encephalitis Lethargica."[4] It was reported by Netter in Paris in 1917[3]. Later, it spread to England, America, and to all known parts of the world. It occurred in epidemic proportions in this country in 1919-25, inclusive. At the present time it is endemic throughout the world. It is the winter type of encephalitis. It is called either lethargic encephalitis or encephalitis, Type A.

Epidemics of summer type of encephalitis have occurred in Japan since 1871. Altogether the Japanese have reported 13 separate epidemics. The last was reported in 1929[6].

The first epidemic in 1871 affected mainly older people. The second, in 1873, was small, but the mortality was reported as 90 per cent. The third occurred from July to October, 1901, a large one affecting mainly older people. The 1903 report was predominantly a meningeal type occurring from August to November. The fifth in 1907, and the sixth occurred m a i n l y in Tokyo. The seventh was another epidemic occurring from August to October, 1912. In 1916, another large epidemic occurred with a fatality rate of 61.5 per cent. In 1917, another epidemic attacked younger individuals from 15 to 20 years of age, but with a fatality rate of 10 per cent.

During the outbreak of 1919, the Japanese concluded they were not dealing with an epidemic meningitis, as they had thought until this time, but that this was a meningo-encephalitis of a special kind.

In 1924, they had their largest outbreak, 7,000 cases were reported with a fatality rate of 60 per cent. Seventy-six per cent of their cases were over 40 years of age. In 1927 and again in 1929, they had epidemics. The latter was the larger—2,000 with a fatality of 63 per cent[7-8].

The largest epidemic in Japan occurred in 1924, at the end of an unusually hot and dry summer. We have previously noted that our epidemic of 1933 occurred during comparable weather conditions, but to a less degree than in 1937. These observations cause much speculation regarding the influence of the weather in the production of the illness. It is well known that the wet, cold, bad months are conducive to epidemic meningitis, therefore, hot dry months may favor the dissemination of epidemic encephalitis.

Encephalitis of the summer type has also been reported from Australia. In January to April, 1917 (the late summer in the southern hemisphere), and again in 1918, a mysterious d i s e a s e was reported by Breinl and called the Australian X disease[9]. About 100 cases were reported that carried a fatality of 70 per cent. The interesting thing about this epidemic is that cases were reported from remote out of the way places, hundreds of miles from metropolitan areas, but all of these widely scattered areas possessed a hot, dry climate. A similar epidemic was reported t h e r e in 1925, but of smaller proportions[10].

No summer type of encephalitis has been reported in E u r o p e, South America or Africa.

The 1933 epidemic in St. Louis was preceded by 27 cases occurring in Paris, Ill., in 1932, during the months of August and September[11].

Since 1933, we feel the disease had been endemic in St. Louis. One of us (A.B.J.) saw in consultation in St. Louis and in nearby towns an occasional case of epidemic encephalitis in 1934. None was seen in 1935. One case was seen at the Barnes Hospital late in 1936.

Chart I shows the age and sex of our 134 cases, the youngest was 18 months, the oldest 94 years. In one instance more than one case occurred in the same family. This was in twin boys, age five. They were admitted to the hospital four days apart.

CHART I
Total Number of Patients 134

Age	0-5	5-10	10-20	20-30	30-40	40-50	50-60	60-70	70-80	80-
Number of each	2	9	9	16	10	13	20	32	17	6
*Number of females	1	1	3	9	7	7	8	17	6	4
†Number of males	1	8	6	7	3	6	12	15	11	2
Colored Patients	0	0	0	2	1	0	1	0	0	2

*Female patients 60 per cent.
†Male patients 40 per cent.

Earlier in the s u m m e r we, now and again, were making the diagnosis of epidemic encephalitis, St. Louis type. The first case occurred in May. These sporadic cases were admitted with a variety of diagnoses. Due to the presence of meningeal symptoms, the absence of other cases of encephalitis and the spinal fluid findings, we often diagnosed them, tentatively, tuberculous meningitis. Rapid recovery necessitated a change in the diagnosis to encephalitis. In the l i g h t of subsequent events (1937 outbreak) we know these cases were epidemic encephalitis, St. Louis type.

The first cases of the 1937 epidemic were reported to the County Health Department on July 12th, to the City Health Department, August 27th. By September 1st, a total of 11 to 13 cases were being reported daily until October 1st. Then there was a drop in the daily case report until October 7th, when again the number reported was 13. The fall and rise in the number of cases reported was concomitant with a cold snap with some precipitation the last days of September and the first few days of October. On October 5th, the weather became very warm again. Then after October 7th there was a rapid decline in the daily occurrence, the last case was reported on October 20th.

As in the previous epidemic, post mortem examinations here were attended by representatives from the Department of Pathology of Washington University Medical School. Dr. McCordock again recognized the etiological agent as being a filtrable virus, that was neutralized when mixed with the serum of a recovered p a t i e n t, either of this or the '33 epidemic [12-12A].

Even though this St. Louis type is qualitatively the same as the Japanese type B, the work of Webster and Fite[13] show that the sera of Japanese B Type patients do not neutralize the St. Louis virus[14]. Webster and Fite have further shown that Epidemic of Encephalitis in Kansas City, Mo., in 1933, Paris, Ill., in '32, St. Louis in '33 and occasional cases in New York in 1933 were all of the same etiology, but cases reported in Indianapolis, Ind., in '33, were not of this category[15].

Pathological sections revealed significant changes only in the central nervous system, except for chronic changes in kidneys, heart, etc., found among the older age groups.

On gross examination were noted varying degrees of congestion of the meningeal and intracerebral v e s s e l s. The microscopic changes consisted of cellular infiltration, vascular congestion, haemorrhage and nerve cell degeneration.

The most striking microscopic change is a perivascular round cell infiltration, described as perivascular "cuffing." In scattered areas of the brain substance, focal collections of mononuclear cells could be seen. Often these focal areas contained some polymorphonuclear leukocytes and a degenerated n e r v e cell. These changes were present practically in every part of the brain. In some of the older individuals small foci of hemorrhages were seen with associated encephalomyelacia.

The protean n a t u r e of the disease is exemplified by a study of the prodromata, Chart II.

CHART II
PRODROMALS

Symptom	No. of Cases	% of Cases
Headache	99	73.1
Fever	74	55.2
Anorexia	5	3.7
Stupor	18	13.4
Dizziness	19	14.1
Head Cold	4	2.9
Delirium	5	3.7
Chills	14	10.4
Photophobia	1	.8
Staggering	2	1.4
Vomiting	23	17.1
Stiff Neck	21	15.6
Backache	6	4.47
Sleeplessness	3	2.2
Partial Paralysis	5	3.7
Nausea	8	5.9
Abdominal Pain	8	5.9
Lethargy	16	11.9
Diplopia	1	0.8
Ringing in ears	1	0.8
Pain in eyes	1	0.8
Sore throat	3	2.2
Syncope	1	0.8
Joint Pain	3	2.2
Post Partum	1	0.8
Incontinent	4	2.9
Coma	5	3.7
Dysphagia	1	0.8
Muscle pain	7	5.2
Twitchings and tremors	11	8.2
Drowsy	31	23.1
General stiffness	2	1.49
Diarrhea	2	1.4
General weakness	6	4.4
Convulsions	1	0.8

The prodromals of the 134 cases show that 73 per cent complained of headaches and 55 per cent of fever. Stupor occurred with the onset in 13 per cent of the cases. Lethargy occurred from the onset in 12 per cent of the cases. This speaks for the severity of the disease and the necessity of ruling out an epidemic form of meningitis. Another early common s y m p t o m was twitching with rigidity of muscles setting in rapidly, especially among the older age groups.

CHART III
NEUROLOGICAL FINDINGS

Symptoms	No. of Cases	% of Cases
Stiff neck	113	84.4
Koernig	51	38.
Brudzinski	8	5.9
Absent Abdom.	101	75.3
Absent cremasters	38	28.3
Absent K. K.	33	24.6
Absent ankle jerks	60	44.7
Spontaneous movements	15	11.2
Rigidities	72	53.6
Tremors	39	29.
Lethargy	75	55.9
Coma and stupor	62	46.25
Retention	7	5.2
Incontinent	51	38.
Paralysis	9	6.7
Diplopia	2	1.5
Strabismus	1	.7
Nystagmus	4	2.9
Absent biceps	4	2.9
Gordon	11	8.2
Oppenheim	12	8.9
Babinski	6	4.4
Hoffman	1	.7
Chaddock	1	.7

The neurological findings (Chart III) were quite varied, however, a stiff neck and absent abdominal reflexes were among the most common findings being manifest in 85 per cent and 75 per cent of the cases respectively. Lethargy was present in 56 per cent of the cases with coma and stupor in 46 per cent. T r e m o r s involving the tongue, face, chin and lips as well as the hands and at times the entire arms, occurred in 29 per cent of the cases. Often these t r e m o r s were similar to those of Parkinson's Disease. Rigidity of the upper and lower extremities were noted in 54 per cent of the cases. Disturbance of the urinary bladder was often seen, 38 per cent of our patients being incontinent and five per cent showing acute retention. In those cases having weakness of an extremity we were always able to elicit tendon jerks. A child may not move an arm or a leg or both arms and both legs on admission, but if the extremity was raised by the examiner and released it did not fall like a flail, nor did the hands or feet lie in positions of flaccidity or limpness as in poliomyelitis. Foot and toe drop were absent. More frequently the thigh was externally rotated, slightly flexed, with the foot at right angles with the leg. There were no t r o p h i c

changes. Within 48 to 96 hours the patient was using hands to feed itself, or walking around in the crib.

Laboratory work was of extreme importance in m a k i n g a diagnosis. As is shown in Chart IV, 92 per cent of the cases showed a white blood cell count of between 5,000 and 15,000.

CHART IV
WHITE CELL COUNTS OF 134 CASES

Counts	No. of Cases	% of Cases
5,000 to 10,000	43	32.08
10,000 to 15,000	80	59.74
15,000 to 20,000	5	3.7
20,000 and over	5	3.7

The spinal fluid was always found to be under increased pressure. Chart V, shows only 15 per cent of the cases having a total spinal fluid cell count of over 200 cells per cu.m.m. Cell counts recorded over 300 we considered an error, red cells probably.

CHART V
SPINAL FLUID CELL COUNT, TOTAL OF
131 CASES

Counts	No. of Cases	% of Cases
* 0- 10	9	6.8
10- 20	10	7.6
20- 40	18	13.7
40- 60	23	17.5
60- 80	14	10.6
80-100	17	12.9
100-200	22	16.7
200-300	9	6.8
†300-	11	8.3

*Counts of 0-100 cells found in 91 cases or 69.1%.
†Five counts were between 1,000-2,000 cells—none over.

Differential cell c o u n t s of the spinal fluid Chart VI, showed 122 cases of 98 per cent, with 50 to 100 per cent lymphocytes. Only two cases showed a polymorphonuclear count of greater than 50 per cent.

CHART VI
LYNPHOCYTES IN SPINAL FLUID, TOTAL OF
124 CASES

% of Lymphs	No. of Cases	% of Cases
0- 20	0	.0
20- 50	2	1.6
50- 80	25	20.1
80-100	97	78.3

In Chart VII, the Pandy test is shown to be positive in 77 per cent of the cases.

CHART VII
PANDY TESTS OF 128 CASES

	No. of Cases	% of Cases
Positive	99	77.3
Negative	21	16.4
Questionable	8	6.3

Spinal fluid sugars were done routinely with blood sugars. In practically all cases the spinal fluid sugar was not diminished, being 50 per cent or more of the blood sugar as is shown in Chart VIII.

CHART VIII
SPINAL FLUID SUGAR IN MG. PER CENT
TOTAL OF 127 CASES

Mg. %	No. of Cases	% of Cases
0- 15	0	.0
15- 30	1	.8
30- 45	7	5.5
45- 60	37	29.1
60- 75	39	30.7
75- 90	23	18.1
90-105	10	7.8
105-115	10	7.8
115-up	0	.0

The mortality is listed for age groups in Chart IX, with a total mortality of 22.38 per cent for all ages. It is interesting to note the tremendous mortality in the older individuals. However, one death occurred in the five to ten age group and one in the 20 to 30 age group.

A total of 86, or 64 per cent of our patients left the hospital normal; 14 per cent with residuals. A total of 80 per cent of these residuals were mental dullness found especially a m o n g the older age groups (Chart X).

Two of our children were discharged with muscle weakness. One of these was a twin mentioned above. The twins were recently examined (four months after discharge) and were f o u n d to be entirely without residuals. The other child discharged with weakness of the left arm and leg still shows a limp in the left leg, but power in the left arm has returned. The muscle tone in the left arm and leg is subnormal. The eight-year-old boy discharged with the eye muscle paralysis showed no evidence of strabismus four months later. The eye movements were entirely normal. He is wearing glasses for correction of an astigmatism.

Epidemic encephalitis, St. Louis Type, is an a c u t e infectious systemic disease,

caused by a filtrable virus, that has a predilection for the nervous system, particularly for the brain and meninges. Probably a great number of cases show the systemic phase only. Either the infection is so mild or the resistance of the patient is so great that neurological signs do not appear. However in these cases, invasion of the nervous system has been demonstrated by the presence of lymphocytes, globulin, and other changes in the spinal fluid.

The disease occurs chiefly in the late summer and early fall (July, August and September). As in epidemic meningitis, weather conditions appear to be a factor in precipitating the disease.

In the 1937 outbreak the onset of the illness was less abrupt than in the 1933 epidemic[16]. The prodromal p e r i o d on the whole was much longer and the total duration of the disease in the main covered a longer period of time. In 1933, it was not unusual to see an abrupt fall in the temperature, or a near crisis. In all our cases

CHART X
STATE ON DISCHARGE

SYMPTOM	No. of CASES	% of CASES
NORMAL	86	64.1
MENTALLY DULL	11	8.6
PSYCHOSIS	1	
MUSCLE WEAKNESS	2	
RETENTION	1	
GAIT DIFFICULTY	1	14.1 % with residuals
EYE MUSCLE PARALYSIS	1	
TWITCHING	1	
INCONTINENT	1	
DEATH	30	

CHART IX
MORTALITY

Age	0-5	5-10	10-20	20-30	30-40	40-50	50-60	60-70	70-80	80-
*Deaths per age group	0	1	0	1	0	2	3	7	11	5
Per cent of deaths per age group	0	11.11	0	6.5	0	15.38	15	21.87	64.7	83.33
Number male deaths	0	1	0	1	0	0	2	5	8	3
Number female deaths	0	0	0	0	0	2	1	2	3	2
†Negro deaths	0	0	0	1	0	0	0	0	0	1

*Total deaths 30, or 22.38 per cent.
†Total colored admitted 6, or 4.47 per cent of total admissions.

in 1937, the fever persisted for a longer period of time, falling by lysis. But, as in the 1933 epidemic, the duration and severity of the illness was extremely variable, from a few days to two or three weeks. The most common type of case was one giving h i s t o r y of generalized headache, fever, nausea and vomiting, and some mental disturbance that had been present from one to 14 days. On admission temperatures varied from 102 to 105; pulse rate from 80 to 120; stiff neck and Koernig sign; drowsiness, stupor or confusion. Lumbar puncture in such cases revealed the findings as in Charts IV, V, and VI.

However, many c a s e s had such complaints as pronounced malaise, anorexia, chills or chilly sensation, grippal aches all over or excruciating pains in the back and legs. Examination revealed some or all of the neurological signs. This is the type of case with a long period of invasion. It was not unusual for such a type of case to have a tentative diagnosis of typhoid fever on account of the relatively high temperature, slow pulse and moderately low leukocyte count with a slight shift to the left.

General rigidity of the body, spontaneous movements, tremors, lightening-like m o v e m e n t s of the eyes, weakness to paralysis of an extremity or extremities were more commonly seen and a more prominent feature than in the epidemic of 1933. One of our more severe cases to recover did not have headache at any time during the illness. The onset was rather sudden, with fever, terrific backache, pains and a feeling of weakness in the thighs and legs. By the fourth day of the illness her temperature reached 106, pulse rate varying from 80 to 120. After three days the temperature gradually fell by lysis with an increase in the pulse rate. In only one case was the illness ushered in by a convulsion. This is in c o n t r a s t to its frequency, especially in children, in the 1933 epidemic.

The neurological signs were inconstant, Chart X. In the milder cases, aside from headache, there may be neurological findings. Stiff neck, Kernig sign, absent abdominal reflexes and absent ankle jerks are the common findings. All of these may be present in the same case or there may be only a stiff neck with any one or more of the neurological findings. Wax-like rigidity of all the muscles was a frequent finding. Any or all combinations of the neurological findings enumerated in Chart X may have been present at one time or another. In other words, there is no pathognomonic neurological p i c t u r e diagnostic of this disease.

In the milder cases there was no disturbance in the sensorium. Some clouding of consciousness, disorientation for short periods of time, muttering and picking at the bed clothes were present in the moderately severe cases. In the more severe cases, stupor and c o m a, with complete amnesia for many days of the illness were common. Especially in the older patients, even after the temperature had returned to normal, many appeared bewildered or confused; they were dull, did not initiate conversation, answered hesitantly in monosyllables. There were a few cases of psychoses characterized by confusion, disorientation, illusions, delusions and poor retentive memory lasting for a few days to two or three months.

Typical case histories are as follows:

Case I

D. C. A 24-year-old white female admitted on 9-12-37 with the history of being perfectly well until 9-8-37 when she developed a terrific generalized headache. The following day she developed a stiffness of the neck and became drowsy. Her temperature was 101° F. She was admitted to City Hospital No. 1 on 9-11-37 and transferred here the following day. On admission she still complained of her headache, appeared slightly drowsy, temperature was 98° F., pulse normal. Neurological examination revealed a bilateral Kernig, absent abdominal reflexes, sluggish patellars, absent right ankle jerk and sluggish on the left. The neck was definitely stiff. On 9-13-37 temperature went to 100.6° F., but by 9-15-37 she was entirely temperature free and symptom free and remaining so until discharge. Laboratory findings on admission showed the spinal fluid to be under increased pressure, but clear, only 28 cells being present with 95 per cent of these being lymphocytes. Spinal sugar was 73 mg. per cent and blood sugar 107 mg per cent. Pandy was positive, Kahn negative, spinal fluid culture showed no growth, W.B.C. count was 10,800 differential was St. 4, Segs. 60, Ly. 32, Mon. 4.

Case II

M. W., age 65, white female admitted 8-27-37 with a history of onset with general malaise and aches and pains lasting four days occurring two weeks before admission. These symptoms were replaced by a "pressure headache" ("head in a vise") and fever. Her neck became stiff and has remained so ever since. She had been nauseated for one week and vomitted daily until day of admission. For three days she had a urinary retention but had been voiding for two days previous to her admission. On admission her temperature was 102-4° F., pulse 96. Rational and conscious. Neck was moderately stiff, abdominal reflexes absent, Kernig was positive bilaterally. A bilateral Oppenheim and Gordon was present and Babinski on the right. The headache and nausea persisted along with a temperature that fluctuated to a 102-6° F. daily until

9-4-37 when her symptoms started subsiding and was normal by 9-6-37. On admission her laboratory work showed W.B.C. 11,650, spinal revealed an increase in pressure, fluid clear with 31 cells being 100 per cent lymphocytes. The spinal sugar was 55 mg. per cent, the blood sugar 98 mg. per cent, spinal fluid showed no growth, urine negative. She was discharged 9-9-37, symptom free.

Case III

H. K., age 67, white female, admitted 8-31-37 with a history of being perfectly well until Saturday night, 8-28-37, when she developed a chill and a severe headache. Generalized aching and weakness followed. On admission, she appeared stuporous but restless. Her musculature showed a slight rigidity of the extremeties. Tremors of the tongue and chin were marked. Her neck was not stiff. Abdominal reflexes, ankle jerks and patellar reflexes were all absent. Her temperature remained elevated as can be seen by the accompanying graph. Rales and an irregular pulse developed, but following digitalization these cleared. Following her return to a normal temperature, her tremors disappeared. Reflexes were all present on discharge. She was sent out on a maintenance dose of digitalis and asked to report to the Cardiac Clinic at City Hospital No. 1. Laboratory findings on admission showed the spinal fluid to be clear but under slight increase in pressure. Three hundred and fifty cells were present, 80 per cent being lymphocytes. Pandy was positive, spinal fluid sugar was 32 mg. per cent, the blood sugar was 75.5 mg. per cent, the Kahn negative, spinal fluid culture revealed no growth. W.B.C. were 11,050, St. 10, Seg. 79, Ly. 8, and Eos. 2.

Case IV

A. H., white male, age 71, admitted 9-4-37 with a history of an acute onset one week before ad-

mission with malaise, chills, fever. He became rapidly stuporus and coma being progressively deeper for two days previous to admission. The day of admission he had a convulsion and a stiff neck was noted at that time. On admission he was in a deep coma, his temperature 104.4° F., pulse was 80. Neck stiff. Moisture in both lung bases. Koernig positive bilaterally, abdominal and cremasterics absent, but all other reflexes present. He seemed to improve somewhat with temperature coming down slowly, but on 9-9-37 a most peculiar movement of the eyes was noted. This "nystagmus" had a vertical, lateral and rotatory component. The above mentioned pulse, temperature ratio persisted as well as lethargy, "nystagmus" and the neurological findings previously mentioned. The patient expired on 9-14-37. Laboratory work on admission revealed the spinal fluid clear and under moderate pressure. Eighty-eight cells were present, 85 per cent being lymphocytes. Pandy was negative, spinal sugar 72 mg. per cent, blood sugar 175 mg. per cent, urine negative, W.B.C. 9,600, J. 1, St. 8, Seg. 58, Ly. 32, Mon. 1, cultures were negative, Wasserman of blood and spinal fluid were negative. We might add here that this peculiar movement of the eyes was seen in a total of three cases. Two recovered.

Diagnosis. An examination of the charts readily indicates a lack of pathognomonic diagnostic criteria either as to symptoms, signs, blood picture, spinal fluid changes or course of the illness. The diagnosis must be built as a house, stone by stone, putting those together that fit and eliminating others. In the differential diag-

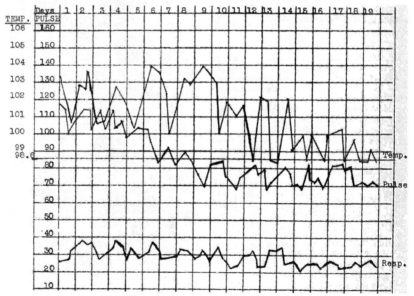

CHART XI
CLINICAL CHART—TYPICAL TEMPERATURE—PULSE—RESPIRATORY CHART

nosis one must eliminate influenza, malaria, typhoid fever, tuberculous meningitis and other forms of encephalitis, including the erroneous admission diagnoses mentioned above.

Prognosis. In the usual case, recovery was surprisingly rapid and complete. In the majority of the cases the temperature was normal within 12 to 18 days of the onset and the patient by that time was obviously well on the road to recovery. In the milder abortive cases within a much shorter period of time, three to seven days, the patient was quite well again or nearly so. When death occurred, it was the death of an overwhelming toxemia. More than 50 per cent of the deaths in our series occurred within the first seven days of the illness.

Age influenced the prognosis more than any other single factor. Pre-existing organic diseases such as nephritis, heart disease or debilitated state generally were factors tending towards a fatal termination.

No single sign or symptom was of much prognostic significance. The development of bronchial pneumonia was a grave prognostic sign.

Treatment. The treatment was entirely symptomatic. Practically all of the lethargic and stuporous patients had to be restrained. Strange as this statement may appear, without warning these patients often would get out of bed and walk about in an aimless manner. Hypertonic glucose (20 per cent) was used daily on all patients so long as lethargy and coma persisted. All o t h e r supportive measures such as digitalization and oxygen were instituted when necessary. The initial lumbar puncture often relieved headache and other symptoms. Subsequent punctures were done infrequently, and only when there was evidence of increased intracranial pressure which intravenous glucose would not control. Sedatives were rarely used. Among the older patients, we preferred large doses of strychnine sulphate to bromides and barbiturates.

BIBLIOGRAPHY

1. The Encephalitis Epidemic in St. Louis City and County in 1933. Statistical Report of St. Louis City Health Department.
2-6. Unted States Public Health Bulletin No. 214.
8-10. Report of the St. Louis Outbreak of Epidemic Encephalitis.
3. Longuet (R) La Nona. Semaine Med., Par, 1892, XII, 275-278.
4. Von Economo: Verin f. Psych. u. Neur. in Wien, Apr. 17, 1917.
5. Netter: Soc. Med. des Hopitaux de Paris, March 22, Apr. 12, 19, 26, May 3, 1918.
7. Encephalitis in St. Louis. J. P. Leake, M.D., J.A.M.A. 101.1 1933, 928-929.
Kaneko, R.: Japan M. World 5:237 (Sept.) 1925.
Kaneko, R.: and Aoki, Y.: Ergebn. d. Inn. Med. u. Kinderh 34:342, 1928.
9. Breinl: Med. Jour. of Australia, March 16, 1918.
11. Houston H. S. Paris, Ill. Report. Ill. Health Quart. 1932 VI, 174.
12. Muchenfuss, R. S., Armstrong, C., McCordock, H. A. Encephalitis: Studies on Experimental Transmission, Public Health Report 1933 — XLVIII 134-1843.
12-A. Personal Communications.
13. Webster, L. T., Fite, G. L., St. Louis Encephalitis, Science 1934 LXXIX 254.
14. Webster, L. T., Fite, G. L. Virus encountered in study of material from cases of Encephalitis in St. Louis and Kansas City Epidemics in 1933. Science 1933 LXXVIII 463-465.
15. Webster, L. T., Fite, G. L., Contributions to the etiology of encephalitis by protective tests. Proc. Soc. Exper. Biol. and Med., 1933 XXXI, 344.
16. Jones, A. B., The Encephalitis Epidemic in St. Louis City and County in 1933. J.A.M.A. 103:827-828, Sept. 15, 1934.

---o---

Effects of 'Benzedrine Sulfate' on Problem Children

Bradley (Am. J. Psych. 94:577, Nov., 1937) reports on the effects of "Benzedrine Sulfate" (benzyl methyl carbinamine sulfate, S.K.F.) administered to a group of 30 "problem" children, aged five to 14 years, under very favorable conditions.

The children chosen for the study manifested various behavior disorders, ranging from specific educational disabilities to the retiring schizoid type and the aggressive egocentric epileptic. They were observed, without subjective questioning, by a special psychiatric nurse for a period of three weeks. Each child received a daily morning dose of "Benzedrine Sulfate" during the second week, the first and third weeks being regarded as control periods. Twenty mg. was the usual dose, but this varied according to the individual.

Although these children had been receiving the usual intensive training available at the Bradley Home, 14 of them, or 47 per cent, promptly "responded in a spectacular fashion" to "Benzedrine Sulfate" therapy, showing marked improvement in speed of comprehension and accuracy of performance, together with a keen desire for accomplishment. Eight others showed some improvement. In all cases improvement disappeared the first day therapy was discontinued.

In emotional response, 15 children, or 50 per cent, became subdued. Seven of these were of the erratic and aggressive type, and the author suggests that "Benzedrine Sulfate," by stimulating the higher centers, may increase voluntary control in such cases. Seven other children reported a definite euphoria. The remaining eight had varied responses. One case of agitation and two cases of anxiety were observed.

In spite of the "attractive results obtained . . . and the apparent low toxicity of the drug," the author concludes that it is too early definitely to recommend "Benzedrine Sulfate" in the general treatment of pediatric behavior problems, and that additional studies should be made in this field.

Summer Diarrhea In Babies

Casec (calcium caseinate), which is almost wholly a combination of protein and calcium, offers a quickly effective method of treating all types of diarrhea, both in bottle-fed and breast-fed infants. For the former, the carbohydrate is temporarily omitted from the 24-hour formula and replaced with eight level tablespoonfuls of Casec. Within a day or two the diarrhea will usually be arrested, and carbohydrate in the form of Dextri-Maltose may safely be added to the formula and the Casec gradually eliminated. Three to six teaspoonfuls of a thin paste of Casec and water, given before each nursing, is well indicated for loose stools in breast-fed babies. Please send for samples to Mead Johnson & Company, Evansville, Indiana.

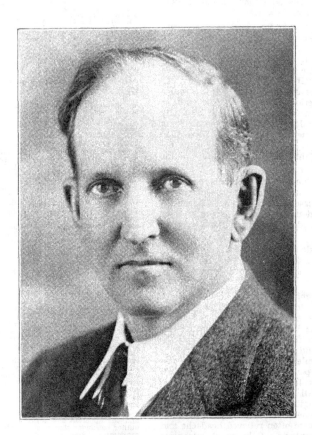

PRESIDENT, 1938-39

Doctor Henry Kirvin Speed

Born, 1884

*Graduated from the University of Texas School of Medicine,
Galveston, 1906*

Engaged in the Practice of General Medicine

THE JOURNAL

OF THE

Oklahoma State Medical Association

Issued Monthly at McAlester, Oklahoma, under direction of the Council.

Copyright, 1938, by Oklahoma State Medical Association, McAlester, Oklahoma.

Vol. XXXI	MAY, 1938	Number 5

DR. L. S. WILLOUR.................................Editor-in-Chief
McAlester, Oklahoma

DR. T. H. McCARLEY.................................Associate Editor
McAlester, Oklahoma

Entered at the Post Office at McAlester, Oklahoma, as second-class matter under the act of March 3rd, 1879.

This is the official Journal of the Oklahoma State Medical Association. All communications should be addressed to The Journal of the Oklahoma State Medical Association, McAlester Clinic, McAlester, Oklahoma. $4.00 per year; 40c per copy.

The editorial department is not responsible for the opinions expressed in the original articles of contributors.

Reprints of original articles will be supplied at actual cost provided request for them is attached to manuscripts or made in sufficient time before publication.

Articles sent this Journal for publication and all those read at the annual meetings of the State Association are the sole property of this Journal. The Journal relies on each individual contributor's strict adherence to this well-known rule of medical journalism. In the event an article sent this Journal for publication is published before appearance in The Journal the manuscript will be returned to the writer.

Failure to receive The Journal should call for immediate notification of the Editor, McAlester Clinic, McAlester, Oklahoma.

Local news of possible interest to the medical profession, notes on removals, changes of addresses, births, deaths and weddings will be gratefully received.

Advertising of articles, drugs or compounds unapproved by the Council on Pharmacy of the A. M. A., will not be accepted.

Advertising rates will be supplied on application.

It is suggested that wherever possible members of the State Association should patronize our advertisers in preference to others as a matter of fair reciprocity.

Printed by News-Capital Company, McAlester.

EDITORIAL

In the April issue of the Journal the Secretary-Treasurer-Editor's r e p o r t was published. It was delivered to the Council and House of Delegates and discussed. In this report are shown the activities of the State Association during the past year and there are some outstanding features. One being that we have liquidated $2,000.00 of our indebtedness, this in spite of the fact that we loaned the Legislative Committee $3,800.00 from the General Fund. The Council has appropriated $2,000.00 this year for carrying on our Post Graduate program in Obstetrics. This was made possible by the work of our Committee on Post Graduate Medical Teaching and being able to acquire funds from Federal Appropriations to the State Health Depart-

ment and a large contribution from the Commonwealth Fund.

For the first time in the history of the publication of our Journal it has been possible to pay the expense of publication from funds acquired from our advertisers and we will probably be able next year to slightly increase the amount of reading material in each issue of the Journal. This increase in income from advertising has not been accomplished by taking any questionable advertisements, as there is nothing advertised in the Journal, or exhibited at our Annual Meetings which has not been acted favorably on by the Council of the American Medical Association.

It is to be hoped that much will be accomplished by the H o u s e of Delegates during the Annual Meeting and a report of the proceedings will be published in the June issue, it being impossible to get the m a t e r i a l in shape for publication this month.

We will look forward to a year of even greater accomplishment and with the continued cooperation of our officers and committee members there is no evident reason why our new President should not have a very satisfactory administration.

————————o————————

Editorial Notes—Personal and General

At the meeting of the Board of Regents of the University of Oklahoma on the 4th instant, the following promotions and appointments were made upon the recommendation of the Dean of the Faculty of Medicine:

Appointments:

Carl William Lindstrom, assistant in obstetrics.
Joseph Fife Messenbaugh, assistant in surgery.
Paul Jack Birge, assistant in surgery.
Raymond Delbert Watson, assistant in surgery.
Neil Whitney Woodward, assistant in surgery.
Tom Lyon Wainwright, assistant in surgery.
Virgil Roy Jobe, assistant in surgery.
Cannon Armstrong Owen, assistant in surgery.
Everett Baker Neff, assistant in surgery.
Louis Najib Dakil, assistant in medicine.
Charles Andrew Smith, assistant in medicine.
Harry Linnell Deupree, assistant in medicine.
William Knowlton Ishmael, assistant in medicine.
Joe Henry Coley, assistant in medicine.
Harry Cummings Ford, assistant in oto-rhino-laryngology.
Melvin Phillip Hoot, assistant in oto-rhino-laryngology.
August Malone Brewer, assistant in urology.
Minard Friedberg Jacobs, instructor in medicine.
Dan Roy Sewell, lecturer in surgery.
Austin Halloway Bell, lecturer in surgery.

Changes in rank and title:

Hull Wesley Butler, assistant in histology and embryology to associate in medicine and associate in histology.
James Patton McGee, assistant professor of oph-

thalmology to associate professor of ophthalmology.

Bert Fletcher Keltz, instructor in medicine to associate in medicine and supervisor of clinical clerkships.

Walker Morledge, instructor in medicine to associate in medicine.

Elmer Ray Musick, instructor in medicine to associate in medicine.

James Floyd Moorman, instructor in medicine to associate in medicine.

Frederick Redding Hood, instructor in medicine to associate in medicine.

James Garfield Binkley, instructor in obstetrics to associate in obstetrics.

Francis Asbury DeMand, instructor in obstetrics to associate in obstetrics.

Floyd Gray, instructor in obstetrics to associate in obstetrics.

George Harry Garrison, instructor in pediatrics to associate in pediatrics.

Ben H. Nicholson, instructor in pediatrics to associate in pediatrics.

Louis Harry Charney, instructor in medicine to associate in medicine.

Herman Fagin, instructor in medicine to associate in medicine.

Nesbitt Ludson Miller, instructor in medicine to associate in Medicine.

William Ward Rucks, Jr., instructor in medicine to associate in medicine.

Wilbur Floyd Keller, instructor in medicine to associate in medicine.

Joseph C. Macdonald, assistant professor of oto-rhino-laryngology to associate professor of oto-rhino-laryngology.

Ephriam Goldfain, instructor in neurology to associate in neurology.

Francis Edward Dill, instructor in gynecology to associate in gynecology.

Joseph Willard Kelso, assistant professor of gynecology to associate professor of gynecology.

Ellis Moore, instructor in urology to associate in urology.

Robert Howe Akin, instructor in urology to associate in Urology.

Stanley Francis Wildman, instructor in urology to associate in urology.

Donald Wilton Branham, instructor in urology to associate in urology.

Patrick Sarsfield Nagle, assistant in surgery to lecturer in surgery.

Fenton Almer Sanger, assistant in surgery to lecturer in surgery.

Oscar White, assistant in surgery to lecturer in surgery.

Clifford Cannon Fulton, assistant in surgery to lecturer in surgery.

Jesse Duval Herrmann, assistant in surgery to lecturer in surgery.

George Henry Kimball, assistant in surgery to lecturer in surgery.

John Powers Wolff, assistant in surgery to lecturer in surgery.

Carl A. Bunde, research fellow in physiology to instructor in physiology.

Dr. Bert Fletcher Keltz, associate in medicine, was advanced from an associate to full Fellowship in the American College of Physicians at the meeting held in New York City, April 4th to 8th, 1938.

Robert U. Patterson, M.D.,
Dean and Superintendent.

SOUTHEASTERN Oklahoma Medical Association had an all-day session at Durant, Tuesday, April 26, the meeting being called to order promptly at 10 a.m. Morning and afternoon programs had been prepared and were carried out as follows: Scientific Program—10 a.m., "The Management of Empyemia," Dr. J. T. Wharton, Durant, Okla.; 10:45 a.m., "Urinary Complications of Pregnancy," Dr. A. R.

Russell, McAlester, Okla.; 11:30 a.m., "The Acute Abdomen as Seen by the General Practitioner." Dr. Earl M. Woodson, Poteau, Okla. Luncheon, 12:15 p.m. at First Methodist church. Program resumed at 1:30 p.m.: 1:30 p.m., "Invocation," Rev. W. L. Broome, Pastor, First Methodist church, Durant, Okla.; "Welcome Address," Dr. Jas. L. Shuler, Durant, Okla.; "Response to Welcome Address," Dr. J. L. Fulton, Atoka, Okla.; 2:00 p.m., "President's Address," Dr. E. H. Shuller, McAlester, Okla.; 2:15 p.m., "Modern Conception of Arthritis with Lantern Slides," Dr. N. D. Buie, Marlin, Texas; 3:15 p.m., "State and National Medical Legislation," Dr. Louis H. Ritzhaupt, Guthrie, Okla.; 4:15 p.m., Annual Election of Officers.

The Chamber of Commerce, Ketchum, Oklahoma, advises that there is a good opening for a young physician to engage in practice in that town and area. They estimate that from 10,000 to 15,000 people will be located in that town within the next six months. At the present time the population is 1,500. Ketchum is located sixteen (16) miles from Vinita, Oklahoma.

Dr. HENRY TURNER, of Oklahoma City, presented a preliminary report on "The Clinical Use of Male Sex Hormones" before the American Therapeutic Society in New York, April 1-2. He was also guest speaker of the St. Joseph Clinical Society, St. Joseph, Missouri, on April 14, addressing the Society on "The Diagnosis and Treatment of Endocrine Disorders."

DOCTOR PAUL C. COLONNA, Professor of Orthopaedic surgery in the University of Oklahoma School of Medicine and Orthopaedic Surgeon to the University and Crippled Children's Hospitals, Oklahoma City, will read a paper before the American Orthopaedic Association in Atlantic City, New Jersey, May 3rd, 1938, entitled "Operative Procedure for Congenital Dislocation of the Hip." He will also read a paper entitled "Reconstruction Operation for Ununited Fractures of the Hip" before the New York State Medical Society in New York City, May 10th, 1938.

Dr. J. Samuel Binkley, formerly of Oklahoma City, who now has a Fellowship in Memorial Hospital, New York City, appeared on the program of the American Association for Thoracic Surgery on April 4th at Atlanta, Georgia. His subject was "Aspiration Biopsy of the Lung," discussed by Dr. Singer, St. Louis; Dr. Dan Elkins, Atlanta; Dr. Jerome Head of Chicago, and a number of others.

---o---

News of the County Medical Societies

CARTER County Medical Society met at Colvert Auditorium, Ardmore, Monday night, April 25, 1938. The program of the evening consisted of talks by physicians, as follows: "Peptic Ulcer," Dr. R. C. Sullivan, Ardmore; "Sulfanilamide," Dr. Fred Perry, Healdton; "Physical Therapy Correlated with Medical Treatment of Arthritis," Dr. William A. Ishmael, Oklahoma City; "Orthopedic Correction of the Deformed Joints in Arthritis," Dr. Howard B. Shorbe, Oklahoma City.

OKMULGEE-OKFUSKEE County Medical meeting was held at the Okemah Hotel, Okemah, Monday evening, April 18, 1938, with dinner at 6:30 p.m. The speakers were Dr. Wendell Long, Oklahoma City, whose subject was "Practical Aids in Pelvic Examinations," and Dr. Basil A. Hayes, Oklahoma City, on "Changes in the Upper Urinary Tract Due to Pelvic Pathology."

News Notes of Woman's Auxiliary

Women's Auxiliary to Woodward County Medical Society

The counties of Woodward, Ellis, Harper, Beaver and Dewey are organized under the name of the Woodward County Medical Society.

The Auxiliary meetings are held at the same time and place as that of the Medical Society.

Beginning with February, meetings are held each alternate month in the year, the August meeting being an annual picnic on Crystal Beech Lake in Woodward.

The Advisory Board to the Women's Auxiliary is: Dr. John L. Day, Supply, Dr. C. W. Tedrowe, Woodward, and Dr. J. C. Duncan, Forgan.

The February meeting was held in the Baker Hotel in Woodward, members paid dues, elected the following officers for the ensuing year: Mrs. D. W. Darwin, Woodward, president; Mrs. T. S. Leachman, Woodward, vice-president; Mrs. C. W. Tedrowe, Woodward, recording secretary; Mrs. H. K. Hill, Laverne, corresponding secretary, and Mrs. O. C. Newman, Shattuck, treasurer.

Other business was omitted and after a turkey dinner both groups were entertained by an interesting and instructive paper on Socialized Medicine read by Dr. C. J. Fishman of Oklahoma City: Dr. Basil Hays, also of Oklahoma City, gave an illustrated lecture on Urology. Several of the doctors present commented on these lectures.

The April meeting was held in Laverne. The Ladies Aid served a chicken dinner in the dining room of the Masonic Hall, after which the Auxiliary retired to the lobby of the hotel. The president, Mrs. D. W. Darwin, brought before the group a number of leading policies in which Auxiliaries can be of service to the Medical Societies.

These projects were discussed by the members. It was voted to maintain a Speakers Bureau. These speakers are to be appointed by the Advisory Board and are to be members of the Woodward County Medical Society. Through their public relations with clubs, Parent Teachers Association and other organizations, the Auxiliary members hope by this method to bring directly to many persons much valuable health instruction, which they otherwise would have no opportunity to receive.

Mrs. F. C. Camp of Buffalo was appointed chairman of Philanthropy committee, Mrs. C. E. Williams of the Hygeia, and Mrs. Hardin Walker, Rosston, chairman of Public Relations and Health Education.

Mrs. N. E. Duncan, Forgan, Press and Publicity and Mrs. O. C. Newman of Shattuck, Historian.

Delegate to the State Meeting in May Mrs. N. E. Duncan, alternate Mrs. John L. Day.

RESOLUTIONS

Jackson County Medical Society, March 28, 1938
Dr. R. H. Mays

WHEREAS our friend and esteemed co-worker, Dr. R. H. Mays has been called by the Great Physician, and

WHEREAS for many years he was a prominent and active member of our Society and our profession, and

WHEREAS his professional achievements, and sterling qualities were known and admired both within and without the profession,

Therefore, Be It Resolved, by the Jackson County Medical Society that we record our sadness and in his untimely going, holding in memory his splendid skill and wonderful personality as a professional man, a loving and generous husband and father, an active leader, a high class citizen and withal, kindly and generous, and

Be It Further Resolved, That a copy of these resolutions be spread upon the minutes of the Jackson County Medical Society and that a copy be sent to the members of the family, and that official copies be sent to the Journal of the Oklahoma Medical Association.

Respectfully submitted,
Edw. A. Abernethy, M.D.,
J. B. Hix, M.D.,
Raymond H. Fox, M.D.,
Committee on Resolutions.

Doctor William Irwin Joss

Whereas, Our fellow member and friend, Dr. William Irwin Joss, of Erick, Okla., who was a highly respected member of the Beckham County Medical Society, was called from us on February 23rd, 1938, and;

Whereas, Dr. Joss for many years has been a member of organized medicine and a valued member of our society, and has rendered most valued service to his profession, and has been recognized by the doctors of this county and state as one of the most beloved members of the medical profession.

Therefore be it resolved, that we extend to his family our deepest sympathy and assure them of our sincere desire to share with them this burden of loss, and

Be it further resolved, that we receive this information with deep sorrow and regret, realizing our loss in both counsel and advice, and Be it further resolved, that a copy of this resolution be made a part of the minutes of this meeting, and be published in the Journal of the Oklahoma State Medical Association, and that a copy be sent to the family.

Signed, G. H. Stagner and P. J. Devany, committee.

---o---

Books Received and Reviewed

THE MANAGEMENT OF THE SICK INFANT AND CHILD, By Langley Porter, B.S., M.D., M.R.C.S. (Eng.), L.R.C.P. (Long.), Dean, University of California Medical School and Professor of Medicine; Formerly, Professor of Clinical Pediatrics, University of California Medical School; Visiting Pediatrician, San Francisco Children's Hospital; Consultant to the San Francisco Department of Public Health, San Francisco, California. AND, Dr. William E. Carter, M.D., Director, University of California Hospital Out Patient Department; Formerly, Chief of Children's Clinic, University of California Hospital, San Francisco; Attending Physician, San Francisco Hospital; Attending Physician, Los Angeles County Hospital, San Francisco, California. Fifth Advised Edition. Price $10.00. The C. V. Mosby Co., St. Louis, 1938.

This is the fifth edition of a well known book on the management of the sick infant. Some of the methods of management applicable to older children as well as to infants have been added.

Part I deals mainly with symptoms, vomiting, diarrhea, constipation, nutrition, hemorrhage, pain and tenderness, convulsions and syncopes, fever, cough and prematurity. Part II deals with diseases of the different systems of the body. Part III deals with methods, formulas and recipes, drugs and poisons. The methods are well illustrated by pictures.

This is one of the better books on pediatrics and should be of great help to the pediatrician, general practitioner and medical student in their work.

ABSTRACTS : REVIEWS : COMMENTS
and CORRESPONDENCE

SURGERY AND GYNECOLOGY
Abstracts, Reviews and Comments from
LeRoy Long Clinic
714 Medical Arts Building, Oklahoma City

Ulcerating Stenosis of the Pylorus and Its Complications (La Stenose Ulcereuse du Pylore et Ses Complications). By J. E. Dube, Medecin de l'Hotel Dieu, Montreal. L'Union Medicale du Canada, April, 1938.

A plasterer 26 years of age was admitted to hospital January 24, 1938, because of grave digestive troubles (des troubles digestifs graves) beginning about December 15, 1937. He was pale, emaciated, weak, able to take only a little liquid food because of bad digestion and abundant vomiting (a cause de sa mauvaise digestion et de vomissements abondants).

Palpitation of the epigastric area was accompanied by splashing (clapotage). A stomach tube was followed by the escape of a large quantity of dirty fluid containing particles of undigested food.

There was a history of "stomach trouble" for about a year before the grave attack beginning in December, 1937. There had been pyrosis and epigastric pain an hour or two after food and sometimes vomiting. At first alkalies or small quantities of food brought relief. Every few months there were exacerbations in connection with overwork.

After an investigation, including an X-ray G. I. series and various laboratory tests, there was a diagnosis of stenosis of the pylorus with retention due to an old ulcer. This period of investigation covered about a week, and then he was sent to surgery for operation. At this time there was an Hgb. of 58 per cent, R. B. C. 3,840,782. It was decided to do a gastro-enterostomy the next morning, but during the night there was collapse with abundant sweating, a pulse of 158 and a tendency to faint (tendance syncopale). A blood count the next day or two showed Hgb. 25 per cent, R. B. C. 2,989,845, W. B. C. 10,155. There were repeated transfusions of blood, but the course was relentlessly downward. On February 11, 1938, Hgb. 20 per cent, R. B. C. 1,750,000. On February 14, 1938, Hgb. 18 per cent, R. B. C. 1,675,000.

Then it was decided to operate because it was reasoned that only an operation would offer a last chance. ("Le malade parait voue a une mort certaine. Faut-il l'operer quand meme? Certes si l'on veut lui offrir une derniere chance.") Operation—gastroenterostomy—was done February 15. He was kept alive until February 22. The last blood count on February 21 showed Hgb. five per cent, R. B. C. 775,000.

Autopsy confirmed the preoperative diagnosis, and, in addition, there was a ramification of arteries in the ulcerating area, all of them filled with thrombi (une grosse ramification arterielle thrombosee).

Comments: This article is abstracted, not because the situation is very uncommon, but because important lessons are to be learned from it, to-wit:

1. When the pathology is so clear and the patient in fair condition would it not be the better part of wisdom to decide to operate as soon as the necessity for operation is obvious? Not within a week, but within a day or two. The author speaks of this, and indicates that there was unnecessary delay in connection with the radiographic examination. In the practice of medicine we ought to strive to develop a fine and accurate discrimination touching the promptitude with which service is rendered in the case of a patient manifestly in immediate need of saving management.

2. Following the collapse a week after admission there were repeated transfusions of blood in addition to the intravenous employment of other fluids. Notwithstanding these intravenous injections there was rapid depletion. Why? Because there was bleeding at the site of ulceration. Doubtless there were attempts at thrombosis in the bleeding vessels, but the thrombi were broken down by temporarily raising the arterial tension through the use of the intravenous fluids. In such a desperate situation would it not be far better to give the patient enough morphine to keep him perfectly comfortable and perfectly quiet, discontinuing intravenous fluids altogether?

·3. Is it wise to undertake an intra-abdominal operation, or any other major operation, for that matter, where the Hgb. is 18 per cent and the R. B. C. 1,675,000 due to hemorrhage unless there is every reason to believe that bleeding can be controlled by the operative procedure? With the operation planned for this purpose—i.e, the control of hemorrhage—then it would be wise to accompany the operation by an intravenous infusion of normal saline solution to temporarily hold up arterial tension, and to follow the operation by transfusion of blood to maintain arterial tension.

LeRoy Long.

Continent Gastrostomy and Cardiospasm (Gastrostomie Continente et Cardiospasme). By Francois De Martigny, chirurgien consultant, hospital Sainte-Jeanne-D'Arc, Montreal. L'Union Medicale du Canada, April, 1938.

Remarking that the average case of cardiospasm yields to medical treatment, and deploring the bad results following the dangerous surgical operation usually advised in a rebellious case, the author is convinced that the pathology is represented by ulceration or fissures in the cardiac opening—i.e., at the junction of oesophagus with stomach—and he likens the lesions to anal fissures.

The thesis of the author is that the ulcerations or fissures will heal if relieved of irritation by the passage of food or other material over them. Acting upon this hypothesis, he conceived the plan of performing a "continent" gastrostomy so that food might be introduced directly into the stomach, the gastrostomy permitting, at the same time, the introduction of antiseptic and analgesic agents. In this way both the oesophagus and the cardia are placed at complete rest.

There are two case reports:

1. A blacksmith who complained of dysphagia, regurgitations and vomiting when the least food was swallowed, pains, and a weight loss of 50 pounds, all these symptoms gradually but progressively developing over a period of about two years. Emaciation extreme, skin dry and scaly, earthy

complexion, sunken eyes, pains on palpation over solar plexus area (douleurs a la palpation au point solaire).

A continent gastrostomy (gastrostomie a lambeau tubulee) was done under ether anesthesia, a "radio knife" (bistouri electrique a ondes entretenues) being employed.

There was rapid improvement. Within a short time there was tentative feeding by mouth. The gastrostomy opening closed between two and three years after operation, and the patient was well and strong.

2. An unmarried woman of 48 came complaining of digestive disturbances and of attacks of regurgitation at irregular intervals (elle souffre de l'estomac avec des crises de regurgitations a intervalles irreguliers) following carbon monoxide poisoning two years before. She had had an examination some months before at another hospital where a gastroscopy was done, the report being that visualization did not disclose any evidence of important pathology. She had never had intense pain, but there had been vomiting of small quantities of blood for some days following the gastroscopy, and there had been great loss of weight.

Radiographic examination after the ingestion of an opaque meal disclosed evidences of obstruction in the lower third of oesophagus, and the radiologist reported cancer of the inferior third of oesophagus. This diagnosis was rather reluctantly accepted by the author. The next day a continent gastrostomy was done under local anesthesia. This was followed by a high caloric diet (milk, malted milk, yolk of egg) per gastrostomy tube, and anyodol was given by mouth in doses of several drops at a time. A month later there was increase of weight and she was able to drink milk and Vichy water without difficulty. Three months later the condition was transformed, there not being any more regurgitation. Vegetable puree and cereal gruels were added to the diet by mouth, they being swallowed without trouble. At the end of another month there had been a gain in weight of 48 pounds.

Another radiographic examination showed that there was still slight narrowing of lower part of oesophagus, but there were no irregularities of oesophagus or about the oesophageal opening into stomach. The radiologist (the same who had made the first interpretation) now reported: "The lesion formerly demonstrable, of irregular aspect, has completely disappeared." ("La lesion anterieurement constatee, d'aspect irregulier, est completement disparue.")

Two years later the patient was able to eat and to swallow normally, and the condition was good in every respect. It was quite clear that the radiographic diagnosis of cancer was an error.

In the comments following these reports the author takes pains to say that continent gastrostomy is not a panacea for cardiospasm. At the same time the different methods of treatment heretofore proposed are briefly reviewed, and in the review attention is directed to the uncertainty and danger attendant upon the blind introduction of sounds; to the harm that is reportedly done in attempts at manual or instrumental dilatation per gastrostomy opening; and to the extreme danger in connection with incisions and sharp dissection about the gastro-oesophageal area. The dangers are contrasted with the relatively small danger associated with gastrostomy.

Comments: This is a very practical, very reasonable and a very valuable contribution. While, as the author, himself, indicates, the exact pathology in the cases reported was not proved, the reasoning employed is sound and leads to the logical conclusion that the suggested analogy between cardiospasm and the pains of anal fissure is altogether apt.

LeRoy Long.

Identical Cancers in Identical Twins. By R. B. Phillips, Fellow in Surgery, Mayo Foundation. Proceedings of the Staff Meetings of the Mayo Clinic, April 6, 1938.

There is a reference to a paper by McFarland and Meade on "The Genetic Origin of Tumors, supported by their simultaneous and symmetrical occurrence in homologous twins," published in 1932. "Their studies seemed to indicate that if a tumor develops in an identical twin in a given organ at a given time, then the same kind of tumor will develop in the other twin in the corresponding organ at the same time or within a reasonable time thereafter."

In the contribution by Phillips there is a sharp distinction between "true identical twins" and twins that are not identical. It is estimated that about 25 per cent of all twins are identical.

It is the conclusion that homologous (identical) twins are the product of one ovum and one spermatozoon which splits in early embryonic life, giving to each half "an amount of chromosome and gene structure approaching as nearly as possible to half of the original whole."

There is a report of the case of one identical twin who developed a carcinoma in the right breast for which operation was done. Ten years later she developed ovarian papillary adenocarcinoma, bilateral, the treatment being hysterectomy and roentgen therapy.

Three years after the development of the carcinoma of the right breast in the first twin the second twin developed a carcinoma of the right breast. It was treated by surgical operation and roentgen therapy.

There is a reference to an editorial in a recent issue of Surgery, Gynecology and Obstetrics by Holman where "he cited six so-called cancer families and suggested that it would be well worth while to have a central library where cases of cancer with definite genetic aspects could be collected for further study."

In discussing the contribution by Phillips, A. C. Broders, Division of Surgical Pathology, Mayo Clinic, referred in a very direct way to the "famous studies on the relationship of heredity to spontaneous cancer" by Maud Slye who in her work has performed necropsy on 140,000 mice, observing more than 100,000 cancers. "She contends that malignancy is transmitted as a localized recessive character and that each type of malignancy is a unit character capable of suppression by a dominant." "According to Maud Slye's investigation, susceptibility and non-susceptibility to spontaneous neoplasms in mice depend absolutely upon genetic factors."

In his discussion Broders refers to "cancer families." In that connection attention is directed to a remarkable cancer family about which Warthin made a report in 1913 and another report in 1925. In 1936 Hauser and Weller made a still later report about this particular family. The paternal founder of the family died about 1856 at the age of 60 with what was thought to be cancer of the stomach or intestine. After that through several generations of his descendants there is a startling repetition of the development of cancer. For example, a son had 11 children, five of them developing cancer.

In closing the discussion Broders said, "The most outstanding evidence in support of the contention that the susceptibility and site of neoplasia in man are controlled by genetic factors is the occurrence either synchronously or asynchronously of cancer and other neoplasms in corresponding organs of identical or homologous twins, as exemplified in this interesting report by Dr. Phillips."

LeRoy Long.

The Bacterial Flora of Clean Surgical Wounds; Ives and Hirshfeld; Annals of Surgery, April, 1938; page 607.

Infection is known to occur in five per cent of all clean surgical wounds even though they are made with due regard to all the principles of aseptic surgical technic.

The paucity of information in the literature upon the bacteriology of surgical wounds and its importance in relation to the problem of wound infection made the authors feel that it would be of importance to carefully culture a series of wounds during the actual operation. They decided to:

1. Take cultures of the skin after it had been prepared for operation.

2. Expose blood agar plates to the air of the operating room during the course of the operation.

3. Take cultures of a series of clean wounds during the actual operative procedure.

4. Follow the healing of the wounds that had been cultured.

5. Review the infections that had occurred in clean wounds on the Surgical Service of the New Haven Hospital during the last three years to determine the incidence of the various types of organisms and their relation to those found in the air, on the skin, and in the wounds at operation.

A study of their figures and of those they were able to collect from the literature justified the conclusion that well over 50 per cent of post-operative wound infections are caused either by Staphylococcus aureus or Staphylococcus albus. It has been shown that these organisms are present in the air of the operating room and on the skin of the patient. They unquestionably contaminate wounds during the operations, and they may be recovered from the wounds by suitable culture methods. If contamination of wounds by these bacteria from the air and skin could be eliminated, the incidence of infected wounds would be much lower.

W. F. Wells and his collaborators in 1933 and 1934, working at the Harvard School of Public Health demonstrated that many of the common pathogenic bacteria are capable of surviving in the air for considerable length of time. Staphylococcus aureus, a common invader of clean wounds, if sprayed into the air according to the technic of Wells, may be recovered after as long as three days. Not only are many bacteria able to live for several days in the air, but when they are sprayed into the air from an atomizer or from the throat by coughing, sneezing or talking, the majority do not settle out quickly but remain suspended almost indefinitely. The air currents waft them about and disseminate them widely.

Wells (Journal A. M. A., November 21, 1936) has discussed the effect of ultraviolet radiation upon bacteria suspended in the air and has stated that it may be possible to sterilize the air of public buildings with radiant energy in conjunction with other methods such as filtration.

D. Hart (Professor of Surgery at Duke University) has attempted to sterilize the air in his operating room with ultraviolet light. He tried this because of the high percentage of staphylococcal infections that were occurring in his thoracoplasty wounds. No source other than the operating room air could be found for these bacteria and after an ultraviolet lamp capable of sterilizing the air about the operating table was installed, a prompt decrease was noted in the incidence of infections.

Gudin (Presse Medicale, March 4, 1936) has emphasized the importance of contamination by bacteria from the air as a cause of wound infection. He was so disturbed by the number of infections occurring in his clean cases that he carefully reviewed all phases of his technic. Despite the strictest attention to the usual details of aseptic technic he was unable to reduce the incidence of

wound infection. The air of the operating room seemed to be the only possible source of the bacteria. In order to eliminate this avenue of contamination, he devised an air-tight operating room ventilated only by air which had been chemically sterilized. The members of the operating team were required to change into sterile gowns in an adjoining room so they would not contaminate the sterile air with bacteria from their skin and clothing. Although Gudin presents no statistics, he states that infection practically disappeared and the wounds healed with surprisingly little reaction after adoption of the sterilized air technic.

Unfortunately, today, the methods which have been used to sterilize air in the operating room are clumsy and difficult to employ.

The authors summarize their findings as follows:

1. A review of the literature reveals that about five per cent of clean surgical wounds become infected.

2. Cultures of a series of wounds taken during the actual operations showed all of them to be extensively contaminated with bacteria, among which Staphylococci predominated.

3. Most of the bacteria which were recovered from the wounds at operation come from the skin of the patient or the air of the operating room.

4. The majority of postoperative wound infections are caused by bacteria similar to those which were isolated from the wounds at operation.

5. Any improvement in surgical technic which will decrease the contamination of operative wounds by bacteria from the air of the operating room or the skin of the patient should result in a decrease in the postoperative wound infection.

LeRoy Downing Long.

The Value of Hormonal Findings in Hydatidiform Mole and Chorionepithelioma; S. A. Cosgrove; American Journal of Obstetrics and Gynecology; April, 1938; Page 581.

This author quotes the conclusions drawn by Fels and Rossler in 1929 which have received practically universal acceptance. They follow.

1. That in hydatid mole and chorionepithelioma there is much more prolan secreted than in normal pregnancy.

2. The quantitative estimation of this hormone is an actual guide to diagnosis in that

3. Presence of increased hormone for more than two weeks after normal pregnancy, or more than eight weeks after the extrusion of hydatid, is proof of chorionepithelioma.

4. Persistence of positive test for this hormone after operation and removal of chorionepithelioma is proof of metastasis.

The author then reviewed 15 cases of hydatid mole which occurred in the Margaret Hague Maternity Hospital prior to March, 1936. During the same space of time 20,450 living babies were delivered in this hospital.

Twelve of the cases of hydatid mole were treated conservatively, mostly by dilatation and curettage. In all instances where the Friedman test was employed, a negative test was received within seven weeks after the extrusion of the mole, except in the three cases of chorionepithelioma which he reports in detail.

Three of the cases with hydatid mole, which were followed carefully by Friedman tests, had persistent positive Friedman tests and were subjected to complete hysterectomy in the 68th, 49th, and 55th days after the extrusion of the mole respectively. Following complete hysterectomy, all patients maintained a negative Friedman test, have remained well, and have shown no evidences of recurrence or metastases.

The author points out that in one patient in

particular exploratory curettage would probably not have identified the chorionepithelioma and that it was only by the positive hormonal test, that effective treatment was instituted early enough to effect a cure.

The author also adds a word of warning in the following quotation: "As indicated above, laboratory findings must not be regarded as wholly determinative in these cases. If they are positive they confirm the significance of the clinical behavior. Negative findings, however, cannot be implicitly relied upon as in all departments of medicine but, the principal basis of diagnosis and treatment must continue to depend upon history, course, clinical findings, and the common sense and surgical training of the attendant."

Comment: As stated by this author, hydatid mole is an uncommon disease and chorionepithelioma a rare one. On the other hand, chorionepithelioma is a very malignant neoplasm, metastasizing early and extensively. It is therefore evident that, in order to obtain cures from chorionepithelioma, the earliest possible positive diagnosis is essential. The continued use of the Friedman test following the extrusion or removal of a hydatid mole is not only an extremely valuable adjunct to clinical course and finding, but in many instances it is the only means of instituting the proper radical treatment early enough to be effective in producing a cure. It, therefore, seems quite evident that all instances of hydatid mole should be followed meticulously and routinely with Friedman tests, preferably in variable dilutions.

Wendell Long.

How Long Does It Take For a Large Carcinoma of the Stomach to Develop? Report of Two Instructive Cases; Staff Meetings of the Mayo Clinic, March 9, 1938; M. W. Comfort and W. L. Butsch.

Every physician sooner or later has the experience of examining a patient carefully and finding nothing in the stomach to account for vague gastrointestinal symptoms, only to have the patient return in a few months with a large gastric carcinoma. In such situations a physician must say to himself, "Did I miss the growth at the time of the first examination or has the growth developed in this short time?" To those who have had such an experience it will be comforting and reassuring to read the reports of two cases given in this article. These reports show that sometimes large carcinomas can develop within a few months.

Three years ago Alvarez, Judd, Wilbur, and Baker were interested in this question as to how long it takes for a large carcinoma of the stomach to grow. They presented at that time a case, showing that a lesion of a low grade of malignancy can grow for at least three years without becoming inoperable, that symptoms can disappear for months at a time and that the blood may be unaffected by the disease so long as there is little oozing from the growth.

The two cases reported by the authors in this article give another answer to the same question. In the first case, at the first admission, although thickening was present it did not appear to be malignant on gross examination or on microscopic examination of a specimen taken for biopsy; within 15 months extensive, multiple, polypoid carcinomas had developed, the largest measuring 4 cm. in diameter. In the second case, at the time of the first operation at Mayo Clinic, the only demonstrable lesion was a slight amount of thickening of the gastric wall, near the posterior suture line of the previous gastro-enterostomy. The stomach was opened but no evidence of disease could be found in the mucosa. Symptoms of obstruction developed within four months and when exploration was carried out eight months after the first exploration, a carcinoma measuring 12 by 15 cm., with extensive involvement of lymph nodes, was removed.

It is evident that a carcinoma of the stomach can reach a large size within a few months.

A negative roentgenologic examination of the stomach may not mean that a cancer has been missed in those cases in which cancer of the stomach is found after the passage of a few months. A growth may be in its precancerous stage or a carcinoma may be too small for demonstration by roentgenologic means. A roentgenologic examination that does not disclose cancer of the stomach should not be allowed to lead to a sense of false security, especially if the patient is in the cancer age, if the symptoms are of recent development, and if the concentration of gastric acids is low. The patient should remain under observation and further roentgenologic examinations of the stomach should be carried out. It is possible that examination with the gastroscope may become most important in the early diagnosis of carcinoma of the stomach. (There is an enlightening report from the London Hospital contained in the 1937 Year Book of Surgery giving results of examinations with the gastroscope).

Konjetzny expressed the belief that hyperplastic gastritis about a gastro-enteric stoma may be the precursor of carcinoma in cases where symptoms persist following gastro-enterostomy. There is a growing mass of evidence pointing to chronic gastritis (accumulation of lymphocytes with faulty regeneration of the mucous cells) as a precursor of carcinoma of the stomach just as is ulcer. Konjetzny stated that carcinoma arises, in the majority of cases, on this basis. The conception that chronic gastritis is the soil in which cancer develops in a large percentage of cases, if finally accepted, will influence greatly the methods used in the prophylaxis and early diagnosis of cancer.

LeRoy D. Long.

EYE, EAR, NOSE AND THROAT
Edited by Marvin D. Henley, M.D.
911 Medical Arts Building, Tulsa

Vitamins in Treatment and Prevention of Ocular Disease. Arthur M. Yudkin, M.D., New Haven, Conn. Archives of Ophthalmology, March, 1938.

Osborne and Mendel and McCollum and Davis, 1913, showed by animal experimentation, that an absence of Vitamin A from the diet resulted in ocular inflammations. Investigators concluded that xerophthalmia and keratomalacia and many similar diseases were caused by an improper diet— namely lack of some one particular vitamin as for instance vitamin A.

The work of Fraudsen on hemeralopia is reviewed. Similar observations have been made on persons presenting a clinical picture of neurasthenia and hysteria. The retinal disturbance may be the same in these conditions. Many of these persons have blond fundi and are very sensitive to light.

A corneal lesion occurring in adults is described. Ordinary routine methods of treating the breaking down of the cornea are usually ineffective. The lesion is often designated as a catarrhal ulcer. There is little if any accompanying inflammation. It appears as if the cornea had been injured but the history for such is negative. Floaters are present in the aqueous humor and Decemets membrane may have many deposits present. Some of these patients showed improvement when cod liver oil was added to their diet. As the response was not universal it was evident that there were some other factors involved. The intestinal tract was suspected as being at fault. The cod liver oil was continued but in addition Vitamin B complex was given before each meal. Most of the ocular and general symptoms improved or disappeared entirely.

The author suggests an early regime of a diet high in vitamin content to retard retinitis pigmentosa. Chorioretinal disorders are also influenced favorably by a diet including vitamin A and brewer's yeast powder. The University Clinic (Yale) policy is to treat the general condition occurring at the same time with the eye condition. Focal infections are not removed until the general health of the patient is improved.

Vitamin B is recommended in anorexia of dietary origin, in securing optimal growth of infants and children, in beriberi, vomiting of pregnancy, several forms of neuritis and in toxic amblyopia due to excessive alcohol and tobacco.

If there is a focus of infection suspected of being the cause of ocular inflammation, then a both A and B vitamin complex is recommended.

Cataract is not associated with scurvy in humans so the relation of vitamin C to cataract formation is enigmatic. Intravenous vitamin C decreases the coagulation of the blood. The author prefers the use of lemon juice to Vitamin C in retinal and vitreous hemorrhages. To an adult showing early lenticular changes the author gives the following advice: an adequate intake of calories, the juice of one lemon before breakfast and dinner, vitamin B complex (or teaspoonful potent brewers' yeast) twice daily before meals; be sure there is no uncompensated cardiovascular condition.

Treatment of Simple Chronic Laryngitis. Louis H. Clerf, M.D., Philadelphia. Archives of Otolaryngology, March, 1938.

Kyle's dictum: laryngeal changes often are a "local manifestation of a systemic condition."

The change of tissue depends on character of the lesion and the intensity and duration of the inflammatory reaction and the individual. Some individuals tend toward excessive proliferation of fibrous tissue; follows hyperemia, cellular infiltration, inflammatory exudate and increase in connective tissue elements. The entire larynx may be involved. Where there is the most activity, there is usually the most involvement, namely — vocal cords — ventricular bands — interarytenoid space. Treatment has two phases: relieve tissue change which interferes with laryngeal function and eliminate the causative factor.

Etiologically there are infections, irritative conditions and systemic disorders. Infections include diseases of the upper air and food passages and of the tracheobronchial tree. Irritative conditions are smoke, dust and gases, excessive use or abuse of the larynx. Systemic conditions are effects of alcohol, defective elimination, gout, hepatic or cardiorenal disease and hypertension. Syphilis, tuberculosis and carcinoma give a chronic laryngitis.

Immediate alleviation of symptoms is the important factor to the patient. This must be taken into consideration by the laryngologist while he is attempting to detect and remove the predisposing cause. All conditions that might erroneously be called chronic laryngitis must be excluded.

Treatment should decrease the chronic congestion present in the larynx. "Don't talk; don't smoke; don't use alcohol." This many times will be sufficient. Additional measures include medication by inhalation, application or instillation. Inhalation of compound tincture of benzoin with probably a little menthol from a vaporizer is advocated. Instillation of an oily solution is an aid. Direct application to the vocal cords traumatizes the mucosa. The author does not use silver nitrate, zinc chloride or ferric chloride solutions. This procedure will usually give symptomatic relief.

Health, habits, occupation and environment of the patient should be investigated. Voice abuse is the most common cause of chronic laryngitis—shouting—cheering—speaking—singing—and incorrect training for singing. These produce an acute laryngitis which is not given ample time to subside before another acute attack is precipitated and so gradually the condition becomes chronic.

Any obstruction of the nose and pharynx should be removed. Any focus of infection of the upper air passages, the ears, the mouth, the teeth and the gums should be located and removed. Faucial and lingual tonsils should not be overlooked. Direct extension of an infection from the nasopharynx or oropharynx to the larynx may occur. Overflow of secretions and food during sleep from an organic stenosis of the oesophagus, cordiospasm or a pharyngeal diverticulum, may produce a chronic laryngitis or tracheitis. Many other probable causes are mentioned. Not always does removing the exciting factor produce a noticeable improvement immediately. As a whole, however, recovery depends on finding the cause and effecting its removal or correction.

Deafness From Drugs and Chemical Poisons. Dr. H. Marshall Taylor, Jacksonville, Fla. The Laryngoscope, September, 1937.

Some drugs and chemicals have a selective action for the VIIIth nerve and the auditory apparatus. Some of the ways that such may affect the auditory apparatus are: "A toxic action on the ganglion cells of the cochlea and associated nerve fibres; cause a change in the endothelium of the smallest capillaries or a contraction of the blood vessels of the internal ear, ischemia, loss of nutrition and anoxemia, degeneration atrophy of the ganglion cells and nerve fibres in the basal coil of the cochlea; a diminution in the endolymphatic pressure, with a resulting collapse of the membrana corti."

An unsuspected susceptibility to some drug possibly might be an etiological factor in nerve deafness. The placenta acts as a dialyzer for certain drugs. Certain drugs may be found in the foetal circulation as well as the maternal circulation, in approximately the same strength. A child is probably 2½ to three years old before a diagnosis of nerve deafness is made. Prenatal history is usually forgotten by this time. Instead of a hereditary deafness it may be the result of an injury to the organ of hearing inutero from administering some particular drug to the mother. This calls for closer cooperation between the otologist and the obstetrician.

Of these drugs quinine is the chief offender being used therapeutically as an abortifacient, in the induction of labor and many other diseases that occur concurrently with pregnancy. Other drugs mentioned are: tobacco, arsenic, salicylates, alcohol, lead, phosphorus, carbon monoxide, carbon disulphide, oil of chenopodium, mercury, morphine and anilin dyes.

Interesting Cases of Lateral Sinus Thrombosis. Henry M. Scheer, F.A.C.S., F.I.C.S. The Eye, Ear, Nose and Throat Monthly, March, 1938.

This article is an interesting discussion of the question in addition to case reports. The author's own conclusion is as follows:

A great amount of data can be assembled from the study of this series of interesting cases, each of which revealed some details not referred to in the typical textbook presentation of this serious intracranial complication.

1. We find it is not essential to have had exposed lateral sinus, either pathological or accidental, to have lateral sinus thrombosis present.

2. Typical "sawtoothed" septic temperatures may or may not be present, preceded or not by chills.

3. The complication may arise early in the course of an acute middle ear infection, though it occurs most frequently during the course of an O.M.P.C.

4. Lateral sinus thrombosis may occur at any age from childhood to old age.

5. In certain cases, no evidence of chronic mastoid disease may be elicted subjectively until the acute clinical picture appears, indicating the presence of acute lateral sinus thrombosis. This most frequently occurs during the course of an O.M.P.C.

6. In certain cases no evidence of the complication may be present subjectively or objectively, until perforation of the lateral sinus occurs during the lateral sinus thrombosis.

7. Eye fundus changes may or may not be present.

8. Metastatic foci may occur early or late in the course of the complication, or not at all.

9. Operations may be done under local anesthesia.

10. Occlusion of the lateral sinus without ligation of the internal jugular vein will give successful results, when the pathology in the lateral sinus is high, and blocking can be performed in the normal region of the lateral sinus, below the site of pathology.

11. To depend upon positive laboratory findings before proceeding surgically in many cases will delay the proper treatment unduly.

12. Laboratory results at times may even mislead and delay.

13. Toby-Ayres cerebrospinal fluid pressure test is not fool-proof.

14. When indicated, investigation of both lateral sinuses may be done with safety to determine which is thrombosed.

15. The wounds after blocking of the sinus should not be sutured, but allowed to granulate in.

16. In an effort to prevent further inward involvement into the lateral sinus where perisinus abscess is present at the time of the mastoidectomy, the normal sinus should be exposed surrounding the pathological area involving the lateral sinus.

17. The patient should be left in the care of a thoroughly trained assistant or nurse, who should be able to recognize and report or even treat untoward symptoms.

18. Application of keen diagnostic acumen and judicious surgical judgment, with early operation for sinus thrombosis, will unquestionably give the patient a better opportunity for complete and uneventful recovery.

19. To prevent intracranial complications, lateral sinus thrombosis or others, O.M.P.C. should be avoided by properly treating O.M.P.A. Every O.M.-P.A. should be followed until a dry middle ear exists, whether treatment be conservative or surgical.

---o---

ORTHOPAEDIC SURGERY
Edited by Earl D. McBride, M.D., F.A.C.S.
717 North Robinson Street, Oklahoma City

Spurs of the Os Calcis. Arthur Steindler and Albert R. Smith. Surg. Gyn. & Obst., March, 1938, Vol. 66, No. 3.

After discussing briefly the fact that the association of painful heels with calcaneal spurs is comparatively recent, the authors describe both the conservative and the radical treatment and give results following treatment. Only cases in which the calcaneal spur could be seen by X-ray were used. A total of 71 painful heels was treated. The age varied from 18 to 75 years. Trauma other than walking was of etiological significance in only nine heels, and gonorrheal urethritis was positively associated in only two instances.

Conservative treatment consisted of an insole,

either felt or solid leather, with a hole cut out over the point of the spur. Soft rubber sponge was sometimes inserted over the spur. In addition to these measures, some of the feet were treated by posterior wedge in the heel of the shoe, to relieve further the stress on the tuber of the os calcis.

With conservative treatment in 71 cases, or 71 heels, 46 per cent received complete and permanent relief, and 54 per cent received slight or no relief. Sixteen of these feet that received no relief were operated by simple excision of the spur. Of this group 44 per cent received complete and permanent relief and 56 per cent slight or no relief.

A rotation osteotomy of the os calcis is described, which consists primarily of a lateral incision, a transverse division of the os calcis; the incision extending across the bone with the osteotomy anterior to the heel cord and also anterior to the insertion of the plantar muscles. A wedge of bone is removed and after lengthening the heel cord, the os calcis is rotated so that the spur points superiorly rather than in a position for allowing pressure on this spur. This is held in place by an ivory peg or metal wire. Eight of these cases were operated with a total of 75 per cent complete and permanent relief, and 25 per cent with slight or no relief. This last operation is rather formidable and should be undertaken only in those cases where conservative therapy has failed, or where the spur has recurred.

Newer Concepts in the Treatment of Injuries to the Ligaments of the Knee Joint: an Evaluation of the Mauck Operation. M. Thomas Horwitz, and Authur J. Davidson. Surgery, March, 1938. Vol. 3, No. 3.

The authors point out first that it has been proved definitely that stable knees may follow severe dislocations of the knee joint treated conservatively; also many surgeons disregard or excise torn crucial ligaments with good results and several observers have shown that repair of the collateral ligament, without repair of the crucial, may result in good stable knees.

The authors wish to show (1) that the clinical and experimental results they have obtained confirm the above contingence and (2) to emphasize that the Mauck operation is of definite value in injury to the knee joint with associated injuries to the crucial and collateral ligaments. They point out anatomically the attachment of the anterior crucial and the posterior crucial ligaments and state that the integrity of the knee joint depends not only on these ligamentous structures but upon the posterior oblique ligament, the muscular aponeuroses and tendons about the joint, and to a less extent the capsule and menisci.

The lateral ligaments become taut in full extension, thus checking hyperextension, lateral motion, and rotation. In flexion they become relaxed and the knee joint is loose, permitting slight lateral and rotatory motion.

Experimentally the authors noted in observations on cadavers and on large dogs, (1) that with the knee fully extended, section of the anterior crucial ligament, posterior crucial ligament, or both, did not disturb the stability of the knee. There was no undue lateral or rotatory motion and only very slight anteroposterior motion present. (2) With the knee in full extension, the collateral ligaments severed, and the crucial ligaments intact, definite anteroposterior, lateral, and rotatory motion existed, which became greatly exaggerated with severance of the crucial ligaments. (3) With the knee flexed, if the anterior crucial ligament was severed, anteroposterior motion became evident; but this was greatly increased, as was also the range of abduction and rotation of the tibia on the femur with the knee flexed, when the internal collateral ligament was severed. (4) With the knee flexed, with the anterior crucial ligament intact, severance of the internal ligament resulted in definite "rocker" motion, or anteroposterior motion, with increase in abduction and rotation of the tibia on the femur. (5) In two cadavers, with the pelvis fixed and the knee flexed, the leg was forcefully abducted on the femur. The internal lateral ligament was torn from its tibial attachment in each case, and with the abducting force continued, marked stress was placed upon both crucial ligaments, the greatest strain being exerted on the anterior when the leg was internally rotated and on the posterior when the leg was externally rotated. In this position the internal meniscus, its anterior and posterior attachments intact, became displaced into the knee joint, but no actual tear was seen to occur, p o s s i b l y due to the absence of superincumbent weight.

The authors then left a number of clinical studies which confirm the anatomical studies. These were made by a number of different observations.

Treatment of this type of injury, either as actual tears or stretching of the internal collateral ligament is next described. Methods advocated by different surgeons are described, and finally the authors describe Mauck's operation for relaxation of the internal collateral ligament.

This operation is indicated after conservative regime has been carried out. The operation is performed by an exposure of the inner aspect of the knee joint with a slightly anterior curved incision, extending from the adductor tubercle of the femur to four inches below the joint line. Using a broad chisel the inner side of the tibial head with the internal lateral ligament, is removed and reflected upward. The capsule is incised and the internal meniscus is removed. At this time the knee joint may be thoroughly inspected. The medial lateral ligament is shortened by mortising the piece of bone previously chiseled off with its attached ligament, into the tibia at a lower level. The leg is fully extended and strongly adducted at this time, so that all the correction possible is obtained. The capsule is plicated if necessary and the subcutaneous tissue and skin closed. The knee is immobilized in plaster in full extension for six weeks. However, it is hinged at the knee at the end of two weeks to allow early flexion and extension, preventing any adduction or abduction.

This technique has been employed by the authors, and in one detail differs in that the bone flap was implanted somewhat forward as well as downward to increase the obliquity of the anterior fibers, to act as an additional check against forward movement of the tibial head of the femur. This, of course, was in cases of anterior crucial ligament tear.

In conclusion, the authors feel that the less extensive operative procedure, as outlined by Mauch, is suitable for treating extensive tears of the medial collateral ligament with associated crucial ligament rupture.

———————o———————

PLASTIC SURGERY
Edited by
GEO. H. KIMBALL, M.D., F.A.C.S.
404 Medical Arts Building, Oklahoma City

Aseptic Uretero-Intestinal Anastomosis. James I. Farrell, M.D., F.A.C.S., and Yale Lyman, B.S., Evanston, Ill. S. G. & O., March, 1938, Vol. 66, Number 3.

The authors have prepared a very clear cut article on the subject, "Aseptic Uretero-Intestinal Anastomosis." The principal interest in this article is the technique employed.

Procedure: A portion of the sigmoid is grasped between two Allis clamps and an incision is made longitudinally in the serosa. The longitudinal muscle of the bowel is separated until the circular muscle is exposed. The circular muscle is not cut, but is separated from the submucosa at the lowermost portion of the incision. The submucosa is then grasped with a small mosquito forceps and brought out through the opening made in the circular muscle. The ureter is approximated to the submucosa by a continuous suture of No. oo chromic catgut. A small vein clamp is placed on the ureter above the site of anastomosis. A curved needle enters the lumen of the bowel opposite its insertion into the ureter. A second suture of catgut is used to approximate the ureter to the bowel. The silk thread is now used to make the opening between the ureter and bowel. This is done by a sawing motion with the thread. When the thread is removed, a second suture line is placed along the point of the ureterosigmoidal junction.

A clamp is now placed on the ureter between the site of anastomosis and the bladder; if any point of leakage occurs it can be seen and closed. The ureter is ligated and cut. The cut end of the ureter is then buried in the bowel wall between the submucosa and the circular muscle. No attempt is made to close the circular muscle since it forms a sphincter at entrance of ureter into the bowel. The longitudinal muscle is approximated with sutures over the ureter.

The resulting anastomosis is completed in one operation. Urine appears in the bowel almost immediately. The ureter is securely anchored to the submucosa thereby preventing it from becoming detached. Side-to-side anastomosis allows for a large longitudinal opening in the ureter, which prevents a contraction of its orifice. The circular muscle of the bowel surrounds the intramural portion of the ureter there by forming a closure mechanism which prevents regurgitation of intestinal contents in the ureter. Because of the ease of doing a side-to-side anastomosis, a water tight anastomosis is made. This is most important because a leak from the bowel usually causes a fatal peritonitis. It is much safer to do this type of anastomosis than to insert the end of the ureter through an opening in the bowel. Leakage is more likely to occur when the ureter is inserted into the bowel.

Experimental Data: Seven dogs had an anastomisis of both ureters and the sigmoid. These dogs were allowed to survive for six months, then four of the animals were sacrificed to study the end-results. One dog died at the end of four months, and autopsy was performed. Two dogs are alive and well after an eight-month period.

(There are numerous photographs and drawings which show technique of procedure and autopsy specimens of kidneys and bowel of dogs.)

Advantages of Technique: The transplantation of the ureters into the bowel is a physiological problem, in which one must adhere to fundamental principles. First, if an anastomosis is to be done between the ureter and sigmoid, it must be an airtight and water tight anastomosis. The escape of urine, fecal material, or gas into the peritoneum, after the completion of the operation, is certain to cause peritonitis. The method of transplantation, described as the side-to-side type, makes it possible to test the anastomosis after its completion.

Second, the maintenance of the original size of the ureteral opening into the bowel is important. Stricture of the ureter following transplantation is often due to the large number of sutures taken in the circumference of the ureter. This is obviated in our operation by the suture of the side of the ureter to the side of the bowel, instead of implanting the cut end of the ureter. In the Higgins technique the uretero-sigmoidal opening c l o s e s spontaneously, if the ureter remains connected with the bladder over a period of six to eight weeks.

In attempting to construct a valve-like action at the site of anastomosis, we have cut no muscle in the bowel wall. The ureter is transplanted so that it traverses the longitudinal and circular muscle layers in the bowel and ends just beneath the mucosa of the bowel lumen. The ureter does not project into the lumen of the bowel. We feel that this is a factor in preventing postoperative blocking of the ureter during the healing process.

Anastomosis of the ureter and sigmoid, without opening either structure in the peritoneal cavity, certainly tends to prevent peritonitis, which is a danger in other procedures. The use of the sawing ligature in blood vessel surgery has long been known. We feel that its use in uterosigmoidal anastomosis is worth while.

Conclusions: The authors apparently have made some improvement in technique in uretero-intestinal anastomosis. The principle of the cutting silk ligature is ingenuous. The principles employed have been previously employed in blood vessel surgery. Anyone attempting this operation should be familiar with the old as well as the new technique. This is one branch of work that has not kept pace with other surgery in this section of the country.

———————o———————

INTERNAL MEDICINE

Edited by Hugh Jeter, M.D., 1200 North Walker. Oklahoma City

The following editorial from the American Journal of Clinical Pathology, March, 1938, seems worthy of serious consideration on the part of Clinicians because they are not and cannot be expected to be familiar with the problems of the laboratory in their routine daily work. Where practical work leaves off and research work begins is something the director of every laboratory must determine and regrettably so in many instances because we have had the experience of having to reject work, new tests or procedures, regrettably for two reasons: First, that the clinician had presented an interesting test and secondly, that we too are eager to invade realms of unknown fields and establish new tests.

The following editorial is quoted in part because an abstract would hardly represent the thought of the editor satisfactorily.

"Clinical Pathologist or Magician?"

"There was a time when the 'laboratory' and its 'staff,' if not entirely overlooked, were regarded with amusement; now they enjoy the mixed blessings of such diverse emotions as contempt, respect, mistrust, confidence, depreciation, and even awe. Of course, opinion is divided, but often even the same individual shuttles back and forth from one attitude to its opposite.

"All in all, however, there is a sufficient number who feel that the laboratory is perhaps of some little use after all, a place in fact where magic of a sort is performed. Some may even look upon the clinical pathologist as something of a magician, though obviously not quite on the same high plane as the allergist or endocrinologist.

"If we consider the fact that a few drops of blood may be made to disclose the condition of a patient's carbohydrate metabolism, a few more reveal the function of his kidneys, and that 5 cc. of urine injected into the ear vein of a rabbit may decide whether she 'is' or she 'isn't,' and contemplate further the number and variety of problems (anatomical, hematological, serological, bacteriological and chemical) left at the door of the laboratory for solutions, it may lead to the conclusion that perhaps this much-berated institution has some little reason for existence. Such a concession often carries the proviso that the laboratory must never err and that it must be capable of performing pretty nearly everything on a moment's notice.

"Clinical pathologists, and very good ones, have confided that one of their major difficulties is the determination of lead in excreta. Somehow at the end of their efforts they are left cold, uncertain as to whether the analysis was really accurate. After several attempts they are often forced to the point of admitting their inability to undertake the procedure. Offhand it may seem that the determination should be easy, but on closer inspection the difficulties become obvious. Usually the necessary equipment is not available even in fairly good laboratories. Besides, the laboratory may be in such close proximity to offices, wards, private rooms and clinics that the fumes and stenches incurred in such an analysis would immediately bring down upon the laboratory the wrath of all, particularly the one who requested it. In a laboratory organized and equipped to do many such analyses, the procedure soon becomes a matter of routine and presents no problem, but the condition is altogether different if a request for a lead degermination comes but once in a long while. It means that someone, usually the director, must drop everything else in order to prepare or restandardize the reagents and conduct the analysis, which may consume several days. I recently inquired from the head of the chemical laboratory in a large eastern teaching hospital whether he encountered any difficulty with the determination of lead. His reply was that the analysis was more trouble than it was worth. After a little discussion, we came to the conclusion that it might be more practical and economical if the various hospitals in this large city cooperated in maintaining a laboratory in one of the institutions where this analysis, and such others as the determination of bismuth, arsenic and mercury, might be more satisfactorily conducted.

"There are many similar examples and also others of a somewhat different type. As a second illustration reference may be made to the work of several groups of investigators on the changes in blood iodine in thyroid disease. Comparison of the values obtained before and after thyroidectomy may be illuminating. It may be very interesting that in a case of hyperthyroidism the blood iodine may rise, let us say from 5r per cent before the operation to over 100r per cent after the operation. It must be conceded that in presenting such a case before a group of students or fellow-clinicians, data of this sort may be legitimately used in illustrating certain aspects of the pathological physiology of the gland. But is this a diagnostic procedure that can be undertaken under ordinary circumstances by the private, or even the hospital laboratory? It is not. Irrespective of how well trained a man may be as a chemist, he must devote many days to the preparation of the necessary reagents, and many more days to acquiring the requisite technical precision. Moreover, the reagents once prepared must be scrupulously watched, protected from the slightest contamination and frequently restandardized, or renewed. It is one thing for a group of three or four investigators restricting themselves to the problem of blood iodine, equipping a laboratory specifically for this purpose, removing it sufficiently from wards and dispensaries where there is always iodine in the air, and performing their work day after day until it becomes a routine. It is a totally different thing to find, some fine morning, a 5 cc. specimen of blood with the request 'Please determine the iodine content.'

"Some time ago a friend of mine came with the proposal that in a certain proportion of his patients it would be very desirable to analyze the urine, and perhaps even the blood, for estrogenic and gonadotropic hormones. A good idea and perhaps even clinically relevant, but imagine setting up a dozen benzene extractors daily, separating the hormones from everything else, injecting the products into series of mice and rats, taking time out for vaginal examination at 96, 104 and 128 hours, and later autopsying and exploring these animals. And where are these mice and rats to come from, who will feed them, and where and how will they be kept? That such studies, conducted under proper auspices, may be of the utmost value cannot be disputed, and it may even be granted that the technic now available may be applied in special instances to clinical diagnosis, but is it a procedure for the general laboratory of a hospital?

"From the foregoing it is not to be concluded that I advocate the avoidance of newly acquired technical procedures. On the contrary progress must continue and it is often for the laboratory to set the pace. But it must be stressed that if there is to be expansion, it must be along sound and practical lines. A laboratory doing 5,000 examinations a month can usually take on an additional 200 without much inconvenience. However, if the 200 additional requests for laboratory work involve unusual and difficult manipulations, the situation becomes different. It may represent an additional load, not of 4 per cent, but of 100 per cent, or even more, and call for unavailable reagents, equipment, room and especially skilled workers.

"If a member of a hospital staff, or a clinician in private practice, wishes to test new laboratory methods, or to follow a legitimate problem, there should be some provision for such pursuits, however fantastic they may seem. But this should not be at the expense of the general laboratory, or of its routine work. Special projects need to be turned over to competent assistants. Many laboratory directors would be willing to act in an advisory capacity without arrogating themselves any part of the credit that might accrue from such work."

———————o———————

UROLOGY

Edited by D. W. Branham, M. D.
514 Medical Arts Building, Oklahoma City

Sulfanilamide Therapy in Gonorrhea and Its Complications—Edwin P. Alyea, Walter E. Daniel, and Jerome S. Harris, D u r h a m, North Carolina. Southern Medical Journal, April, 1938.

The authors discuss their experiences with sulfanilamide therapy in the treatment of gonococcal urethritis. They report that 86 per cent of their cases were cured when they were treated with the drug. Of particular interest to them, so far as its relation to the success and failure in treatment was the blood concentration of sulfanilamide. Through blood determinations they found no significant relation between the amount of the drug concentrated and whether a good or bad result was obtained.

The average cured case showed 6.2 mg. sulfanilamide per 100 c.c. of blood while the average unimproved case presented only slightly less amounts of the drug (4.8 mg. per 100 c.c.). Many of the patients who showed good results had a concentration as low as 2.5 mg. to .3 mg. per cent, however, some patients who did not respond favorable to the lower dose did react to an increased amount which raised their blood concentration level. In spite of this observation some cases showing failure had concentrations as high as 10 mg. to 13 mg. per 100 c.c. In view of these observations they felt that blood concentration is not the important factor that determines whether there will be a success or failure in treatment.

Comment: No drug has received as much publicity the past few months as sulfanilamide in the treatment of gonorrhea. Nobody disputes the fact that it is an extremely potent preparation useful in the cure of this infection, but the only question to be settled is how efficient it is. The literature is full of papers where 75 to 95 per cent cures are reported. Despite such optimistic reports, it is my belief the average practitioner is not obtaining such good results and certainly I am personally not seeing such success. Even increasing the amount of drug, given to 80 and even 100 grains daily at the beginning of treatment I have not been able to show more than 30 per cent cures in the ambulatory patient who has acute gonorrhea. It must be understood that by cure, I mean absence of discharge, shreds, and pus in the urine, freedom from prostatic infection by examination of the secretion repeatedly and most important of all failure to provocate the infection by appropriate measures. All such criteria of successful cure should be present not later than two to three weeks following the onset of the infection and initiation of treatment.

Because of such a difference in views as regards the efficacy of sulfanilamide, I would welcome correspondence of a statistical nature from individual physicians over the state detailing their experience with this drug as far as it is related to the treatment of gonorrhea. Only by large number of case records obtained from many individual doctors may we clarify in our minds the therapeutic status of the remarkable medicine. Such information will be compiled to be used for future publications in the Journal. In your replies it is only necessary to state the number of cases treated, the percentage of successes or failures, and the number of toxic reactions encountered.

The authors of this article have contributed much to our knowledge of the drug by these observations on blood concentration of sulfanilamide. I believe that we will utilize blood determination more in the future in order to be assured that an adequate concentration of the drug is being obtained during treatment.

———————o———————

Simplified Analgesia In Urology
Joseph E. F. Laibe

(Assoc. Clin. Prof. of Urol., Loyola Univ. School of Med., Chicago.) Ill. Med. Jour., 73:224 (March) 1938.

The analgesic state should be deep enough to allow the surgeon to carry on the operation, but, when practical, less of the anesthetic or analgesic should be used to at least partly eliminate some of the operative risk. A dose of 1/32 to 1/20 grain Dilaudid plus 1/150 to 1/100 grain scopolamine given about one-half an hour before cystoscopy has been found to produce a satisfactory analgesic effect with adequate relief of pain within a shorter time than with morphine. In general, this combination holds these patients so well that other analgesics are not required. Patients weighing 120 pounds or less are given the smaller doses while the larger amounts are reserved for larger patients.

For major surgery, Dilaudid, 1/20 grain, and atropine, 1/150 to 1/100 grain are given about 45 minutes before the operation, which is usually done under ethylene or nitrous oxide. In general, Laibe found Dilaudid a satisfactory opiate for pre or post-operative use, as well as in such conditions as renal colic, bladder spasm, etc. In concluding his report he states:

"1. Adequate analgesia for cystoscopies is often obtained by using morphine, grain 1/6 to 1/4, or Dilaudid, grain 1/32 to 1/20, with scopolamine, grain 1/150 to 1/100, depending on the weight and irritability of the patient. If such a procedure is used the risk of depression is not as great as when inhalation or spinal anesthesia are used.

"2. Dilaudid has proved to be a more satisfactory opiate than morphine for the relief of pain in cystoscopies or other surgical cases, in renal colic, tumors, etc., since there is practically no nausea or other evidence of stimulation accompanying its use, and there is less necessity for post-operative catheterization."

THE JOURNAL

OF THE

OKLAHOMA STATE MEDICAL ASSOCIATION

| VOLUME XXXI | McALESTER, OKLAHOMA, JUNE, 1938 | Number 6 |

Syphilis of the Eye*

F. T. GASTINEAU, M.D.

VINITA, OKLAHOMA

One has but to look at our insane hospitals and schools for the blind to realize that the present campaign against syphilis is timely indeed. Of the new admissions to the Eastern Oklahoma Hospital during the past five years, 12.14 per cent have been infected with syphilis. The mental condition of 8.38 per cent was due to syphilis alone, while the infection in the other 3.76 per cent was incidental to some other form of insanity. The incidence of syphilis among the males was 13.6 per cent in contrast to 9.92 per cent among the females. Syphilis alone was the cause of the mental trouble in 10.43 per cent of the males and in 4.73 per cent of the females. For some unknown reason, possibly due to an immunity p r o d u c e d by menstruation and child bearing, the syphilitic female is less likely to develop neuro-syphilis than the syphilitic male.

I have recently completed an ocular examination of 100 males suffering from general paresis. Bilateral Argyll Robertson pupils were found 22 times while the monocular type was found three times. There were three cases of doubtful classification, in which the pupils would react slightly to light but would almost immediately dilate again. In one patient, this type of pupil was associated with an Argyll Robertson pupil in the other eye. Ten others had very sluggish pupils that could have been classed as of the Argyll Robertson type had the loose classification been used. Two of the Argyll Robertson pupils were

about five mm in diameter and were associated with a typical Argyll Robertson pupil in the other eye; the remaining pupils were three mm or less in diameter. The pupils were unequal in 18 cases, two of which were of the Argyll Robertson type. Choroiditis was found in eight patients, binocular in two and monocular in six. Signs of a previous iritis were found in five cases, one binocular and four monocular. Optic neuritis, manifested by a slight swelling of the nerve head, was present eight times; binocular in three and monocular in five. Lens opacities were present in five cases, binocular in three and monocular in two. Optic atrophy was found in two cases, both of which were binocular. The most common defect was the atypical response to a cycloplegic, as 50 per cent reacted imperfectly to homatropine. In only about 25 per cent of the patients were the eyes free from manifest disease.

Syphilis has been called the great imitator. The truth of this statement is well demonstrated in the eye, for no part of this delicate organ is immune from the ravages of the spirochete.

A recent survey by Dr. Conrad Berens of New York revealed that 5.3 per cent of the blindness among children in schools for the blind is due to syphilis, as is also about 15 per cent of all blindness. This does not take into consideration the much larger number of individuals who are suffering to a lesser degree.

Congenital syphilis can be prevented to a great extent by treating, during preg-

*Read before the Eye, Ear, Nose and Throat Section of the Oklahoma State Medical Association at Muskogee, Oklahoma, May 11, 1938.

nancy, every woman who has been unfortunate enough to contract syphilis at any time during her life. This should be done regardless of the reaction of the blood and spinal fluid at this time. All too often a walled off focus of infection exists in treated cases even though the serology is negative. A case illustrating this point has been reported by Dr. F. Bruce Fralick of Ann Arbor. A man, hospitalized because of gonorrheal arthritis, during his stay in the hospital developed iritis, which he said had been recurrent at irregular intervals for a period of ten years. He denied any luetic infection, and since his blood and spinal fluid were both negative, the condition was considered of gonorrheal origin. Still suspicious, Dr. Fralick made a Kahn test on the aqueous of the infected eye, found it positive, and confronted the patient with this evidence. The patient then admitted having had an infection 11 years previously, followed by supposedly adequate treatment. While this case reported is in a male it could be equally true in the female. Thus we see such a focus of infection may lie dormant in any part of the body, producing few if any symptoms, becoming active during pregnancy, with the usual disastrous results.

The danger is too great, and the consequences are too grave to omit treatment during these periods of pregnancy. I wish, therefore, to repeat: every woman who has been unfortunate enough to contract syphilis at any time in her life should be treated during periods of pregnancy. This should be done regardless of the present reaction of the blood and spinal fluid. It has been estimated that this procedure alone would reduce the incidence of blindness due to syphilis by 50 per cent.

Any obscure disease of the eye is an indication for a blood test. The first sign of neuro-syphilis is frequently observed in the eye. Degenerative changes of the brain frequently parallel those in the eye, therefore, the more suggestive conditions, such as paralysis of the extra-ocular muscles, Argyll Robertson pupils, and optic atrophy, call for a complete physical and neurological examination as well as thorough laboratory tests on the blood and spinal fluid.

Interstitial keratitis calls for the same complete examination as the degenerative diseases, for it is usually caused by congenital syphilis. This form of keratitis may be associated with a negative blood and spinal fluid, in which case other signs of congenital syphilis should be sought. Tuberculosis may be the causative agent in, perhaps, 10 per cent of the cases. Dr. Berens lists eight other causes of interstitial keratitis. (These are smallpox, influenza, mumps, nephritis, meningococcemia, epidemic encephalitis, malaria, and dental sepsis.) When the blood and spinal fluid are negative and the stigmata of congenital syphilis are a b s e n t, a thorough search should be made for other causes. The nature of the treatment will, of course, depend upon the cause. Under proper treatment 60 per cent will regain useful vision.

In abnormalities of the extra-ocular muscles, one will often notice the peculiar position in which the head is carried. Turning the head in the proper position will lessen the strain on a weakened muscle and often prevent diplopia. The patient soon learns the position that gives him most relief and assumes his characteristic pose. Thus the first symptom noticed in a destructive process of the sixth nerve would be an exophoria caused by the inflammatory stimulation. This possibly might be followed by a short period of e x t e r n a l strabismus. When the destruction of the nerve is complete, however, the paralysis of the external rectus will result in an internal strabismus. It is during the various stages of this destructive process that the patient may get relief by carrying his head so that he is able to look to one side.

Modern methods of diagnosis and treatment have greatly reduced the incidence of acute ocular syphilis. Dr. Hans Barker of San Francisco reports, in the California and Western Medical Journal of July, 1936, that such clinical material was abundant 25 years ago. Today he finds it difficult to demonstrate cases of syphilitic iritis, papillitis, or fresh chorioretinitis to the Stanford medical students. Even interstitial keratitis is decreasing in frequency. If acquired syphilis is adequately treated we may expect uveal tract involvement in about four per cent during the secondary stage, if inadequately treated the expectation increases to eight per cent.

Choroiditis is often a very disabling disease, especially if the lesion is in the macular region, in which case, central vision is lost. When syphilis is the causative agent, there is an associated retinitis. The fresh lesions have hazy, poorly defined, buff colored borders, and are produced by an infiltration of leucocytes with a throwing out of exudates. As the disease becomes chronic, the exudates are absorbed, the choroid and retina become atrophic over the diseased areas, pigment migrates from the choroid to the margin of the lesions, and contrasts sharply with the white sclera below. These scars remain as a permanent record. The lesions may range from the salt and pepper type to the larger sharply outlined atrophic spots resembling retinitis pigmentosa.

Since degenerative changes in the brain closely parallel those in the eye, one is able to look at a case of choroiditis and visualize a similar condition that may be taking place in the brain. Treatment may cause these exudates to be absorbed, but if the brain cells are destroyed they never regenerate. Some part of the mental symptoms of a paretic may be caused by the infiltration of leucocytes with the resulting inflammatory exudate. As the exudate is absorbed under the influence of treatment, mental improvement results only in so far as the symptoms were caused by the exudate. The patient does not regain that mentality lost by destruction of n e r v e tissue.

The v i t r e o u s may be involved, being filled with many dust like particles in contrast to the larger opacities found in association with other causes. Yet do not be deceived, syphilis may be the cause also of some of the larger opacities.

Subjectively, there is no pain unless the iris or ciliary body is involved. Objects may appear distorted because of the uneven surface of the retina, and flashes of light may appear because of retinal irritability. Scotomas are present corresponding to the involvement.

Because choroiditis and associated lesions are frequently caused by diseases other than syphilis, the ophthalmoscope is not a reliable m e a n s of differential diagnosis. Laboratory help is essential.

In 1869, Argyll Robertson, a Scotch physician, published a paper entitled "Four cases of Spinal Miosis with Remarks on the Action of Light on the Pupil." In his remarks he named five points which he said were characteristic of this phenomenon; namely, (1) The retina is sensitive to light. (2) The pupils are miotic and (3) do not react to light, but (4) react readily to accommodation and convergence, and (5) they dilate imperfectly with atropine. This phenomenon has been called the Argyll Robertson Pupil in honor of its discoverer. Dr. Robertson also stated that pupils conforming in every particular to t h i s description are peculiar to syphilis. Since that time many others have found similar reactions differing only in regard to the size of the pupil. Believing that the two similar reactions should be classed together, they have insisted on cataloguing them with the Argyll Robertson pupil. Dr. R. Lindsay Rea of London defines the Argyll Robertson pupil as one with an absence or *gross diminution of the reaction to light,* but with the preservation of the reaction to accommodation and convergence. Others continue to insist, however, on the original definition. From my search of the literature, I believe the majority of writers are agreed that the definition as now accepted does not restrict the size of the pupils. Those who dogmatically state that it is diagnostic of syphilis usually insist on the definition as originally stated by Dr. Robertson. W h a t constitutes a miotic pupil is another point where agreement is lacking. Some writers contend that to be classified as miotic a pupil should be two mm or less in diameter; others are willing to accept a three mm p u p i l as miotic.

There is likewise much controversy over the site of the lesion that produces the Argyll Robertson pupil. It is believed by some to be in the c i l i a r y ganglion; by others in the cervical cord. The weight of evidence seems to indicate the location to be in the mid-brain somewhere near the n u c l e u s of the third nerve; but many writers feel that it cannot be definitely located. Bernheimer's chart is an excellent aid in localizing many nerve lesions affecting the eye.

In support of the opinion that the lesion is located somewhere near the nucleus of the third nerve, we might say that since the pupil is active to accommodation and convergence, the efferent part of the arc must be intact. The site of the lesion therefore would seem to be in the afferent pathway. Since vision is not disturbed, the lesion must be located in the afferent reflex fibers after they have separated from the visual tract. The reflex fibers leave the visual tract near the external geniculate body and travel to the nucleus of the third nerve by a route, the whole course of which has not been determined. Fibers from the third nerve complete the reflex arc. If miosis is present it must be either paralytic or spastic. Since it continues for a long period of time, the spastic type can be ruled out, and we are safe in saying that the contracted pupil is caused by a destruction of the sympathetic n e r v e s which s u p p l y the radiating or dilating muscles of the iris. Since the a f f e r e n t pupilomotor fibers, or those fibers that carry the light stimulus to the nucleus of the third nerve, and the sympathetic or pupilodilator fibers run t o g e t h e r for short distance in the mid brain near the nucleus of the third nerve, it is conceivable how one lesion in this location would produce both a miosis and a reflex iridoplegia.

Before the discovery of the Wasserman reaction in 1907, clinicians were inclined to assign syphilis as the cause of many obscure conditions. This disease was blamed for many things of which it was not guilty. If the physician was unable to find any other cause, syphilis was a very convenient diagnosis, and no one could disprove it.

All of you remember the old s a y i n g "When in doubt give KI." Since the discovery of the Wasserman reaction we have of necessity abandoned the habit of ascribing syphilis as the cause of all obscure pathology. The p r e s e n t day laboratory procedures help us not only to confirm or deny the presence of syphilis, but they help us to diagnose many other diseases. We may discover, by use of the X-ray, an abscessed tooth or an infected sinus that is causing the disease, when previously syphilis would have received the blame. For this reason, many of the observations concerning the Argyll Robertson p u p i l made before the development of the Wassermann test are of doubtful value.

While all are a g r e e d that the Argyll Robertson pupil is found more frequently in syphilis than in any other disease, all are not agreed that it is found exclusively in syphilis. Observations m a d e over a period of years have found this phenomenon in (1) epidemic encephalitis, (2) multiple sclerosis, (3) cerebral tumors, (4) syringiomyelia, (5) chronic alcoholism, (6) traumatism, (7) cerebral hemorrhage, (8) arterio-sclerosis, (9) diabetes, a n d (10) Freidreichs disease. Any thing that will produce a lesion in that vulnerable part of the brain will produce an Argyll Robertson pupil.

Treatment of syphilis no matter where the focus of infection is found, is for the most part systemic. It must be remembered that each patient may react differently to treatment, and no hard and fast rules can be made. Because of the delicate mechanism of the eye, a Herxheimer reaction, following large initial doses of arsenicals, may prove disastrous to vision. Treatment should commence with bismuth or mercury, preferably bismuth; and after a few doses of this, one may begin with small doses of a trivalent arsenical. This may be given in gradually increasing doses along with the bismuth for a period of 20 weeks. At the beginning, the treatment should be given at shorter intervals and the length of the interval increased as the size of the dose is increased. The maximum dose can be reached usually within three or four weeks. When the eye becomes quiescent, the remaining treatment should be considered from the standpoint of the body as a whole.

When there is even the slightest possibility that the existing eye disease could be caused by syphilis, a blood test should be made. If the disease is of the degenerative type, a test of the s p i n a l fluid should be made without fail. The presence of a positive Wasserman test does not mean necessarily that the eye lesion is caused by syphilis. Infected teeth, tonsils, and. sinuses should be searched for, and if found, cared for as though they were the cause of the disease. In addition to this treatment of syphilis should be instituted at once. In case operative interference is advisable it is well to postpone it until the patient has had sufficient anti-luetic treatment to render him a safe operative risk.

The ophthalmologist should not regard the eye as an isolated organ, but as an integral part of the body influenced by the general health of the patient. It is his duty to society in general and to the patient in particular, to diagnose those systemic diseases whose signs may be manifested in the eye. The first evidence of neuro-syphilis is frequently discovered in the eye, therefore we owe it to our patients to diagnose this condition before irreparable damage is done.

If the campaign against syphilis is to be successful it must be twofold; first, the spread of the disease must be prevented; second, those having the disease must be discovered and treated. A high percentage of those afflicted are unaware of the fact. Some know they have been infected, but they have taken a few shots and have been told they were cured. Having unlimited faith in their physician, and being blissfully ignorant of the dangers of the infection, they have been coasting along through life believing themselves cured. As a result of this belief they frequently deny a previous infection, because they think their past is none of our business. Others having a mild lesion have failed to consult a physician, and therefore n e v e r have been aware of their infection. There are still others who have been treated for an innocent appearing sore by a well meaning but misguided druggist. Syphilis of the innocent is not uncommon. No one, regardless of his station in life, should be above suspicion. The one who is least suspected is frequently the one who is most neglected, because f a m i l y physician and specialist alike take it for granted that he is free of syphilis.

I wish to urge that you become syphilis conscious, that you think of the probability of syphilis as a causative agent in obscure conditions. WHEN IN DOUBT MAKE A WASSERMAN.

BIBLIOGRAPHY

Berens, C., Syphilis in Relation to Prevention of Blindness. J.A.M.A., Sept. 4, 1937.

Lennarson, V. E., Congenital Syphilis of the Eye. Am. J. Syphilis, Gonor. & Ven. Dis., January, 1937.

Barkan, H., Ocular Syphilis and Blindness. Cal. & West. Med., June, 1936.

Culler, A. M., Artificial Fever Therapy in Cases of Ocular Syph. Arch. of Ophth., April, 1936.

Klien, B. A., Acute Metastatic Syphilitic Corneal Abscess. Arch. of Ophth., October, 1935.

Drake, R. L., Ocular Syphilis. Arch. of Ophth., October, 1934.

Carris, L. H., Preventing Blindness through Social Hygiene Cooperation. National Society for Prevention Blindness. Pub. No. 138.

Fralick, F. B., The Kahn Reaction in the Aqueous Humor, its Relation to Syphilis of the Eye. Arch. of Ophth., December, 1933.

Drake, R. L., Ocular Syphilis, III. Arch. of Ophth., February, 1933.

Greene, M. L., Constitutional Treatment of Ocular Lues. Jour. Missouri, Med. Assn., February, 1933.

Klauder, J. V., Ocular Syphilis, II. Arch. of Ophth., February, 1932.

Cary, E. H., Ocular Lesions in Syphilis, with discussion of other aspects of the disease. Texas State Journal, October, 1930.

Bane, W. M., Syphilis of the Eye. Col. Med., May, 1930.

Friedenwald, J. S., Ocular Lesions in Fetal Syphilis. Bulletin Johns Hopkins Hos., February, 1930.

Cary, E. H., Syphilis, its Presence and Eye Ravages. Nat. Soc. for Prev. of Blindness, Prac. 1929, Conf.

Rodin, F. H., Eye Lesions in Patients with Positive Wasserman Reactions. J.A.M.A., August 3, 1929.

Meyer, S. J., Chancre of Conjunctiva with Parenchymatous Keratitis. Med. Jour. & Record., June 16, 1926.

Berens, C. B., The Eye in Syphilis. Journal of Social Hygiene, November, 1936.

Merritt, H. H., and Moore, M. The Argyll Robertson Pupil. Arch. of Neur. & Psych., 30:357, August, 1933.

Adie, W. J., Argyll Robertson Pupils, True & False. British Med. Jour., 2:136, July 25, 1931.

McAndrews, L. F.: Argyll Robertson Pupil. Arch. of Ophth., 10:520, 1933.

Beigelman, M. N.: Syphilis & Blindness. Calif. & West. Med., June, 1936, 44:497.

Masters, Robt. J.: Lessons Learned from a Blind School Survey. Ill. Med. Journal, October, 1937, 72:309.

Culler, A. M., & Simpson, W. M.: Artificial Fever Therapy in Cases of Ocular Syphilis. Arch. of Ophth., 15:624, April, 1936.

---o---

Syphilis and Public Health*

CHAS. M. PEARCE, M.D.
OKLAHOMA CITY, OKLAHOMA

In public health discussions the subject of syphilis is usually presented only as one of venereal disease. A program designed as control of syphilis is usually designated as a venereal disease program. However, the actual procedures of most venereal disease programs are concerned chiefly with syphilis. Syphilis is probably the major public health problem of today.

In an absence of s p e c i f i c vaccination against the disease, it would appear that syphilis control must depend upon systemized social action. The particular factors that make it necessary for society, prob-

*Read before the Section on Genito-Urinary Diseases and Syphilology, Annual Meeting, Oklahoma State Medical Association, Muskogee, Okla., May 11, 1938.

ably through government, to take this action are as follows:

1. Syphilis is a communicable disease.

2. It affects a large proportion of the population, not only those exposing themselves with the carelessness characteristic of human beings.

3. The cost for treatment of syphilis is greater than can be borne by most of the individuals that have it.

4. That these people caught the disease through their carelessness and violation of the moral code from a public health standpoint is entirely out of the question.

5. Public health education is essential to the necessary syphilis control program, and public health education can be brought about through careful planning and continuous effort.

6. In other countries, notably in Sweden, systemized action has produced satisfactory results.

Mortality figures give no indication as to the magnitude of this problem. Certainly the 12,000 deaths reported as being due to syphilis in the United States in 1935 cannot be considered as an actual number of deaths which occurred during this year. Perhaps the reason for this is that unless syphilis stands out clearly as the cause of death, it is not likely to be reported by the physician. The disease rarely causes death during its early and easily recognizable stages. The disease is frequently diagnosed as something else. Many physicians fail to take routine Wassermans on general examinations.

It is said that the public does not like to hear or talk about anything connected with syphilis. In my own experience in initiating this program in Oklahoma, I do not think this is true. The public appears to be quite interested in it and willing to hear and talk about it, but it is not willing to be embarrassed or incriminated. Unfortunately, however, the public has obtained rather an amazing mass of information about the disease. The average layman is more likely to be afraid of toilet seats and drinking glasses than of casual exposure. He is more likely to think of syphilis in

terms of a "sort of rash" than of a long continuous chronic infection. Before sound information can be conveyed to the public, this misinformation must be gotten rid of.

The objective of the State Health Department of Oklahoma is to put the consideration of syphilis on the same basis as that of any communicable disease. The individual member of society may as the result of observation of moral code, or because of having received instructions in sex protection himself on syphilis, and this is helpful from the standpoint of the public health program.

On the other hand, health agencies have not in the past been successful and there is no reason to believe they will be more so in the future in attempting to bring about syphilis control through a moral approach, or one based upon sex hygiene information to individuals. Syphilis is a communicable disease and on this basis must the program be subjected and carried out.

Up until the past two years the means of approach was very questionable. Broadcasting stations would not allow this subject to be discussed on the air. A few of our leading newspapers carried small editorials about syphilis, but most of them dared not discuss the problem openly. But today the subject is discussed in most of our newspapers, in pulpits, civic groups and discussed freely over the radio. This has largely been accomplished through the efforts of the Surgeon General of the United States Public Health Service, Thomas Parren.

During my 14 years experience in Public Health work, I have formed several firm convictions. First, that syphilis is easily the most prevalent of the major communicable diseases. That directly and indirectly it cost the taxpayer more than any other infectious disease. That there are already available weapons with which it might be partially if not entirely stamped out, and so reduced to a minor problem. That though these weapons have been available for a decade or more, we are progressing not forward but backward. Syphilis in this country is increasing, not decreasing. The blame for this, in my opinion, is largely due to failure of the physicians to report those cases with which they come in contact. Many of our hospitals and clinics report only the acute cases of syphilis and disregard altogether the chronic cases. A few of the states are sufficiently equipped with trained personnel to check the sources of contact and source of infection, which, I think, is one of the primary factors in ridding the country of this disease. The irregularity in treatment is perhaps the greatest weakness in the handling of known cases of syphilis. Personally, I think, this is due to the following: First, the individual is mislead by his improvement after a little treatment, and if he has to pay for this treatment is quite likely to discontinue as soon as he feels better or the sore and rash disappear. S e c o n d, w h e n the individual discontinues treatment, it is not always possible for the Health Department to l o c a t e him, even though he has a name and address on the date of his original report. Third, actual prosecution for failure to continue treatment until the infectious stage is passed is so unusual as to make it a personal persecution. If an individual is finally carried to court the prosecution must be prepared to prove that he, or she, is in an infectious stage. Unless there is a visible evidence of syphilis, the judge and jury are not likely to give serious consideration to the defendant's potentiality of infecting others. The health officer will naturally be guided by the law under which he is operating, with the character of the case in question, and by his own common sense. Prosecutions are unusual except with the prostitutes. Most of our states have laws, whereby ample drugs are furnished for those individuals who have syphilis, and are unable to pay a private physician for treatment.

Though a case of syphilis is less dramatic to the public than a case of diphtheria and from society's standpoint disgraceful and to be condemned, at present there is greater necessity for making these drugs easily available than supplying diphtheria antitoxin or toxoid. The rural health officers distribution of this material depends largely on the policies of the State Health Department, or upon the local Health Department and supplies available.

I consider syphilis the most urgent public health problem in this country today. In the first place, so many people have it and when this d i s e a s e is untreated, or not properly treated, these results are dangerous to them and costly to the community. In the second place, it is contagious. In its untreated earliest stage, each person who has it is dangerous to those with whom he associates and, finally, syphilis tops the list of public health problems, because we know how to be rid of it, yet we are doing very little about it. The whole h e a l t h problem in the control of syphilis comprises two main elements. First, every infected person must take treatment and, second, facilities for diagnosis and treatment must be made freely available. First and foremost is the need of adequate facilities for diagnosis and treatment. This method has been the backbone of European control.

Knowing the method for control, we have but to proceed with our campaign intensively. Contributions to effective treatment have been made in many instances. The cooperation and proper attitude of the various components of the medical profession, plus free and complete education of the general public, will help considerably in the solving of our p r o b l e m of venereal infection.

Treatment for every person needing it is available and can be arranged for irrespective of the individual's circumstances. The State Health Department does not sponsor free clinics, but exercises every effort to see that every case receives proper and full attention.

Why is it then that scientific treatment is not utilized by everyone who is so unfortunate as to contract venereal disease? Many who should be under treatment are quite ignorant that they are infected, some who do know that they are infected are ashamed to admit it and therefore receive care usually from quacks. This is the direct result of the wide-spread belief that nice people do not have it, and that nice people should not have anything to do with those who have syphilis. There exists the foolish notion that the disease is a "mark of guilt" and therefore that the victims deserve what they get. This destructive attitude is all the more unchangeable because it is so utterly false. ' Not every sufferer of syphilis is guilty of anything except misfortune.

Although the U. S. Public Health Service has a national program of venereal disease control, there is a tendency on the part of that unit to rely upon the different states to initiate programs in accordance to their own judgment and to fit their particular needs. In this state a test has been made along these lines by contacting C o u n t y Medical Societies and outlining to them our state policy of desiring that patients with syphilis, or venereal disease of any type, are to be treated by their own doctor. To this end we have set out to educate the people on the hazard of venereal infection, and what part these infections play in social life.

Upon request, the state furnishes any physician with the necessary arsenicals, mercury and bismuth, and any such other drugs as are needed. Therefore, we must m a k e k n o w n throughout the land the knowledge which we have and our willingness to dispense it liberally in order to prevent injury to countless people having a disease which modern science can control.

We cannot escape the following facts:

1. There are at least six and one-half million people in the United States that have syphilis.

2. Two per cent of the children of the nation have congenital syphilis.

3. It is responsible for 15 per cent of all blindness.

4. Syphilis causes at least 10 per cent or 15 per cent of all the known types of insanity.

Lastly, it has been estimated that the cost of caring for and treating all of our veneral disease patients in the United States is in excess of three billion dollars.

The Management of Early Syphilis*

DAVID V. HUDSON, M.D.
TULSA, OKLAHOMA

The subject of early or acute syphilis is very extensive. This paper will be confined to a resume of findings and recommendations of the Cooperative C l i n i c a l Group as outlined by Moore followed by a discussion of some of the difficulties encountered in the effective treatment of early syphilis.

Under early syphilis is included not only primary and secondary syphilis but early latency of less than four years duration. In other words the term is used to denote those infections where there is favorable c h a n c e for complete or biological cure under continuous, intensive treatment.

The principles of treatment of e a r l y syphilis according to Moore are:

1. The aim of treatment is radical cure.

*Read before the Section on Genito-Urinary Diseases and Syphilology, Annual Meeting, Oklahoma State Medical Association, Muskogee, Oklahoma, May 11, 1938.

2. Study of the patient before treatment to determine
   a. Complications of syphilis
   b. Other complicating diseases
   c. Base l i n e physical findings, to compare with subsequent examinations.

3. Examine contacts.

4. To secure maximum treponemicidal effect, use
   a. Old arsphenamine (606) in place of other arsenicals
   b. Bismuth in place of mercury.

5. Treatment must be continuous—no rest periods.

6. Use the arsphenamines and heavy metals in alternating courses—not in combination.

7. Utilize serologic control — b l o o d

Wassermann and cerebrospinal fluid to determine duration of treatment.

8. Prolong continuous treatment for one full year after blood Wassermann and cerebrospinal fluid become and remain permanently negative.

9. Follow treatment with rigidly controlled year of probation.

10. Thereafter, follow patient for his lifetime with periodic physical and serologic examinations.

SCHEME OF TREATMENT

The treatment outlined by Moore consists of alternating courses of arsphenamine and bismuth. The first arsphenamine course consists of eight injections and subsequent courses six. The first bismuth courses comprises four injections given simultaneously with the first four arsphenamine injections. The second bismuth course of four weekly injections follows the first arsphenamine course and each subsequent course is increased by two injections, until a total of ten is reached. Seronegative primary syphilis r e q u i r e s four courses of arsphenamine followed by bismuth in alternation if the Wassermann is consistently negative whereas seropositive primary and early secondary syphilis s h o u l d h a v e at least five courses of arsphenamine. If neoarsphenamine is used Moore recommends 10 to 12 maximal doses 0.9 gram. The Wassermann reaction is recommended at the beginning and end of each course of arsenic and routine spinal fluid examination between the second and third courses of arsenic. During the year of probation monthly Wasserman reactions are recommended if possible and at least every two months. At the end of this year of probation the patient should have a complete physical and neurological examination, spinal fluid test and if possible, fluoroscopic examination of the cardiovascular stripe.

Moore gives the actual average duration of treatment in the various types of early syphilis as follows:

Seronegative primary syphilis — Nine months, provided the blood Wassermann remains negative throughout. If the blood cannot be examined at the time of each arsphenamine injection to rule out the presence of a provocative Wassermann a full year of treatment should be given.

Seropositive primary and e a r l y secondary syphilis — Fifteen to 18 months. Treatment should be continued for one year after the Wassermann becomes and remains negative. This reversal usually takes place at the start of or during the second arsenic course.

Delayed or late secondary s y p h i l i s — Eighteen months to two years.

Thomas Parran states that persistent and continuous treatment will produce the following percentage of cures:

In sero negative primary stage......86.4% of cases
In seropositive primary stage..........64.3% of cases
In secondary stage..............................81.5% of cases

Thus it is obvious that the patient who has an early diagnosis as soon as possible after the appearance of the primary lesion has the best chance for a complete or biological cure. D a r k f i e l d examinations should be made on all suspicious lesions and in spite of negative findings the patient should be kept under observation until there is no doubt as to the presence or absence of syphilis. So many persons have used ointments or caustics before applying for examination that darkfield determination of the presence of treponema has been consistently fruitless and eventually serological tests establish the diagnosis. It is necessary to f o l l o w negative darkfields with Wassermann reactions until all doubt is removed. Some individuals, especially women, may have such slight secondary manifestations that this stage is missed and unless instructed to report back for rechecking at a specified time may be entirely ignorant of the existence of the disease.

Serological examinations are not made as frequently as they should be. All patients treated for gonorrhea should be carefully examined for primary syphilitic lesions and a Wassermann reaction employed at some time during the course of treatment despite absence of signs of syphilis. When a patient brings up the question of the advisability of serologic examination it is well to follow this through and secure the serologic test before the patient becomes indifferent to the possibility of a luetic lesion.

DIFFICULTIES ENCOUNTERED IN THE TREATMENT OF EARLY SYPHILIS

With the knowledge that continuous, persistent treatment a f f o r d s a very good chance of cure it would appear that there should be little difficulty in clearing up most of these cases of early syphilis which come to us. This is, however, not the case. For every case that comes to me directly for treatment after diagnosis either in this office or elsewhere I have two or more individuals who have begun treatment elsewhere, usually under good men, and allowed themselves to neglect regular treatment or who have dropped all treatment entirely before securing anything like an adequate amount. These individuals will probably be a problem as long as syphilis is treated. They are concerned about their condition immediately after diagnosis, begin treatment, but soon lose all sense of the dangers involved and take advantage of the slightest excuse to postpone or discontinue treatment. I know of no way to handle this group other than to state that there is no short cut to cure and insist on the maximum treatment in hopes that they will have had at least minimal treatment before getting away.

Finances play an important part in the treatment. It is impossible to expect a patient to continue treatment when the charges are beyond his means but every patient has his financial level and when the treatment is adjusted to this he can take all the treatment necessary without undue financial strain. I am opposed to free treatment where the patient can pay even a small amount, since with no investment in the treatment he minimizes its value and tends to neglect seeing it through to completion.

Reactions are encountered at some time by practically all men treating syphilis. Probably the most frequent is the nausea following intravenous injections and while not important in itself frequently causes the patient to avoid treatment. Moore expects his patients to have some nausea in a considerable proportion of cases and tells them to anticipate and make allowance for it. I find it difficult to give the larger doses of neoarsphenamine to a considerable number of my patients who find the attending discomfort interferes with their work to such an extent that they lose time from their job and fear loss of employment.

Changing from one brand to another or cutting down the dose frequently controls this. Some favor mapharsen, but in my experience I find practically the same reactions to that drug as neoarsphenamine although a patient may react to one and not the other.

Tuberculosis in the patient with syphilis complicates the picture and frequently only the heavy metals may be used with occasional patients who tolerate small doses of arsenic cautiously administered. Relatively good results are secured with bismuth alone and the individual not infrequently not only secures satisfactory reversal of the Wassermann but gains weight and improves in general health.

Where reversal of the Wassermann is delayed spinal fluid examination is important. The patient then may be treated with tryparsmide or fever therapy where indicated after increasing the amount of arsenic. Those patients who miss treatment during the first and especially the second course of arsenic are most apt to have neuro-recurrence.

SUMMARY

Continuous intensive treatment produces favorable results in early syphilis, especially in the seronegative primary stage. Treatment should be continued without interruption for one full year after the blood Wassermann and cerebrospinal fluid become negative and remain permanently negative.

BIBLIOGRAPHY

Moore, Joseph Earle: The Modern Treatment of Syphilis.
Parran, Thomas: Shadow on the Land.

Syphilis in Pregnancy*

F. A. DeMand, M.D.
OKLAHOMA CITY, OKLAHOMA

At the present time, when only lately we have had so much p u b l i c education about syphilis, we find a considerable portion of the public rather syphilis conscious. But still, the surprise shown by some when in the routine antepartum examination a positive Wasserman is obtained proves the ignorance of the existing condition. Why, because no clinical evidence has s h o w n itself. Cooke suggests that these mothers are free from clinical symptoms because they have acquired the spirochtaetal infections from their husbands through his semen. The spirochaeta have been lying dormant in the testicles from an initial early infection, and thus are transmitted to the mother to lie in some organ in an attenuated or dormant state and no clinical signs show themselves. Serologically, however, the existence of the disease may manifest itself.

The plea then, is for a routine Wasserman in each and every case. Only by such routine can we give the mother, and most particularly her child the best chance of survival. Only by a routine serological investigation can we hope to cut down the appalling number of infants dying in utero from the disease, and reduce the number of clinical cases manifesting themselves later in the child's life.

Most incidences of syphilis in children have been acquired congenitally and cases have been known where congenital syphilis has not shown itself serologically or clinically until the eighteenth year of the individuals' life.

A positive Wasserman in a mother should call for a test of the father and, also of any children born previously, to the couple. Many indeed, of the offspring will be found clinically or serologically positive. The obstetrician can and should play a great part in the fight against syphilis. Twenty-

*Read before the Section on Obstetrics & Pediatrics, Annual Meeting, Oklahoma State Medical Association, Muskogee, Okla., May 10, 1938.

five thousand fetal deaths a year, in the United States from syphilis, is too high, and the observant pains-taking obstetrician is the one to reduce this number.

Three to four per cent of syphilis in the country today has been acquired congenitally. The early diagnosis of syphilis in pregnancy is imperative. In a group of cases in which the mothers were known to be syphilitic and received no treatment, 17 per cent of the children came through unscathed. Whereas, 83 per cent were either aborted, stillborn or born with some congenital defect or serologically or clinically positive.

Colles law states that a woman may carry a luetic child and become immune to syphilis herself and remain so. Profetas said that a healthy child can come from a luetic mother and be immune from syphilis. Syphilologists today claim that all children from syphilitic parents and all parents of syphilitic children are infected and that the disease will become manifest sooner or later. An occasional case will support the theory of direct infections of the child by the father, the mother escaping. However, the majority of these mothers observed over a period of time will be found later to have developed p o s i t i v e clinical or serological evidence of the disease.

The mode of transmission of the spirochetes from the mother to the child is by way of the placenta. Therefore, syphilis thus acquired by the child is congenital and not hereditary. When the initial infection of the mother is acquired at the beginning or during pregnancy, the extensive spirochetemia occurring during the primary and secondary stages of the disease always infects the placenta and then the fetus. Transmission is dependent on active spirochetes in the mother's blood stream. There are transient periods of spirochetemia in cases of latent lues, and these periods of spirochetmia become less frequent as time passes on, but if at any time during a pregnancy a period of spirochetemia occurs, then the fetus becomes infected. Single spirochetes may pierce a vessel wall and enter the blood stream of the fetus without producing visible defects in the placenta. When, however, large numbers produce a rupture of the blood vessel walls, then we find the resultant infarcts in the substance of the placenta. The old contention that the placenta acts as a filter, so to speak, against the infection reaching the child from the mother, is at present discredited.

Spirochetal manifestations in the fetus depends upon two factors. First, the duration of the mother's syphilis and second, the stage of development of the fetus. If the infection of the mother takes place a short time before conception the fetus is almost certain to die in utero. The longer the mother has had syphilis before conception, the more probable is the birth of a still-born child, a macerated fetus, a premature child or a living child with latent syphilis.

The diagnosis of syphilis in pregnancy is many times rather difficult. As to its incidence, it is found on the average of six per cent in clinical cases and one per cent in private cases. In the majority of cases, 82 per cent, according to Zangmeister, there are no clinical symptoms of syphilis in pregnancy. This tallies fairly well with the figures found in the non-pregnant state. In the remaining 18 per cent h o w e v e r, where definite manifestations of the disease exist, we can note certain variations. Generally speaking, all l o c a l syphilitic lesions are more marked in pregnancy because of the increased vascularity of the pelvic tissues. Chancres take longer to heal, and there is a tell-tale induration of tissues and lesions present. D i a g n o s i s should usually not be diffcult especially when lesions are presenting themselves in the cervix during pregnancy, for the normally soft cervical tissues contrast so clearly with the luetic induration. Cervical chancres are usually of the erosive type, being oval in shape and forming fissures which radiate toward the cervical canal.

In color they appear redder than the surrounding bluish tissues, are friable and bleed easily. The dark secondary manifestations undergo e a r l y suppuration. Eroded papules develop rapidly, undergo progressive hypertrophy and often constitute veritable granulating tumors, which invade and deform the entire vulva.

Opinions differ as to the effect of syphilis on the general condition of the gravida. Moore and Solomon express the view that pregnancy, through metabolic changes, in a large measure protects the central nervous system from the spirocheta and lessens the severity of syphilis as it affects the patient generally. Davies holds that aggravation of the disease in pregnancy is the exception and pregnant women suffer less from s y s t e m i c disturbances than nonpregnant women. It is known that in many cases, no evidence of syphilis is apparent d u r i n g pregnancy. Its presence being diagnosed only when the new-born shows unmistakably its existence in the mother. Gellhorn states that he has yet to note in any syphilitic g r a v i d a, that exuberant feeling of good health, that blossoming out into intensified well-being, which we so often find in normal pregnancy. On the contrary, syphilitics often show aggravated subjective discomforts c o m m o n to the pregnant state, and in addition, frequently complain of headache, loss of hair, insomnia, and neuralgias in various parts of the body. They are anemic, lose weight and have more or less persistent fever. Renal complications are not usually found while eclampsia is rare because syphilis usually causes premature termination of the pregnancy.

Some authorities believe that the Wasserman reaction of a pregnant w o m a n cannot be relied upon with the same degree of assurance as otherwise. Moore reports three pregnant women with active secondaries, whose respective Wassermans were negative. Belding believes that in the blood serum of pregnant women the formation of anti-complimentary and nonsyphilic fixation substances is eight times as frequent as in the non-pregnant women. He believes that the serum of pregnancy has a tendency to become anti-complimentary.

L. Kolbe found the flocculation reactions of Kiss and Kahn particularly well suited for pregnancy cases in that the detection of latent syphilis was more frequent when they were used. Fordyse and Rosen do not consider a weakly positive Wasserman in the pregnant woman shortly before delivery as diagnostic of syphilis. The majority of syphilologists agree that a strongly positive blood in pregnancy, verified on repetition, as diagnostic of syphilis.

The labors of syphilitic women may be perfectly normal and differ in no way from those of healthy women. However, abnormal presentations are comparatively common, because of prematurity or maceration of the fetus. Such cases usually produce precipitate labors. On the other hand, full term labor with the child in normal position often shows weak uterine contractions. In some cases, c e r v i c a l tissue changes from local lesions result in marked resistance to dilatation to the degree of actual dystocia, with marked tendency to cause deep lacerations at delivery. If a syphilitic granuloma is present, it may cause enough obstruction to block delivery, while condylomata lata usually cause such friability of the perineum that it tears like wet blotting paper. Some authorities insist that repairs in syphilitic women should not be done primarily, but be allowed to heal by granulation and r e p a i r e d later after successful anti-luetic treatment. Of the more rare complications encountered during luetic labor may be mentioned rupture of the heart, aneurism of the uterine artery and exhaustion of the adrenal system with fatal result.

It is unnecessary to urge that early, energetic, systematic and more or less continuous anti-luetic treatment must be the rule throughout the full term of pregnancy, for only thereby, can we hope for the survival of the child. It was formerly thought that the greatest loss occurred during the first four months of the fetal life. Now it is known that most deaths occur after the sixteenth week. From then on the child's life is in constant danger. The tremendous toll of infant life, which syphilis exacts is appalling. Some authorities found that habitual abortions accounted for 20 per cent. Late abortions and premature births of macerated fetuses occur in more than 60 per cent of the cases. Only 15 per cent of infected children r e a c h full term. Of these 67.5 per cent either are still-born, or die within the next few days. It is evident that the earlier in pregnancy treatment is instituted the better chance the child has of surviving. However, no matter how late in pregnancy m a t e r n a l syphilis is recognized, intensive, systematic treatment must be given.

Dr. Soule suggests the following outline of treatment for luetic pregnancy. Make an attempt to administer as vigorous treatment as the mother will tolerate safely. P r e n a t a l care must be given weekly through the duration of the treatment with special attention to urinalysis and blood pressure readings. If nephritis appears, treatment must be postponed temporarily at least. Give weekly injections of .15 gm. neoarsaphenamine gradually increasing the dosage to .3 gm. or .45 gm. From nine to 12 such doses are given consecutively. A few days following each intravenous of bismuth injection, starting about the third or fourth week, an intramuscular injection is given, and continued for four weeks following the last dose of Neo. If the patient tolerates the treatment well, the above routine is repeated at once or after a short interval. An attempt should be made to so calculate the treatment that the patient arrives at term u n d e r neoarsaphenamine alone on the basis that the arsenicals are less irritating to the kidneys than the compounds of bismuth. Eighteen weeks of treatment is considered a reasonable course of treatment to protect the life of the child.

Most authorities insist that the maximal amount of neo per dose should not be over .3 gm. to .45 gm. The treatment should be mild and light, but continued the maximal length of time and more or less continuously.

Latent and Somatic Syphilis*

JAMES STEVENSON, M.D.

TULSA, OKLAHOMA

I. — LATENT SYPHILIS

Following the acute symptoms of primary and secondary syphilis, there is, in the otherwise healthy individual, a period when the immunological resistance factors of the body temporarily or permanently balances the virulence of the invading organism. That syphilis is often a benign disease was first emphasized by Bruusgaard, who s t u d i e d a fairly large group of syphilitics who had never received any treatment. He found that 27 per cent of these people had apparently completely eliminated their d i s e a s e by their own powers of immunity.

The clinical diagnosis of latency can be made only when the cerebro-spinal fluid is normal, and a careful physical examination reveals no lesions attributable to syphilis. Such an examination should include:

1. Cardio-vascular system, including X-ray for aortic enlargement.
2. Fundus Oculi.
3. Viscera.
4. Nervous system.
5. Osseous system.
6. Mucous membranes. (Occasionally, as O'Leary observes, leucoplakia may be the only clinical evidence of active syphilis.)

The only evidence on which to base a diagnosis of latency are the positive blood serology, a clear history of infection, a necropsy, or the birth of a syphilitic child.

Cannon, Stokes and Busman, and others, believe that a positive serology means an active infection, and the observations of Warthin also bear out this point. Practically, however, many people with a positive Wassermann live to a r i p e old age without showing clinical complications. It seems probably true, that in many such

*Read before the Section on Genito-Urinary Diseases and Syphilology, Annual Meeting, Oklahoma State Medical Association, Muskogee, Oklahoma, May 11, 1938.

patients, that the immunological mechanism is so effective, that while microscopic damage may be done, it is so insignificant that no clinical symptoms arise. The report of the Cooperative Clinic group emphasizes the observations of Bruusgaard. They found that if a group of latent syphilitics were observed for ten years the results would be as follows:

1. Spontaneous cure, 25 to 35 per cent.
2. Wassermann fasts, 25 to 35 per cent.
3. Late syphilis of skin, mucous membrane, or bones, 10 to 15 per cent.
4. Cardio-vascular syphilis, 10 to 15 per cent.
5. Syphilis of central nervous ssytem or viscera, 1 to 3 per cent.

The number of latent syphilitics is constantly increasing, due to the routine use of the blood Wassermann and other serological tests in hospital, industrial, and private practice. Today, the treatment of this t y p e of patient confronts the physician nearly as often as the treatment of him with early syphilis. The patient is interested in his prognosis. The spinal fluid examination is of great value in this connection—in latent syphilis a normal spinal fluid means that neuro-syphilis will almost never develop. If the spinal fluid becomes positive, neuro-syphilis is probable.

In the treatment of latent syphilis, the golden rule is to treat the patient and not the Wassermann reaction. In the early years of latent syphilis the arsenicals may be used liberally, and in the later years, sparingly. O'Leary states that in latent syphilis more than four years old, bismuth should be used largely. In women with latent syphilis the possibility of pregnancy complicates the problem of treatment. In cases of pregnant women with late latency, 17 per cent result in syphilitic children. In such patients, treatment may be as vigorous as the physical condition would warrant.

It is known that nearly all the serious sequelae of syphilis are clinically manifest 12 to 18 years after the primary infection. A patient past this p e r i o d, with latent syphilis, may be "paroled," without treatment. His positive Wassermann may be ignored, if he reports annually for physical examination, especially of the cardio-vascular system.

In conclusion, one may be reasonably optimistic regarding the future of a patient, if he reaches the latent stage, even if inadequately treated, if he shows no tendency to clinical relapse, and if his spinal fluid remains normal. Such a patient's death certificate will not be adorned with the word "syphilis."

* * * *

II. — SOMATIC SYPHILIS

Stokes believes the routine use of the Wassermann test in young a d u l t s with bone, joint and muscle symptoms would reveal a considerable number of cases of early syphilis. While the characteristic features of the bone changes in early and recurrent syphilis is nocturnal pain, exaggerated by heat, and relieved by movement of the affected part, these are not at all constant. The diffuse headache of the secondary stage is due in part, probably, to bone changes, as are the sternalgia and pleurodynia. Early syphilitic periostitis is not uncommon, involving chiefly the long bones, especially the tibia. This is a localized process, usually recognized by palpating an extremely tender elevation of the bone.

Probably few syphilitics e s c a p e some pathological changes in the osseous system in the course of their disease. The roentgenological studies of the bones in pre-natal syphilis of McLean, and Pendergrass, Gilman and Castleton, suggest that in the future more careful X-ray studies of the bones will be made in acquired syphilis. McLean, in his classical article, gives a number of roentgenological pictures practically pathognomonic of pre-natal syphilis. In this aspect of the disease osteochondritis (i.e., lesions at the diathysoepiphyseal junctions) is the typical pathological finding in the first few months of

life. Later periostitis, osteo-myelitis, and Parrot's pseudo-paralysis may be found. In l a t e r childhood bone manifestations most often occur between the fifth and twelfth year, involving usually the tibia and ulna. While in infancy osteo-periostitis affects mainly the ends of long bones, the tendency here is to involve chiefly the shaft, probably because trauma plays an important role in selecting the site for the pathological changes. There is some pain, often nocturnal, in these cases, often described as "growing pains," but comparatively little functional disability. Later an osteo-myelitis may develop, but more often the typical bone deformities, such as the markedly bowed saber tibiae. Clutton's joints are highly characteristic of pre-natal syphilis, and this symptom is notably associated with interstitial keratitis. Clutton's joints, usually involving the knees or elbows, is a symmetrical, painless, chronic synovitis, with almost no functional disability.

Neisser found the spirochoeta pallida in the bone marrow within a few hours after it had entered the body. Bone syphilis may, therefore, be considered an early infection of the medulla, later spreading by the blood vessels in the Haversian Canals to the cortex and periosteum. The extent of the pathology then depends on the virulence of the organism and the resistance of the bony structure. The young, actively growing bone of infants and young children is naturally less resistant to all types of infection than adult bone, and it follows that the osseous pathology in pre-natal syphilis is much more severe than that which occurs in acquired syphilis. The changes that occur in bone in syphilis, as in osteo-myelitis are preponderantly constructive, that is, there is a tendency to new bone formation, while in tuberculosis and malignancy the tendency is towards bone destruction. By keeping this fundamental pathology in mind, the roentgenologist is frequently of great aid in diagnosing bone and joint syphilis, and it is important to remember this, as the blood serology is not invariably positive.

The treatment of skeletal syphilis yields satisfactory results in 90 per cent of cases if arsphenamine and bismuth are used for at least a year. In early cases the treat-

·ment should be continuous, but in very late cases such as a tibial osteo-myelitis rest periods to increase the general resistance is better. In lesions of the palate and nasal septum great resistance to treatment is often encountered, and after thorough use of arsphenamine and bismuth, mercury and iodides may need to be used for years. There are certain lesions, notably gummatous osteitis of the s k u l l, osteo-myelitis of the long bones with sequestra, and the charcot joint which will require the assistance of surgery.

Contrary to prevalent opinion, syphilis has little or no deleterious influence in the healing of fractures. The reason for this harmonizes with the p a t h o l o g y before discussed — bone responding to syphilitic infection by bone production. Even in the case of gummata accompanying the destructive process, there is always also active reproduction.

---o---

New Director of State Health Laboratories Announced by Dr. rearce

We wish to announce that we have secured the service of Wm. D. Hayes, Dr. P.H., as director of the State Health Department laboratories.

Doctor Hayes is an outstanding man in laboratory work having been director of the laboratories of the State Board of Health in Kentucky; presiaent of the State Board of Health of Iowa for two years; director of the State Board of Health Laboratories of Florida; member of the State Board of Health of Iowa for six years; director of laboratories City of Sioux City, Iowa; assistant bacteriologist for the State of Iowa; taught in medical school in Iowa and taught hygiene and sanitation while connected with the laboratory.

We are very fortunate in securing a man of Doctor Hayes' ability to direct our laboratories and it is our desire that you use the State Laboratories at any and all times.

We have one central laboratory located at Oklahoma City and three branch laboratories, one at Tahlequah, one at Talihina and one at Elk City.

Chas M. Pearce, M.D.,
Commissioner of Health.

---o---

OBITUARIES

Doctor James C. Reynolds

Dr. James C. Reynolds, 57 years of age, pioneer physician of Frederick, died May 14th, following a short illness.

He was born January 1, 1881, at Fulton, Mississippi. After graduation from Fulton High school he attended Memphis Medical College, receiving his degree in 1904. Dr. Reynolds had lived in Frederick since 1920, when he moved there with his family from Wynn, Arkansas, where he had practiced for 17 years, after his graduation from Tulane University.

Dr. Reynolds is survived by his widow, one daughter and two sons.

Interment was in the Frederick Cemetery.

MacLEOD'S PHYSIOLOGY IN MODERN MEDICINE, Edited by Philip Bard, Professor of Physiology, John Hopkins University School of Medicine, with the collaboration of Henry C. Bazett, Professor of Physiology, University of Pennsylvania; George R. Cowgill, Associate Professor of Physiological Chemistry, Yale University School of Medicine; Harry Eagle, Passed Assistant Surgeon, United States Public Health Service and Lecturer in Medicine Johns Hopkins University School of Medicine; Chalmers L. Gemmill, Associate in Physiology, Johns Hopkins University School of Medicine; Magnus I. Gregersen, Professor of Physiology, College of Physicians and Surgeons, Columbia University; Formerly Professor of Physiology, University of Maryland School of Medicine; Roy G. Hoskins, Director of Research, Memorial Foundation for Neuro-endocrine Research; Research Associate in Physiology, Harvard Medical School; J.M.D., Olmsted, Professor of Physiology, University of California; Carl F. Schmidt, Professor of Pharmacology, University of Pennsylvania. Eighth Edition, The C. V. Mosby Company, St. Louis, 1938.

This is the eighth edition of a well known book on Physiology. The greater part of the book has been entirely rewritten. There are nine contributors, including the editor. Each major subdivision is the work of a writer who is actively engaged in the study of some phase of the subject he treats.

Small type is used in the description of methods; for data judged to be of secondary importance to the student; for treatment of matters which are at present largely controversial; and for considerations which are chiefly of clinical interest.

The book is divided into nine parts: 1. The Neuromuscular and Central Nervous Systems. 2. The Special Senses. 3. The circulation. 4. The respiration. 5. The Physiology of the Alimentary Tract. 6. Metabolis and Nutrition. 7. The Endocrine Glands. 8. The Distribution and Regulation of water in the body. 9. The Kidney.

There are many fine illustrations throughout the book, totaling 355 in all. This book should be a welcome addition to any physician's or medical student's library.

---o---

Opportunities For Practice

Mr. Fred Fleming, City Treasurer, Oakwood, Oklahoma, advises there is an excellent opening for a young physician in his city. Oakwood is on Highway 270. This notice is published for the information of those who may be interested.

There is an excellent opportunity for practice in Odessa, Texas, and surrounding territory — in the heart of one of the largest oil fields in Texas. The closest modernly equipped medical office is 120 miles away in El Paso. A well qualified physician is needed badly.

The Lions Club at Wakita, Oklahoma (in Grant County), advises there is an excellent opportunity for a qualified young medical man to practice in that area. Wakita is about eight miles from the Kansas line and 37 miles north of Enid. The population of the town itself is about 500, but there is a large farming territory in the area which raises the available practice in population to treble that number.

Anyone interested should communicate with Mr. R. H. Guthrie, Secretary of the Lions Club, Wakita, Oklahoma.

THE JOURNAL
OF THE
Oklahoma State Medical Association

Issued Monthly at McAlester, Oklahoma, under direction of the Council.

Copyright, 1938, by Oklahoma State Medical Association, McAlester, Oklahoma.

Vol. XXXI	JUNE, 1938	Number 6

DR. L. S. WILLOUR............................Editor-in-Chief
McAlester, Oklahoma

DR. T. H. McCARLEY...........................Associate Editor
McAlester, Oklahoma

Entered at the Post Office at McAlester, Oklahoma, as second-class matter under the act of March 3rd, 1879.

This is the official Journal of the Oklahoma State Medical Association. All communications should be addressed to The Journal of the Oklahoma State Medical Association, McAlester Clinic, McAlester, Oklahoma. $4.00 per year; 40c per copy.

The editorial department is not responsible for the opinions expressed in the original articles of contributors.

Reprints of original articles will be supplied at actual cost provided request for them is attached to manuscripts or made in sufficient time before publication.

Articles sent this Journal for publication and all those read at the annual meetings of the State Association are the sole property of this Journal. The Journal relies on each individual contributor's strict adherence to this well-known rule of medical journalism. In the event an article sent this Journal for publication is published before appearance in The Journal the manuscript will be returned to the writer.

Failure to receive The Journal should call for immediate notification of the Editor, McAlester Clinic, McAlester, Oklahoma.

Local news of possible interest to the medical profession, notes on removals, changes of addresses, births, deaths and weddings will be gratefully received.

Advertising of articles, drugs or compounds unapproved by the Council on Pharmacy of the A. M. A., will not be accepted.

Advertising rates will be supplied on application.

It is suggested that wherever possible members of the State Association should patronize our advertisers in preference to others as a matter of fair reciprocity.

Printed by News-Capital Company, McAlester.

EDITORIAL

Those who attended the Muskogee Meeting are certainly well repaid for their time and effort. The local Committee on Arrangements had everything properly synchronized and there was not a hitch in the entire program. Every courtesy was shown the visitors by the Muskogee profession.

The registration at this meeting was exceptionally good, there having been 430 doctors registered.

It was, of course, impossible to give to our exhibitors under the conditions at Muskogee, as good accommodations as we would have liked, however, every doctor who registered had to visit the exhibits, but it was impossible to make a loafing place as it might have been under different circumstances.

The Council, as you will observe from the minutes, which are published in this issue of the Journal, accomplished considerable work. They tried in every way to respond satisfactorily to the action of the House of Delegates and gave, I believe, a comprehensive report of last year's work. It appeared to be the consensus of opinion of the House of Delegates that the employment of a lay executive secretary is urgent and important. In fact, it is so urgent that the House of Delegates made a request that every County Medical Society contribute at least $5.00 per member to defray the expense of the executive secretary from now until the 1939 dues are paid, and then to continue his employment, the State dues were raised, by the unanimous approval of the House, to $12.00 per year, beginning January 1, 1939.

This is without question an important step and will mean much in accomplishing a more satisfactory understanding between the organization and the doctors of the State as well as between organized medicine and the laity.

Committee reports to the House of Delegates were quite complete and showed all Committees of the Association taking a very a c t i v e interest in their respective duties.

There was, of course, some political talk and the consensus of opinion of the House of Delegates seemed to be that it is the duty of every doctor in the State to see to it that the officials, for whom he votes, are pledged to the support of the legislative program of the Medical Association. It is also the opinion that if this is done legislation, which will protect the health of our citizens, will be enacted and there will be no interference with the regulations governing the practice of medicine in this State.

The Scientific program was unusually good. Our guest speakers, Doctors Neff, Middleton and Ochsner, presented valuable material and their presentation was much appreciated by all who could attend these Sessions. Not only were these guests excellent speakers but they added much to the social and fraternal features of the meeting. We have received from them, since their return home, very friendly greetings and expressions of appreciation of the treatment they were rendered by our Association.

The secretary has suggested s e v e r a l times that a change be made in the time of meeting of the House of Delegates so that the officers and delegates can attend the General Sessions on Tuesday morning. The suggestion is that the first meeting of the House be held the first day at 3 p.m. and the second meeting at 8 p.m. This would complete this part of the work the first day and leave the Delegates free to attend the Scientific Session the morning of the second day. What is your reaction to this change?

Next year we go to Oklahoma City and can look forward to another large meeting with many excellent features that Oklahoma City has to offer.

---o---

Editorial Notes—Personal and General

The Oklahoma City Academy of Ophthalmology and Otolaryngology held its last meeting of the season, May 31, at the Oklahoma Club.

There was no scientific program and the meeting was held in honor of Dr. E. S. Ferguson, Professor of Ophthalmology of the State University Medical School. Dr. W. Albert Cook was the guest speaker.

DR. HENRY TURNER, Oklahoma City, was guest speaker of the Jackson County Health Forum in Kansas City, Mo., Wednesday evening, May 18th. His subject was "The Facts About our Glands."

DR. E. A. CANADA, Ada, has been appointed on the surgical service of Bellevue Hospital in New York City for a period of three or four months.

DR. CHAS. ED WHITE, who has been in St. Louis for the past six months doing post graduate work, was the guest of his mother, Mrs. E. P. White of Muskogee, and attended the meeting of the Oklahoma State Medical Association in May. Dr. White returned to Muskogee the first of June where he will continue his practice.

DR. and MRS. W. J. WHITAKER, Pryor, have returned from Rochester, Minn., where Dr. Whitaker took post graduate work at the Rochester Clinic.

Dr. Hermon S. Major announces that Dr. Henry S. Millett is associated with him in The Major Clinic at 3100 Euclid Avenue, Kansas City, Missouri.

Dr. Millett received his degree of Doctor of Medicine at the University of Kansas in 1928, interned at the Kansas City General Hospital in 1928 and 1929 and was engaged in the general practice of medicine in Kansas City, Missouri, from 1929 to 1930. Following this, he was associated with Dr. T. Klingman in neurology and psychiatry at the Mercywood Sanitarium and St. Joseph Hospital at Ann Arbor, Michigan, from September, 1930, to March, 1932. Later he was Resident in neurology at the Neurological Institute, New York City, from March, 1932, to March, 1934. Assistant in neurology

at Columbia University from March, 1932, to June, 1935, and at the same time neuropathology at Columbia University from September, 1933, until March, 1934. Assistant in neurology at New York University, New York City, on the neurological wards of Bellevue Hospital from March, 1934, to May, 1938. Assistant Physician at Brooklyn State Hospital from March, 1934, until May, 1938, and Instructor and Assistant Clinical Professor of neurology at the Long Island College Medical School, Brooklyn, New York, from September, 1936, until May, 1938.

Dr. Millett is a lieutenant in the United States Naval Reserve and is a member of the Metropolitan Psychiatric Society, New York City. He is married, has a little daughter four months of age, and lives at the Locarno Apartments, 235 Ward Parkway, Kansas City, Missouri.

The Oklahoma City Clinical Society announces that it is joining with the Southern Medical Association of a great meeting to be held in Oklahoma City, November 15 to 18 inclusive. It is hoped you will be able to attend this meeting which will be the most outstanding medical conference in the history of Oklahoma.

The Oklahoma City Clinical Society will continue its regular annual sessions in the fall of 1939.

DR. JAMES STEVENSON, Tulsa, was appointed Councilor of District No. 6, filling the unexpired term of Dr. W. A. Howard, Chelsea.

DR. L. B. WOODS, Ardmore, has returned from New York where he has completed a post graduate course in Obstetrics and Gynecology at the New York Polyclinic Medical School and Hospital.

DR. L. H RITZHAUPT, Guthrie, was the guest speaker at the meeting of the Creek County Medical Society held at Bristow in May. His subject covered the legislative status of things medical, both state and national.

DR. and MRS. MERL CLIFT, Blackwell, are spending the next three months in Europe, with Dr. Clift doing post graduate work in surgery at the University of Edinburgh, Scotland.

The Hospital owned by Dr. Geo. H. Stagner, Erick, was destroyed by fire May 8th, while the doctor was attending the State Medical Meeting in Muskogee. Fire was said to have started when a hot water tank exploded in the basement. Fortunately there was no loss of life or patients injured.

The Clinton News announces that the State Board of Affairs opened bids, May 19th, on an estimated $30,000.00 project of remodeling the north building of the Western Oklahoma Charity hospital at Clinton.

Funds will be taken from a $60,000.00 surplus remaining after $115,000.00 was spent in acquiring the new institution from Dr. McLain Rogers, former owner, last December.

The extensive remodeling program, which will increase the capacity of the north wing to more than 100 patients and the total capacity of the hospital to more than 150 patients, is expected to get underway in early summer.

Dr. H. K. Speed, Jr., superintendent of the hospital, said he had not been informed officially of the Board's intention to do the work by contract but added he presumed the contract would call for installation of a new heating plant and laundry in addition to the remodeling.

DR. H. J. NELSON, Granite, and DR. J. M.

ALLGOOD, Altus, are attending the post graduate course at the Vanderbilt School of Medicine at Nashville, Tennessee.

---o---

TRANSACTIONS OF THE FORTY-SIXTH ANNUAL SESSION OF THE OKLAHOMA STATE MEDICAL ASSOCIATION, MUSKOGEE, MAY 9, 10, 11, 1938

THE COUNCIL
May 9, 1938, 3 P.M.

Meeting of the Council called to order by the President, Dr. Sam A. McKeel, with the following members present: Drs. McNeill, Speed, Fulton, Aisenstadt, Walker, Howard, Templin, Kuyrkendall and Willour.

The minutes of the meeting of the Council on November 3, 1937, were read by Dr. Willour and approved.

The matter of publishing Dr. Edward H. Ochsner's address was discussed and it was decided to give Dr. Ochsner the privilege of having it published by anyone he chose.

The bills receivable next p r e s e n t e d to the Council, were gone over in more or less detail, the aggregate being $612.75; showing a decrease over previous years.

The matter of the balance, which Mr. Clearman claims, $164.64, was discussed by the Council and was allowed to carry over until the Auditing Committee had completed the audit of the Secretary's accounts. Action to be taken at the next meeting of the Council.

The Council next considered the expenditures of the Legislative Committee during the past year, the expense having been incurred as a result of the Initiative Petition No. 166 and the bills of the attorney, hand writing experts, et cetera, were gone over.

On motion of Dr. Willour, seconded by Dr. Howard, and which unanimously carried, an Auditing Committee was appointed, with Drs. L. C. Kuyrkendall, Chairman; E. Albert Aisenstadt, and O. E. Templin.

The proposition of employing a full time executive secretary was discussed by the Council and after going over the expense for the past year, taking into consideration the fact that $2,000.00 from this year's dues was paid on our indebtedness, and $2,000.00 being appropriated for Post Graduate Medical Teaching, it was thought that it would be impossible for the Council, under present conditions, to finance the employment of such a secretary, unless increased income could be obtained.

Dr. Pearce advised that the $2,000.00 for Post Graduate Medical Teaching had to be paid when due otherwise both the State Health Department and the Commonwealth Fund would withdraw their aid.

The proposition of selling our bonds, which are hypothecated, in order to liquidate a portion of our indebtedness was presented by Dr. Speed. This was discussed by Drs. Howard and Fulton and on motion of Dr. Fulton, seconded by Dr. Templin, it was decided not to sell the bonds at this time.

The Secretary presented the matter of financing the Journal and showed that our advertising income for the past year had exceeded the printing of the Journal by about $1,500.00. This being the first time that the Journal had been completely self supporting. It was also called to the attention of the Council that the Cooperative Medical Advertising Bureau had treated this Journal very fairly, giving us our full quota of national advertising. The Cooperative Medical Advertising Bureau has increased their rates and the Journal increased their rates to all advertisers and in view of this fact we have lost practically none of our advertising business.

Dr. McNeill discussed the cost of publication of the Journal and said he had consulted with five different publishing companies in Oklahoma City and found it impossible to obtain as good a contract as the present one.

Mead Johnson & Company had communicated with the Secretary and their communications were presented to the Council relative to the Council endorsing the picture "Birth of a Baby." The matter was discussed and it was finally decided, on motion of Dr. Willour, seconded by Dr. Aisenstadt, that decision be withheld until a showing of the film could be had. Carried by vote of 7 to 2.

The Council, having heard some criticism relative to the discharge of Jess Harper as executive secretary, recommended that in the report to the House of Delegates they be given the reason for this discharge—that reason being lack of funds with which to pay him.

On motion, duly seconded, the Council adjourned.

THE COUNCIL
May 10, 1938, 3 P.M.

The meeting was called to order by Dr. Sam A. McKeel, and the following were present: Drs. Aisenstadt, Fulton, Howard, McNeill, McKeel, Speed, Templin, Walker and Willour.

The question of raising money for the employment of a full time executive secretary, in compliance with the resolution adopted at the meeting of the House of Delegates, was discussed and their qualifications were considered, the probable amount necessary to finance their salary and expenses.

Dr. James Stevenson, Tulsa, who was a guest of the Council, discussed the work of a full time executive secretary in Tulsa County, as well as in the State of Kansas.

On motion of Dr. Willour, seconded by Dr. Walker, and unanimously carried, the President-Elect, Dr. Speed, was authorized to appoint a committee of three, the majority of them to be members of the Council, to accept applications and investigate applicants for this position of full time executive secretary. This committee to report back to the Council. The following were appointed: Drs. J. D. Osborn, Jr., Chairman; Phil M. McNeill, and James Stevenson.

Dr. E. Albert Aisenstadt, for the Auditing Committee, reported that the accounts of the Secretary were found correct and moved the audit submitted be accepted. Duly seconded, this motion carried unanimously.

On recommendation of the Auditing Committee, a motion was made by Dr. J. A. Walker, seconded by Dr. O. E. Templin, that in view of that fact that Mr. Clearman had received a check in the amount of $146.64, marked payment in full to date, properly endorsed by him, and inasmuch as the audit revealed excessive expense accounts during his stay in Oklahoma City, and inasmuch as no service has been rendered by him since the date of the above mentioned check, the Secretary is instructed to issue no additional checks on this account.

Motion carried by vote of nine to two.

There being no further business the Council adjourned.

HOUSE OF DELEGATES
May 9, 1938, 8 P.M.

The meeting called to order by the Speaker of the House, James D. Osborn, Jr.

Dr. Starry, Oklahoma City, moved that the reading of the minutes of the last meeting be dispensed with as they were published in the June, 1937, issue of the Journal. Seconded by Dr. Fulton, unanimously carried.

Dr. Fulton, Atoka, was recognized and said "Before we take up any business, I would like to call your attention to one thing. There is a member who is not here tonight and will not be here tomorrow, although we have expected him, a man who has been a member of the Association in Indian Territory and of the Oklahoma State Medical Association for about 45 years. He has always been in attendance. He has been an active man. I am speaking of our friend, Dr. LeRoy Long, of Oklahoma City, who has had an attack of sickness, coronary thrombosis, I understand. I therefore move you that our Secretary be authorized to extend to Dr. Long our sympathy in his sickness." The motion was seconded and carried, and the Secretary sent a telegram of sincere regret to Dr. Long.

The Speaker then called upon the President, Dr. Sam A. McKeel:

"Mr. Speaker and Gentlemen of the House of Delegates I am the first man to have the honor of addressing the Speaker in this body for the purpose of making an address. This is a change in our State Association that I am sure will be very acceptable. My purpose in talking to you this evening is to inform you of some things that I would like to see done after my term of office expires.

Socialized medicine is being debated all over the nation—in the high schools, colleges and even in the Congress of these United States. I don't know the number of people that have called on me, students asking me to help them arrange or get up data on socialized medicine. Some of them are in favor and some against it. I do not feel that I am competent to discuss the question fully, but I am against socialized medicine or any other form of medicine that takes away from the doctor his individuality. I am opposed to State Hospitals scattered over the State, except for the care of the insane and the tubercular. Institutions are being advocated by every one of our law-makers. It is things of this kind I am opposed to, and I don't think I should raise my voice against a thing like that unless I felt I had something to offer in its place. I believe it would be better for the indigent sick and for the medical profession if a tax were levied in each County, sufficient to take care of the indigent in that County. I think it could be done with less taxation than it can be done to have a hospital in each district. I mean that we do owe it to the indigent sick to take care of them and we owe it to them to let them select the doctor who treats them. There is an old adage that 'beggars cannot be choosers.' That might be all right except for the sick, but I for one do not want to treat anyone that does not want me, even if I had a State appointment.

In view of this I have a resolution to present for your approval or rejection."

(This resolution was referred to the Resolutions Committee and never brought back to the Floor of the House of Delegates.)

Dr. Lealon Lamb, Clinton, then presented another resolution, which was referred to the Resolutions Committee and was not returned to the floor of the House of Delegates.

Dr. Ned Smith, Tulsa, then requested a report of the Credentials Committee before any further vote was taken.

Dr. W. A. Howard, Chelsea, Chairman of the Credentials Committee, reported 71 Delegates present and voting.

On motion of Dr. McNeill, seconded by Dr. Aisenstadt, which carried unanimously, our State Health Commissioner was extended the privilege of the floor.

On motion of Dr. Fulton, Atoka, seconded by Dr. Cook, Tulsa, carried, Dr. James L. Shuler, Durant, was extended the courtesy of the floor.

The Speaker then ruled that a quorum would be 25 and then called Dr. H. K. Speed, for his address, who said, in part: "Dr. McKeel, if I do as good a job as you have done, I will be entirely satisfied. Gentlemen, I have never approached a job with as much concern as I do this. I feel that most of you are my friends. I had a job similar to this three years ago and I thought then being President of the State Medical Association would be about the best job in the world. I am going to expend every effort in trying to salve our trouble, because I believe there are as many different ideas and different views as there are members in this Association. I will listen to everybody's advice, and invite all of you to give me advice and I will take all I can take and disregard the rest, and hope there will be a friendly relationship when I leave this place. We have too many grudges in this Association. Let's get them out of our system. We are all medical men and have a job to do; we accomplished a little last year and most of you know what that job was, how it was outlined before we started. You didn't know who was going to carry out your wishes when you voted to do certain things. Those things were done seriously, and some have not been satisfactory. It makes no difference to me whether anybody is satisfied. I have committed no offence for which I am sorry. If I have been wrong it has been through ignorance and I have no apology to make. But, Gentlemen, let's forget all that has gone and try to accomplish something in the next 12 months. I am for organized medicine altogether. What you do with the hospital situation will be entirely satisfactory to me, because I am first, last and always for the best interest of my profession. It is my way of making a living.

I am going to ask you gentlemen in no uncertain terms to contact your candidates for office and see them before they go down to the capitol next January, so that our Legislative Committee will not have an impossible job before them. I beseech you, do not endorse any candidate or condemn any candidate without knowing his views first. We must be in position to expect a fair deal from anybody that might be elected to office. If we have several candidates in the different counties to represent us in the House and Senate I think it not unwise to put these gentlemen on the spot and see just where they stand on our proposed program. Had this been done previously we would not have had so much trouble with our Basic Science Law. I think it is our duty to our profession, to ourselves and to our state in general to try to get these gentlemen committed, and it is every man's duty to get behind this method of procedure."

On motion of Dr. Cliff Logan, Hominy, seconded by Dr. R. M. Adams, Hobart, an appeal was made from a ruling of the Chair as to presentation of resolutions, Dr. Logan insisting that the resolutions be discussed immediately by the House and not referred to the Resolutions Committee.

This motion, requiring two-thirds majority to carry, was defeated.

The report of the Council to the House of Delegates was then presented by the Secretary:

"The Council of the Oklahoma State Medical Association hereby submits its report to the House of Delegates as authorized by the Constitution and By-Laws of this organization:

"There has been much business to come before the Council at meetings during the past year, however, they have not been as frequent as in the previous year. The principal thing which has made it necessary for our meetings has been the work of the Legislative Committee, in their endeavor to defeat the Initiative Petition No. 166, which you all know would destroy our Medical Practice Act. The Legislative Committee has carried on as active a campaign as possible with the amount of funds available—as their report will indicate.

"At one meeting of the Council $2,000.00 annually

for two years, was appropriated for Post Graduate Medical Teaching, this to be used in conjunction with an appropriation from the Commonwealth Fund and money from Congressionally appropriated funds to the State Health Department, and we are delighted to see this work already inaugurated.

"The Council, in considering the appropriation, had reason to believe that much would be accomplished. FIRST, there would be an improvement in the practice of obstetrics throughout the state; SECOND, as the full time Instructor would be available to appear before lay groups, he would be able to 'sell' organized medicine to the groups of Oklahoma; THIRD, if the doctors see that the State Medical Association is really doing something to advance their professional interests, the membership of the State Medical Association would thereby be increased.

"The Council has heard some criticism from the membership because Mr. Harper was discontinued as executive secretary, and we feel that the House of Delegates is entitled to know that our reason for discontinuing his service was because we did not have sufficient funds to meet the expense.

"The Delegates will notice the fact that the Journal of the Association, during the past year, more than made expenses, the audit showing a profit of about $1,500.00. It would be fortunate if this amount could be increased, however, it probably cannot be, as we are now carrying all of the advertising that a Journal of this size can expect to acquire. Our amount of advertising is largely based upon two factors: the size of our Journal and the number of subscriptions, and we are informed that we are now carrying as much advertising, through the Cooperative Medical Advertising Bureau, as any other Journal of our size.

"If the same profit can be maintained in the future, the Editor has proposed that the basic contract be increased eight pages for each issue. Our basic contract at this time is for 56 pages and we would like to increase it to 64.

Respectfully submitted,
Sam A. McKeel, President."

On motion of Dr. Fulton, seconded by Dr. Cook, the report of the Council was adopted.

The Speaker then called for report of Committees, these reports, which were published in the Journal, were presented by the Secretary and in all instances were adopted.

Dr. Turner, Chairman of the Committee on Post Graduate Medical Teaching, submitted a supplement verbal report as follows: "We have 85 per cent attendance in the northeastern part of the state. Letters went out last Thursday to the southeastern part, and we had six registrations come in Monday morning. That is excellent, I believe. I would like to express the appreciation of the Committee personally to Dr. Pearce for his fine cooperation. He is saving us lots of money by mimeographing our letters. Dr. Patterson of the School of Medicine allowed us to use some of his equipment, which would have been very expensive. That is saving the State Association, for their Post Graduate Teaching, a great deal of money."

Dr. Byrum, Chairman of the Committee on Public Policy and Legislation, said "of the 1,349 who are members of the Association 625, or less than half, responded to the Committee's appeal for funds. Part of this was spent in printing the Petition which you have in your hands at this time; other money was spent in preparation of the case before the Secretary of State, and more expense was necessary to appeal this to the State Supreme Court. A motion is now pending in the Supreme Court to dismiss this bill. If the Supreme Court acts favorably on that motion then our troubles are ended. If this matter comes to a vote the campaign must be diligently prosecuted and it is

my opinion that the doctors of the state must arouse themselves to greater activity than ever before."

On motion of Dr. McNeill, seconded by Dr. Walker, the report of this committee was unanimously adopted.

The election of Honorary Members was next taken up and on motion, duly seconded and carried, the following were elected: Doctors Caroline Bassman, Claremore; J. C. Bushyhead, Claremore; W. T. Ray, Gould; D. D. McHenry, Oklahoma City; G. W. West, Eufaula.

The Speaker then called for report of the Resolutions Committee, and Dr. Ewing, Chairman, requested further time, which was granted.

Dr. McNeill presented the following amendment to the By-Laws, which was accepted and will be voted upon at the next meeting of the House of Delegates.

Chapter VII — Committees

Section 1. The Standing Committees of this Association to be appointed by the President, shall be as follows:

1. A Committee on Scientific Work.
2. A Committee on Public Policy and Legislation.
3. A Committee on Medical Defense of the Council.
4. A Committee on Medical Education and Hospitals.
5. A Committee on Medical Economics.
6. A Committee on Public Health.

Each of these committees, except the Public Health Committee shall consist of three members, each of whom shall serve for a term of three years. One member of each of these Committees, except the Public Health Committee, shall be appointed annually by the President; one member shall be appointed for a term of three years; one for two years, and one each for a year. The Public Health Committee shall consist of one member from each Councilor District to be appointed as follows: Three members for three years; three members for two years; and four members for one year, and continuing in this manner, maintaining a Committee of ten (10) members. The President may appoint such other Committees as may be deemed necessary for special occasions.

Section 2, Section 3, Section 4, Section 5, and Section 6, as is.

Section 7, Change: "The Committee on Public Health shall study the problems of Public Health of the State of Oklahoma and advise with the Commissioner of Public Health as to an acceptable program."

Section 8, (Present Section 7).

* * *

Dr. Starry, Oklahoma City, presented an amendment to the Constitution:

Article VI — Council Members

The Council shall be the Board of Trustees of this Association. The Council shall have full authority and power of the House of Delegates between annual sessions, unless the House of Delegates shall be called into session, as provided in the Constitution and By-Laws. It shall consist of the (1) Councilors, (2) the President, (3) President-Elect, (4) Secretary-Treasurer-Editor, (5) Speaker of the House of Delegates, and (6) the Vice Speaker of the House of Delegates. The quorum shall consist of eight members.

This amendment was accepted by the House of Delegates and will be voted upon at the 1939 meeting.

Dr. Wendell Long, Oklahoma City, was recognized by the Chair, and presented the following discussion as to the report of the Committee on Control of Cancer:

"I am Chairman of the Committee on Control of Cancer. We are getting through rather early and I hesitate to speak about it, but apparently many of the members of the State Medical Association missed some of the masterpieces in our State Journal. In that State Journal was a report of our Committee in March or in April, which outlined the Women's Field Army activities. I call attention to it so that the members may read that report as applying to Oklahoma. I call attention to that report, because in Oklahoma, we have taken the greatest care to establish the policy so that the doctors in each County will have full control of the activities within that County, not only full control of the medical activities, but full control of the Women's Field Army activities within that County. The second thing I would like to suggest is that this is the only scheme of which I know in which lay education is attempted by organized medicine, and controlled by organized medicine as such. You can judge it on its merits whether that is a desirable way to have contact with the lay public. The third point is the fact that the American Society for the Control of Cancer has been most liberal in giving out material and in giving funds for the establishment of this program in this state, and up until the first of April all of the County Societies had been informed and material sent to them, and the Women's organization over the state had been formed with total expenditure, including some 80,000 pieces of literature, 12 projection machines, 60 film scripts, and our office expense in Oklahoma City, of $960.00. All the women worked for nothing and the doctors did the same thing. Mr. Speaker, I thank you for the privilege of presenting these additional points."

House adjourned.

* * *

HOUSE OF DELEGATES
May 10, 1938, 8 A. M.

Meeting called to order by Speaker of the House.

Dr. C. P. Bondurant, Oklahoma City, appointed Sergeant-at-Arms and asked that none be admitted but Delegates and Members of the State Medical Association.

Report of the Credentials Committee by Dr. Howard.

Speaker asked for nominations for President-Elect.

Dr. Ewing presented the name of Dr. W. A. Howard, Chelsea. Nomination seconded by Dr. Ritzhaupt.

On motion of Dr. Adams, seconded by Dr. Fulton, which unanimously carried, nominations were closed and the Secretary was instructed to cast the entire ballot for Dr. Howard as President-Elect. The Secretary complied with the motion.

The newly elected President-Elect addressed the House of Delegates, saying "I appreciate this honor you have conferred upon me. I am just an ordinary country doctor and practitioner. I know the record that has been set by my predecessors and shall endeavor to merit this confidence you have placed in me. I have one object in view and that is to forward a constructive program for organized medicine in Oklahoma."

The speaker called for nominations for Secretary-Treasurer-Editor and the name of Dr. Willour was presented by Dr. McCarley seconded by Dr. Walker and Dr. Fulton.

On motion of Dr. Harris, Wilburton, seconded by Dr. Cook, the nominations were closed and Dr. Howard was instructed to cast the vote of the House of Delegates for Dr. Willour. Dr. Howard complied.

Nominations for Councilors were then called for and the following: Doctors Risser for District No. 3;

McNeill for District No. 4; Hardy for District No. 5; and Stevenson for District No. 6, were named.

On motion of Dr. Willour, seconded by Dr. Logan, and unanimously carried, the above named doctors were elected Councilors from their respective Districts.

Dr. H. C. Weber, member of the Committee on Post Graduate Medical Teaching then presented Dr. Edward N. Smith, full time Instructor on Post Graduate Medical Teaching in Obstetrics, who expressed himself as being pleased to meet the members of the House of Delegates, and saying in part "We have been underway for about five weeks and the attendance seems to be between 95 and 98 per cent. I have answered about 50 requests for consultation, ranging from ectopic pregnancy to a little matter of malpractice. One doctor has to drive 70 miles to attend this course and all of these things are very gratifying. I feel there is a definite need for this work. This is really a great responsibility that you have placed on me and whether or not your County Societies and I meet that responsibility had better be talked about next year."

The Speaker then called for nominations for Delegates to the American Medical Association.

Dr. Searle, Tulsa, placed the name of Dr. Cook, Tulsa, which was seconded by Dr. McNeill, Oklahoma City.

The Secretary then explained that our quota had been reduced from three to two Delegates and explained that they would have to be elected in alternate years.

Dr. Ewing then asked the question "When do the Delegates' term begin and end?"

The Secretary stated "Drs. Cook and Reed were elected for the years 1939 and 1940. It has been the custom of the State Medical Association that Delegates begin their terms of office one year from time of election."

Dr. Ewing then asked where the authority for this could be found.

Dr. Willour replied: "There is no authority but it has been a matter of custom since the organization of this Association and the Constitution and By-Laws do not specify as to this particular point."

In view of the complicated situation Dr. Cook requested the privilege of the floor and tendered his resignation as Delegate. This was followed by Reed's resignation.

The Speaker said, before ruling upon the question, "I would like to read a letter from Dr. Wm. C. Woodward of the Legal Department of the American Medical Association." This he did and after some discussion presented the following ruling: "THAT Dr. McLain Rogers, Clinton, is the duly elected Delegate for 1938 and we will proceed with the election of one Delegate."

Dr. Phil McNeill made a motion that we appeal from the ruling of the Chair. This was duly seconded, but two-thirds being required, the motion was lost upon vote.

Dr. Searle then nominated Dr. Cook, Tulsa.

Dr. Lealon Lamb, Clinton, nominated Dr. Reed, Oklahoma City.

Dr. Ritzhaupt, Guthrie, nominated Dr. Fulton, Atoka.

The ballot was then spread and the tellers reported Dr. Fulton 29 votes, Dr. Cook 21, and Dr. Reed 20.

The Chair then ruled that it took a majority to elect, and Drs. Fulton and Cook having the largest number of votes, were voted upon and the ballot was reported showing Dr. Cook received 38 and Dr. Fulton 36.

On motion of Dr. Fulton, duly seconded, Dr. Cook was unanimously elected as Delegate.

Dr. I. W. Bollinger, Henryetta, placed the name of Dr. Edwards, Okmulgee, as alternate for Dr. Cook.

Dr. Turner, Oklahoma City, placed the name of

Dr. Reed as alternate for Dr. Rogers.

On motion, duly seconded, these alternates were unanimously elected.

The Speaker then called for nominations for a Meeting Place for 1939.

Dr. Dale Collins, Oklahoma City, invited the Association to that City for 1939.

On Motion duly seconded their invitation was unanimously accepted.

Dr. Willour read the amendment to the By-Laws, presented at the last meeting of the House of Delegates (May 9th, 1938). On motion of Dr. Bondurant, seconded by Dr. Ritzhaupt, this amendment was unanimously adopted.

Report of the Resolutions Committee was then called for and Dr. Ewing, Chairman, presented the following:

RESOLUTION

"WHEREAS, there has been introduced by Congressman Drew of Pennsylvania, a bill which would place osteopaths on the same plane with qualified doctors of medicine, under the United States Employees' Compensation Act, and

"WHEREAS, it is our opinion that osteopathy is not a safe method of diagnosis and treatment of disease or injury,

"THEREFORE BE IT RESOLVED that we advise our Senators and Members of Congress to oppose this measure."

The above resolution was duly seconded and adopted.

* * *

The following resolution was presented and Dr. Ewing moved its adoption:

"WHEREAS, the business activities of the Oklahoma State Medical Association are increasing in volume and in importance, and

"WHEREAS, the constitution of the Oklahoma State Medical Association provides for the employment of an Executive Secretary, and

"WHEREAS, we believe that the best interests of this State Association would be served through the employment of a full-time Executive Secretary,

"THEREFORE BE IT RESOLVED, that the House of Delegates recommends that the Council employ an Executive Secretary at the earliest practicable time."

This resolution was discussed by Drs. Ned Smith and James Stevenson of Tulsa. In their discussion they laid great stress upon the employment of this executive secretary, at the earliest possible moment, not later than Jan. 1st, 1939. Various methods of raising sufficient funds to comply with the above resolution were discussed, i.e., raising the dues, voluntary contributions, or assessments. **On motion of Dr. Ned R. Smith, seconded by Dr. J. S. Fulton, unanimously carrying, the annual dues will be $12.00 beginning January 1, 1939.**

* * *

Dr. Aisenstadt made a motion that the President of the Association be authorized to appoint a committee of three to have charge of the revision of the Constitution and By-Laws, and submit their report at the next meeting of the House of Delegates. Seconded.

An amendment was offered by Dr. Ritzhaupt, providing for a Committee of three, appointed by the Speaker, approved by the Council, and authorized to secure legal talent, if necessary, to assist in carrying out this work. This was accepted by Dr. Aisenstadt and unanimously adopted.

Dr. Reed suggested that the Judicial Council of the American Medical Association be called upon to assist in this matter. The amended motion was there voted upon and unanimously carried.

Dr. Ritzhaupt then presented the following legislative program: "I move that the House of Delegates approve the legislative program which follows and instruct the President, Councilors and Legislative Committee of the Oklahoma State Medical Association to prepare in detail and diligently try to fulfill it.

"1. Authorizing the State Board of Medical Examiners to annually register each physician in the state who has been examined or registered under the Medical Practice Act of the State of Oklahoma.

"2. To resist and defeat any legislation that would destroy or lower the standard as set out in the Medical Practice Act of the State of Oklahoma.

"3. To encourage such legislation which will make it mandatory for the County Commissioners of the several counties in the state to set aside sufficient funds to provide hospitalization, medical and surgical care for the 'medical needy.'

"4. To ethically and professionally endeavor to preserve such statutes as now exist for the protection of the public health and welfare of the citizenship of Oklahoma."

On motion by Dr. Ritzhaupt, seconded by Dr. Willour, and adopted, that it become the Legislative Program of the State Association.

On motion of Dr. Byrum, seconded by Dr. Ritzhaupt and unanimously carried, the Secretary was instructed to write the Secretary of each County Medical Society to the effect that it is the request of the House of Delegates that each County Society will be expected to make a contribution equal to $5.00 per member, this for the purpose of paying the expenses of the full-time Executive Secretary, until the payment of dues for 1939.

Dr. Garrison, Oklahoma City, presented the following communication from the Women's Auxiliary and said "The purpose is that this may be a help to you in the situation which we have discussed most of the morning. The purpose behind it is correct; therefore, I move you the sentiment expressed in this communication be approved by the House of Delegates:"

"To the House of Delegates,
Oklahoma State Medical Association,
Muskogee, Oklahoma.

"Gentlemen: The Women's Auxiliary to the Oklahoma State Medical Association, with a membership of 400, feels that it may be of great potential service to the State Association in matters of public education.

"With this in mind we wish to present for your consideration—

"First—That the Auxiliary be given an associate membership on the Public Policy and Legislation Committee, without vote but for the purpose of correctly informing the Auxiliary membership concerning legislative matters.

"Second—That we wish to offer our services to the County and State Associations for such organized lay-education as the Associations may direct.

> Signed: The Executive Board
> Mrs. Hugh Perry, President
> Mrs. Geo. H. Garrison, President-Elect.
> Mrs. Frank L. Flack, Secretary
> Mrs. W. S. Larrabee, Treasurer."

The above was seconded by Dr. Bondurant and unanimously carried.

On motion of Dr. Bondurant, seconded by Dr. Lamb, and carried unanimously, our Delegates to the American Medical Association are to go uninstructed as to future meeting place.

Dr. J. A. Morrow, Sallisaw, addressed the House of Delegates, insisting that they use every effort to see to it that the newly elected Senate and House are favorable to our legislative program and that we not wait until the January election, but before we vote, ascertain definitely their attitude toward Organized Medicine and their problems.

House adjourned.

NECROLOGY COMMITTEE

The following report of the Necrology Committee was presented at the Memorial Service:

Each year at the time of our annual meeting it is indeed fitting that we pause and pay our respects to the members of our profession who have been called from the activities of life into the mysteries of the great hereafter.

Year by year we miss the faces of our friends with whom we have associated in the activities of this Association. Those of us who participated in the organization meeting at Oklahoma City in 1906 have seen many changes. There are but few now active who participated in this meeting. The ones who laid the foundation for this structure and so well planned for its development and progress have with a few exceptions passed on, and others have taken their places and will carry on the work. Those of us who belong to the Old Guard mourn today the loss of our old friends; we have lived to see many changes. Years of connection with this organization and its individual members have generated within us an affection and loyalty that makes loss or error strike to our very hearts.

The passing of an old associate or any misconduct of the Organization arouses within us a feeling of sadness or regret. We have our extra curricular hobbies, we have our golf or bridge buddies, we have our business and dinner club associates, but for our old and most intimate friends we come back to our profession and the men with whom we have worked as Doctors in the relief of suffering and the effort to raise the standard of the practice of medicine in Oklahoma.

May the members of this Association from generation to generation ever keep in mind the pioneer work which has been necessary to make possible this progressive organization. Never forget the old fashioned Doctor with his old fashioned and high ideals. Respect him, honor him, and sometimes mention him, that his reflection on this structure may not grow so dim as to be forgotten.

During the past year the Great Reaper has stretched forth His hand and taken from our membership about the usual number; their faces, their presence and their wise counsel we miss today. They have finished the course, they have kept the faith, and leave with us the memories of pleasant association and broken ties of friendship. Let us revere their memory, and so conduct ourselves both as individual Doctors and as an Association as to reflect no discredit upon their cherished memories.

The following list of deceased members have been reported to us during the past year:

Bagby, Oliver, Vinita, Craig.
Callahan, Hubert W., Tulsa, Tulsa.
Caton, Charles, Wynona, Osage.
Chambers, M. E. Vinson, Greer.
Clifton, G. M., Norman, Cleveland.
Cox, Charles P., Ninnekah, Grady.
Crawford, Gwen W., Bartlesville, Washington.
Fannin, Frank, Muskogee, Muskogee.
Friedeman, Paul, Stillwater, Payne.
Garabedian, G. A., Tulsa, Tulsa.
Hammer, John E., Kiowa, Kansas, Woods.
Harris, H. A. McAlester, Pittsburg.
Hinson, T. B., Enid, Garfield.
House, Chas. F., Walters, Cotton.
Howell, Chas. H., Meeker, Okfuskee.
Jacobs, J. C., Miami, Ottawa.
Joss, Wm. Irwin, Erick, Beckham.
Lain, L. C., Oklahoma City, Oklahoma.
Leonard, John D., Wagoner, Wagoner.
Mays, R. H., Altus, Jackson.
McCallum, C. L., Sapulpa, Creek.
Milroy, Joseph A., Okmulgee, Okmulgee.
Phillips, I., Miami, Ottawa.
Stooksbury, Jacob M., Shawnee, Pottawatomie.

Werner, John W., Newkirk, Kay.
West, A. A. Guthrie, Logan.
Wiley, G. A., Norman, Cleveland.

---o---

News Notes of Woman's Auxiliary

MRS. L. S. WILLOUR, McAlester, retiring president of the Women's Auxiliary of the Pittsburg County Medical Society, was elected State Vice-President at their meeting at the convention of the Oklahoma State Medical Association in Muskogee, in May.

The silver tray, awarded to the outstanding unit each year, was won by the Oklahoma County auxiliary.

---o---

The Management of the Septic Patient With Otitis Media

J. H. Maxwell, Ann Arbor, Mich. (Journal A. M. A., May 7, 1938), employs the expression "the septic patient with otitis media" rather than "the patient with otitic sepsis" in order to emphasize the frequently forgotten fact that the otitis media may be an incident in the course of an infection elsewhere in the body responsible for the patient's sepsis. In the present discussion those patients have been considered septic in whom, during the course of an otitis media, leukocytosis has developed with intermittent fever rising to 103 F. or higher at least once daily and who have continued to manifest such evidence of illness without abatement for five days or longer. A septic patient with otitis media may fall into one of three rather clearly defined groups: In the first group there is an infectious process, local or general, producing the clinical picture of sepsis antedating the otitis media. Unless a careful and detailed history is obtained the otologist may be led to performing a mastoidectomy or ablation of a sigmoid sinus when the source of the sepsis is extra-aural. The second group of cases is that in which there develops during the course of an acute suppurative otitis media an intercurrent infection which in itself is responsible for the appearance of sepsis. Because of this possibility, one never should be hasty in performing a mastoidectomy on a septic patient without careful attention to a complete physical examination. The third group of cases represents those of real otitis sepsis in which the infection of the middle ear and mastoid is responsible for the whole picture. These cases require truly individualized management, both medical and surgical. In such a patient one may be dealing with a toxemia or with a true septicopyemia, which may or may not be related to actual phlebitis or thrombosis of the sigmoid sinus.

---o---

Undulant Fever: Its Treatment With Sulfanilamide

Brucella melitensis, originally known as Micrococcus melitensis, is pleomorphic, its morphology in part determined by the culture medium or the preparation used for its study. Morphologically it is considered variously by several authors on bacteriology to be a coccus, a bacillus or a coccobacillus. On this basis, with the effect of the drug in question established against certain other pathogenic bacterial forms, Robert L. Stern and Ken W. Blake, Los Angeles (Journal A. M. A., May 7, 1938), working independently, gave sulfanilamide in therapeutic doses to each of three private patients suffering from clinically and serologically established undulant fever. Highly satisfactory and prompt results with clinical cure followed. The maximal dosage according to present standards appears to be necessary.

ABSTRACTS : REVIEWS : COMMENTS
and CORRESPONDENCE

SURGERY AND GYNECOLOGY
Abstracts, Reviews and Comments from
LeRoy Long Clinic
714 Medical Arts Building, Oklahoma City

Segmental Enteritis; Richard Lewisohn; Surgery, Gynecology and Obstetrics; February, 1938.

The subject of so called regional or as the author prefers to call it, segmental enteritis, is being widely discussed at present. A large number of papers on this subject have appeared in the last four years. Opinions differ not only as to the pathogenesis of these interesting lesions but also as to the best method of surgical treatment.

Undoubtedly a few years will elapse until we arrive at fairly definite views concerning the etiology of this disease and the best form of treatment for these lesions.

The author's conclusions are as follows: 1. Segmental or regional enteritis is not a rare disease. 2. Opinions differ widely not only as to the pathogenesis of these interesting lesions, but also as to the best method of surgical treatment. 3. This lesion is encountered most frequently in the terminal ileum. However, it may occur in any part of the gastro-intestinal tract. 4. It is doubtful whether segmental ileitis and ileocolitis are clinical entities. They may represent an attenuated form of acute ulcerative colitis and ileitis. 5. Perianal fistulas are frequently encountered. 6. Ileocolostomy with division of the ileum may effect a complete cure. 7. In the presence of fistulous communications with other parts of the intestinal tract primary resection becomes mandatory.

LeRoy D. Long.

Malignant Disease of the Small Intestine, Delayed Anastomosis Following Resection in Chronic Obstruction; P. K. Gilman; Western Journal of Surgery, Obstetrics and Gynecology; May, 1938.

Conditions found in the small bowel differ considerably from those in the large bowel. There is an almost complete absence of abrupt angulation associated with fluidity of alkaline contents in the former but no real basic difference to account for the rarity of malignant growths of the small gut compared with the rest of the canal.

This freedom of the small bowel applies not alone to growths primary in type, but, as is well illustrated in the duodenum, to invasion by extension. Carcinoma is rarely found at autopsy. Formerly death from intestinal obstruction undoubtedly included cases of cancer of the small bowel. Sarcoma is apparently found more frequently in the small than in the large bowel. Malignancy in the small bowel apparently manifests itself twice as frequently in men as in women.

The earlier in the disease the diagnosis of obstruction is made and exploration done the better prognosis. At best the prognosis is poor for malignant tumors whether operable or inoperable.

Intra-intestinal fluid levels and gas in the distended bowel shown in the X-ray plates denotes obstruction.

Tumors of the small bowel cause no characteristic symptoms. Symptoms present are usually those of intermittent partial obstruction.

Delayed anastomosis after resection where great disparity in size and physical condition between the resected ends exists would seem to be indicated. The procedure followed in one of the author's cases caused no more shock than would have followed enterostomy with a later resection and anastomosis and it resulted in lessened morbidity.

LeRoy D. Long.

Pilonidal Cysts; Surgery, Gynecology and Obstetrics; Stephen A. Zieman; February 1, 1938.

Pilonidal cysts are by no means rare. Numerous theories have been proposed in explanation of the etiology and pathology. Subjectively, pilonidal cysts are without symptoms unless infection sets in with the usual sequelae of inflammation.

There is considerable discussion regarding the treatment of pilonidal cysts. Summarily, the many methods may be condensed to: 1. Primary closure with suture after excision of tract. 2. Transplantation (Lahey method). 3. Excision with or without the use of the cautery knife and packing.

A recent article by L. K. Ferguson and P. M. Mecray in American Journal of Surgery, 1937, sponsors the primary suture method. An article by H. Rogers and M. G. Hall in the Archives of Surgery in 1935 leads one to believe that this sort of operation may be performed under the ordinary conditions of office practice. It is difficult to see how one can consider the treatment of pilonidal cyst a routine office procedure. No one can predict the extent, direction, or involvement of adjacent structures of these sinus tracts, and consequently, it appears to be as rash to perform an excision of a pilonidal sinus in the office as it is to resort to an equally dangerous practice of injecting with sclerosing material. Surgeons are unanimous in claiming that primary closure never should be done in recurrent cases, nor in the presence of apparent inflammation. Under these conditions, there is no election; excision and packing is the operation of choice. It is the author's belief that careful dissection can be done only under a general anesthetic with preparation commensurate with the uncertainty apparent in the handling of this type of case.

He thinks that excision with the cautery knife and cauterization of the epithelial sinus tract are likewise fraught with several dangers, not the least of which is the collection of serum that follows a burn. Primary closure, consequently, under these conditions appears contra-indicated.

He feels that the method of excision with open pack and permitting granulation from below is time tried, and in his hands, 100 per cent effective. The objection of long debilitation following such operation with protracted stay in the hospital and subsequent dressings is not substantiated in fact; nor is the criticism of a resulting large tender scar. The average days in the hospital for the writer's series of cases have been two, while the subsequent period of dressing has extended from six to 12 weeks, a favorable comparison with the other methods. The patient is not restricted from work for longer than one week. An interesting observation is that wide excision in this region is associated with little pain or discomfort. He feels that even if there were as much pain as one might expect, the extremely low recurrence should offset any of the above objections. Success is judged by the ultimate criterion of recurrence; assuredly, then, the last method is by far the one of choice.

The procedure followed by the author in pilonidal cyst excision consists in the administration of a gas anesthetic while the patient is flat on his stomach. The usual sterile preparation of the operative field having been completed, injection of methylene-blue-hydrogen-peroxide into the sinus opening is done. He prefers hydrogen-peroxide to ethereal mixtures, or simple water, in as far as the ethereal mixtures are fat solvents and may lead to spurious tract excursions, while the plain water has very little penetration power. Wide excision of approximately two inches on each side of the midline is then done and ligation of the bleeding points accomplished by double No. 0 plain catgut. Occasionally currettement of the presacral fascia is required. With this sacrifice of tissue, one is not likely to overlook a remnant of epithelial structure. Wide excision also gives a large area for complete inspection. An iodoform pack is allowed to remain in the defect for a period of 24 hours. Thereafter, simple vaseline gauze and mercurochrome constitute the bi-weekly dressings. At each dressing, the small bands of adhesions across the midline are ruthlessly destroyed, and the wound permitted to granulate, filling in from below only.

LeRoy D. Long.

Non-invasive Potential "Carcinoma" of the Cervix. By Charles Summers Stevenson, Baltimore, Md., and Elemer Scipiades, Jr., Budapest, Hungary. Surgery, Gynecology and Obstetrics, May, 1938, Volume 66, Page 822.

This is a study based upon examination of all the cervical tissue in the files of the gynecological pathological laboratory of Johns Hopkins Hospital covering 4,000 cases with 10,000 microscopic sections of cervical tissue.

The purpose of this review was the isolation of instances of what they prefer to call non-invasive potential "carcinoma" of cervix and what Schiller considers and treats as definite early carcinoma.

The characteristics of this condition are anoplasia of the epithelial cells, hyperchromatic nuclei, heterogenous confusion of the epithelial cells, and a sharp border between the normal epithelium and the "carcinoma," usually oblique but no projection or invasion of the epithelium into the sub-epithelial structures.

In their study these authors were able to find 18 cases of this nature and they have studied their case histories in an attempt to correlate these pathological findings with actual carcinoma of the cervix.

In one patient the "carcinoma" remained non-invasive for eight years and one month following which it developed into a clinical carcinoma and caused the death of the patient.

A second patient died of pernicious anemia three years after the first biopsy examination had revealed a non-invasive potential "carcinoma." At autopsy serial sections of this cervix revealed that invasion had taken place shortly before death.

"The original pathological diagnosis in nine cases was 'epidermoid carcinoma of cervix,' while in seven it was 'chronic cervicitis'; both polyps were called benign. As far as we were able to determine, from making serial sections of all available tissue on these cases, all of the growth was apparently removed with the specimen in four of the five trachelorrhaphies, the two amputations, and the one panhysterectomy. In nine of the 11 other patients subjected merely to biopsy, sectioning of the remaining available tissue did not allow us to make up our minds definitely on this point, although in one instance it might well have all been removed." Therefore, in seven of their cases they felt that all of the lesion was apparently removed when the specimen was obtained and would therefore have no significance in the development of a subsequent clinical carcinoma.

Five of the remaining nine cases were recognized as "carcinoma" and were given adequate radium treatment so that they too are of little assistance in establishing the relationship of this condition to clinical carcinoma.

Of the four remaining patients two were given thorough cervical cauterization following biopsy and have had no subsequent clinical carcinoma.

Of the two remaining patients one has not been followed but the other was alive and well when last seen in July, 1936.

The authors therefore present this material feeling that they cannot say definitely that the invasive carcinoma developed as a true growth continuity in any of their patients but that it was highly suggestive and they feel that other studies should be attempted so as to combine it with such as this one in order to ascertain whether or not this non-invasive potential "carcinoma" of the cervix will eventually produce invasion of the stroma and clinical carcinoma.

Comment:

These authors have done a very laborious piece of work and have arrived at no definite conclusion. They are not willing to call this condition definite carcinoma and do not feel that they have justification for establishing a true continuity between this lesion and clinical carcinoma.

However, it must be evident to all that the earliest possible diagnosis of malignancies of the cervix is essential to a high rate of cure and it is equally evident that the lesion is probably present without symptoms for some time before it is even clinically evident upon the basis of present interpretations. It is therefore such work as this that will lead us into a proper appreciation of clinical findings and their correct correlation with pathological courses. It has the additional value of making doctors conscious of such early lesions, difficult to diagnose but relatively easier to cure.

Wendell Long.

The Treatment of Gonococcic Vaginitis with the Estrogenic Hormone. By Richard W. Te Linde. Baltimore, Md. Journal of the American Medical Association, May 14, 1938, Vol. 110, Page 1633.

This is a report of the cure of 175 cases with gonococcic vaginitis by amniotin.

There is a review of the previous work of Te Linde and Brawner published in October, 1935, and abstracted in this department at that time. In their previous work Te Linde and Brawner treated patients with gonococcic vaginitis by oral, hypodermic and vaginal administration of amniotin with results indicating that daily administration of vaginal suppositories containing 600 international units of amniotin was by far the preferable means of treatment.

In their previous series all showed the vaginal epithelial response in an average time of 13 days and the smears became permanently negative in 18 days, though treatment was continued over an average total time of 26 days.

The present routine of treatment adopted by Dr. Te Linde is well given in the original article and is here summarized. One suppository of amniotin containing 1,000 international units is introduced daily at bed time by the mother. The patients are brought back to the clinic at weekly intervals when vaginal smears and washings are made, the washings being made with a small medicine dropper. After the first negative smear the treatment is continued for two more weeks. In the average case the entire treatment extends over about one month. Earlier discontinuation of treatment is associated with recurrences. The children are brought back to the clinic one and two months after discontinuing treatment for routine washings and smear.

The first 100 patients treated have been followed for a much longer time and of them 98 were well at the time of last examination, indicating a high degree of permanence of cures as there is a distinct possibility that the two who were not cured were probably subjected to re-infection.

They have been unable to find any clinical evidence of harm due to the treatment and the laboratory investigations quoted confirm this observation.

There is a rather long discussion of the importance of the increased acidity produced in the vagina as a factor in the cure of these patients.

Dr. Te Linde's summary is quoted below:

"We have reported the cure of 175 patients with gonococcic vaginitis. All, except 16 of those to whom the product was given hypodermically in oil, were cured by the use of amniotin vaginal suppositories. We have yet to encounter a patient who failed to get well by this method of treatment, and we consider it a very satisfactory way of dealing with the disease. A follow-up of our first 100 patients, from three months to two and one-half years after the last treatment, showed 98 of them well. We saw no clinical evidence of harm due to the treatment, and laboratory investigations confirm this observation. We feel that the increased acidity brought about in the vagina by the action of the estrogen is a factor in overcoming the infection, but, since our results were not nearly so good when another acidifying suppository was employed, we believe that amniotin introduces an additional factor. We are inclined to think that this other factor is the covering of the vagina with thick epithelium, which prevents reinfection of the subepithelial tissues and thus permits the inflammatory process in them to subside. Our clinical observations and biopsies have indicated that the essential lesion of gonococcic infection of the lower part of the genital tract in female children is vaginitis."

Comment:

This is an excellent piece of work in stabilizing the treatment of a condition which was, until a few years ago, a most annoying and intractable type of disease. There is no question in my mind but that the proper treatment for gonococcic vaginitis in children is administration of estrogenic substances by vaginal suppositories. The results are satisfactory and convincing.

Wendell Long.

PLASTIC SURGERY
Edited by
GEO. H. KIMBALL, M.D., F.A.C.S.
404 Medical Arts Building, Oklahoma City

Breast Deformities; Anatomical and Physiological Considerations in Plastic Repair. Jacques W. Maliniac, M.D., New York City. American Journal of Surgery, January, 1938.

The author points out that successful repair of the breasts demands complete familiarity with the anatomy and physiology of the structures involved. Also that hypertrophic breasts may be malignant.

Physiology: Embryonic development: Traced from its embryonal origins, the breast first appears as an epidermal ridge extending from the axilla to the groin. Certain points of this ridge are thickened, forming the mammary glands. When the so-called "milk spots" (which are believed to derive from the sweat glands) develop unduly, accessory breasts appear at different points on the site of the epidermal ridge.

Infancy: At birth the breasts consist of epithelial

columns without lumens, but they soon undergo change. The ducts assume definite cylindrical form and a milky fluid may be produced. These characteristic alterations occur in boys as well as girls. The process is completed during the first or second week of life and the epithelium returns to a quiescent state. Until puberty there is no further change. The gland measures about 2 cmm. in diameter and 1 cmm. in thickness.

Puberty: At puberty the female breast begins to develop, reaching adult form and proportions within a varying period of time. The normal breasts are made up principally of connective tissue, with comparatively little fat and glandular tissue. This gives it a characteristic resilience. At this period of life, the breast is usually a firm hemisphere which varies little with change of position, for the connective tissue bands which control its form have not yet sustained the repeated congestion produced by mammary function.

Pregnancy and lactation: Omitting the periodic changes of menstruation (when the tissue is oedematous, the fiber thicker and the epithelium becomes taller and stains more deeply) the next great alteration in the breast occurs during pregnancy. Its volume increases, especially after the third month, and the functional growth of the gland causes a diminution in fibrous tissue, with the result that the breast loses its hemispherical form. The skin covering is stretched and may show distension scars (striae) similar to those which appear on the abdominal wall. With lactation there is a further increase in volume and weight; the breast becomes still more distended and the tendency to pendulousness is heightened. As function ceases, a retrogression of glandular tissue occurs, but the pendulousness frequently remains because of the inability of the skin and supporting ligaments to regain their former elasticity. This is particularly true after repeated pregnancies, the extent of the process varying with the individual.

Senility: The final senile involution of the breast, in which the glandular structure disappears, begins at the menopause. As a rule, this involution involves the skin, fat and fibrous tissue as well as the gland. The result is a small, atropic mamma.

Anatomy:

The author points out that the fixation of the breast is two fold. Number (1) is the skin and number (2) is the retro-mammary fascia. I believe that the skin is the principal means of support. When the skin releases or elongates the pendulous breast develops.

In the plastic repair it is necessary to secure fixation of the transposed breast by using sutures placed against the pectoral fascia.

Blood Supply:

The blood supply must be preserved during reconstruction of the breasts. The breast derives its blood supply from three sources:

1. The thoracic lateral artery (branch of the axillary artery).

2. The internal mammary artery (branch of the subclavicular).

3. Perforant branches deriving from the third to the seventh intercostal arteries.

Surgical Procedure of Choice:

Whenever large amounts of fat and glandular tissue must be removed, the risk of interfering with the blood supply exists. To minimize this the author has employed for many years a two-stage procedure. The nipple is transposed with most of the blood supply intact and secondary resection is postponed until after the "take" of the ventral portion of the gland is complete.

This does not complicate or prolong the repair to any extent. Aside from the risk of necrosis, it is contraindicated to perform a complete reconstruction of two breasts in one stage. Speed is not the primary consideration where form and symmetry and the avoidance of scars are essential elements in a good end-result. Since a one-stage operation must be highly protracted to accomplish all of these aims, it is more advisable to employ the two-stage procedure, which removes all risk to the blood supply and lessens the operative strain on the patient.

Summary:

Fixation of the breast is provided by the skin through multiple fibrous prolongations (Cooper's Ligament) into the gland and by the retro-mammary fascia which provides a suspensory ligament attached to the clavicula. A marked increase in the weight of the breast, from any cause, overtaxes this apparatus and produces ptosis.

In mammary reconstruction, the transposed gland should be firmly attached to the pectoral fascia to simulate normal fixation. This is done by means of a circular row of non-absorbable sutures, which must not be permitted to involve large amounts of gland or fat.

In reducing the gland, the central portion should be left intact to preserve the blood supply to the nipple and to retain such function as exists in the main central ducts. In glandular hypertrophy of the breast, a rare condition bordering on malignancy, the entire breast gland should be removed. Circulation: Circulation in the breast is derived from the (1) thoracic lateral, which supplies the external half and skin; (2) the internal mammary, which is the principal source of supply of the internal half, including the central portion of the gland and the nipple; and (3) several perforant branches of the intercostal arteries which also supply the deep and central portions of the gland. There is little anastomosis between these, so the main blood supply must be carefully preserved in each part.

Since the thoracic lateral does not supply the nipple, the large amounts of glandular structure may be removed from the external quadrant without impairing the "take" of the transposed nipple. Great care must be taken in the excision of excessive fat and glandular structures in the area of the nipple and areola. Although the circular incision in the areola does not endanger the blood supply it should be superficial so as not to injure the underlying circular muscle fibers or interfere with the surrounding vascular plexus.

As the blood supply comes through the deep portion of the gland, there is always risk of interfering with the blood supply when large quantities of fat and glandular tissue must be removed. The author employs a two-stage procedure to minimize this risk. The nipple is transposed with most of the blood supply preserved and secondary resection is postponed until after the "take" of the central portion of the gland is complete.

Comment: I believe that Dr. Maliniac has the soundest plan so far advanced for reconstruction of pendulous breasts. The two-stage plan minimizes the impairment of circulation as well as infection. Recent experience of my own has proved to me that the plan is practical. It is well to remember that all breasts presented are not suited for plastic repair. When the indications are presented there are few operations that give such satisfactory results both to the surgeon and to the patient.

---o---

UROLOGY

Edited by D. W. Branham, M.D.
514 Medical Arts Building, Oklahoma City

Fundamentals In Water Balance. Walter G. Maddock; The Journal of Urology; April, 1938.

A normal adjustment between fluid intake and output to keep the water content of the body at a constant level of 70 per cent of body weight is necessary to good health. More than half the total daily supply of water is obtained from the food partaken. Each gram of food furnished 0.9 gm. of water, the resultant total amounting to 1,000 to 1,500 c.c. daily.

Water excretion concerns itself with two functions. 1. Excretion of waste material in solution by the kidneys. 2. The dissipation of body heat. The feces play no part normally so far as loss of water is concerned. Water for vaporization to dissipate heat may be thought of as having "preferential rights" on available fluid in the body.

In determining the amount of fluid required by the average patient having undergone a surgical operation one must compute the amount of water necessary for vaporization, the loss of fluid through hemorrhage, vomiting, etc., in conjunction with the amount of water necessary for excretion of 0.35 gm. of waste material by means of the urine. The average patient requires 1,000 to 1,500 c.c. of water daily for vaporization and providing the kidneys are in normal condition will necessitate 500 c.c. for excretion. However, if the kidneys are unable to concentrate the urine satisfactorily twice or three times this amount is needed. As there is always some abnormal loss of fluid content of the body incident to the operation this too must be added to the total. It will be observed that approximately 2,500 c.c. of fluid is absolutely necessary in the average non-septic patient undergoing an operation. If the patient is septic an extra 1,000 c.c. should be added to take care of the increased fluid loss incident to excessive vaporization, vomiting and excretion. Dehydrated patients obviously require an excess of water over this figure.

In regards to the parenteral administration of fluid it has been found that excess sodium chloride will result in retention of fluid in the tissue. As the normal salt intake is only 5 to 6 grams daily, large amounts of saline solution given parenterally will result in chloride retention. Where diuresis is desired the type of fluid given should be glucose solution in low concentration, while in the treatment of dehydration normal saline is preferable.

Comment: This is an excellent article which should be carefully read by every surgeon, especially those who do urological surgery. An adequate fluid intake is absolutely essential to the s m o o t h convalescence of all patients undergoing surgery, the amount of water to be administered dependent on the several factors outlined above. It is my belief that a standard post-operative order for all surgical patients should be a measure of all the fluid intake and especially the output. No post-operative patient should have less than a liter output of urine for the first few days following surgery and if the specific gravity has been found to be low before surgery this minimum requirement must be increased. Strict attention to the maintainance of a proper water balance is an absolute essential in the care of surgical patients.

Is Sudden Emptying of the Chronically Distended Bladder Dangerous? C. D. Creevy; The Journal of Urology, April, 1938.

The author has reviewed the literature on this controversial question and he states that he has failed to find evidence to support the generally accepted view that it is a hazardous procedure. By critical analysis and a review of cases of deaths from prostatism who had been treated by both methods he has developed the following conclusions:

Conclusions: The idea that sudden emptying of the chronically distended bladder is dangerous is firmly fixed in the literature.

A classification of the theories explaining these dangers is presented.

The theories fail to withstand critical analysis, because:

At autopsy no lesions ascribable to sudden emptying of the chronically distended bladder can be distinguished from those due to infection in the absence of residual urine.

Eighty per cent of the patients who die after catheterization sucumb to pyelonephritis, either acute or chronic; 20 per cent succumb to infections outside the urinary tract.

Sudden death after catheterization may be due to coincidental coronary thrombosis or pulmonary embolism.

The phenomena usually ascribed to s u d d e n emptying of the bladder can be produced by pyelonephritis.

Gradual decompression of the distended bladder did not reduce the mortality in a series of 120 cases when compared to a similar series in which sudden emptying was practised.

Gradual decompression should be abandoned. Doing so has not produced any untoward reactions in my experience.

Comment:

No teaching has been so firmly intrenched in the minds of the medical profession as this one. It has been handed down from generation to generation as to practically become an urological dogma. This seems strange when it is considered the paucity of proof which it rests on. Dr. Creevy has shown courage in facing the problem and joins a growing group who are of the opinion that no harm can result from the procedure.

Personally it is my belief that in practically all cases the quicker the bladder is emptied and kept empty the better for the patient. With him I agree the greatest danger lies in a super imposed infection incidental to the first catheterization. Because of this the initial catheterization should be accomplished with as little trauma as possible and the greatest care should be taken in preventing bacterial contamination. The prostatic case who is suffering from a long standing urinary retention preferably should be hospitalized before subjecting them to the first catheterization and subsequent treatment.

--------o--------

EYE, EAR, NOSE AND THROAT
Edited by Marvin D. Henley, M.D.
911 Medical Arts Building, Tulsa

Intracapsular Cataract Extraction. O. M. Duthie, M.D. British Journal of Ophthalmology, January, 1937.

The author agrees that this is a highly controversial subject and cites Appleman with a series of 100 cases who regards it as an ideal procedure, however de Grasz thinks further results of the intracapsular removal must be followed up for many years, while Duke-Elder think that before a worthwhile opinion can be formed, the end results of the operation must be examined more carefully.

Sinclairs' method is used by the author with minor deviations, i.e. extraction of the lens by "tumbling"—grasping the anterior capsule below and delivering the lower pole first which dislocates the upper pole backward.

The series reported in this article is made up of 100 consecutive cases—43 mature and 57 immature cataracts.

The modifications of Sinclair procedure are: The author uses a retro-ocular injection 20 minutes before operation. This reduces tension and lessens

the chance of losing vitreous. Elsching agrees with this but Knapp does not deem a preliminary softening necessary. The author inserts retraction sutures painlessly with local anaesthesia at the junction of the middle and inner, and the middle and the outer thirds of the margin of the upper lid. No speculum or lid elevator is used. He likes a large corneal section made completely with a Graefe Knife if possible, ending with a small conjunctival flap. If the globe is not softened preoperatively, there is danger of dislocating the lens if a very large section is made with the knife. In extracting, the anterior capsule must be grasped well down as near the level of the pupillary margin below as possible. Going slowly the lens is rocked gently until it is dislocated below and then with the forceps guiding the lens through the wound, the lens is delivered with the aid of pressure exerted on the globe below. It is quite important that the operator have a forceps that is suitable. Postoperatively the lids are kept closed by strapping the upper lid sutures on to the cheek for 24 hours. A peripheral iridectomy with a firm closure of the wound after operation is the ideal procedure.

In order to prevent prolapse and ultimate eccentric pupil, some of the cases were kept on pilocarpine for 48 hours after operation. These had a tendency to develop iritis. If the section is large, you have the attending danger of a prolapse.

In the complications there were 28 hyphaemas, seven iritis, eight iris prolapse, four loss of vitreous at operation, two loss of vitreous after operation and one each of corneal blood staining, detached choroid and detached retina.

If cases are excluded where vision was reduced as a result of the other eye being diseased (not related to the operation) then the author claims 6/6 or better in 77 per cent and 6/9 - 6/12 in 19 per cent visual acuity.

The Management and Treatment of Otogenic Meningitis. Samuel J. Kopetzky, M.D. The Annals of Otology, Rhinology and Laryngology, March, 1938.

This is the Presidential Address, delivered before the Western Section meeting of the American Laryngological, Rhinological and Otological Society, Santa Barbara, California, January 29, 1938. It is an unusually interesting paper that does not lend itself well to abstracting. The author's conclusions are as follows:

1. In conclusion, I would say that the surgical drainage of the meninges does not answer the problem presented by mastoiditis, because the lesion is usually a multiple one consisting of many foci of active infection spreading along the route of many pial vessels. The problem is more concerned with keeping the brain tissue alive. To accomplish this, results of the brain-tissue-cell activity must be removed from the region of the brain cells, and the desired means of doing this is in keeping the cerebrospinal fluid circulating. Any procedure which stops the circulation of the fluid defeats the objectives which are in view. Brain cells naturally function best and their deleterious products are removed best when they are surrounded by cerebrospinal fluid whose chemistry is maintained as nearly normal as possible. The repeated small blood transfusion has in my hands accomplished this purpose better than any other method, and in all the cases which I have here sketched, stoppage has not occurred, and I think this is due to the prompt institution of transfusion with the first advent of the case in my care, and the continuous use of this means, irrespective of other therapy.

2. Study of healed cases from literature showed that cured cases seemed to be obtained where the clinical picture is not so stormy and the symptom complex may be described as weak, and where

pressure signs predominate over signs of toxicity. Repeated taps with a study of the pressure each time helps to control this pressure by giving an intimation of how promptly the pressure falls and how long it remains low.

3. The removal of the surgical bone focus cannot be too strongly stressed. In exposing the dura surrounding the temporal bone the procedure to do this breaks the contiguity of the penetrating skeletal dural vessels and interrupts the progress along these vessels of an infection from the bone to the dura, and helps healing the meningeal lesion.

In the examination of the cerebrospinal fluid, the following factors all need evaluation in summing up a clinical picture; the physical characteristics of the fluid; the pressure under which it is obtained; its biochemistry; its cytology; and finally its bacteriology.

4. Chemotherapy, especially sulfanilamide, has given me better results than any I have obtained by any other drug, sera or vaccine. It is demonstrable in the blood and in the cerebrospinal fluid when given by mouth. Combined with small transfusions it is the best means to date which I have employed.

In giving sulfanilamide it is well to make periodic examinations to watch for the formation of metahemoglobin, a pathological by-product sometimes found in the administration of this drug. The formation of metahemoglobin must be avoided. Its marked presence constitutes a danger sign indicating stoppage of the drug. The simultaneous administration of the transfusions helps to hold this by-product within bounds and enables us to continue it longer than otherwise.

5. Rosenthal found sulfanilamide a potent therapeutic agent in experimental pneumococcal infection with virulent strains, in mice, rabbits and particularly in rats. The curative action was most evident with Type III pneumococcal infections. Rosenthal concluded that "up to the present time no other compounds have been found as effective against pneumococcic infections as sulfanilamide."

Gross and Cooper also obtained favorable results with the use of sulfanilamide in Type III pneumococcal infections in rats.

Long and Bliss reported that, our experience in the treatment of clinical pneumococcal infections in human beings has been primarily limited to those of the middle ear and mastoid. Our observations tend to show that sulfanilamide has about one-half the chemotherapeutic effect in pneumococcal infections that it has in hemolytic streptococcal infections of the middle ear and mastoid."

Mertins and Mertins recently reported a case of unclassified Type IV meningitis of otitic origin which recovered following sulfanilamide therapy.

The mode of action of sulfanilamide is still mooted. Rosenthal believes that "the bacteriostatic and bactericidal action of sulphonamide on pneumococci in vitro is adequate to explain its chemotherapeutic effect in animals. The nature of this action in vitro is unusual in that the drug is not an antiseptic in the usual sense." Long and Bliss, however, hold that a change takes place in the organism which renders them susceptible to phagocytosis, but the nature of this change is still unknown.

6. When a meningitis has run its course, and the fluid tends to become normal, and the symptoms present themselves suggestive of a brain abscess, it is well to perform ventriculography before accepting a diagnosis of brain abscess. If the fluid can be kept circulating, and the pressure kept down, otogenic hydrocephalus has a tendency to heal, as the three cases cited by me all tend to demonstrate.

7. Handled in this logical way, we are in a position to say, that otogenic streptococcic meningitis is on the way toward coming under therapeutic control, and the prognosis heretofore invariably grave, gives better promise now than formerly that more recoveries will be accomplished.

Differential Diagnosis of Bacterial Meningitis of Aural and of Nasal Origin. Joseph C. Yaskin, M.D., Philadelphia. Archives of Otolaryngology, April, 1938.

This is a comprehensive statistical report on the etiological factors of bacterial meningitis. This disease occurs frequently and ranks as one of the most important acute infections of the central nervous system. While it occurs most frequently as an independent infection it frequently complicates ear and nose infections. Hospital statistics from the more densely populated areas show meningococci and tuberculous meningitis most common. In the author's series of 123 cases of bacterial meningitis, a different picture is indicated. These 123 cases occurred between 1920 and 1937 and were from all causes. Ninety-six cases were from the Graduate Hospital of the University of Pennsylvania. "In 54 of these cases the condition was not a complication of any frank infection of the ear or nose; in 37 it was a complication of disease of the temporal bone; in 21 a complication of disease of the paranasal sinuses, and in 11 a sequala of cranial trauma." The organisms most frequently present in the infection resulting from nose or ear infections were streptococcus, pneumococcus and staphylococcus.

Some factors enumerated which irritate the meninges are: exogenous poisoning, systemic toxemia, virus and bacterial intoxication and infection, epidural infection in the brain and spinal cord and certain types of tumor of the brain. Common signs and symptoms are headache, dizziness, vomiting, rigidity of the neck and Kernig's and Brudenski's sign. Changes in the spinal fluid tell the type and cause of the meningeal irritation. The differential diagnoses includes conditions not due to invasion by known bacteria such as cervical adenitis, retropharyngeal abscess, meningismus, virus diseases, hemorrhagic conditions, acute syphilitic meningitis and aseptic meningitis and also other forms of bacterial meningitis, most commonly meningococcic and tuberculous.

Each case presents a problem in itself. All the signs and symptoms are rarely present in one case; many have a paucity of signs and symptoms; many are atypical. The clinician must be ever alert in giving due consideration to the entire picture presented in one of these cases if the best results are to be obtained.

The author states he has never had a recovery in a case of tuberculous meningitis.

The Clinical Picture of Diseases of the Labyrinth Wall. Dr. Edmund Prince Fowler, New York. The Laryngoscope, March, 1937.

Correlation of clinical, laboratory and autopsy findings presupposes progress in the understanding of any disease.

Anatomically the author describes the labyrinthine walls as "a bony capsule surrounding the static and auditory membranous labyrinths." There are present entrances and exits for lymph, blood vessels and nerves; the two cochlea windows for pressure and vibrations; the labyrinth walls have in them many spaces which contain tissue juices, arterioles, veins and neural structures which by their action have to do with the bony structure both in health and disease.

The bone of the labyrinthine capsule differs in structure from ordinary bony formation. Haversian systems are not present, except in the very aged. Basophilic islands which are ordinarily found only in the embryo are normally present in the adult labyrinthine capsule. Route of invasion may be by any or all of the following: the middle ear, mastoid, labyrinth and cranial cavities, sheaths of the nerves, the lymph channels, and lumen or sheaths of the vessels.

Suppurative disease of the capsule may cause death. The signs and symptoms are variable. All medical and surgical procedures intrinsically are preventive. Heredity is a factor to be considered in disease of the capsule. Total loss of function may ensue following an infection. This depends upon "the extent, virulence and position of the lesions and upon adjacent or distant coincidental or contributing factors."

Some symptoms simulating labyrinthine wall disease which may lead one to making a wrong diagnosis are: Deep-seated pain, diminished hearing or complete deafness, tinnitus, vertigo or other disturbances of equilibrium, nausea, vomiting, positive fistula test, spontaneous or abnormally induced nystagmus and past pointing, and facial paralysis. Differential diagnosis includes evidence of rickets, osteitis dystrophia fibrosa, asteomalacia, von Recklinghausen's and Paget's disease, unhealed fractures and new bone formations. Osteomyelitis does not occur here as there is no marrow in the capsule.

The author is of the opinion that otosclerosis is not wholly due to a general disease since the pathology in the bony capsule of the labyrinth is not found any other place in the body.

Stereoscopic Roentgenograms if read carefully and accurately are a great help in arriving at a correct diagnosis. Every available means and method must be employed if a minimum of incorrect diagnoses are made. Most to be relied upon is "the correlation of the history and repeated neurological, hearing and labyrinthine tests, with X-ray and laboratory findings."

If there is a suppurative disease present, drainage must be established. This is a radical procedure and the preservation of function is of secondary importance.

The Effectiveness of Therapeutic Measures after Poisoning with Sublethal and Lethal Dosages of Barbital in the Rabbit. O. W. Barlow, (Dept. of Pharmacology, Western Reserve Univ. School of Medicine). J. of Lab. & Clin. Med., 23:601 (March, 1938).

It is well known that resuscitation measures are symptomatically more effective against the short acting hypnotics of the pentobarbital, amytal, or avertin type than against barbital itself. The generally unfavorable prognosis clinically in barbital poisoning suggested the need for this study, which was partially supported by the Council on Pharmacy and Chemistry of the American Medical Association.

"Symptomatic control of the effects of barbital sodium poisoning in rabbits appears to be best accomplished by means of frequent medication with two central convulsants—picrotoxin and Metrazol, the judicious administration of a vasopressor agent, ephedrine, and the administration of fluids intravenously preferably in the form of five per cent glucose. . . . Medication should be continued at short intervals at the outset of the poisoning as judged by the symptoms present, and at longer intervals as the depth of hypnosis diminishes.

"The administration of picrotoxin results in a submaximal stimulation of respiration, and reactions become maximal only after a latent period. The product in these respects is inferior to Metrazol for emergency purposes. However, the duration of action of picrotoxin, which ranges from 30 to 180 minutes, depending on the depth of hypnosis, is superior to that of Metrazol. On the other hand, picrotoxin is not wholly free of undesirable side actions, in that significant secondary depressant effects may develop after excessive dosages.

"The respiratory stimulant effects of Metrazol

were definitely superior to those of other agents tested. . . . This product is best suited for emergency purposes under conditions of respiratory failure. On numerous occasions spontaneous respiratory movements have been initiated with Metrazol intravenously in the presence of continued heart action, one or two minutes after cessation of respiration.

"Ephedrine . . . has a definite place in the antidotal sequence against hypnotic or narcotic poisoning. . . . Larger dosages of ephedrine are prone to produce a heart block of greater or less degree and an embarrassment of respiration due to the development of pulmonary edema.

"The administration of fluids by vein relieves the anuric effects of barbital, accelerates the urinary excretion of barbital slightly, maintains a more normal water balance, and very probably reduces the tendency for the development of acidosis. . . . Optimal results are obtained when fluids are administered in conjunction with picrotoxin, Metrazol, and ephedrine.

"Coramine, strychnine, and caffeine were of questionable value in the treatment of even lighter grades of barbital sodium poisoning. The order of observed efficiency corresponds to that in which the compounds are listed, as a matter of fact, the data obtained indicate undesirable effects, such as secondary depression from effective dosages, and, in the case of caffeine, these toxic effects were additive with those of the hypnotic."

The Chemistry of Vitamin A and Substances Having a Vitamin A Effect

L. S. Palmer, St. Paul (Journal A. M. A., May 21, 1938), gives a brief discussion of the chemistry of vitamin A and the substances having similar effects. In a previous vitamin symposium in The Journal, the perplexing question as to why the yellow-red plant pigment carotene exhibits vitamin A activity although the familiar vitamin A of liver oils is essentially a colorless substance had been answered by the discovery that carotene is convertible in the body to vitamin A. The chemical basis for such a relationship has been established by Karrer and his associates, who had determined the chemical constitution both of plant carotene and also of vitamin A from fish liver oil. The first complete structural formula for carotene has since turned out to be that of B-carotene which is by far the most important and widely distributed of the known coloring matters which have vitamin A activity. The final step in this chemical story is the synthesis of the pure vitamin in vitro. Recent reports indicate that this has been accomplished. The isolation of the crystalline natural vitamin has also been reported.

Drainage of Cerebrospinal Fluid in Treatment of Hydrocephalus, Syringomyelia and Syringobulbia

The shrinkage of the brain on the ipsilateral side suggested to N. D. Royle, Sydney, Australia (Journal A. M. A., April 16, 1938), that the operation of superior thoracic ganglionectomy might be used in the treatment of hydrocephalus. He has thus treated two patients in this manner. The operation of superior thoracic ganglionectomy causes an increase in the rate of capillary flow in the cervical region of the spinal cord and of the brain. The operation of lumbar sympathectomy increases the rate of drainage on the ipsilateral side of the cord in the lumbar region. Both operations provide an outlet for the cerebrospinal fluid where they tap the spinal circulation. In contrast to the other methods of draining the cord, this method has the virtue of permanence. Epinephrine has little effect after sympathetic denervation.

ROSTER

Oklahoma State Medical Association
1938

ADAIR

CHURCH, R. M. ....Stilwell
GREENE, E. P. ....Westville
MEYERS, WM. A. ....Stilwell
SELLARS, R. L. ....Westville

ALFALFA

BEATY, C. SAM ....Cherokee
BUTTS, A. J. ....Cherokee
CLARK, Z. J. ....Cherokee
DUNNINGTON, W. G. ....Cherokee
HARRIS, G. G. ....Helena
HUSTON, H. E. ....Cherokee
LANCASTER, L. T. ....Cherokee
SLATON, F. K. ....Helena

ATOKA

BRIGGS, THOS. HIRAM ....Atoka
CLARK, J. B. ....Coalgate
CODY, R. D. ....Centrahoma
FULTON, J. S. ....Atoka
HIPES, J. J. ....Coalgate

BECKHAM

BAKER, L. V. ....Elk City
DENBY, J. M. ....Carter
DEVANNEY, P. J. ....Sayre
JONES, C. F. ....Erick
JOSS, WM. I. ....Erick
KILPATRICK, E. S. ....Leedy
McCREERY, R. C. ....Erick
McGRATH, T. J. ....Sayre
SPEED, Jr., H. K. ....Clinton
SPEED, Sr., H. K. ....Sayre
STAGNER, G. H. ....Erick
STANDIGER, O. C. ....Elk City
TISDAL, V. C. ....Elk City
TISDALL, W. C. ....Clinton

BLAINE

BARNETT, J. S. ....Hitchcock
BROWNING, J. W. ....Geary
BUCHANAN, R. F. ....Canton
COX, A. K. ....Watonga
GRIFFIN, W. F. ....Watonga
HOLCOMB, GEORGE ....Okeene
LEISURE, J. B. ....Watonga
MURDOCK, L. H. ....711 Medical Arts Bldg.,
                                                Oklahoma City
MILLIGAN, E. F. ....Geary
WIGGINS, C. W. ....Canton

BRYAN

BAKER, ALFRED ....Durant
CAIN, P. L. ....Albany
COKER, B. B. ....Durant

(continued)

COLWICK, O. J. ....Durant
COLWICK, J. T. ....Durant
DeLAY, W. D. ....2245 Palmetto Ave., Daytona
                                                Beach, Fla.
FUSTON, H. B. ....Bokchito
HAYNIE, JOHN A. ....Durant
HAYNIE, W. KEILER ....Durant
McCARLEY, W. H. ....Colbert
MOORE, B. H. ....Perrine Bldg., Oklahoma City
MOORE, CHAS. F. ....Durant
PRICE, CHAS. G. ....Durant
RUSHING, G. M. ....Durant
SAWYER, R. E. ....Durant
SHULER, JAS. L. ....Durant
TONY, S. M. ....Bennington
WELLS, A. J. ....Calera
WHARTON, J. T. ....Durant

CADDO

ANDERSON, P. H. ....Anadarko
CAMPBELL, GEO. C. ....Anadarko
COOK, ODIS A. ....Anadarko
HASLAM, G. E. ....Anadarko
HAWN, W. T. ....Binger
HENRY, J. WORRELL ....Anadarko
HUME, CHAS. R. ....Anadarko
INMAN, E. L. ....Apache
JOHNSTON, R. E. ....Bridgeport
KELLEAM, E. A. ....Sells, Arizona
KERLEY, W. W. ....Anadarko
McCLURE, P. L. ....Ft. Cobb
MILES, J. B. ....Anadarko
TAYLOR, A. H. ....Anadarko
WILLIAMS, R. W. ....Anadarko

CANADIAN

ADERHOLD, THOS. M. ....El Reno
BROWN, HADLEY C. ....El Reno
CLARK, FRED H. ....El Reno
CRADEN, PAUL J. ....El Reno
DEVER, HARVEY K. ....El Reno
FUNK, G. D. ....El Reno
GOODMAN, GEO. LEROY ....Yukon
HEROD, PHILLIP F. ....El Reno
JOHNSON, ALPHA L. ....El Reno
LAWTON, W. P. ....El Reno
MILLER, W. R. ....Calumet
MYERS, PIRL B. ....El Reno
PHELPS, JOS. T. ....El Reno
PHELPS, MALCOM E. ....El Reno
RILEY, JAS. T. ....El Reno
RICHARDSON, D. P. ....Union City
STOUGH, Sr., D. P. ....Geary
TOMKINS, JOHN E. ....Yukon
WARREN, CHESTER ....Yukon

CARTER

BOADWAY, F. W. ....Ardmore
CANTRELL, Jr., D. E. ....Wilson

CANTRELL, D. E. ....Healdton
CANTRELL, EMMA J. ....Wilson
CARLOCK, J. HOYLE ....Ardmore
EASTERWOOD, A. Y. ....Ardmore
HARDY, WALTER ....Ardmore
HATHAWAY, W. G. ....Lone Grove
HIGGINS, H. A. ....Ardmore
JACKSON, T. J. ....Ardmore
JOHNSON, C. A. ....Wilson
JOHNSON, G. E. ....Ardmore
JOHNSON, WALTER ....Ardmore
LOONEY, MacDONALD ....Marietta
PARRISH, R. M. ....Ardmore
PERRY, FRED T. ....Healdton
POLLOCK, J. R. ....Ardmore
SAIN, W. C. ....Ardmore
SULLIVAN, R. C. ....Ardmore
VEAZEY, L. C. ....Armore
VEAZEY, J. H. ....Ardmore
VON KELLER, F. P. ....Ardmore
WOODS, L. B. ....Ardmore

CHEROKEE

ALLISON, J. S. ....Tahlequah
BAINES, SWARTZ ....Tahlequah
BARNS, HARRY E. ....Tahlequah
JOHNSON, J. J. ....Moody
MASTERS, HERBERT A. ....Tahlequah
MATHEWS, G. F. ....Tahlequah
MEDEARIS, P. H. ....Tahlequah

CHOCTAW

HARRIS, G. E. ....Hugo
JOHN, W. N. ....Hugo
JOHNSON, E. A. ....Hugo
WATERS, FLOYD L. ....Hugo
SWITZER, FRED D. ....Hugo

CLEVELAND

ATKINS, W. H. ....Norman
BOBO, C. S. ....Norman
BUFFINGTON, F. C. ....Norman
COOLEY, B. H. ....Norman
DORSEY, ELIZABETH ....Norman
FOWLER, W. A. ....Norman
GABLE, J. J. ....Norman
GRIFFIN, D. W. ....Norman
HADDOCK, Jr., J. L. ....Norman
HOOD, J. O. ....Norman
HOWELL, O. E. ....Norman
KNISELY, H. B. ....Norman
LAMBERT, J. B. ....Lexington
MAYFIELD, W. T. ....Norman
MERRITT, I. S. ....Norman
NIELSON, GERTRUDE ....Norman
PROSSER, M. P. ....Norman
RAYBURN, C. R. ....Norman
REICHERT, R. J. ....Moore
REIGER, J. A. ....Norman
SCHMIDT, ELEANORA ....Norman
STEEN, CARL ....Norman
STEPHENS, E. F. ....Norman
THACKER, R. E. ....Lexington
TURLEY, L. A. ....Norman
WICKHAM, M. M. ....Norman
WILEY, G. A. ....Norman
WILLARD, D. G. ....Norman
WILLIAMS, G. H. ....Norman

COMANCHE

ANGUS, DONALD ....Lawton
ANGUS, H. A. ....Lawton
ANTONY, JOS. T. ....Lawton

BARBER, GEO. S. ....Lawton
BROSHEARS, JACKSON ....Lawton
DUNLAP, E. B. ....Lawton
FOX, FRED ....Lawton
FERGUSON, L. W. ....Lawton
GOOCH, L. T. ....Lawton
HAMMOND, F. W. ....Lawton
HATHAWAY, E. P. ....Lawton
JOYCE, CHAS. W. ....Fletcher
KERR, GEO. E. ....Chattanooga
KNEE, L. C. ....Lawton
LUTNER, THOS. R. ....Lawton
MALCOLM, J. W. ....Lawton
MARTIN, CHAS. M. ....Elgin
MITCHELL, E. BRENT ....Lawton
PARSONS, O. L. ....Lawton
VAN MATRE, REBER M. ....Lawton

COTTON

BAKER, G. W. ....Walters
COTTON, W. W. ....Walters
HALSTEAD, A. B. ....Temple
JONES, M. A. ....Walters
SCISM, MOLLIE F. ....Walters

CRAIG

ADAMS, F. M. ....Vinita
BAGBY, LOUIS ....Vinita
BRADSHAW, J. O. ....Welch
DARROUGH, J. B. ....Vinita
GASTINEAU, F. T. ....Vinita
HAYS, P. L. ....Vinita
HERRON, A. W. ....Vinita
JOHNSON, L. G. ....Vinita
LEHMER, ELIZABETH ....Vinita
MARKS, W. R. ....Vinita
McPIKE, LLOYD H. ....Vinita
MITCHELL, R. L. ......Veterans Hospital, Muskogee
STOUGH, D. B. ....Vinita
SANGER, PAUL G. ....Vinita
SANGER, WALTER B. ....Vinita
WALKER, C. F. ....Grove

CREEK

BISBEE, W. G. ....Bristow
COPPEDGE, O. S. ....Depew
COWART, O. H. ....Bristow
CROSTON, GEO. C. ....Sapulpa
CURRY, J. F. ....Sapulpa
HAAS, H. R. ....Sapulpa
HOLLIS, J. E. ....Bristow
JONES, ELLIS ....Sapulpa
KING, E. W. ....Bristow
LAMPTON, J. B. ....Sapulpa
LEWIS, P. K. ....Sapulpa
LONGMIRE, W. P. ....Sapulpa
McDONALD, C. R. ....Mannford
NEAL, WM. J. ....Drumright
REESE, C. B. ....Sapulpa
SCHRADER, CHAS. T. ....Bristow
SISLER, FRANK H. ....Bristow
SMITH, WENDELL L. ....Drumright
STARR, O. W. ....Drumright
WELLS, JOHN M. ....Bristow
WHITE, EDW. E. ....Oilton
WILLIAMS, J. CLAY......208 Philcade Bldg., Tulsa

CUSTER

ALEXANDER, C. J. ....Clinton
BOYD, T. A. ....Weatherford
CUNNINGHAM, CURTIS B. ....Custer City
CUSHMAN, HARRY B. ....Clinton
DEPUTY, ROSS ....Clinton
DOLER, C. ....Clinton

FRIZZELL, J. T. ....Clinton
GAEDE, D. ....Weatherford
GOSSOM, K. D. ....Custer City
HINSHAW, J. R. ....Butler
LAMB, ELLIS ....Clinton
LAMB, LEALON ....Clinton
LINGENFELTER, PAUL ....Clinton
LOYD, E. M. ....Taloga
McBURNEY, C. H. ....Clinton
NEWLIN, WM. H. ....Clinton
PAULSON, A. W. ....Clinton
ROGERS, McLAIN ....Clinton
RUHL, N. E. ....Weatherford
VIEREGG, FRANK R. ....Clinton
WILLIAMS, GORDON D. ....Weatherford
WOOD, J. G. ....Weatherford

GARFIELD

BAGBY, E. L. ....Enid
BAKER, R. C. ....Enid
BRADY, J. H. ....Fairview
CHAMPLIN, PAUL B. ....Enid
COPPAGE, O. W. ....Enid
DUFFY, FRANCIS M. ....Enid
GILL, W. W. ....Enid
GREGG, O. R. ....Enid
FEILD, JULIAN ....Enid
FRANCISCO, GLENN ....Enid
FRANCISCO, J. W. ....Enid
HARRIS, D. S. ....Drummond
HAMBLE, V. R. ....Enid
HOPKINS, P. W. ....Enid
HUDSON, F. A. ....Enid
HUDSON, H. H. ....Enid
HYER, J. V. ....Garber
JACOBS, R. G....610 N. W. 9th St., Oklahoma City
KENDALL, W. L. ....Enid
MAYBERRY, S. N. ....Enid
McEVOY, S. H. ....Enid
MERCER, J. WENDALL ....Enid
METSCHER, ALFRED JOHN ....Enid
MILES, G. O. ....Enid
NEILSON, W. P. ....Enid
NEWELL, W. B. ....Enid
PIPER, A. S. ....Enid
REMPEL, PAUL H. ....Enid
RHODES, W. H. ....Enid
ROBERTS, C. J ....Enid
ROBERTS, D. D. ....Enid
ROSS, GEORGE ....Enid
ROSS, HOPE ....Enid
RUDE, EVELYN ....Enid
SHANNON, H. R. ....Enid
SHEETS, MARION E. ....Enid
TALLEY, EVANS E. ....Enid
VANDEVER, H. F. ....Enid
WALKER, JOHN R. ....Enid
WATSON, J. M. ....Enid
WILKINS, A. E. ....Covington
WOLF, E. J. ....Waukomis

GARVIN

ALEXANDER, ROBT. M. ....Paoli
CALLAWAY, JOHN R. ....Pauls Valley
GREENING, W. P. ....Pauls Valley
GROSS, J. T. ....Lindsay
JOHNSON, G. L. ....Pauls Valley
LINDSEY, RAY H. ....Pauls Valley
MONROE, HUGH H. ....Lindsay
PRATT, CHAS. M. ....Lindsay
ROBBERSON, JR., MARVIN E. ....Wynnewood
ROBBERSON, M. E. ....Wynnewood
SHI, A. H. ....Stratford
SHIRLEY, EDWARD ....Pauls Valley
SULLIVAN, C. L. ....Elmore City

GRADY

BARRY, W. R. ....Alex
BAZE, ROY E. ....Chickasha
BAZE, W. J. ....Chickasha
BONNELL, W. L. ....Chickasha
BOON, U. C. ....Chickasha
BYNUM, TURNER ....Chickasha
COOK, W. H. ....Chickasha
DOWNEY D. S. ....Chickasha
EMANUEL, L. E. ....Chickasha
EMANUEL, ROY ....Chickasha
GERARD, G. R. ....Chickasha
LEEDS, A. B. ....Chickasha
LITTLE, AARON ....Minco
LIVERMORE, W. H. ....Chickasha
MARRS, S. O. ....Chickasha
MASON, REBECCA H. ....Chickasha
McCLURE, H. M. ....Chickasha
McMILLAN, J. M. ....Chickasha
MITCHELL, C. P. ....Chickasha
PYLE, OSCAR S. ....Chickasha
RENEGAR, J. F. ....Tuttle
WOODS, L. E. ....Chickasha

GRANT

HARDY, I. V. ....Medford
HARRIS, FRANK M. ....Medford
LAWSON, E. E. ....Medford
LIVELY, S. A. ....Wakita

GREER

BORDER, G. F. ....Mangum
HOLLIS, J. B. ....Mangum
LANSDEN, J. B. ....Granite
LOWE, J. T. ....Mangum
MEREDITH, J. S. ....Duke
NELSON, H. J. ....Granite
OLIVER, W. D. ....Mangum
PEARSON, LEB. E. ....Mangum
POER, E. M. ....Mangum
RUDE, JOE C. ....Collis P. Huntington Memorial
                              Hosp., Boston, Mass.

HASKELL

CARSON, WM. S. ....Keota
HILL, A. T. ....Stigler
THOMPSON, W. A. ....Stigler
TURNER, T. B. ....Stigler
WILLIAMS, N. K. ....McCurtain

HUGHES

BENTLEY, J. A. ....Allen
BUTTS, A. M. ....Holdenville
DAVENPORT, A. L. ....Holdenville
DIGGS, G. W. ....Wetumka
MAYFIELD, IMOGENE BUTTS ....Holdenville
McCARY, D. Y. ....Weleetka
FORD, R. B. ....Holdenville
FREY, HARRY ....Holdenville
HAMILTON, S. H. ....Non
HICKS, C. A. ....Wetumka
HOWELL, H. A. ....Holdenville
MORRIS, R. D. ....Allen
MUNAL, JOHN ....Holdenville
PRYOR, V. W. ....Holdenville
TAYLOR, W. L. ....Holdenville

JACKSON

ABERNETHY, EDW. A. ....Altus
ALLGOOD, JOHN M. ....Altus
BERRY, THOS. W....CCC Camp, Winnsboro, Texas
BIRD, JESSE ....1545 N. W. 44th, Oklahoma City
BROWN, R. F. ....Altus

CROW, E. S. ....Olustee
ENSEY, J. E. ....Altus
FOX, RAYMOND H. ....Altus
HIX, JOSEPH B. ....Altus
MABRY, EARL W. ....Altus
McCONNELL, L. H. ....Altus
RAY, W. T. ....Gould
REID, JOHN R. ....Altus
STARKEY, WAYNE ....Altus
TAYLOR, ROBT. Z. ....Blair

JEFFERSON

ANDRESKOSKI, W. T. ....Ryan
BROWNING, W. M. ....Waurika
COLLINS, D. B. ....Waurika
DERR, J. I. ....Waurika
EDWARDS, F. M. ....Ringling
HOLLINGSWORTH, J. I. ....Waurika
MAUPIN, C. M. ....Waurika
McCALIB, D. C. ....Ringling
MINGUS, F. M. ....Loco
WADE, L. L. ....Ryan

JOHNSTON

LOONEY, J. T. ....Tishomingo

KAY

ARMSTRONG, W. O. ....Ponca City
ARRENDELL, C. W. ....Ponca City
BARKER, W. JACKSON ....Ponca City
BEATTY, J. H. ....Tonkawa
BERRY, G. L. ....Blackwell
BROWNE, H. S. ....Ponca City
CLIFT, M. C. ....Blackwell
CURRY, JOHN R. ....Blackwell
GARDNER, C. C. ....Ponca City
GHORMLEY, J. G. ....Blackwell
GIBSON, R. B. ....Ponca City
GORDON, D. M. ....Ponca City
GOWEY, H. O. ....Newkirk
HOWE, J. H. ....Ponca City
HUDSON, J. O. ....Braman
KREGER, G. S. ....Tonkawa
MATTHEWS, DEWEY ....Tonkawa
McELROY, THOMAS ....Ponca City
MILLER, D. W. ....Blackwell
MOORE, G. C. ....Ponca City
MORGAN, L. S. ....Ponca City
NEAL, L. G. ....Ponca City
NIEMANN, G. H. ....Ponca City
NORTHCUTT, C. E. ....Ponca City
NUCKOLS, A. S. ....Ponca City
OBERMILLER, R. G. ....Ponca City
PETERS, M. L. ....Blackwell
RISSER, A. S. ....Blackwell
SANGER, W. W. ....Ponca City
VANCE, L. C. ....Ponca City
WAGGONER, E. E. ....Tonkawa
WAGNER, J. C. ....Ponca City
WALKER, I. D. ....Tonkawa
WHITE, M. S. ....Blackwell
WRIGHT, L. L. ....Blackwell
YANDELL, HAYS R. ....Ponca City

KINGFISHER

LATTIMORE, F. C. ....Kingfisher
TAYLOR, J. R. ....Kingfisher

KIOWA

ADAMS, J. L. ....Hobart
ADAMS, RICHARD ....Hobart
ANDERSON, H. R. ....Mountain View
BONHAM, J. M. ....Hobart

BRAUN, J. P. ....Hobart
FINCH, J. WM. ....Sentinel
HATHAWAY, A. H. ....Mountain View
MOORE, J. H. ....Hobart
PIERSON, DWIGHT D. ....Hobart
WALKER, F. E. ....Lone Wolf
WATKINS, B. H. ....Hobart

LATIMER

HARRIS, J. M. ....Wilburton

LE FLORE

BAKER, F. P. ....Talihina
BOOTH, G. R. ....LeFlore
COLLINS, E. L. ....Panama
DEAN, S. C. ....Howe
FAIR, E. N. ....Heavener
HARTSHORNE, G. E. ....Spiro
HENRY, M. L. ....Heavener
JONES, L. D. ....Talihina
MINOR, R. W. ....Williams
ROGERS, G. A. ....Talihina
SHIPPEY, W. L. ....Poteau
SKEMP, FRANK S.   846 Garfield, Denver, Colo.
WOODSON, E. M. ....Poteau
WOODSON, O. M. ....Poteau
WRIGHT, R. L. ....Poteau

LINCOLN

ADAMS, J. W. ....Chandler
BAILEY, C. H. ....Stroud
BAUGH, HAROLD ....Meeker
BROWN, F. C. ....Sparks
BURLESON, NED ....Prague
DAVIS, W. B. ....Stroud
HURLBUT, E. F. ....Meeker
JENKINS, H. B. ....Tryon
MARSHALL, A. M. ....Chandler
NICKELL, U. E. ....Davenport
NORWOOD, F. H. ....Prague
ROBERTSON, C. W. ....Chandler
ROLLINS, J. S. ....Prague

LOGAN

BARKER, C. B. ....Guthrie
BARKER, E. O. ....Guthrie
BARKER, PAULINE ....Guthrie
BUSSEY, H. N. ....Mulhall
CORNWELL, N. L. ....Coyle
DRESBACH, H. V. ....Mulhall
FIRST, F. R. ....Crescent
GARDNER, P. B. ....Marshall
GOODRICH, E. E. ....Crescent
GRAY, DAN ....Guthrie
HAHN, L. A. ....Guthrie
HILL, C. B. ....Guthrie
LARKIN, W. H. ....Minco
LE HEW, Jr., J. L. ....Guthrie
MILLER, WM. C. ....Guthrie
PETTY, C. S. ....Guthrie
PETTY, JAMES ....Guthrie
REDDING, A. C. ....Coyle
RINGROSE, R. F. ....Guthrie
RITZHAUPT, L. H. ....Guthrie
SOUTER, J. E. ....Guthrie
TRIGG, F. E. ....Guthrie
WOLF, EUGENE ....Marshall

MAJOR

SPECHT, ELSIE ....Fairview

MARSHALL

HOLLAND, J. L. ....Madill
LOGAN, J. H. ....Lebanon
YORK, J. F. ....Madill

MAYES

ADAMS, SYLBA ....Hayward, Wis.
BRYANT, W. C. ....Choteau
COPPEDGE, O. N. ....Disney
HERRINGTON, V. D. ....Pryor
HOLLINGSWORTH, J. E. ....Strang
MORROW, B. L. ....Salina
PUCKETT, CARL ....22 W. Sixth, Oklahoma City
RUTHERFORD, S. C. ....Locust Grove
WERLING, E. H. ....Pryor
WHITAKER, W. J. ....Pryor
WHITE, L. C. ....Adair

McCLAIN

COCHRANE, J. E. ....Byars
DAWSON, O. O. ....Wayne
KOLB, I. N. ....Blanchard
McCURDY, W. C. ....Purcell
ROYSTER, R. L. ....Purcell

McCURTAIN

BARKER, N. L. ....Broken Bow
CLARKSON, A. W. ....Valliant
MORELAND, J. T. ....Idabel
MORELAND, W. A. ....Idabel
OLIVER, R. B. ....Idabel
SHERRILL, R. H. ....Broken Bow
SIZEMORE, PAUL ....Broken Bow
WILLIAMS, R. D. ....Idabel

McINTOSH

JACOBS, L. I. ....Hanna
LITTLE, D. E. ....Eufaula
STONER, RAYMOND WARD ....Checotah
TOLLESON, W. A. ....Eufaula
WOOD, JAS. L. ....Eufaula

MURRAY

ANADOWN, P. V. ....Sulphur
BURKE, RICHARD M. ....Sulphur
FOWLER, Jr., A. ....Sulphur
LUSTER, J. C. ....Davis
ROSE, ERNEST ....Sulphur
SADLER, F. E. ....Sulphur
SLOVER, GEO. ....Sulphur

MUSKOGEE

BALLANTINE, H. T. ....Surety Bldg.
BERRY, W. D. ....Barnes Bldg.
BLAKEMORE, J. L. ....Barnes Bldg.
BRUTON, L. D. ....Commercial Natl. Bldg.
COACHMAN, E. H. ....Manhattan Bldg.
DIVINE, DUKE G. ....Wagoner
DORWART, F. G. ....Barnes Bldg.
EARNEST, A. N. ....Barnes Bldg.
EWING, F. W. ....Surety Bldg.
FITE, E. H. ....Barnes Bldg.
FITE, W. P. ....Barnes Bldg.
FRYER, S. J. ....Surety Bldg.
FULLENWIDER, C. M. ....Barnes Bldg.
HAMM, S. G. ....Haskell
HOLCOMB, R. N. ....Surety Bldg.
JOBLIN, W. R. ....Porter
KAISER, GEO. L. ....562 No. Sixth
KLASS, O. C. ....Surety Bldg.
KUPKA, J. F. ....Haskell

McALISTER, L. S. ....Barnes Bldg.
MOBLEY, A. L., Vets. Facility, Albuquerque, N. M.
NEWHAUSER, MAYER ....Vet. Administration
NEELY, S. D. ....Commercial Natl. Bldg.
NICHOLS, J. T. ....Equity Bldg.
NOBLE, JOS. G. ....1400 E. Okmulgee
OLDHAM, Jr., I. B. ....426 North Sixth
OLDHAM, Sr., I. B. ....426 North Sixth
RAFTER, J. G. ....Manhattan Bldg.
SCOTT, H. A. ....Commercial Natl. Bldg.
SWEET, L. K. ....
THOMPSON, M. K. ....Surety Bldg.
TILTON, W. B. ....Vet. Hospital, Muskogee
WALKER, JOHN H. ....1620 W. Okmulgee
WARTERFIELD, F. E. ....Commercial Natl. Bldg.
WEAVER, W. N. ....Barnes Bldg.
WHITE, CHAS. ED ....2430 Boston
WHITE, J. H. ....Surety Bldg.
WOLFE, I. C. ....426 North Sixth
WOODBURN, JOEL T. ....Surety Bldg.

NOBLE

CAVITT, R. A. ....Morrison
COOKE, C. H. ....Perry
EVANS, A. M. ....Perry
FRANCIS, J. W. ....Perry
RENFROW, T. F. ....Billings
WIGNER, R. H. ....Marland

NOWATA

KURTZ, R. L. ....Nowata
LANG, S. A. ....Nowata
PRENTISS, H. M. ....Nowata
ROBERTS, S. P. ....Nowata
SCOTT, M. B. ....Delaware

OKFUSKEE

BLOSS, C. M. ....Okemah
BOMBARGER, C. C. ....Paden
BRICE, M. O. ....Okemah
COCHRAN, C. M. ....Okemah
JENKENS, W. P. ....Okemah
KEYES, ROBERT ....Okemah
LUCAS, A. C. ....Castle
MELTON, A. S. ....Okemah
PEMBERTON, J. M. ....Okemah
PRESTON, J. R. ....Weleetka
SPICKARD, L. J. ....Okemah

OKLAHOMA

ADAMS, ROBT. H. ....501 Ramsey Tower
AKIN, R. H. ....400 West Tenth St.
ALFORD, J. M. ....Medical Arts Bldg.
ALLEN, E. P. ....1200 North Walker
ALLEN, GEO. T. ....100 North Walker
ANDREWS, LELIA E. ....1200 North Walker
ARRINGTON, C. T. ....805 North Walnut
BAILEY, WILLIAM H. ....301 West Twelfth St.
BAIRD, Sr., W. D. ....2519½ South Robinson
BAIRD, Jr., W. D. ....2519½ S. Robinson
BALYEAT, RAY M. ....1200 North Walker
BARB, THOS. J. ....240 West Commerce
BARKER, CHAS. E. ....505-13 Osler Bldg.
BATCHELOR, J. J. ....Medical Arts Bldg.
BATES, C. E. ....Vet. Admin., Wichita, Kans.
BELL, A. H. ....300 West 12th St.
BEYER, M. R. ....State Health Department
BERRY, CHAS. N. ....119 No. Broadway
BINKLEY, J. G. ....119 No. Broadway
BINKLEY, J. SAM ....Memorial Hospital,
                                    New York City
BLACHLEY, C. D. ....2752 N.W. 18th
BLACHLEY, LUCILLE ....2752 N.W. 18th
BOATRIGHT, LLOYD C. ....Perrine Bldg.
BOGGS, NATHAN ....Perrine Bldg.

BOLEND, REX ....Medical Arts Bldg.
BONDURANT, C. P. ....Medical Arts Bldg.
BONHAM, WM. L. ....Medical Arts Bldg.
BORECKY, GEORGE L. ....Ramsey Tower
BOWEN, RALPH ....1200 North Walker
BRADLEY, H. C. ....Perrine Bldg.
BRANHAM, D. W. ....Medical Arts Bldg.
BREWER, A. M. ....Perrine Bldg.
BROWN, G. W. ....Medical Arts Bldg.
BRUNDAGE, C. L. ....1200 North Walker
BURTON, JOHN F. ....Osler Bldg.
BUTLER, H. W. ....1200 North Walker
CAILEY, LEO F. ....Medical Arts Bldg.
CAMPBELL, COYNE H. ....Medical Arts Bldg.
CANADA, J. C. ....216½ West Commerce
CATES, ALBERT ....Medical Arts Bldg.
CAVINESS, J J. ....Medical Arts Bldg.
CHARNEY, L. H. ....Medical Arts Bldg.
CLARK, ANSON L. ....Medical Arts Bldg.
CLOUDMAN, H. H. ....Medical Arts Bldg.
CLYMER, CYRIL E. ....Medical Arts Bldg.
COLEY, A. J. ....Hightower Bldg.
COLOPY, PAUL J. ....State Health Department
COLLINS, H. D. ....Medical Arts Bldg.
COOPER, F. M. ....Medical Arts Bldg.
COSTON, TULLOS O. ...First National Bank Bldg.
COTTRELL, W. P. ....1706 S.E. 29th
DAILY, H. J. ....Medical Arts Bldg.
DANIELS, HARRY A. ....Medical Arts Bldg.
DAVIS, E. P ....1601 N.W. 25th
DEMAND, F. A. ....1200 North Walker
DERSCH, WALTER H. ....Medical Arts Bldg.
DEUPREE HARRY L. ....St. Anthonys Hosp.
DICKSON, GREEN K. ....1200 North Walker
DOUGHERTY, VIRGIL T., Gorei, Abyssinia, Africa
DOWDY, THOS. W. ....Medical Arts Bldg.
EASTLAND, WM. E. ....Medical Arts Bldg.
ELEY, N. P. ....400 West Tenth St.
EMENHISER, LEE K. ....Washington Univ.
                                      St. Louis, Mo.
EPLEY, C. O. ....418 Osler Bldg.
ESKRIDGE, J. B. ....1200 North Walker
ERWIN, F. B. ....Medical Arts Bldg.
FAGIN, HERMAN ....400 West Tenth St.
FARIS, BRUNEL D. ....Medical Arts Bldg.
FELTS, GEO. R. ....Osler Bldg.
FERGUSON, E. G. ....Medical Arts Bldg.
FERGUSON, E. S. ....Medical Arts Bldg.
FISHMAN, C. J. ....132 West Fourth St.
FITZ, R. G., Taming Fu Hoppi, Prov. No. China
FLESHER, THOS. H. ....Edmond
FOERSTER, HERVEY A. .....119 North Broadway
FORD, HARRY C. ....Medical Arts Bldg.
FRIERSON, S. E. ....Medical Arts Bldg.
FRYER, S. R. ....119 West Fifth St.
FULTON, CLIFFORD C. ....Medical Arts Bldg.
FULTON, GEO. S. ....American Natl. Bank Bldg.
GARRISON, GEO. H. ....1200 North Walker
GEE, O. J. ....Medical Arts Bldg.
GIBBS, ALLEN G. ....Ramsey Tower Bldg.
GLOMSET, JOHN L. ....621 Osler Bldg.
GOLDFAIN, E. ....Medical Arts Bldg.
GOODWIN, R. Q. ....Medical Arts Bldg.
GRAHAM, ALLISON T. ....26 S.W. 25th
GRAY, J. WORTH ....1315 South Agnew
HALL, CLARK H. ....Medical Arts Bldg.
HANEY, A. H. ....Perrine Bldg.
HAMMONDS, O. O. ....623 North East 18th St.
HARBISON, FRANK ....Terminal Bldg.
HARBISON, J. E. ....Terminal Bldg.
HARRIS, HENRY H. ....1200 N. Walker
HASKETT, PAUL E. ....Hales Bldg.
HASSLER, GRACE CLAUSE ....Med. Arts Bldg.
HATCHETT, J. A. ....Medical Arts Bldg.
HAYES, BASIL A. ....625 North West 10th St.
HAYGOOD, CHAS. W. ....Municipal Bldg.
HAZEL, O. G. ....Medical Arts Bldg.
HEATLEY, JOHN E. ....Medical Arts Bldg.
HERRMANN, JESS ....Medical Arts Bldg.

HETHERINGTON, A. J. ....2014 Gatewood Ave.
HICKS, F. B. ....Medical Arts Bldg.
HIRSHFIELD, A. C. ....Medical Arts Bldg.
HOLLIDAY, J. R. ....1200 North Walker
HOOD, F. REDDING ....1200 North Walker
HOOT, M. P. ....301 West 12th St.
HOWARD, R M. ....Osler Bldg.
HUGGINS, J. R. ....Medical Arts Bldg.
HULL, WAYNE M. ....800 N.E. 13th
HYROOP, GILBERT L. ....Medical Arts Bldg.
ISHMAEL, WM. K. ....717 North Robinson
JACKSON, A. R. ....2528½ South Robinson
JACOBS, MINARD F. ....Medical Arts Bldg.
JANCO, LEON ....10 West Park Place
JETER, HUGH ....1200 North Walker
JOBE, VIRGIL R. ....717 North Robinson
JOLLY, W. J. ....615 West 14th St.
JONES, HUGH ....Medical Arts Bldg.
KELLER, W. F. ....Medical Arts Bldg.
KELLY, JOHN F. ....Medical Arts Bldg.
KELSO, JOSEPH W. ....Medical Arts Bldg.
KELTZ, BERT F. ....Medical Arts Bldg.
KERNODLE, S. E. ....First Natl. Bldg.
KIMBALL, G. H. ....Medical Arts Bldg.
KUHN, JOHN F. ....Medical Arts Bldg.
KUHN, Jr., JOHN F. ....Medical Arts Bldg.
LACHMANN, ERNST ....801 East 13th St.
LAIN, E. S. ....Medical Arts Bldg.
LAMB, JOHN H. ....Medical Arts Bldg.
LAMBKE, PHIL M. ....605 North East 28th St.
LaMOTTE, GEORGE A. ....Colcord Bldg.
LANGSFORD, WM. ....323 N.E. 11th
LANGSTON, WANN ....Medical Arts Bldg.
LAWSON, PAT ....119 N. Broadway
LEE, CLARENCE E. ....Hightower Bldg.
LEMON, C. W. ....119 No. Broadway
LEWIS, A. R. ....Hightower Bldg.
LINDSTROM, W. C. ....Medical Arts Bldg.
LINGENFELTER, F. M. ....1200 North Walker
LITTLE, JOHN R. ....Ramsey Tower
LONG, LEROY ....Medical Arts Bldg.
LONG, LEROY D. ....Medical Arts Bldg.
LONG, WENDELL ....Medical Arts Bldg.
LOWRY, DICK ....1200 North Walker
LOWRY, TOM ....1200 North Walker
LOY, C. F. ....Perrine Bldg.
LUTON, JAMES P. ....Medical Arts Bldg.
McCABE, R. S. ....Medical Arts Bldg.
MacDONALD, J. C. ....300 West Twelfth St.
MARGO, E. ....717 North Robinson St.
MARTIN, HOWARD ....Ramsey Tower
MARTIN, J. T. ....1200 N. Walker
MASTERSON, MAUDE M. ....119 No. Broadway
McBRIDE, Earl D. ....717 North Robinson
McGEE, J. P. ....404 Osler Bldg.
McHENRY, D. D. ....508 North West 15th St.
McHENRY, L. C. ....Medical Arts Bldg.
McKINNEY, MILAM ....Medical Arts Bldg.
McNEILL, PHIL M. ....Medical Arts Bldg.
MECHLING, GEO. S. ....Osler Bldg.
MELVIN, JAMES H. ....119 No. Robinson
MESSENBAUGH, J. F. ....Colcord Bldg.
MILES, W. H. ....Municipal Bldg.
MILLER, NESBITT L. ....119 No. Broadway
MILLS, R. C. ....Hightower Bldg.
MOFFETT, JOHN A. ....University Hospital
MOORE, C. D. ....Perrine Bldg.
MOORE, ELLIS ....Medical Arts Bldg.
MOOR, H. D. ....800 East Thirteenth St.
MOORMAN, FLOYD ....1200 North Walker
MOORMAN, L. J. ....1200 North Walker
MORGAN, C. A. ....First Natl. Bldg.
MORLEDGE, WALKER ....Osler Bldg.
MORRISON, H. C. ....807 North West 23rd St.
MULVEY, BERT M. ....Medical Arts Bldg.
MURDOCH, R. L. ....Medical Arts Bldg.
MUSICK, ELMER R. ....Medical Arts Bldg.
MUSICK, V. H. ....Medical Arts Bldg.
MUSSILL, W. M. ....Medical Arts Bldg.

MYERS, RALPH E. ....1200 North Walker
NAGLE, PATRICK ....Medical Arts Bldg.
NEFF, EVERETT B. ....1200 No. Walker
NICHOLSON, B. H. ....301 N.W. 12th
NOELL, ROBT. L. ....Medical Arts Bldg.
O'DONOGHUE, D. H. ....Medical Arts Bldg.
OWEN, CANNON A. ....311 N.W. 9th
PATTERSON, ROBT. U. .....801 North East 13th St.
PAULUS, D. D. ....301 West Twelfth St.
PENICK, GRIDER ....Colcord Bldg.
PHELPS, A. S. ....Medical Arts Bldg.
PINE, JOHN S. ....Medical Arts Bldg.
POSTELLE, J. M. ....Medical Arts Bldg.
POUNDERS, CARROLL M. ....1200 North Walker
PRICE, J. S. ....1200 North Walker
RECK, J. A. ....Colcord Bldg.
REED, HORACE ....Osler Bldg.
REED, JAMES ROBERT ....Medical Arts Bldg.
REICHMANN, RUTH S. ....124 North West 15th St.
RIELY, LEA A. ....Medical Arts Bldg.
RILEY, J. W. ....119 West Fifth St.
ROBINSON, J. H. ....301 West Twelfth St.
RODDY, JOHN A. ....Ramsey Tower
ROGERS, GERALD ....Osler Bldg.
ROSENBERGER, P. E. ....Perrine Bldg.
ROUNTREE, C. R. ....1200 North Walker
RUCKS, Jr., W. W. ....300 West Twelfth St.
RUCKS, W. W. ....300 West Twelfth St.
SADLER, LEROY H. ....Osler Bldg.
SANGER, F. A. ....Key Bldg.
SANGER, F. M. ....Key Bldg.
SANGER, WINNIE M. ....Key Bldg.
SEIBOLD, GEO. J. ....1200 N. Walker
SERWER, MILTON ....1200 North Walker
SEWELL, DAN R. ....400 North West Tenth St.
SHELTON, J. W. ....Medical Arts Bldg.
SHEPPARD, MARY V. S. ....1200 North Walker
SHORBE, HOWARD B. ....Medical Arts Bldg.
SIMON, BETTY HARRIS ....1000 N.W. 40th
SMITH, CHAS. A. ....Medical Arts Bldg.
SMITH, D. G. ....First National Bank Bldg.
SMITH, RALPH A. ....443½ North West 23rd St.
SNOW, J. B. ....1200 North Walker
STANBRO, GEO. E. ....Medical Arts Bldg.
STARRY, L. J. ....1200 North Walker
STILLWELL, ROBT. J. ....American Natl. Bldg.
STONE, S. N. ....Edmond
STOUT, M. E. ....209 West Thirteenth St.
STRADER, S. ERNEST ....Hightower Bldg.
SULLIVAN, ELIJAH S. ....Medical Arts Bldg.
SULLIVAN, ERNEST ....Hightower Bldg.
TABOR, GEO. O. ....First National Bldg.
TAYLOR, C. B. ....Medical Arts Bldg.
TAYLOR, W. M. ....1200 North Walker
THOMPSON, W. J. ....1200 N. Walker
TOOL, DONOVAN ....Edmond
TOWNSEND, CARY W. ....Medical Arts Bldg.
TURNER, HENRY H. ....1200 North Walker
UNDERWOOD, E. L. ....2604 No. Shartel
VALBERG, ERNEST ....Perrine Bldg.
VON WEDEL, CURT ....610 N. W. 9th St.
WAILS, T. G. ....Medical Arts Bldg.
WAINWRIGHT, TOM ....Medical Arts Bldg.
WARMACK, J. C. ....1615 No. Robinson
WATSON, I. N. ....Edmond
WATSON, O. ALTON ....1200 N. Walker
WATSON, R. D. ....Britton
WEIR, MARSHALL W. ....Ramsey Tower
WELLS, EVA ....Medical Arts Bldg.
WELLS, WALTER W. ....Medical Arts Bldg.
WEST, W. K. ....1200 North Walker
WESTFALL, L. M. ....Medical Arts Bldg.
WHITE, ARTHUR W. ....Medical Arts Bldg.
WHITE, OSCAR ....1200 North Walker
WHITE, PHIL E. ....Perrine Bldg.
WILDMAN, S. F. ....Medical Arts Bldg.
WILKINS, HARRY ....Medical Arts Bldg.
WILLIAMS, L. C. ....Osler Bldg.
WILLIAMSON, W. H. ....Hightower Bldg.

WILSON, KENNETH J. ....Medical Arts Bldg.
WOLFF, J. P. ....Osler Bldg.
WOODWARD, NEIL W. ....1200 North Walker
WRIGHT, HARPER ....240 West Commerce

OKMULGEE

ALEXANDER, ROBT. L. ....Okmulgee
BOLLINGER, I. W. ....Henryetta
BOSWELL, H. D. ....Henryetta
CARLOSS, T. C. ....Morris
CARNELL, M. D. ....Okmulgee
COTTERAL, J. R. ....Henryetta
EDWARDS, J. G. ....Okmulgee
GLISMANN, M. B. ....Okmulgee
HOLMES, A. R. ....Henryetta
HUBBARD, RALPH ....1501 E. 11th, Okla. City
HUDSON, W. S. ....Okmulgee
KILPATRICK, G. A. ....Henryetta
LESLIE, S. B. ....Okmulgee
MABEN, CHAS. S. ....Okmulgee
MATHENEY, J. C. ....Okmulgee
McKINNEY, G. Y. ....Henryetta
MING, C. M. ....Okmulgee
MITCHENER, W. C. ....Okmulgee
NELSON, J. P. ....Beggs
RAINS, H. L. ....Okmulgee
RANDEL, D. M. ....Okmulgee
RANDEL, H. O. ....Okmulgee
RODDA, E. D. ....Okmulgee
SIMPSON, N. N. ....Henryetta
SMITH, C. E. ....Henryetta
TORRANCE, L. B. ....Okmulgee
VERNON, W. C. ....Okmulgee
WALLACE, V M. ....Morris
WATSON, F. S. ....Okmulgee

OSAGE

AARON, W. H. ....Pawhuska
ALEXANDER, EVERETT T. ....Barnsdall
BAYLOR, R. A. ....Fairfax
DALY, J. F. ....Pawhuska
DOZIER, B. E. ....Snidler
GOVAN, T. P. ....Pawhuska
GUILD, C. H. ....Shidler
HEMPHILL, G. K. ....Pawhuska
HEMPHILL, P. H. ....Pawhuska
KARASEK, M. ....Shidler
KEYES, EDW. C. ....Shidler
KIMBALL, MELVIN C. ....Webb City
LIPE, E. N. ....Fairfax
LOGAN, C. K. ....Hominy
RAGAN, T. A. ....Fairfax
RUST, M. E. ....Pawhuska
SMITH, R. O. ....Hominy
SULLIVAN, B. F. ....Barnsdall
WALKER, G. I. ....Hominy
WALKER, ROSCOE ....Pawhuska
WEIRICH, C. R. ....Pawhuska
WILLIAMS, CLAUDE W. ....Pawhuska
WORTEN, D. ....Pawhuska

OTTAWA

AISENSTADT, E. ALBERT ....Picher
BARRY, J. R. ....Picher
BUTLER, V. V. ....Picher
CANNON, R. F. ....Miami
CHESNUT, W. G. ....Miami
CRAIG, J. W. ....Miami
COLVERT, G. W. ....Miami
CONNELL, M. A. ....Picher
COOTER, A. M. ....Miami
CUNNINGHAM, P. J. ....Miami
DeARMAN, M. M. ....Miami
DeTAR, G. A. ....Miami
DOLAN, W. M. ....Picher

HAMPTON, J. B. ....Commerce
HETHERINGTON, L. P. ....Miami
HUGHES, A. R. ....Wyandotte
JACOBY, J. S. ....Commerce
KERR, W. C. ....Picher
LANNING, J. M. ....Picher
LIGHTFOOT, J. B. ....Miami
McKAY, ED. D. ....Miami
McNAUGHTON, G. P. ....Miami
MILLER, H. K. ....Fairland
PERSLEY, TURNER ....Pitcher
RALSTON, B. W. ....Commerce
RITCHEY, H. C. ....Picher
RUSSELL, RICHARD ....Picher
SAYLES, W. JACKSON ....Miami
SHELTON, B. W. ....Miami
SIEVERS, CHAS. M. ....Picher
SMITH, W. B. ....Fairland
WORMINGTON, F. L. ....Miami

PAWNEE

BERNSTEIN, MAXWELL ....Pawnee
BROWNING, R. L. ....Pawnee
JONES, R. E. ....Pawnee
LeHEW, ELTON W. ....Pawnee
LeHEW, J. L. ....Pawnee
SADDORIS, M. L. ....Cleveland
SPALDING, H. B. ....Ralston

PAYNE

ADAMS, JAMES E. ....Cushing
BASSETT, C. M. ....Cushing
CLEVERDON, L. A. ....Stillwater
DAVIS, BENJ. ....Cushing
DAVIDSON, W. N. ....Cushing
FRY, POWELL E. ....Stillwater
HACKLER, JOHN W. ....Stillwater
HARRIS, E. M. ....Cushing
HERRINGTON, D. J ....Cushing
HOLBROOK, R. W. ....Perkins
LEATHEROCK, R. E. ....Cushing
MANNING, H. C. ....Cushing
MARTIN, EMMETT O. ....Cushing
MARTIN, JOHN F. ....Stillwater
MARTIN, J. W. ....Cushing
MITCHELL, L. A. ....Stillwater
OEHLSCHLAGER, F. KEITH ....Yale
PERRY, D. L. ....Cushing
RICHARDSON, P. M. ....Cushing
ROBERTS, R. E. ....Stillwater
SMITH, A. B. ....Stillwater
STRAHN, EVA ....Stillwater
WAGGONER, ROY E. ....Stillwater
WALTRIP, J. R. ....Yale
WILHITE, L. R. ....Perkins

PITTSBURG

BARTHELD, F. T. ....McAlester
BAUM, F. J. ....McAlester
BRIGHT, J. B. ....Kiowa
BUNN, A. D. ....Savanna
COLLINS, GLENN J. ....McAlester
DORROUGH, JOE ....Haileyville
GEORGE, L. J. ....Stuart
GREENBERGER, E. D. ....McAlester
KIES, B. B. ....Wetumka
KILPATRICK, G. A. ....McAlester
KLOTZ, W. F. ....McAlester
KUYRKENDALL, L. C. ....McAlester
LIVELY, CLAUDE E. ....McAlester
McCARLEY, T. H. ....McAlester
MILLER, F. A. ....Hartshorne
MUNN, J. A. ....McAlester
NORRIS, T. T. ....Krebs
PARK, J. F. ....McAlester

PEARCE, C. M., State Capitol Bldg., Oklahoma City
PEMBERTON, R. K. ....McAlester
RAMSAY, W. G. ....Quinton
RICE, O. W. ....McAlester
RUSSELL, ALLEN R. ....McAlester
SAMES, W. W. ....Hartshorne
SHULLER, E. H. ....McAlester
THOMAS, ERNEST ....McAlester
WAIT, WILL C. ....McAlester
WILLIAMS, C. O. ....McAlester
WILLOUR, L. S. ....McAlester
WILSON, HERBERT A. ....McAlester

PONTOTOC

BRECO, J. G. ....Ada
BRYDIA, CATHERINE ....Ada
BURROWS, L. I. ....Ada
CANADA, E. A. ....Ada
CRAIG, JOHN R. ....Ada
COWLING, ROBT. E. ....Ada
CUMMINGS, ISHAM L. ....Ada
DEAN, W. F. ....Ada
EVANS, R. ERLE ....Ada
FRY, MELVIN ....Stonewall
GULLATT, E. M. ....Ada
HINES, SIDNEY, J. T. ....Fittstown
LEWIS, E. F. ....Ada
LEWIS, MILES L. ....Ada
MAHON, GEO. S. ....Ada
McDONALD, GLEN W. ....Ada
McKEEL, SAM A. ....Ada
McNEW, M. C. ....Ada
MILLER, OSCAR H. ....Ada
MOREY, JOHN B. ....Ada
NEEDHAM, C. F. ....Ada
PETERSON, WM. G. ....Ada
ROSS, SAMUEL P. ....Ada
RUTLEDGE, JAS. A. ....Ada
SUGG, ALFRED R. ....Ada
WEBSTER, M. M. ....Ada
WELBORN, ORANGE E. ....Ada
YATES, JUNE ....Ada

POTTAWATOMIE

ANDERSON, R. M. ....Shawnee
APPLEWHITE, G. H. ....Shawnee
BAKER, M. A. ....Shawnee
BALL, W. A. ....Wanette
BAXTER, GEO. S. ....Shawnee
BLOUNT, W. T. ....Maud
BROWN, R. A. ....Prague
BYRUM, J. M. ....Shawnee
CAMPBELL, H. G. ....St. Louis, Okla.
CARSON, F. L. ....Snawnee
CORDELL, U. S. ....McComb
CULBERTSON, R. R. ....Maud
CULLUM, J. E. ....Earlsboro
FORTSON, J. L. ....Tecumseh
GALLAHER, F. C. ....Shawnee
GALLAHER, PAUL ....Shawnee
GALLAHER, W. M. ....Shawnee
GASTON, JOHN I. ....Shawnee
GILLICK, D. W. ....Shawnee
HUGHES, H. E. ....Shawnee
HUGHES, J. E. ....Shawnee
IRBY, J. P. ....Maud
KAYLOR, R. C. ....McCloud
KEEN, FRANK M. ....Shawnee
MATTHEWS, W. F. ....Tecumseh
McADAMS-WILLIAMS, ALPHA ....Shawnee
McFARLING, A. C. ....Shawnee
NEWLIN, FRANCES P. ....3748 Cambridge,
                                                  Kansas City
PARAMORE, C. F. ....Shawnee
RICE, E. E. ....Shawnee
ROWLAND, T. D. ....Shawnee
ROYSTER, J. H. ....Wanette

STEVENS, WALTER S., 315 P. O. Bldg., Okla. City
WALKER, J. A. ....Shawnee
WILLIAMS, A. J. ....McLoud

PUSHMATAHA

BALL, ERNEST ....Sulphur
CONNALLY, D. W. ....Antlers
GUINN, E. ....Antlers
HUCKABAY, B. M. ....Antlers
KIRKPATRICK, J. ....Tuskahoma
LAWSON, JOHN S. ....Antlers
PATTERSON, E. S. ....Antlers

ROGERS

ANDERSON, F. A. ....Claremore
ANDERSON, P. S. ....Claremore
ANDERSON, W. D. ....Claremore
BASSMAN, CAROLINE ....Claremore
BESON, C. W. ....Claremore
BIGLER, EARL E. ....Claremore
COLLINS, B. F. ....Claremore
HOWARD, W. A. ....Chelsea
JENNINGS, K. D. ....Chelsea
MELOY, R. C. ....Claremore
NELSON, D. C. ....Claremore

SEMINOLE

BLACK, W. R. ....Seminole
DEATON, A. N. ....Wewoka
GIESEN, A. F. ....Konawa
HUDDLESTON, W. T. ....Konawa
JONES, W. E. ....Seminole
KNIGHT, CLAUDE B. ....Wewoka
KNIGHT, W. L. ....Wewoka
LONG, W. J. ....Konawa
MILLS, N. W. ....Seminole
MOSHER, D. D. ....Seminole
PRICE, J. T. ....Seminole
REEDER, H. M. ....Konowa
STEPHENS, A. B. ....Seminole
TURLINGTON, M. M. ....Seminole
WALKER, A. A. ....Wewoka
WARE, T. H. ....Seminole

SEQUOYAH

MORROW, J. A. ....Sallisaw

STEPHENS

CARMICHAEL, J. B. ....Duncan
COKER, JOHN K. ....Duncan
DOWNING, G. G. ....Lawton
HARGROVE, FRED T. ....Duncan
IVY, W. S. ....Duncan
KING, E. G. ....Duncan
LINDLEY, E. C. ....Duncan
McCLAIN, W. Z. ....Marlow
McMAHAN, A. M. ....Duncan
PATTERSON, J. L. ....Duncan
PRUITT, C. C. ....Comanche
RICHARDSON, R. W. ....Duncan
SALMON, W. T. ....Duncan
SMITH, L. P. ....Marlow
TALLEY, C. N. ....Marlow
THOMASSON, E. B. ....Duncan
WATERS, CLAUDE B. ....Duncan
WEEDN, Jr., A. J. ....Duncan

TEXAS

BLUE, JOHNNY A. ....Guymon
HAYES, R. B. ....Guymon
LEE, DANIEL S. ....Guymon

SMITH, MORRIS ....Guymon
THURSTON, H. E. ....Texhoma

TILLMAN

ALLEN, C. C. ....Frederick
ARRINGTON, J. E. ....Frederick
BACON, O. G. ....Frederick
CHILDERS, J. E. ....Tipton
DAVIS, W. W. ....Davidson
FISHER, R. L. ....Frederick
FUQUE, W. A. ....Grandfield
OSBORN, JR., JAMES D. ....Frederick
'REYNOLDS, J. C. ....Frederick
SPURGEON, T. F. ....Frederick

TULSA

ALLEN, V. K. ....1001 Medical Arts Bldg.
ALLISON, T. P. ....Sand Springs
ARMSTRONG, O. C. ....915 Medical Arts Bldg.
AMENT, C. M. ....305 Ritz Bldg.
ATCHLEY, R. Q. ....507 Medical Arts Bldg.
ATKINS, PAUL N. ....1011 Medical Arts Bldg.
BARHAM, J. H. ....314 New Daniel Bldg.
BEESLEY, W. W. ....501 Medical Arts Bldg.
BEYER, J. W. ....621 McBirney Bldg.
BILLINGTON, J. J. ....404 Medical Arts Bldg.
BLACK, HAROLD J. ....209 Medical Arts Bldg.
BOLTON, J. F. ....211 Medical Arts Bldg.
BRADFIELD, S. J. ....607 Medical Arts Bldg.
BRADLEY, C. E. ....202 Medical Arts Bldg.
BRANLEY, B. L. ....315 Med. Arts Bldg.
BRASWELL, JAS. C. ....1109 Medical Arts Bldg.
BROGDEN, J. C. ....414-15 Medical Arts Bldg.
BROOKSHIRE, J. E. ....313 Ritz Bldg.
BROWN, WALTER E. ....1923 S. Utica
BROWNE, HENRY S. ....615 Medical Arts Bldg.
BRYAN, Jr., W. J. ....801 Medical Arts Bldg.
CALHOUN, C. E. ....Sand Springs
CALHOUN, WALTER H. ....405 Daniels Bldg.
CAMERON, PAUL B. ....604 S. Cincinnati
CAMPBELL, W. M. ....10½ North Lewis
CARNEY, A. B. ....402 Atlas Life Bldg.
CHALMERS, J. S. ....Sand Springs
CHARBONNET, P. N. ....206 Med. Arts Bldg.
CHILDS, D. B. ....1226 South Boston
CHILDS, HENRY C. ....1226 South Boston
CHILDS, J. W. ....1226 South Boston
CLINTON, FRED S. ....823 Wright Bldg.
CLULOW, GEO. H. ....410 McBirney Bldg.
COHENOUR, E. L. ....1102 Medical Arts Bldg.
COOK, W. ALBERT ....1006 Medical Rrts Bldg.
COULTER, T. B. ....1011 Medical Arts Bldg.
CRAWFORD, WM. S. ....1228 Exchange Bank Bldg.
CRONK, FRED Y. ....801-05 Medical Arts Bldg.
DAILY, R. E. ....Bixby
DAVIS, A. H. ....710 Medical Arts Bldg.
DAVIS, B. J. ....Sand Springs
DAVIS, T. H. ....404 Medical Arts Bldg.
DEAN, W. A. ....610 Medical Arts Bldg.
DENNY, E. R. ....1105 Medical Arts Bldg.
DUNLAP, ROY W. ....808 Medical Arts Bldg.
EADS, CHAS H. ....607 Medical Arts Bldg.
EASON, K. K. ....401 Atlas Life Bldg.
EDWARDS, D. L. ....203 Philcade Bldg.
EVANS, HUGH J. ....303 Medical Arts Bldg.
FARRIS, H. LEE ....303 Medical Arts Bldg.
FLACK, F. I. ....Natl. Bank of Tulsa Bldg.
FORD, H. W. ....417 Oklahoma Natl. Bank·Bldg.
FRANKLIN, S. E. ....Broken Arrow
FULCHER, JOSEPH ....417 Medical Arts Bldg.
*GARABEDIAN, G. ....15 West 13th St.
GARRETT, D. L. ....701 Medical Arts Bldg.
GILBERT, J. B. ....307 Roberts Bldg.

*Deceased.

GLASS, FRED A. ....404 Medical Arts Bldg.
GODDARD, R. K. ....Skiatook
GOODMAN, SAMUEL ....603 Medical Arts Bldg.
GORRELL, J. FRANKLIN, 610 Medical Arts Bldg.
GRAHAM, HUGH C. ....1307 So. Main St.
GREEN, HARRY ....1116 Medical Arts Bldg.
GROSSHART, PAUL ....302 Medical Arts Bldg.
HALL, G. H. ....427 McBirney Bldg.
HARALSON, CHAS. H. ......816 Medical Arts Bldg.
HARRIS, BUNN, ...Box 356, Jenks
HART, M. M. ....1232 South Boulder
HART, M. O. ....1232 South Boulder
HASKINS, THOS. M. ....814 Daniels Bldg.
HAYS, LUVERN ....Med. Arts Bldg.
HENDERSON, F. W. ....304 Medical Arts Bldg.
HENLEY, M. D. ....911 Medical Arts Bldg.
HENRY, G. H. ....801 Medical Arts Bldg.
HILLE, H. L. ....Collinsville
HOKE, C. C. ....207 Philtower Bldg.
HOOPER, J. S. ....Heavener
HOOVER, WILKIE D. ....201 Philcade Bldg.
HOUSER, M. A. ....606 Beacon Life Bldg.
HOTZ, CARL J. ....604 South Cincinnati
HUBER, WALTER A. ...1113-14 Medical Arts Bldg.
HUDSON, MARGARET G., 411 Medical Arts Bldg.
HUDSON, DAVID V. ....215 Medical Arts Bldg.
HUMPHREY, B. H. ....Sperry
HUTCHISON, A. ....Bixby
HYATT, EMRY G. ....604 South Cincinnati
JACKSON, L. T. ....206½ South Main
JOHNSON, CHAS. D. ....1117 Medical Arts Bldg.
JOHNSON, E. O. ....206 Medical Arts Bldg.
JOHNSON, R. R. ....Sand Springs
JONES, W. M. ....204 Medical Arts Bldg.
JUSTICE, H. B. ....303 Roberts Bldg.
KEMMERLY, H. P. ....902 Medical Arts Bldg.
KRAMER, A. C. ....415 Medical Arts Bldg.
LARRABEE, W. S. ....411 Medical Arts Bldg.
LAWS, J. H. ....Broken Arrow
LEE, J. K. ....212-14 Medical Arts Bldg.
LeMASTER, D. W. ....902 Medical Arts Bldg.
LHEVINE, MORRIS B. ......1007 Medical Arts Bldg.
LONEY, W. R. R. ....301 Medical Arts Bldg.
LOWE, J. O. ....402 Atlas Bldg.
LYNCH, T. J. ....201 Philcade Bldg.
MacDONALD, D. M. ....1739 South Utica
MARKLAND, JAMES D. ....Medical Arts Bldg.
MARGOLIN, BERTHA ....214 Medical Arts Bldg.
MAYGINNIS, P. H. ....505 Palace Bldg.
McCOMB, L. A. ....801 Medical Arts Bldg.
McDONALD, J. E. ....310 Medical Arts Bldg.
McGILL, RALPH A. ....1010 Medical Arts Bldg.
McGUIRE, H. J. ....910 Medical Arts Bldg.
McKELLAR, MALCOLM ......604 South Cincinnati
McLEAN, B. W. ....Jenks
McQUAKER, MOLLY ....1648 East 13th St.
MILLER, GEORGE H. ....206 Atlas Bldg.
MINER, J. L. ....810 Medical Arts Bldg.
MISHLER, D. L. ....604 S. Cincinnati
MOHRMAN, S. S. ....604 Daniels Bldg.
MUNDING, L. A. ....516 Medical Arts Bldg.
MURDOCK, H. D. ....1011 Medical Arts Bldg.
MURRAY, P. G. ....506 Medical Arts Bldg.
MURRAY, SILAS ....501 Medical Arts Bldg.
MYERS, F. C. ....502 Daniels Bldg.
NEAL, JAMES H. ....1944 North Denver Place
NELSON, I. A. ....1107 Medical Arts Bldg.
NELSON, F. J. ....603 Medical Arts Bldg.
NELSON, F. L. ....Atlas Life Bldg.
NELSON, M. O. ....307 Medical Arts Bldg.
NESBITT, E. P. ....917 Medical Arts Bldg.
NESBITT, P. P. ....917 Medical Arts Bldg.
NORMAN, G. R. ....17½ North Lewis
NORTHRUP, L. C. ....410 McBirney Bldg.
OSBORN, GEO. R. ....1105 Medical Arts Bldg.
PAVY, C. A. ....801 Medical Arts Bldg.
PEDEN, J. C. ....612 Medical Arts Bldg.
PERRY, HUGH, ...416 McBirney Bldg.
PERRY, JOHN C. ....618 McBirney Bldg.

PIGFORD, A. W. ....1001 Medical Arts Bldg.
PIGFORD, CHARLES ....Medical Arts Bldg.
PIGFORD, R. C. ....1001 Medical Arts Bldg.
PITTMAN, COLE D. ....1009 Medical Arts Bldg.
PORTER, H. H. ....510 Medical Arts Bldg.
PRICE, HARRY ....407 Medical Arts Bldg.
RAMEY, CLYDE ....612 Palace Bldg.
RAY, R. G. ....401 Atlas Bldg.
REESE, K. C. ....1101 Medical Arts Bldg.
REYNOLDS, J. L. ....305 Palace Bldg.
RHODES, R. E. LEE ....509 Medical Arts Bldg.
RICHEY, S. M. ....3830 West 44th St.
ROBERTS, T. R. ....417 Wright Bldg.
ROGERS, J. W. ....407 Medical Arts Bldg.
ROTH, A. W. ....607 Medical Arts Bldg.
RUPRECHT, H. A. ....604 South Cincinnati
RUPRECHT, MARCELIA ......604 South Cincinnati
RUSHING, F. E. ....505 Medical Arts Bldg.
RUSSELL, G. R. ....604 South Cincinnati
SCHRECK, P. M. ....603 Medical Arts Bldg.
SEARLE, M. J. ....202 Medical Arts Bldg.
SHEPARD, R. M. ....306 Medical Arts Bldg.
SHEPARD, S. C. ....706 Medical Arts Bldg.
SHERWOOD, R. G. ....412 Wright Bldg.
SHIPP, J. D. ....Sisler Clinic
SHOWMAN, W. A. ....409 Medical Arts Bldg.
SIMPSON, CARL F. ....502 Medical Arts Bldg.
SINCLAIR, F. D. ....Springer Clinic
SIPPEL, M. E. ....1542 East 15th St.
SISLER, WADE ....807 South Elgin
SMITH, D. O. ....604 South Cincinnati St.
SMITH, N. R. ....703 Medical Arts Bldg.
SMITH, ROY L. ....809 Medical Arts Bldg.
SMITH, R. N. ....1017 Medical Arts Bldg.
SMITH, RONALD R. ....403 Daniels Bldg.
SMITH, W. O. ....203 Philcade Bldg.
SPANN, L. A. ....305 Roberts Bldg.
SPRINGER, M. P. ....604 South Cincinnati
STALLINGS, T. W. ....724 South Elgin
STANLEY, MONT V. ....901 No. Denver
STEVENSON, JAS. ....615 Medical Arts Bldg.
STEWART, H. B. ....2500 East 27th Place
STUART, FRANK A. ....311 Medical Arts Bldg.
STUART, L. H. ....1107 Medical Arts Bldg.
SUMMERS, C. S. ....611 Daniels Bldg.
SWANSON, K. F. ....Springer Clinic
TAYLOR, J. H. ....1304½ West 17th
TRAINOR, W. J. ....1011 Medical Arts Bldg.
TURNBOW, W. R. ....908 Medical Arts Bldg.
UNDERWOOD, D. J. .....414-15 Medical Arts Bldg.
UNDERWOOD, F. L. ....1001 Medical Arts Bldg.
UNGERMAN, ARNOLD H. ....902 Med. Arts Bldg.
VENABLE, S. C. ....1135 South Quaker
WALKER, W. A. ....322 Kennedy Bldg.
WALLACE, J. E. ....914 Medical Arts Bldg.
WALL, G. A. ....902 Medical Arts Bldg.
WARD, B. W. ....823 Wright Bldg.
WEST, T. H. ....612 Medical Arts Bldg.
WHITE, N. STUART ....416 Medical Arts Bldg.
WHITE, P. C. ....312 Medical Arts Bldg.
WILEY, A. RAY ....812 Medical Arts Bldg.
WITCHER, E. K. ....511 Medical Arts Bldg.
WITCHER, R. B. ....910 Medical Arts Bldg.
WOODSON, FRED E. ....908 Medical Arts Bldg.
ZINK, ROY ....807 Daniels Bldg.

WAGONER

BATES, S. R. ....Wagoner
CRANE, FRANCIS S. ....Wagoner
PLUNKETT, J. H. ....Wagoner
RIDDLE, H. K. ....Coweta

WASHINGTON

ATHEY, J. V. ....Bartlesville
BEECHWOOD, E. E. ....Bartlesville
CHAMBERLIN, E. M. ....Bartlesville

CRAWFORD, H. G. ....Bartlesville
CRAWFORD, J. E. ....Bartlesville
CRAWFORD, T. O. ....Bartlesville
DORSHEIMER, G. V. ....Dewey
ETTER, F. S. ....Bartlesville
GENTRY, RAYMOND C. ....Bartlesville
GREEN, O. I. ....Bartlesville
HUDSON, L. D. ....Dewey
KINGMAN, W. H. ....Bartlesville
LeBLANC, WM. ....Ocnemta
PARKS, S. M. ....Bartlesville
REWERTS, F. C. ....Bartlesville
SHIPMAN, W. H. ....Bartlesville
SMITH, J. G. ....Bartlesville
SOMERVILLE, O. S. ....Bartlesville
STAVER, B. F. ....Bartlesville
TORREY, J. P. ....Bartlesville
VANSANT, J. P. ....Dewey
WEBER, H C. ....Bartlesville
WEBER, S. G. ....Bartlesville
WELLS, C. J. ....Bartlesville

WASHITA

BUNGARDT, A. H. ....Cordell
DARNELL, E. E. ....Colony
HARMS, J. H. ....Cordell
JONES, J. PAUL ....Dill
LIVINGSTON, L. G. ....Cordell
McMURRAY, J. F. ....Sentinel
NEAL, A. S. ....Cordell
SULLIVAN, C. B. ....Cordell
TRACY, C. M. ....Sentinel
WEAVER, E. S. ....Cordell
WEBER, A. ....Bessie

WOODS

BENJEGERDES, THEODORE D. ....Beaver
CLAPPER, E. P. ....Waynoka
DOUGAN, A. L. ....Amorita
ENSOR, D. B. ....Hopeton

HALE, ARTHUR E. ....Alva
HALL, RAY L. ....Waynoka
McGREW, EDWIN A. ....Beaver
ROGERS, CHAS. L. ....Carmen
SIMON, JOHN F. ....Alva
SIMON, WM. E. ....Alva
STEPHENSON, ISHMEL F. ....Alva
STEPHENSON, WALTER LOGAN ....Aline
TEMPLIN, OSCAR E. ....Alva
TRAVERSE, CLIFFORD A. ....Alva

WOODWARD

CAMP, E. F. ....Buffalo
DARWIN, D. W. ....Woodward
DAVIS, J. J. ....Higgins, Texas
DAY, J. L. ....Supply
DUER, JOE L. ....Taloga
DUNCAN, J. C. ....Forgan
FORNEY, C. J. ....Woodward
HILL, HARRY K. ....Laverne
JOHNSON, H. L. ....Supply
LEACHMAN, T. C. ....Woodward
NEWMAN, FLOYD ....Shattuck
NEWMAN, MESHECH HASKELL ....Shattuck
NEWMAN, O. C. ....Shattuck
NEWMAN, ROY ....Shattuck
RUTHERFORD, V. M. ....Woodward
SILVERTHORNE, C. R. ....Woodward
TEDROWE, C. W. ....Woodward
TRIPLETT, T. B. ....Mooreland
VINCENT, DUKE W. Vici
WALKER, HARDIN ....Rosston
WEAVER, GLENN A. ....Supply
WILLIAMS, C. E. ....Woodward

A list of the members has been submitted to the Secretary of each County Medical Society for correction. Less than half of these have been returned. If there are errors on this list it is not the fault of the State Secretary.

THE JOURNAL

OF THE

OKLAHOMA STATE MEDICAL ASSOCIATION

| VOLUME XXXI | McALESTER, OKLAHOMA, JULY, 1938 | Number 7 |

Management of the Hypertonic Period of Early Infancy*

FRANK C. NEFF, M.D.
KANSAS CITY, MISSOURI

There are certain features of the infant's first three to six weeks which justify the designation of that time of life as a hypertonic p e r i o d. These manifestations are suggested in many infants and should be regarded as reactions to common environmental influence. While they may be seen during the newly born period, they may be present any time within the early months. The physician is called upon to treat the following three clinical conditions common in this period:

1. "Colic" of early infancy.

2. Cutaneous exudative tendencies.

3. Feeding disturbance w i t h pylorospasm.

I wish to discuss these briefly and to make suggestions for their management and treatment.

1. *Colic of Early Infancy.* Young infants often react to the new environment of the outside world by evidences of excessive and unexplained crying, sleeplessness and motor unrest. This clinical condition has come to be known as colic, a term which has the disadvantage of applying specifically to intestinal and abdominal pain. I feel sure that the disturbance should be interpreted as the response to excitement by a young infant in whose organism inhibitions are as yet undeveloped.

*Read at the Annual Meeting, Oklahoma State Medical Association, Muskogee, May 10, 1938. From the Department of Pediatrics, School of Medicine, University of Kansas, Kansas City, Kansas.

The brain and central nervous system are fresh and plastic. Experiences are beginning to be recorded on the impressionable cells which are as active as the newest fullcharged b a t t e r y. Joseph Brennemann, with his gift for apt description, states in his recent work, the Encyclopedia of Pediatrics, that he has felt that the human infant is born somewhat "underdone."

Have you ever noticed that the visits of the young infant to your office will be accompanied by paroxysms of screaming? This is not due to the sudden development of colic or intestinal pain. I doubt that we have any proof that the well-fed normal young infant is suffering from pain during such paroxysms. These attacks may occur at home, but especially when the infant is disturbed greatly. If you think that he is not affected by conditions in his surroundings try the effect of elevating your voice suddenly; abruptly lifting the child while flexing the head and thighs forward; slamming the door; slapping the side of the crib. You will see the immediate movements of the arms and legs, which has been called the "startle-reflex."

The Startle-Reflex of Moro[1]. At about the sixth day of life a phenomenon may be elicited by striking the infant's bed with one's hand. Instantly there is a response due to startling, likened to an "embrace reaction," in which the infant spreads his arms, then brings them together in a bowed position, sometimes with a clonic vibration of the forearms. The legs are also included in this body startle-reflex. At about one month of age this reaction is at its maximum, but in many infants it still may be brought out for several months. Crying may accompany the disturbance which is evidently a manifestation of startling or frightening. The pattern[2] of the reaction may undergo some changes.

Interpretation of Colic in Early Infancy. Paroxysms of severe crying are produced by frightening, and can well be due to the same mechanism that produces the body-startle-reflex. This early evidence of hypertonus corresponds to the p e r i o d in which the Moro reaction is present. There is another reflex of early infancy known as the suspension-grasp reaction w h i c h may be accompanied by crying. This behavior trait is remarkable in the ability of the infant to grasp a small rod with the fingers of one hand and hold it sufficiently tight that he may be lifted for a few seconds. This might also be regarded as a manifestation of an increased nerve and muscle tonus.

The appearance of restlessness and of outbursts of screaming usually begins in the third or fourth week. This greatly disturbs the mother, who becomes much worried because of her inability to quiet the baby. When the infant cries, there is a similar emotional response from the mother. In the management of the mother and child I believe that the attendants, whether physician, nurse or member of the family, should appreciate the fact that the mother at this period is in a state of emotional imbalance or exhaustion.

The effect of the infant's immoderate crying is to interfere with rest and sleep, the appetite, the milk production, and even the judgment of the mother who believes that the infant is hungry all the time; that she is unable to supply enough food, and that she is therefore a poor mother. She concludes that her milk must be poor in quality, affected by her nervousness. The w h o l e household becomes likewise concerned.

So, changes are made in the intervals of nursing, formulae are begun, laxatives are given to the infant, household remedies are tried—all efforts are without avail. The infant is constantly kept agitated by such m e t h o d s as carrying, shaking, rocking, passing to various members of the family. The long drawn-out daily bath is accompanied by steady crying of the infant. The average home has much noise and confusion, and this helps prevent the infant from sleeping in the late afternoon and the first half of the night.

The physician is perplexed because of his failure to suggest successful methods for quieting the child. He decides in extreme cases that the infant be taken to the hospital. Conditions there are usually bettered, for the nurses are too busy to pay much attention to the infant which is fed, put down in its bed, and let alone.

It is common for families of physicians, of graduate nurses, of college professors, and of higher social levels to furnish many of the cases of hypertonic infants. Recently I talked on this subject in a nearby city and a colored physician told me that he had utilized my advice with good results. I answered that I had not known that "colic" bothered colored infants, but I suggested that the explanation might be in the fact that his wife probably belonged to the intelligentsia. "Yes," he said, "I guess she does belong. My wife has two college degrees."

Management of Environmental Conditions. From what has been stated regarding the exciting cause, it is obvious that conditions in the home must be changed from commotion to complete quiet. Instead of a complex program the schedule should be simple. The number of attendants should be limited to a few who comprehend what is needed, usually the mother and father.

Hours of rest will be increased if the intervals between feedings be lengthened. Breast feeding, complemental feeding, a dietary adequate in food factors and vitamins—when such are given it will rarely be necessary to make radical changes.

Management of Medicinal Treatment. Sedatives are indicated at regular intervals for several days. If relapses of crying occur, the dose may be increased at the time of day when most needed. The drugs which have proved successful and their dosage for the age levels in early infancy are as follows:

Age in Weeks	Phenobarb. Sol.	Atropine Sulf.	Codein Sulf.	Paregoric
2	gr. 1/6	gr. 1/2000	gr. 1/20	gtt. 10
4	gr. 1/5	gr. 1/1500	gr. 1/15	gtt. 15
8	gr. 1/4	gr. 1/1200	gr. 1/12	gtt. 20
12-20	gr. 1/3	gr. 1/1000	gr. 1/10	gtt. 25

The desired dose may be added to any syrup as a vehicle, and given in half or full teaspoonful. It s h o u l d be administered regularly, before each feeding. After a day or two of comfort the dose may be reduced or if it is still difficult to quiet the infant the dose may be continued or increased.

Phenobarbital soluble is nearly always effective, if not it may be advisable to try one of the other sedatives. Atropine and codein may be given together in a vehicle in case either alone does not produce rest. Paregoric seems to be helpful in an emergency and may be made to have a less objectionable taste and appearance by embodying it in a prescription rather than in water.

2. *Exudative Cutaneous Tendencies.* — From the day of birth skin lesions of various types and degrees are common upon the infant, indicating the vulnerability and tendency to exudation. Although during the entire period of infancy the skin is easily inflamed, it is m o r e sensitive in the early months, reacting in as vigorous a way to irritants as does the cerebral behavior to environmental irritation.

Physiological erythema is a simple manifestation of the neonatal days which appears promptly, sometimes with mild desquamation. Some infants have a t o x i c erythema which is probably a variety of physiological erythema, characterized by small areas of reddened skin the center of which is surmounted by a blanched papule resembling a tiny urticarial lesion. Erythema of the newborn is without clinical importance, except for the apparently severe itching. If the child's hands are free the face will be severely scratched and excoriated, or if the child lies upon its abdomen the face will be violently rubbed against the bedclothes. In our nursery the attendants are in the habit of restraining the infant who shows this tendency. This is done by elbow splints and a thin voile mask over the face.

(a) *Intertrigo*[3]. A lesion of importance, very common in the newborn is intertrigo, which may occur in many regions of the body. It is often due to "scalding" from frequent loose acid stools. This may occur any time in early infancy, if the soiled diaper be retained any l e n g t h of time. Highly acid urine sometimes causes a similar dermatitis during the n e w l y born period. It is the retention of the soiled wet diaper that usually causes the intertrigo. For treatment the newly born infant is placed in the knee-chest position, all diapers are discarded and the skin kept clean and dry.

For some unexplained reason ammoniacal decomposition of the urine in the diaper does not occur in the newly born period; and almost never in infants fed on breast milk alone. It comes in the early months with artificial feeding of large amounts of cow's milk. It is a result of urea-splitting of the voided urine in the warm moist diaper through bacterial contamination. Such ammonia burns from urine should not occur with hygienic care and with proper laundering of the infant's c l o t h e s and sheets. It is a d v i s a b l e to reduce the amount of cow's milk during such periods, if it be large.

Predisposed sites for intertrigo are the c o n v e x elevations of the body surfaces such as the buttocks, nates, the vulva, and labiae, the prepuce, meatus and scrotum which become inflamed from protracted c o n t a c t with moist soiled clothes. The chin, tip of nose, prominence of cheeks all show rapid inflammatory lesions from such exposure to dampness such as saliva and regurgigated food. Moisture which persists upon the face of the young infant is the cause of most instances of erythema or r a s h e s. The face stays wet by fingersucking, or contact with mother's wet nipple and breast; also from leakage from bottle, perspiration, delay in cleansing or drying the skin. Cleanliness, dryness and ventilation are the factors in prevention or cure. Excessive amount of clothing especially of heavy material producing overheating, sweating and restlessness h a v e much to do with exudative manifestations in infants.

(b) *Eczema of Early Infancy.* Eczema is often preceded or accompanied by manifestations of restlessness, immoderate crying, constipation or diarrhea. The infant loses sleep, is uncomfortable at all times. Early infancy is especially susceptible. I have purposely placed the discussion of eczema with that of intertrigo. Both develop in the well-fed i n f a n t, sometimes lacking in hygiene and favored by moist, uncleanly environment. Facial eczema in the young infant occurs as a mask on the convex surfaces similar to the sites of intertrigo; also in the bend of the elbow and the knee, where the moist warm surfaces away from air and evaporation permit a sodden state of the skin.

The infant becomes almost frantic from the intolerable itching so that, by scratching, the skin surface is traumatized. The erythema and small papular eruption may be changed into a moist denuded surface.

The Prevention of Eczema in the Young Infant. The relief of the restlessness and frantic traumatizing of the skin is best accomplished by (1) sedatives; (2) immobilization of the h a n d s and arms; (3) the wearing of a light mask or hood; the disease may be prevented, checked or cured if treatment is begun in this way. The hypertonic infant is the potential eczematous subject.

It has been the custom in most obstetrical nurseries to feed the newly born infant skimmed or other cow's milk for several days while awaiting the establishment of milk in the mother's breast. Very few infants in private hospital nurseries are fed breast milk alone and sooner or later infants get on cow's milk exclusively. Raw cow's milk is more apt to sensitize the child than is well boiled milk; even the boiling of evaporated milk should be practiced. For two years the evaporated milk used in our feeding cases in the nursery has been boiled for ten minutes. If there be a reasonable expectation that the mother can nurse the baby, cow's milk should not be started in the nursery but a sugar solution may be used to supplement the b r e a s t feeding.

The attempt should not be made to feed over-amounts of cow's milk simply for the purpose of rapid gain. The history of the feeding in infants who have acquired eczema is one of an over-abundant dietary whether on the breast or bottle. I have seen numerous cases of eczema occur when the quantity of cow's milk has been increased. Therefore sensitization may be quantitative in origin. Babies have gotten as much as 30 ounces of actual milk daily; have gained above the average weight and the bowels have been disturbed either by diarrhea in breast milk feeding or obstinate constipation from too much casein and calcium in the cow's milk. Finally the i n f a n t becomes restless, uncomfortable; sometimes exhibits colic, and a rash appears as a milk crust of the scalp or as an eczema of the cheeks. Early scratching makes it become rapidly worse and it is at this time that prevention of traumatism by restraint with splints and a light voile hood is of the utmost benefit.

Local Treatment of Eczema. In the beginning a bath in bran water may be needed so as to soak off the crusts. The lesions may then be p a i n t e d with tar-acetone-collodion m i x t u r e twice daily with a camel's hair brush. For a whole week this dressing is not removed. Tar is not used on the scalp or over pustules. The latter are drained, kept moist by application of boric acid packs.

Once each week the tar-acetone-collodion dressing is removed with acetone so that results may be observed. One should be sure to get a mild non-irritating preparation of crude coal tar; weaker mixtures of the tar are used in active inflammatory lesions, and stronger concentrations of tar are used in chronic eczema. The following proportions are suggested:

Rx Liquid Crude Coal Tar	gms	2	5	6-15
Acetone	cc	2	5	6-15
Flexible collodion	cc	30	60	90

There is a caution not to be forgotten as to the treatment of severe eczema. The mortality rate is high in severe cases of generalized eczema if the patient acquires intercurrent infection, such as upper respiratory disease. Most deaths occur in February, March and April. It would be better therefore in the winter or spring to treat the child as an outpatient rather than confining in a hospital ward.

Type of Diet in Eczema. In mild cases

one may continue milk but r e d u c e the amount, adding other foods to take the place.

In severe cases, determine the questions as to whether the eczema is being kept active by irritation from a food to which the child is sensitive; whether the eczema persists because of excessive c l o t h e s or bedcovers; whether there is irritation from secretions such as sweat or urination. In nearly every case traumatizing by scratching is the principal cause of exacerbation or chronicity.

Substitute Feeding. It s h o u l d not be necessary to wean a child from the breast for eczema. A reduction in amount if overfed, or if insufficient the addition of other foods s h o u l d be undertaken. Soy bean flour makes a good substitute for cow's milk. It is much similar to milk in its food factors but slightly deficient in carbohydrate. Soy bean milk is used commonly in Asia as the routine artificial bottle feeding. It even contains enough antiscorbutic so that scurvy rarely exists.

		1 pint	1 quart
Rx Soy Bean flour4......Tablespoons		12	24
Water ....Ounces		16	32
Sugar or syrup........Tablespoons		1 to 2	2 to 4

Feed with bottle or spoon in s i m i l a r quantities to milk.

We have not found permanent benefit from feeding goat's milk. Simply changing the species of animal milk would give only temporary relief, as the child soon acquires sensitization to the casein or lactalbumin.

Most eczema gets well or becomes quiescent when excessive amount of milk is discontinued; when additional foods are substituted for part of the milk; when the child is restrained for every minute of the day and night so that traumatization of the skin cannot occur; when a sedative such as phenobarbital soluble is g i v e n sufficiently to produce sleep and rest. The face and body must be dry. If clothing has been too heavy or irritating the skin may be made to return to normal more easily if exposed to warm air and drying.

(3) *Feeding Disturbance with Pylorospasm.* Occasionally one sees a young infant who has not gained well and has had a type of forcible vomiting suggestive of hypertrophic pyloric stenosis. Such infants have always c r i e d frequently and e v e n violently, have had poor appetite, have been immoderately restless. Their vomiting has been unexplainable for it occurred with all types of feeding. There may be evidence of hyperperistaltic waves. However the stools are not of the scanty hunger type seen in pyloric tumor obstruction. Barium given by the mouth passes the pylorus readily and normally. The child exhibits severe paroxysms of crying and may lie with retracted head and stiffened extremities during the screaming. The age incidence is different from that of pyloric tumor; it may begin in the newly born period or not till six weeks or more of age. The clinical picture is that of the hypertonic and neuropathic infant. An infant of eight weeks was sent into the hospital diagnosed as hypertrophic p y l o r i c s t e n o s i s. We found however that his stomach emptied completely in three hours and that there were g o o d stools though peristaltic waves were present. He did not require an operation.

The treatment is sedative, using atropine and codein, or phenobarbital. The dietary c o n s i s t s of milk incorporated in thick c e r e a l such as oatmeal or farina, which makes a concentrated feeding, less easily vomited than ordinary milk mixture.

Conclusion

Three clinical peculiarities common in early infancy may be successfully managed by the methods suggested. Colic is a term which is inappropriate as the infant is restless and startled rather than suffering from pain. The tendency to certain skin lesions, to vomit easily because of pylorospasm at this same period of early life also are disturbances belonging to this same hypertonic period. In all three conditions sedatives are of the greatest value.

Bibliography

1. E. Moro, Des Erste Trimenon, Munch. med. Wchnschr 65:1147-1150, 1918.

2. McGraw, Myrtle B., Ph.D., A. J. D. Children 54, 240-251, 1937.

3. Intertrigo literally means "rubbing between." It has usually been synonymous with the common word "chafing" such as so easily happens in flexor folds and between the thighs. The term is just as appropriate when used in connection with irritation or chafing of convex surfaces.

4. A commercial preparation readily obtainable is known as "Sobee." The mixture needs only to be brought to a boiling point.

Chairman's Address*

M. B. GLISMANN, M.D.
OKMULGEE, OKLAHOMA

As Chairman of the Obstetric-Pediatric Section of the Oklahoma State Medical Association, I welcome every one of you to this meeting, and ask that you each feel free to take part in the discussion of the p a p e r s presented. I am sure that you recognize that this section is unique in that it alone deals not only with the welfare of the individual patient, but also with the future welfare and progress of the nation. It is along this line that I would address you briefly this afternoon, in order that we may more clearly see our problems and our responsibilities, and perhaps, our possibilities.

When we realize that Oklahoma has its full share and more of the 150,000 American homes that are saddened and disrupted each year by the death of the mother or the new-born baby, or both; when we consider the vast number of children who are left motherless, and add to that, the other great group of mothers invalided by childbirth; then when we face the fact that this is our chosen field and that we, as physicians especially interested in obstetrics and pediatrics, have as our goal, a nation of living strong babies, and healthy mothers—we must admit that our gains in this direction, worthy as they are, have fallen far short of our ideals.

We shall hear during this session much of the story of the fight that the medical profession is making against the physical enemies of the mother and the baby, and we can thrill to the victories over the toxemias, tuberculosis, and syphilis. We still have far to go, and the road is a rough one, before we can see our losses brought to the irreducible minimum. We must consolidate our gains, refuse to falter in our preventive and educational program, and press on to extend our field of influence, until every mother and baby may expect

*Read before the Section on Obstetrics & Pediatrics, Annual Meeting, Oklahoma State Medical Association, Muskogee, Okla., May 10, 1938.

and shall profit by the advances of scientific medicine.

Our program, however, does not go far enough, and our concept is not as yet adequate. It is not enough that every conception shall result in a healthy, living baby. Our real problem is to help in the production of useful citizens, men and women who will be a credit and a benefit to society, instead of a burden on and an enemy of society. There are too many incompetents, too many mental and psychopathic inferiors, who owe their lives to our skill, only to have them become a burden, if not an actual danger to the useful members of the community. Most of these individuals are not "sports" or accidental misfits, but are the obvious and to-be-expected fruits, from their family tree.

It seems to me that our path in this field is plain. We cannot restrain the desire to co-habit, which seems especially strong in these uncontrollable personalities, but we can urge sterilization of the obviously unfit—the habitual criminal, the mentally unbalanced, and the degenerate. Gradually we will eliminate from our human herd the blood of this inferior stock, and America will be a safer and a happier place to live.

There is another great group that should engage our attention — the economically unfit. These we have always had with us in Oklahoma—the one-gallus son-of-gun in a two-room h o u s e. This tribe has increased enormously in these past years of depression, repression, the WPA dole and the like. It is possible that a family of this type can rear a family of one, two or even three children, feeding, clothing and educating them, and making of them, worthwhile m e m b e r s of the commonwealth. There comes a time, with the multiplicity of off-spring, however, when the heritage and the environment breeds o n l y dirt, hunger, neglect, lack of mental and moral training — and from this soil comes the anti-social member of the mobs, the hi-jacking gangs, and finally the bulk of our prison population. The dissemination of birth-control information in this g r o u.p, properly conducted by organized medicine, supervised and controlled, will do much to alleviate the hard-ships of this group and elevate the social and living standards of the whole group. Such work is already being started in several of our communities, and should spread throughout the state under the influence and control of the medical profession.

Even among our private patients, we can serve as improvers of the race, if we will but try. Can we not regularly and consistently urge a pre-marital examination, until it shall become a legal pre-requisite for marriage? Thereby we can eliminate most of the diseased, and many of the physically unfit and mental cases. This examination, with an intelligent attempt to give pre-marital advice where possible, p l u s pre-conceptional consultations with those of our families, already m a r r i e d, would do much toward improving the all-round quality of the babies who are born, giving them and their families an opportunity to fill their places in the world adequately. In this field we could give contraceptive advice to those with bad mental backgrounds, or severe constitutional disease. Knowledge of sex and marital hygiene will go far toward making a happy, adjusted home, which is the family background every youngster needs. The mat-ter of family planning should be stressed, and the dangers and results of abortion should be explained. It is easier to prepare the minds of a young couple, when they are planning a family, than convince them when they are faced with an untimely and perhaps unwanted pregnancy.

We shall, never, perhaps, know the biologic laws and the individual histories of the human animal, sufficiently so we can mate them even approximately well. It is doubtful, if we shall even advance very far, in applying the eugenic laws we know, for the human is a complex, and a stiff-necked race, and that goes double for those with the love madness. It is incumbent upon us, who are peculiarly fitted to know the problems, and to proceed logically toward their solutions, ever to t h i n k on these things. I leave for your thought the ideas of pre-marital and pre-conceptional advice. I urge you to work for the compulsory p h y s i c a l examination of those about to get married. Consider the establishment in your community of supervised birth-control clinics for the under-privileged, and be insistant, in season and out of season, for the legal sterilization of the unfit.

Finally, we must never forget the lessons we have learned about the care of the parturient woman, and the protection of the new-born baby, yet our responsibility goes farther than this. We must consistently aim toward the elevation of the physical, mental, and social standards of the human race in our state and nation.

————o————

Analgesia and Anesthesia in Labor*

GEORGE ALLEN, M.D.
OKLAHOMA CITY, OKLAHOMA

In our experience we are satisfied that there is no harmless anesthetic or analgesic. Knowing this and also knowing that most women demand some form of relief during labor, one should, only by constant and intelligent observation of patient and baby administer the v a r i o u s drugs and combination of drugs used in obstetrics today. Some of the more popular drugs are: s c o p o l a m i n e morphine, and its various modifications, the amytals, s o d i u m pentobarbital and scopolamine,

*Read before the Section on Obstetrics and Pediatrics. Annual Meeting. Oklahoma State Medical Association, Muskogee, Oklahoma, May 9-11, 1938.

quin-ether oil, paraldehyde, pantopon and sodium evipal. There are the anesthetic agents: nitrous oxide, ethylene, cyclopropane, ether, chloroform, and local anesthesia.

Every one knows that no one drug acts the same on every p a t i e n t. This fact makes the giving of the various r e l i e f agents a difficult problem in obstetrics. A drug may be ideal for one patient but affect the next in such a manner that she becomes most unruly, not only endangering herself and the baby but even making things quite disagreeable and uncomfortable for the attendants. Such a case is much more difficult to handle than a woman in her right mind who is having the usual labor pains.

Occasionally comparatively small doses of analgesics stop labor pains almost completely. Of course, the labor usually starts again but in the meantime the patient has become quite discouraged, to say nothing of her mother and husband.

There are reports in the literature of maternal deaths due to the administration of any one of the above mentioned drugs. Luckily such cases are rare, yet one death due to improper administration or carelessness w o u l d not be forgotten quite easily.

I am sure most obstetricians would like to dispense with our analgesics and most of our anesthetics altogether, yet when a woman in labor asks for it, we think it is our duty to give some form of relief. We have tried most of the analgesics used in obstetrics today, but have relied upon morphine and scopolamine in by far the greatest number of cases. Occasionally we use nembutal. Nembutal makes pain tollerable, produces a dream state affording almost perfect amnesia and usually does not interfere with progress of l a b o r. The amytals act similarly to the pento-barbital. We have abandoned quin-ether oil mainly on account of the inconvenience of its administration and the irritation it causes to the rectum. We have had no experience with paraldehyde or sodium evipal. Pantopon is used in an occasional case, that is, one sensitive to morphine.

Regardless of what medication one uses and regardless of how careful he is there

will be harmful results either to the baby or to the mother occasionally. All orders for medication used in labor should be written and not given verbally to some nurse. There should be no routine orders for any of the sedatives.

In the normal patient our chief concern is the baby and not the m o t h e r. The mother usually recovers quite satisfactorily following any form of reasonable medication. The baby however is not only subjected to the various depressing effects of the drugs but usually is allowed to be pressed for a longer period of time during the second stage of labor, or if not this, the termination of labor is by use of some forecep operation more difficult and much more dangerous to both the b a b y and m o t h e r than the ordinary prophylactic forcep operation. There are many women unfortunately who are not normal, and their particular condition demands special attention as to the relief of labor pains both in the first and the second stages of labor. In the first place we usually omit our analgesics in a primipara with a contracted pelvis and a floating or high head. We use no drugs in inertia uteri. No sedatives except morphine are given in advanced pulmonary or heart disease. Scopolamine and the barbiturates t e n d to speed up an already too fast pulse. No medication for relief of pain s h o u l d be given if there exists an immediate or prospective indication for the operative termination of labor as in placenta previa, asphyxia in utero, and so forth. Very seldom is any drug given in advanced labor, at least not less than two hours previous to delivery.

Ether may cause a bronchitis and even pneumonia especially in the presence of an acute upper respiratory c o n d i t i o n. Chloroform affects the liver and kidneys and may occasionally lead to an acute yellow atrophy of the liver. Consequently, it should never be used in any pre-eclamptic, eclamptic, or any case with kidney or liver dysfunction. Ether should be used in place of the various gases when it is necessary to operate in heart disease or shock, and when uterine relaxation is required as for version or other intra uterine manipulation.

During the second stage of labor we prefer either nitrous oxide or ethylene, to ether or chloroform. We use nitrous oxide in our practice probably because of some danger of explosion with ethylene anaesthesia. Explosions, of course, are rare yet I have more peace of mind when using a gas with less e x p l o s i v e characteristics. Ethylene has its advantages however. A higher percentage of oxygen may be given with ethylene whereas nitrous oxide requires p a r t i a l asphyxiation to produce anasthesia. Both gases cause a tendency to capillary oozing. We have never used cyclo-propane. In the administration of nitrous oxide the time for giving the gas depends upon how much pre-anesthetic medication has been given to the patient during the first stage of labor. Some patients need no anesthetic until the head is ready to be born or until an episitomy is done or instruments applied for delivery. However, for the patient that has had no, or very little, medication during the first stage; in primiparas we start gas usually at the beginning of the second stage of labor and in multiparas we begin our gas at any time the pain becomes quite severe after dilation has well advanced. The amount of nitrous oxide needed varies with every patient. When giving gas with pains the p a t i e n t must not become cyanotic nor should she lose consciousness until time for delivery. We usually allow water sparingly during this time. This prevents parching of the lips and throat. During the birth of the baby deep anathesia is produced for a few minutes. Immediately after the birth of the baby a few breaths of pure oxygen are given to the mother. As a rule nitrous oxide does not lessen the strength of the uterine contractions appreciably.

In consideration of the baby since one seldom sees a narcotized baby from the administration of nitrous oxide we have depended upon this agent as our chief analgesic during advanced labor. It is not unusual that one patient gets this gas so long as two or three hours. Usually a very high percentage of oxygen with nitrous oxide will satisfy the most difficult patient. This is not the very easiest procedure, yet the end results are most gratifying. During earlier labor we give hypodermics of morphine and scopolamine. The usual doses being one-sixth grain of morphine and one

two-hundredth grain of scopolamine. The first hypodermic in primiparas is given only after labor is well established. In a primipara we may repeat the same dosage of scopolamine once or twice, usually at two or three h o u r intervals. In the average patient a second dose of morphine is not given, yet, we do not hesitate to repeat it if labor is porgressing quite slowly in spite of s e v e r e pains. We think it b e t t e r to give no medication in cases of abnormally prolonged labor. In such a case the baby is already subjected to excessive amounts of pressure and trauma and the addition of any depressing drug may prove fatal. In labors of 24 to 36 hours or longer the pains are usually of such nature that no medication is required. The mother's pulse and the fetal heart should be watched quite closely and body fluids supplied by intra-venous and subcutaneous routes if necessary. As a rule, in multiparas, we give no medication during the first stage of labor. Usually labor is not so long and when sedatives are required, nitrous oxide may be given. One can usually d e p e n d upon a short enough labor for this procedure, however, there are many exceptions. If there is a possibility of prolonged labor and the pains are sufficiently strong then our medications are the same as in primiparas.

If we ever use barbiturates t h e y are used in small doses. This is almost a useless procedure so far as relieving pain is concerned. To relieve pain or produce amnesia with pento-barbital or any of the barbiturates one must use very large doses. As high as five to seven and one-half grains of nembutal must be given at one time. These large doses naturally benumb the respiratory center of both the baby and the mother. The babies after such treatment are usually dopey for several days and take up nursing unwillingly. Never should a barbiturate and m o r p h i n e be given together, as both are powerful respiratory depressants, and may do serious harm to the baby as well as to the mother. It is not our intention to produce complete amnesia for any patient. To most obstetricians a baby born with a lusty, piercing cry is m u c h m o r e satisfying than one which requires five to ten minutes to resuscitate. One can only hazard a guess as to the future life of an individual who has recovered from a period of oxygen want in his brain. It is a well known fact that prolonged cyanosis destroys b r a i n cells and that destroyed brain cells are irreplaceable. It has been suggested that some of the later psychoses observed in children and adolescents, perhaps the problem child, spastic muscles, and so forth, are due not alone to trauma but to the asphyxia so common after hard deliveries.

During the second stage of labor, which is usually prolonged to the detriment of the baby by the administration of any sedative, one must watch the fetal heart tones quite carefully. They fluctuate normally, usually ranging from 80 to 90 beats per minute immediately following and during a pain to 160 or thereabouts between pains There is little cause for alarm unless they remain below or above these figures. In the second stage the irregular heart beat is very significant, especially the irregular slow heart. This certainly is an indication for an immediate forcep delivery. Another

danger sign is the passing of meconium. This usually indicates a distressed baby and again labor should be terminated

Too frequently in obstetrics it is necessary for one to perform a cesarean section. Although a local anesthetic may be used to advantage in many normal deliveries we confine our local anesthesia to cesarean sections. Some patients are given general anesthetics for sections but as a rule only to those patients who are in the very best condition. It would not be a bad procedure to do all cesarean operations with local anesthesia, however. This method of anesthesia proves especially advantageous in all types of complicating heart conditions, acute respiratory infections or in any type of vital organ impairment in which general anesthesia would act as an overload. In toxemias of pregnancy, in which the physiology of the mother is greatly unbalanced with accompanying liver dysfunction, one could hardly think of a better reason for choosing a local in preference to a general anesthetic.

STILLBIRTHS*

P. N. CHARBONNET, M.D.
E. O. JOHNSON, M.D.
TULSA, OKLAHOMA

INTRODUCTION

Too frequently we neglect to find out the etiology of the stillborn or to do autopsies on them because we feel that, even though we have lost the child, we have successfully protected the life of the mother, or prevented lacerations, hemorrhages, trauma, etc., particularly if the labor and delivery were difficult. However, a critical review of the "obstetrical a u t o p s y sheet" seemingly should afford a very effective means of ascertaining our limitations in reducing the i n c i d e n c e of stillbirths as well as reveal many of our mistakes in management and treatment.

*Read before the Section on Obstetrics and Pediatrics, Annual Meeting, Oklahoma State Medical Association, Muskogee, Oklahoma, May 9-11, 1938.

Before we enter into the discussion let us first define "stillbirth."

DEFINITIONS

1. Dorland, The American Illustrated Medical Dictionary, "The birth of a dead fetus." Fetus: "The child in the womb after the end of the third month."

2. De Lee—"Some confusion exists regarding the definition of 'Stillbirth'—the majority of a u t h o r s hold stillborn and dead-born to be identical, which appears to me the simplest way."

3. American Public Health Association: "A stillborn child is one which shows no evidence of life after birth (no breathing, no action of heart, no movements of voluntary muscle). Birth is considered com-

plete when the child is altogether (head, trunk, and limbs) outside the body of the mother, even if the cord is uncut and the placenta still attached."

4. Certificate of Birth, Oklahoma State Board of Health—"A stillborn child is one that neither breathes, nor shows evidence of life after birth."

It is obvious that there are several discrepancies or inadequacies in the above definitions. A satisfactory, complete definition must answer the following points: period of gestation of the fetus, time of death in relation to the birth, what physiological actions of the baby are to be used as criteria of life and death, and a satisfactory uniform definition of birth.

The p e r i o d of gestation is important. Everyone agrees that the expulsion of a fetus before it is viable is an abortion and not a stillbirth. Thus "stillbirth" must include all fetus born dead after they have reached the period of viability, which is generally considered about the 28th week. However, our definitions are not concise on this point, and all stillbirth statistics vary in the duration of gestation in their classification of stillbirths. Gillespie and Dunham included deaths after five months gestation in their stillbirth statistics.

Is the death, two or three weeks before birth, of a fetus of 28 weeks gestation or more classified as a stillbirth the same as a fetus that dies during or at birth? According to our definition of born dead it must be.

The definition of the American Public Health Association is adequate in its description of those actions of the baby which d e n o t e life and what constitutes birth. However, it seems to me that the heart beat should be the only index needed for determining whether the fetus is alive, and much less confusing than trying to detect s l i g h t attempts at respiration, or movements of the limbs. Gillespie recorded among his reports on stillbirths those cases in which the fetus never breathed, even though the heart continued to beat for a few minutes after birth. Such cases, it seems to me, would be better classified as neonatal deaths.

A simple definition which seems to an-

swer the prerequisites which were previously stated is: "A stillbirth is the birth of a fetus of 28 weeks or more gestation which has no heart beat. Birth is considered complete when the child is altogether (head, trunk, and limbs) outside of the body of the mother, even though the cord is uncut and the placenta still attached."

Using the definition one would probably prefer to divide the stillbirths into two groups, in so far as management and treatment is concerned, namely: those that died before the onset of labor, and after onset of labor.

ETIOLOGY OF STILLBIRTHS

About 90 per cent of all dead born fetus can be grouped into one of the following clinical g r o u p s: asphyxia, prematurity, b i r t h trauma, congenital anomalies, and maceration. However, some of the more specific, common causes of fetal death are as follows:

I. *Maternal.*

1. Systemic Diseases — Syphilis, heart disease, toxemia of pregnancy, diabetes, pernicious anemia, pneumonia, t y p h o i d fever, scarletina, measles, malaria, metallic poisonings (lead, phosphorus, coal gas), focal infections and upper respiratory infections(?), septicemia.

2. Anomalies—Bicornate uterus.

II. *Developmental Causes.*

1. Cord anomalies — Short cord, coils about neck, knots, tumors of cord, velamentous insertion.

2. Placental—Premature separation, too small, abruptio, tumors.   .

3. Hydramnios.

4. Fetal—Papyraceous, monsters, hydrocephalus, anencephalus, etc.

III. *Accidents of Labor (T r a u m a, asphyxia, hemorrhage).*

1. Abnormal presentations, difficult deliveries, asphyxia.

2. Intracranial hemorrhage.

3. Trauma to vital centers.

IV. *External Factors.*

1. Anaesthesia, analgesia.

2. Drugs—Quinine, salicylates.

V. *Lethal mutations (maceration).*

DIAGNOSIS

The diagnosis is not made until birth, but sometimes the death of the fetus can be diagnosed before birth, or during labor.

Diagnosis of Death of Fetus Before Onset of Labor.

1. Lack of fetal movements (preceded by hyperactivity).

2. Failure to elicit motion by:

   a. Having mother hold breath several times (Drosin).

   b. Grasping anterior shoulder of fetus pushing up and back (Drosin).

   c. Pressure on fetal head in rectal or vaginal examination (Kanter).

3. Lack of fetal heart sounds.

4. Inability to palpate fetus satisfactorily because of flabbiness. (Spalding's fetal collapse). Softened fetal skull.

5. Decrease in size of uterus since last examination.

6. Increase in uterine souffle.

7. Retrogressive changes in b r e a s t s (Williams), soft, flabby.

8. Maternal systemic symptoms: Chill, nausea, malaise, bad taste and breath, epigastric pain, lower abdominal pains.

9. Laboratory tests:

   a. Ascheim-Zondek.

   b. Drop in B. M. R. (Baer).

   c. Acetonuria (Polak). King refutes this.

   d. Shorter coagulation time of blood (Guirauden).

10. X-ray shows overlapping of skull bones (Horner, Spalding).

11. "Audible silence." (A. D. Horner).

Diagnosis of Death of Fetus After Onset of Labor.

1. With rupture of membranes, f o u l smelling amniotic fluid, colored.

2. Rectal and vaginal examination on feeling crepitant skull bones.

3. Abnormal presentations occur more frequently (Dippel).

4. Absence of cord pulsation if version or intra-uterine manipulation is b e i n g done.

With the perfection of the fetal heart amplifiers which are being used in the delivery room in some clinics, fetal distress may be detected earlier, and death after full dilation may be reduced.

STASTICS

United States—The stillbirth rate in the United States has dropped gradually from 1933 to 1936, the rates for those years being 3.7 and 3.4 per 100 live births respectively. The total number of stillbirths has dropped from 77,059 to 73,735 annually during that time. The total number of live births in 1936 in the United States was 2,144,790, as compared to 77,059 stillbirths for the same year.

In 1936 the states with the highest stillbirth rates were Georgia (5.9 per 100 live births), South Carolina (5.8), Florida and Maryland (4.9). These are all southern states with comparatively large negro population, which probably means many midwives in attendance. However, Wyoming, which is the 48th ranking state in so far as population is concerned, which means that doctors are also probably harder to reach, has the lowest stillbirth rate in the United States, namely 1.4 (1936).

The three states with the greatest number of stillbirths for the years of 1933, 1934, 1935, and 1936 were: N e w Y o r k, 7,221 (1936), Pennsylvania, 5,034 (1936), and Texas, 3,905 (1936). It is rather interesting to note that Texas is the fifth ranking state according to population, yet it has a higher stillbirth rate and number of stillbirths than Illinois and Ohio, which rank third and fourth respectively in population.

Oklahoma—Oklahoma is the 21st ranking state according to population, which was estimated at 2,509,000 in 1935. According to the Bureau of Census of the Department of Commerce, Washington, D. C., Oklahoma had 1,181 stillbirths in 1936, as compared to 41,815 live births, making the stillbirth rate 2.8 per 100 live births.

In 1936 there were 17 other states in the United States which have a lower stillbirth rate than Oklahoma, and two others with the same rate, so that Oklahoma ranks in stillbirth rate about the same position as in population (20th). There are several questions which naturally arise. Does this mean that we have better obstetrics and obstetricians, give better care than the 28 other states which have a higher rate, or does it mean poorer statistical records, inadequate reporting of stillbirths, p o o r e r filing blanks, etc.?

The stillbirth rate for Oklahoma from 1932 to 1936 inclusive has been 2.6, 2.6, 2.8, 2.9, and 2.8 respectively, which is a slight increase. The greatest number of stillbirths was in 1934, with a total of 1,301 for that year.

Let us interpolate the stillbirths in Oklahoma for 1936, which totaled 1,182 into the figures of previous investigators. The excellent reports of Plass, Grulee, Dippel, Gillespie, and Dunham show the various causes of the stillbirths.

According to Grulee and Gillespie the chief causes for stillbirths were: prematurity, intrauterine death (maceration), b i r t h trauma, and asphyxia, which accounted for 65-75 per cent of all stillbirths. These were divided into prematurity (13-16 per cent), asphyxia (33 per cent), trauma at birth (30 per cent), intra-uterine death (16-40 per cent). Congenital defects in the fetus accounted for 5-10 per cent of the stillbirths. Williams (in 1920) reported 302 fetal deaths and ascribed syphilis as the cause of death in almost one-third of them. More recent r e p o r t s from other clinics do not agree with his findings, however. Placing our 1,182 stillbirths i n t o these groups we find the following: trauma at birth, 354; prematurity, 177; intrauterine death, 177 to 472; congenital defects in fetus, 59 to 118; leaving only 60 cases unclassified.

Birth trauma, certain cases of prematurity, asphyxia, and certain cases of intrauterine death can be directly influenced by the obstetrician. Congenital d e f e c t s are problems in eugenics which are affected more by legislation than by the obstetrician, except possibly in an advisory capacity directly to the patients, who seek it. However, we, as obstetricians, have direct influence over the outcome of 50-60 per cent of all stillbirths. Curtis says that about 50 per cent of fetal deaths are due to faulty o b s t e t r i c s, one-fourth due to curable diseases of the mother, and one-fourth unpreventable. This is a direct challenge to the obstetricians, and those doing obstetrics. We must seek the causes, and attempt to correct them.

DISCUSSION

In spite of the fact that the stillbirth rate and total number of stillbirths from 1932 to 1936 in the United States shows no tendency to increase, there are several factors prevalent now which may maintain this level or even cause an increase in the rate. Some of these factors may also influence the neonatal mortality rates. They are: inaccuracies in stillbirth reports and statistics, increase in the use and indications for induction of labor as in toxemia and cases of borderline pelvis, demands for complete relief of pain and amnesia by the patient, and the increasing incidence of operative deliveries.

STILLBIRTH REPORTS

Some states have only one report to be filled out by the physician in cases of stillbirth. In these states, if the newborn child shows very little evidence of life and dies in the first five or ten minutes following delivery, it is much easier for the attending physician to call it a stillbirth and save the time of filling out a death certificate also. Also, if the parents are told that their baby was stillborn, it seems to provoke less questioning of the doctor as to the exact cause than to have to explain why their baby did not live but a few minutes.

Bundesen, in Chicago, has r e c e n t l y pointed out the inaccuracies of the International List of the causes of death for neonatal mortalities, and is endeavoring to get them corrected. A revision of the causes of deaths for stillbirths might not be inapropos at the same time.

INDUCTION OF LABOR

As we are getting better methods and facilities to diagnose disproportion, contracted and borderline pelvis by X-ray encephalometry and pelvimetry, we are attempting to induce labor either early in borderline pelvis or at term to lessen the cases of postmaturity and oversize babies. The textbooks still list techniques of induction which c o n t a i n 20 to 30 gr. of quinine, and large doses of Pituitrin in spite of the fact that Gellhorn, Torland,

and others have reported fetal deaths from their use. Also, there seems to be another pathological condition of the lungs called "congenital pneumonia" which Leff attributed partly to the use of pituitrin during labor.

DEMAND FOR RELIEF OF PAIN

We are all quite aware of difficulties encountered in conducting a painless childbirth, and the increasing demands of our patients for complete relief, after reading articles in the current popular periodicals telling them that they should not only be absolutely free of pain but also have complete amnesia. This demand has placed a tremendous task on the obstetrician, with the threat that if he is unable to satisfy it he will lose his practice to the obstetricians who can. Consequently, heavier doses of analgesia and longer anaesthetics are being used. Eastman has shown that gas (N_2O-O_2) given in proportions of less than 85 to 15 are not harmful to the fetus, but that in concentrations greater than this, definite effects on the fetus can be n o t e d. Everyone of us have seen sleepy babies following the use of Nembutal and other barbiturate analgesics during labor, and I'm sure that I've seen newborns fail to breathe because of their use. This, of course, would a f f e c t the neonatal mortalities chiefly. However, Franklin Snyder of Johns Hopkins has shown that fetal respiration in utero does exist in animals. He has also shown that the administration of Nembutal to the mother animal causes a marked s l o w i n g of the intrauterine respiratory movement of the fetus. Perhaps this will explain some of our stillborns which have asphyxia as the only ascribable cause of death. This question has been brought out by Dr. Eastman.

OPERATIVE DELIVERIES

Plass in Iowa, in a very exhaustive study found the stillbirth rate four times as high in operative as spontaneous deliveries. He noted that the operative incidence among primipara was four times as great as in multipara, and that the stillbirth rate was higher in primipara. He also noted that stillbirths were higher in version and extraction and breech delivery than in any o t h e r operative procedures, including Caesarean sections. Plass concluded that

"the stillbirth rate among full term children increases in proportion to the operative incidence (so that it is highest in urban hospitals where operative intervention is more commonly practiced)." It is generally considered that the incidence of operative procedures is mounting, especially in the larger clinics.

CONCLUSIONS

1. Stillbirth statistics are presented.

2. A uniform definition is needed with revision of the International List of causes of death for stillbirths.

3. Questions for additional information on the certificate of birth or death in cases of stillbirths would aid in this problem in our state.

BIBLIOGRAPHY

1. Curtis. Obstetrics and Gynecology, Saunders Pub. Co., 1934. Vol. 1, page 554.

2. De Lee, Principles and Practice of Obstetrics, Saunders Pub. Co.

3. Plass et al. "Statistical Study of 129,539 births in Iowa with special reference to the method of delivery and the stillbirth rate," Am. J. Obst. and Gyn. Vol. 28, page 293, July-December, 1934.

4. Horner, D. A., "Antepartum Fetal Death," Am. J. Obst. and Gyn., Vol. 32, Page 67, July-December, 1936.

5. Horner, D. A., Roentgenography in Obstetrics, Surg. Gyn. and Obst., Vol. 35, Page 67-71, 1922.

6. Spalding, A. B., "Pathognomonic Sign of Intrauterine Death," Surg. Gyn. and Obst., Vol. 34, Page 754, 1922.

7. Torland, J., "Fetal Mortality of the Induction of Labor by Castor Oil and Quinine," J. A. M. A., Vol. 90, Page 1190, 1928.

8. Williams, J. W., Obstetrics, D. Appleton and Co., pub.

9. Gellhorn. "Can Quinine Kill Fetus in Utero," Am. J. Obst. and Gyn., Vol. 13, Page 779, 1927.

10. Dippel, A. L. "Death of Fetus in Utero," Bulletin of the Johns Hopkins Hospital, Vol. 54, page 24, January-June, 1934.

11. Gillespie, J. B., "Stillbirths," Am. J. Dis. of Child. Vol. 44, No. 1, Page 9, July, 1932.

12. Dunham, E. C., and Tandy, E. C., "The Causes of Stillbirths," South. Med. Journ. Vol. 30, No. 6, Page 643, June, 1937.

13. Grulee, "Fetal and Neonatal Mortality," The Journal of Pediatrics, Vol. 8, No. 1, Page 182, July, 1933.

14. Bundesen, H. N. et al, "Factors Responsible for Failure Further to Reduce Infant Mortality," J. A. M. A., Vol. 109, Page 387-343, July 31, 1937.

15. Eastman, N. J., "Role of Anaesthesia In Asphyxia of the Newborn," Vol. 31, No. 4, Page 563, April, 1936.

16. Baer, J. L. "Basal Metabolism in Pregnancy and the Puerperium." Am. J. Obst. and Gyn., Vol. 2, Page 249, 1931.

17. Williams, J. W., "The Significance of Syphilis in the Prenatal Care and Causation of Fetal Death," Bull. Johns Hopkins Hosp., Vol. 31, Page 141, May, 1920.

18. Eanter, A. E., "Diagnostic Sign for Viability of Fetus," J. A. M. A., 196, 234, Jan. 18, 1936.

19. Leff, M., "Fetal Heart Dilation; Pulmonary Congestion; and Pulmonary Edema Neonatorium, Congenital Pneumonia; Asphyxia," Am. J. Obst. and Gyn. 32:246; Aug., 1936.

20. Vital Statistics—Special Reports, Dept. Commerce Washington, D. C., Vol. 5, No. 18, Page 51, March 3, 1938.

21. Vital Statistics—Special Reports, Dept. Commerce, Washington, D. C., Vol. 3, No. 12, Page 71, April 21, 1937.

22. Vital Statistics—Special Reports, Dept. Commerce, Washington, D. C., Vol. 5, No. 11, Page 29, Jan. 25, 1938.

23. Charbonnet, P. N., and Johnson, E. O., "Congenital Pneumonia," Jour. Okla. State Medical Assoc., Vol. 20, No. 4, Page 120, April, 1927.

24. Williams, Philip F., "The Stillbirth Problem," Am. J. Ob. & Gyn. Vol. 34, No. 6, Page 840, December, 1927.

Birth Control*

GEORGE OSBORN, M.D.
TULSA, OKLAHOMA

I selected this subject when requested by your secretary to present a paper before this section and soon found myself in an embarrassing predicament—"caught in a trap," so to speak, and it all happened because I knew and still know so little about birth control outside of my experience in private practice and seven or eight years conducting a prenatal clinic sponsored by the Tulsa County Public Health Association, and yet it is a subject that intrigues my interest.

In the first place reproduction is a primitive instinct, inherent in all animals.

Man, in the process of evolution, developed an intellect and a will. As these two protuberances of his forebrain developed he found himself, through them, adapted to social intercourse and civilization which, of course, led to organization, government, etc. His life became more complex and he fought his enemies and conquered them; he solved some of the p r o b l e m s that threatened his life, but the impulse to live and reproduce is still dominant although those instincts in the process of civilization have become perverted.

It is trite but true to say that the human male, like the males of most lower animals is, by nature, a polygamous animal. Human laws and social conditions have put restraints and regulations upon him which, through the ages, he has been compelled to acknowledge as right and good.

However, through these same eons of time, changes have taken place in the female of the human species. She ovulates in a more frequent cycle than other animals and submits to sexual relations more frequently than does the female of other species.

Man worries and s t r u g g l e s with the problems of birth control and eugenics; trying to evolve some plan that will supplant the law of the survival of the fittest.

He is as stiff necked as the ox which was one of the first among domesticated animals, and is so imbued with the idea that he can work out his own destiny that he will not junk the notion that he can circumvent, at will, the union of the wily spermatazoid and the coy ovum.

Nature has not lost control of the process of reproduction in man, and it is my conviction that she never will. I realize, however, that telling the world of my personal conclusions will not stop the fight.

Birth control is a social problem and involves economics, religion and all phases of civilization.

If control is essential to the betterment of society and mankind in general, then the medical profession must interest itself to the extent of determining the most scientific and efficient method of control and that alone should be its responsibility. I think the medical profession does sense its responsibility and that it will fall to our lot to teach the social worker that birth control does not mean contraception alone.

These enthusiasts are now fostering and abetting one of the most gigantic commercial rackets of modern times. I refer to the manufacture and sale of so-called contraceptives. We, as medical men, know that this racket has supplanted the patent medicine business as the leader of frauds in the United States. This p r o f i t a b l e racket is becoming a menace to the ethics of our own profession, even greater than the practice of abortion.

I will mention only one device: the so-called gold cap or button pessary with the hairpin spring, inserted in the cervix. I have removed several of these in recent years from cervices where they had become imbedded and, in two instances, have

*Read before the Section on Obstetrics and Pediatrics, Annual Meeting, Oklahoma State Medical Association, Muskogee, Oklahoma, May 10, 1935.

I found them in the cervices of women, one three months and the other five months pregnant.

In every instance these had been placed by so-called reputable physicians. There may be men whose ignorance would be responsible for imperiling the health and life of their patients but it may be done for the fee.

Birth c o n t r o l must be scientifically studied, not with the idea of limiting reproduction but to overcome sterility and spacing pregnancies. Contraception has long been recognized as a phase of preventive and public health medicine. It seems that many present day social workers think birth control or limiting reproduction among the indigent class is a comparatively recent or modern idea.

As proof to the contrary and to substantiate the old saying that there is nothing new under the sun, let me mention a few examples of early knowledge of contraception cited by Norman E. Himes in the Journal of Contraception, May, 1937.

"A few primitive peoples knew a sterile period.

"An Indian tribe living in the northern part of South America possessed a female condom made from a large seed pod.

"In the mika operation used by the Australian natives an artificial hypospadias was created.

"The Ebers papyrus of Egypt, 1950 B.C., mentions the first known chemical contraceptive; viz: tips of acacia intravaginally —under fermentation acacia forms lactic acid.

"Aristotle recommended smearing the os uteri with olive oil and recently Dr. Maric Stopes rediscovered the m e t h o d for the poor of the Orient.

"Soranus' Gynecology in the second century, A.D., lists the greatest array of contraceptive suppositories and pessaries to be found in medical literature for centuries.

"The Biblical reference to coitus-interruptus.

"Fallopius, the Italian anatomist — discoverer of the tubes which bear his name —mentioned the glans condom.

"The vulcanization of r u b b e r in 1840 made effective the diffusion of knowledge of the condom as a preventative."

These examples of early knowledge of contraception show that little progress has been made, either in scientific agents for contraception nor has birth control been very effective in reducing the birth rate among the indigent classes.

This paper has been presented merely to raise the question—What and how much are we, as medical men, going to do about it?

---------------O---------------

Prenatal Care, or the Management of Pregnancy*

G. L. KAISER, M.D.
MUSKOGEE, OKLAHOMA

Prenatal care is the supervision, care and instruction given to pregnant women.

By careful examination and frequent observation, toxemis of pregnancy and other progressive illnesses arising in the pregnant woman may be reduced, and with complete prenatal care eclampsia, our most

*Read before the Section on Obstetrics and Pediatrics, Annual Meeting, Oklahoma State Medical Association, Muskogee, Oklahoma. May 10, 1938.

horrible complication with its high mortality rate can be eliminated.

In addition to reducing and eliminating complications, prenatal care provides a means of accurate determination of the size of the fetus in relation to the pelvis, the type of presentation and position. With this information the probable type of delivery may be planned insuring maximum safety against the accidents of parturition.

In the present day of general obstetrical information and education, the duties of the medical attendant are very definite.

On the first visit of the patient, the doctor should obtain:

1. A short, concise past h i s t o r y embracing the following.

a. The occurrences of family diseases and a malignancy history.

b. A history of childhood diseases, including scarlet fever, diphtheria and particulary if there were any sequelae.

c. A complete menstrual history, the date of onset, cycle, w h e t h e r or not there is any complication, if so, what?

d. A history of operations, their type if any.

2. History of previous pregnancies, their dates, illness during pregnancy, nature of the labor, length of labor and type of delivery.

3. A complete physical examination; in detail of the head, eyes, ears, nose, throat, tonsils and teeth; refer to a good dentist for check up, and if there is any cavity, this should be filled immediately.

Next examine the neck, thyroid and cervical glands; following this the chest; heart and lungs should be examined if any questionable conditions arise, these should be checked by X-ray and other laboratory procedures.

The breast should be examined and the type of nipples determined; show the patient how to evert the nipples and instruct her to do this two or three times daily in order to assure that they will be everted and tough. This procedure will greatly facilitate nursing.

The abdomen should be examined and the condition of the abdominal wall determined. Estimate the height of the fundus, and determine the presence of hernia and rashes.

The Pelvis: Examine for lacerations or other pathological conditions existing.

Measure the pelvic outlet. Take a smear routinely from the cervix. Take the blood pressure and obtain a urinalysis and Wasserman.

Subsequent Visits: The patient should be instructed to return at intervals of three to four weeks bringing a s p e c i m e n of urine. On each of these visits the pregnant woman should be questioned as to her well being, ability to rest and sleep, and any required advice given.

Blood ppressure, urinalysis and weight should be taken and recorded each time.

Diet: It seems reasonable that if the food intake of the mother be restricted the child will be reduced in size and weight, thereby causing an easier delivery. Observation proves this erroneous, s i n c e the child being a true parasitic growth, develops at the expense of the maternal tissues no matter how marked the degree of underfeeding. The nutritional problem as it arises during gestation may be considered as follows:

1. The frequency of abnormal appetite causing pregnant women to overeat with a consequent excessive g a i n in fat and greater strain upon the already laboring excretory organs.

2. The tendency to over indulgence of protein and urea rich foods, with the attendant danger of kidney failure.

3. The various methods by which food intake may be made to regulate the size and weight of the fetus. In regard to the quantity of food eaten it is g e n e r a l l y known that pregnant women over eat. An undernourished patient has a better chance of withstanding the stress of l a b o r and avoiding toxemia than one who is excessively overfed.

In contrast to using a restricted diet it is much more satisfactory to group the foods: The following grouping is very satisfactory:

1. One and one-half pints of milk daily. This may be used in cooked foods.

2. Calcium, (calcimalt or cal gluconate tablets) if the patient prefers the calcimalt may be added to the milk.

3. Cod liver oil.

4. No pork or fatty meats, crisp bacon excepted.

5. Small amounts of lean meats, fish and eggs once daily.

6. No fried or greasy foods, medium portions of fried chicken occasionally.

7. Green vegetables and fresh fruits at

least two at the noon and e v e n i n g
meal and one raw.

8. Starchy foods are to make up the
least part of the diet.

9. Sweets, only small amounts of sweets
and desserts should be taken. An
occasional Coca-Cola or other carbonated water is permissable.

With this grouping p a t i e n t s average
about 20 pounds gain, and rarely gain as
much as 25 pounds.

Maintenance of a balanced diet is required and pregnant women should not be
permitted to reduce arbitrarily during this
time.

Hypotension is encountered in a large
number of patients, a systolic reading of
100 mm. or even less being found very
often. This condition is regarded as of
little significance.

Hypertension is one of the great warning signals of impending toxemia, especially is this true when a pressure apparently normal during the first few months,
steadily rises as pregnancy proceeds. In
these conditions the urine should be examined with the utmost care. The patient
should be considered toxic and treated accordingly.

At the seventh month, the patient should
be completely re-examined, the position
and presentation of the fetus being determined at this time, and again at the
ninth month to recheck the type of delivery that is anticipated.

HYGIENE

Dress: Garments which, while accom-
modating the patient's changing figure,
still retain lines of grace may be obtained.
The usual corset may be worn until about
the fifth month, when a maternity corset
may be adopted.

Shoes should not be c h a n g e d unless
swelling of the feet necessitates the use of
a larger size. One who has been accustomed to wearing high heels should continue to do so and vice-versa.

Exercise: Dancing, golf and walking are
advised. Heavy lifting and arduous labor
should not be permitted. An abundance of
sunshine and moderate e x e r c i s e in the
fresh air are essential.

Bathing: A daily bath, preferably a
shower is desirable. The bath should be
neither hot or cold, but pleasantly warm,
and should be followed by a brisk rub.
Swimming in quiet waters may be moderately practiced.

Automobiling: It has been found that
the strain of resisting road shock, sudden
starting and stopping and rapid turns, is
quite exhausting and too frequently results in debilitating fatigue. There may
be some nerve s t r a i n dependent upon
steady and long continued exposure to the
wind by a rapidly moving vehicle. However the relaxation, change of scene and
fresh air to be obtained through moderate
uses of the motor car are of inestimable
benefit. The patient may drive to about
the sixth month provided reasonable care
as to speed and accident is used.

Regulation of Bowels: Evacuation should
occur daily, if constipation supervenes it
is to be met by gentle laxatives.

Maternal Impressions: Scientific opinion
of the present day denies the possibility of
the direct transmission of a maternal impression upon the fetus. The physician
should be very definite regarding this matter. The strongest emphasis should be
laid upon the fact that the fetus is fully
formed at the end of the sixth week, and
that no mental image created in the mother's mind has any effect whatsoever upon
the child.

Preservation of the Figure: The athletic
girl of today because of her indulgence in
swimming, tennis and other types of exercise, runs but little risk of losing the tone
of her abdominal m u s c l e s as compared
with her languishing sister of a generation
ago. After impregnation there is no longer
time to strengthen the abdominal muscles,
the wearing of corsets should be advised.
The support of the abdomen is of more importance in relaxed multiparae in whom
the abdomen may become so pendulous
that malpresentation quite often occurs.

Coitus may be indulged in cautiously
during pregnancy until about the seventh
month, during the first three months special care should be exercised at about the
time menses would ordinarily take place.

Sleep: Due to s t r a i n and stresses to

which a pregnant woman is exposed, it is imperative that she should have an abundance of sleep to restore her nervous tone. Eight to ten hours, with an hour or so in mid-afternoon.

Morning sickness: This at times is quite annoying causing uneasiness especially if allowed to continue untreated.

Nervous System: Insomnia, restlessness and anxiety are common accompaniments of what is otherwise a normal pregnancy.

Back aches and p a i n s in legs: Back aches are due in most cases to a change in posture produced by the weight of the pregnant uterus, and to sacro-iliac strain; a well fitting abdominal belt gives support and relief of pain. Pains in legs: This condition is often annoying and difficult to manage. It is the result of pressure of the presenting part, and disappears with delivery.

Tingling and numbness of the hands and feet: These seem to be a result of calcium deficiency and will generally respond to calcium therapy.

Determination of Sex: This is still a realm of conjecture and is abused by many of our colleagues, a practice which should be discouraged.

Selection of Nurse: The patient should be instructed to secure the services of the best type of nurse permitted by her financial budget.

Surgical Operations: Surgery is to be avoided if possible, and still stay within the realms of safety.

The Treatment of Poison Ivy*

HERVEY A. FOERSTER, M.D.
OKLAHOMA CITY, OKLAHOMA

The ivy plant is known by the botanical name of Rhus Toxicodendron. The active principal causing the poison ivy dermatitis is a glucoside called toxicodendrol. This active principal can be destroyed by alkalies, less so by acids. So one of the best prophylactics after exposure or suspected exposure to the ivy vine, is plenty of washing with a good strong alkaline soap such as any of the so-called laundry soaps, followed by an alcohol sponging. If this procedure is carried out within an hour or two after exposure, many an otherwise severe case of ivy dermatitis can be prevented.

Children under three years of age are very rarely sensitive to the poison ivy plant and some individuals have a natural immunity. But by constant exposure and contact a sensitivity can be developed. A patient who is very sensitive to poison ivy can be helped or have his resistance increased. This is on the basis of allergic

desensitization. The mechanism is not exactly known, as there is no reagins. The active principal of the Rhus plant can be carried by the blood stream to different areas of the skin and an extreme generalized reaction can be produced.

There are many external irritants that can produce a dermatitis venenata that may stimulate the dermatitis due to Rhus, so that a few w o r d s of caution are advisable; be sure that the dermatitis is due to poison ivy before you use any injections or ivy extracts.

I am going to describe the use of an e a s i l y made extract that I have been using which can be adapted both as a prophylactic and a treatment. The method is not original by me but is one that has been used for a number of years in the East and was developed by the allergic department of the Postgraduate Medical School of Columbia University, by my good friend, Dr. Will Spain, and I want to give him full credit for my knowledge of this method.

*Read before the Section on Dermatology and Radiology, Annual Meeting, Oklahoma State Medical Association, Muskogee, Oklahoma, May 10, 1938.

An extract is made by collecting the leaves of the Rhus plant, dehydrating the leaves in an oven, then crushing the dry leaves to a fine smoking tobacco like size. Next extract with absolute alcohol, in the proportion of 10 grams of the leaf to 100 cc of absolute alcohol. This is extracted for 48 hours then filtered and the filtrate made up into various dilutions from the stock solution, the 1 to 100, 1 to 1,000, and 1 to 10,000 are the strengths most often used.

Now in the desensitization procedure, suppose you have an individual who is highly sensitive to the ivy plant and who wishes to have his immunity built up before the start of the poison ivy season. You test the patient by putting on patch tests (usually on f l e x o r s of the arms or the back) of dilutions of your stock solution of the extract. Start out with the 1 to 10,000 strength. Read the results in 48 hours. If you get no erythema or vesiculation then test with the s t r o n g e r dilutions. The strength of the solution that gives just a slight positive reaction is the one to begin your prophylactic treatment with. Your first dose is 1/20 of a c.c. of the extract diluted with .9 c.c. of normal saline solution injected subcutaneously. I n j e c t once a week increasing the strength of the dilutions until you reach a top strength of 1/20 c.c. of the 1/10 solution. Usually eight doses are required for prophylactic treatment for the season. This should be given in January or February, and repeated each year.

For the treatment of an acute attack of ivy, dermatitis, there are several principles to remember in the local application of drugs. Never put on an oil or ointment, these retain the active principal and will prolong the dermatitis. Wet packs of boric acid solution, normal saline or weak potassium permanganate are the drugs of choice. A nice prescription is: Rx.

Phenol	2.0
Zinc Oxide	15.0
Lime water q.s	250.0

Sig: Sponge on every three hours.

I have seen several cases of tattoo marks left following use of Ferrous Chloride solution, so do not use it in the local treatment. Now the use of the extracts in the treatment of an acute attack: give 1/20 c.c. of

the 1 to 1,000 solution every two days, usually three to five injections are necessary. After the second dose the patient usually shows improvement. If any reaction or exacerbation is encountered then, decrease your dosage or use the 1 to 10,000 dilution.

I find this procedure very satisfactory and in the cases that I have used it, I have had uniform good results.

I would like at this time to mention some of the difficulties in the diagnosis of Rhus poisoning. I recall one dear old lady who had a chronic eczema-venenata dermatitis on the face and hands and as it was during the winter months, ivy was not suspected, she was questioned about contacts, etc., she mentioned that she had some plants that she watered and cared for. On bringing leaves from the plants, one was a poison ivy plant that she had thought was the tame ivy. She had been watering it and caring for it since the fall before. This was proved to be the cause of her dermatitis.

Another individual had an acute dermatitis with vesiculation on the hands. He gave no history of being in the woods or in contact with plants. He worked at a filling station and of course gasoline dermatitis was thought of. He reacted negative to all tests with gasoline, paints and oils. However, on further questioning he remembered an automobile that had been into the station which had tied across the rear fender, oak leaves and branches which the occupants had gathered in the woods. I believe that this was the source of Rhus dermatitis. Occasionally, I have seen individuals w i t h s u c h a sensitivity that, driving through a country road, the Rhus toxicodendrol will be carried by the wind and the left side of the face and left hand alone will be involved if they are driving the car. I have seen several very severe cases where burning leaves and trash in the fall along with ivy vines, and the smoke borne Rhus will penetrate the clothed parts of the body as well as the exposed areas.

In closing, I wish to state that the treatment of ivy poisoning is still far from a satisfactory p r o b l e m and you will hear prescribed and tried by the many patients who have suffered from this dermatitis a host of things. Nearly everyone has a sure remedy, just as they will give advice on treating a cold. I have found the method of treatment I have outlined is a satisfactory one and it is on a rational basis.

The San Francisco Meeting

The following doctors attended the Annual Meeting of the American Medical Association, held in San Francisco, June 13-17, 1938. The Association, was represented in the House of Delegates by Drs. W. Albert Cook, Tulsa, and McLain Rogers, Clinton. Also seated in the House of Delegates, but not voting, were Drs. Horace Reed, Oklahoma City, and L. S. Willour, McAlester, Secretary-Editor. Dr. Earl D. McBride, Oklahoma City, appeared on the program of the Orthopedic Section. Dr. Henry H. Turner, Chairman of the Post Graduate Medical Teaching, attended a conference of those interested in Post Graduate Medical Teaching from various states in the Union.

A report of our Delegates will be published in the August issue of the Journal.

Following is the report of attendance from the state of Oklahoma.

Monday's registration: H. R. Anderson; W. G. Bisbee, Bristow; W. Albert Cook, Tulsa; Lt. Col. William S. Culpepper, Fort Sill; Phil J. Devanney, Sayre; William E. Eastland, Oklahoma City; James G. Edwards, Okmulgee; Roy E. Emanuel, Chickasha; Gallaher, Shawnee; James M. Gordon, Ardmore; George K. Hemphill, Pawhuska; Forrest M. Lingenfelter, Oklahoma City; Paul B. Lingenfelter, Clinton; Wendell Long, Oklahoma City; Earl D. McBride, Oklahoma City; W. R. Marks, Vinita; Warren T. Mayfield, Norman; George S. Mechling, Oklahoma City; William C. Miller, Guthrie; Harry Dale Murdock, Tulsa; Robert Urie Patterson, Oklahoma City; Dwight D. Pierson, Clinton; Horace Reed, Oklahoma City; McLain Rogers, Clinton; H. K. Speed, Jr., Clinton; Wildridge Clark Thompson, Stillwater; W. C. Tisdal, Clinton; L. C. Veazey, Ardmore; Harry Wilkins, Oklahoma City; L. S. Willour, McAlester, and Divonis Worten, Pawhuska.

Tuesday's registration: Wm. H. Bailey, Oklahoma City; A. M. Brewer, Oklahoma City; Anson L. Clark, Oklahoma City; D. W. Darwin, Woodard; Ephriam Goldfain, Oklahoma City; Everett S. Lain, Oklahoma City; John H. Lamb, Oklahoma City; T. H. McCarley, McAlester; Earl Winters Mabry, Altus; L. A. Mitchell, Stillwater; R. L. Murdoch, Oklahoma City; I. A. Nelson, Tulsa; F. S. Newman, Shattuck; R. C. Pigford, Tulsa; H. H. Turner, Oklahoma City, and Raymond D. Watson, Britton.

Wednesday's registration: R. H. Goldwaithe, Fort Sill; A. C. Hirshfield, Oklahoma City; Wayne M. Hull, Oklahoma City; Phil M. Lambke, Oklahoma City, and R. G. Sherwood, Tulsa.

Thursday's registration: L. J. Moorman, Oklahoma City; Marque O. Nelson, Tulsa; Lea A. Riely, Oklahoma City, and Charles B. Taylor, Oklahoma City.

International Goiter Conference

The Third International Goiter Conference will be held at Washington, D. C., September 12th to 14th.

The scientific sessions are open to members of the medical and allied professions who are in good standing.

All meetings are to be held in the ball room of the Mayflower Hotel, conference headquarters.

THE DOCTOR

Sculpticolor of Fildes' Masterpiece Goes to Rosenwald Museum

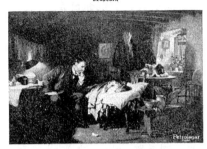

Now In a Permanent Home

The $150,000 reproduction of the Sir Luke Fildes masterpiece "The Doctor" first shown by the Petrolagar Laboratories at Chicago's Century of Progress Exposition in 1933, was recently presented by its owners to the new Rosenwald Museum of Science and Industry in that city.

Following the two World's Fairs, "The Doctor" exhibit went on a tour of 50,000 miles and was viewed by over 5,000,000 people in 18 principal cities throughout the country.

Designed to remind the public of the importance of the family physician, it required the full time of the late Chicago sculptor, John Paulding, and the noted artist, Rudolph Ingerle, and a large corps of assistants, and took nearly a year to complete.

In its new location in the Rosenwald Museum it will be seen by millions of visitors annually.

Additions To 1938 Roster

The following have become members of the State Association since the compilation of the Roster which appeared in the June Journal:

BECKHAM COUNTY

CARY, W. S.	Reyden
DILLARD, J. A.	Hammon
PHILLIPS, G. W.	Sayre
PITTS, D. H.	Elk City

CREEK COUNTY

COFFIELD, A. W.	Sapulpa

CUSTER COUNTY

SEBA, W. E.	Leedy

GARFIELD COUNTY

LAMERTON, W. E.	Enid

HUGHES COUNTY

WALLACE, C. S.	Holdenville

SEMINOLE COUNTY

GRIMES, J. P.	Wewoka
JONES, RUTH	Seminole
VAN SANDT, G. B.	Wewoka
VAN SANDT, M. M.	Wewoka
WHITE, J. H.	Wewoka

TILLMAN COUNTY

BOX, O. H.	Grandfield
COLLIER, E. K.	Tipton
FOSHEE, W. C.	Grandfield
FRY, F. P.	Frederick

Correction

TABOR, GEO. R., Oklahoma City, instead of Geo. O. Tabor.

THE JOURNAL
OF THE
Oklahoma State Medical Association

Issued Monthly at McAlester, Oklahoma, under direction of the Council.

Copyright, 1938, by Oklahoma State Medical Association, McAlester, Oklahoma.

Vol. XXXI	JULY, 1938	Number 7

DR. L. S. WILLOUR..............................Editor-in-Chief
McAlester, Oklahoma

DR. T. H. McCARLEY..............................Associate Editor
McAlester, Oklahoma

Entered at the Post Office at McAlester, Oklahoma, as second-class matter under the act of March 3rd, 1879.

This is the official Journal of the Oklahoma State Medical Association. All communications should be addressed to The Journal of the Oklahoma State Medical Association, McAlester Clinic, McAlester, Oklahoma. $4.00 per year; 40c per copy.

The editorial department is not responsible for the opinions expressed in the original articles of contributors.

Reprints of original articles will be supplied at actual cost provided request for them is attached to manuscripts or made in sufficient time before publication.

Articles sent this Journal for publication and all those read at the annual meetings of the State Association are the sole property of this Journal. The Journal relies on each individual contributor's strict adherence to this well-known rule of medical journalism. In the event an article sent this Journal for publication is published before appearance in The Journal the manuscript will be returned to the writer.

Failure to receive The Journal should call for immediate notification of the Editor, McAlester Clinic, McAlester, Oklahoma.

Local news of possible interest to the medical profession, notes on removals, changes of addresses, births, deaths and weddings will be gratefully received.

Advertising of articles, drugs or compounds unapproved by the Council on Pharmacy of the A. M. A., will not be accepted.

Advertising rates will be supplied on application.

It is suggested that wherever possible members of the State Association should patronize our advertisers in preference to others as a matter of fair reciprocity.

Printed by News-Capital Company, McAlester.

EDITORIAL

WHY SUPPORT ORGANIZED MEDICINE?

The year covered in the report of the Board of Trustees of the A.M.A. has been characterized by a very notable expansion in the activities of the various councils, bureaus and departments of the Association until, at times, available facilities have been seriously strained. A constantly growing interest on the part of the general membership in changing social conditions; increased efficiency of medical organization in counties and states throughout the nation; a more active and intelligent interest on the part of the public in matters pertaining to public health and medical service; legislative activities in the states and in the federal government; the consideration of important questions pertaining to medical education, hospital operations and the extension of public health programs; greater financial and administrative participation on the part of the federal government in public health affairs in states and in communities; proposals for the development of medical and hospital service plans for the benefit of the members of low income groups and actual operation of such plans, and a notable increase in the number of members of the Association together with many other important factors have brought into the headquarters offices a veritable flood of inquiries and demands for information and service. An earnest effort has been made to meet such demands as fully and as helpfully as possible.

The gross earnings of the Association for 1937 were $1,654,203.74; operating expenses were $982,830.10. The operation of the Council, bureaus and departments amounted to $431,635.63. Incidental expenses, including insurance, taxes, building expenses and depreciation, fuel, legal services and special publications amounted to $218,601.19, showing a net income of $122,242.92, of which sum $83,563.74 represents income from investments, so that the actual net operating income was $38,679.18.

The place held by the Journal of the American Medical Association in the field of medical periodicals is now so well established that it is unnecessary to offer comment on this point. In the State of Oklahoma there are 951 subscribers to the Journal; however, there are only 685 Fellows.

The special Journals published by the American Medical Association were published at a loss of $25,958.37 to the Association in 1937, while Hygeia was published at a loss of $31,004.90.

The Cooperative Medical Advertising Bureau earned on advertising contracts secured, $156,705.47, rendering to the participating Journals most valuable service.

The Council on Pharmacy and Chemistry, Foods and Physical Therapy have been closely correlated. The work of the Council on Pharmacy and Chemistry has been greatly increased during the past year on account of the submission of a large number of products by manufacturers and the nature of the investigation made, and for the further reason that the activities of the Council are being more fully supported by the medical profession generally.

An important series of articles dealing with diet, prepared by highly qualified investigators are being published under the auspicies of the Council, these later to appear in book form.

The endocrine principles and new therapeutic substances of various kinds have required prolonged and intensive consideration. The Council on Physical Therapy has established standards for acceptable audiometers and has given careful examination of short wave and diathermy apparatus.

The Council on foods has made every effort to promote truthful advertising of wholesome food products and has had the benefit of the services of a number of distinguished scientists in conducting necessary scientific investigations.

The Chemical Laboratory in the past year carried out an important accomplishment as a result of investigations of the poisonous effects of a product known as Elixir of Sulfanilamide, when it was established that at least 76 deaths were due to this product, and the toxic agent was found to be diethylene glycol. Much work has been done in the laboratory to establish standards for important therapeutic products.

The Bureau of Legal Medicine and Legislation has been very active during the past year supporting the enactment of the National Cancer Institute Act, the Marihuana Tax act, an act authorizing the Bureau of Mines to manufacture and sell helium gas for medical and other non-governmental uses, and an act devolving on the Federal Trade Commission jurisdiction over the advertising of foods, drugs, diagnostic, therapeutic devices and cosmetics. Efforts to arouse interest in the establishment of a Federal Department of Health have been unproductive.

The Council is closely in touch with all Federal Legislation such as legislation pertaining to vivisectionist, social security act, federal income tax act and the legislative problems of the various states.

· The Bureau of Health and Public Instruction has carried on an extensive program throughout the year. The dramatized radio program conducted with the cooperation of the National Broadcasting Company completed its second successful season in 1937. The Bureau has cooperated as fully as possible with official agencies concerned with the protection of scientific research. The Director and the Assistant Director of the Bureau have appeared before a larger number of audiencies than in any previous year. The educational publications issued under the direction of the Bureau have been widely distributed.

The Bureau of Medical Economics is conducting a survey of need for medical care and in this survey it would be necessary that every State and County Medical Society heartily cooperate, as this information will be very necessary to determine the exact need for any change in the plan of medical practice. This Bureau has also investigated the many forms of medical practice, and has made extensive study of group hospitalization and workmen's compensation. They have also looked into the Insurance Medical Directories and advised physicians not to be victimized by publishers of pay-as-you-enter insurance medical directories.

Many articles and abstracts pertaining to medical economic problems have been prepared by the Bureau.

The Bureau of Investigation received and answered from 10,000 to 12,000 communications during the year. This Bureau has continued its cooperation with medical societies and other professional groups, and with Federal, State and City governments.

The Bureau of Exhibits reports that at the Atlantic City session there were 254 exhibits, the largest that has ever been shown. There were special exhibits on fractures and anesthesia, which were outstanding successes. Association exhibits, dealing with the activities of the Association, were sent out on 115 occasions to 33 states. Through exhibits approximately 3,500,000 persons were reached, including the Cleveland and Dallas expositions. The demand for motion pictures has been constant and the new film on syphilis has been received with much favor.

The foregoing sketch from the complete and comprehensive report of the Board of Trustees is being published editorially in your Journal in order that you may develop some idea of what the American Medical Association means to the individual doctor. It would be well if every physician could read the entire report and he would then be convinced that without the A. M. A. and its component organizations the problems of the practitioner of medicine would be even more intricate than they are at present. This parent Association deserves the support of every regular practicing physician and can only be supported by your membership in your County and State Association and Fellowship in the A. M. A. All of the benefits that come from the parent association we take as a matter of course. Some, however, are so thoroughly convinced of the importance of the work done that they subscribe to its support, while in Oklahoma there are some 1,600 doctors who are deriving these benefits and contributing n o t h i n g. In other words they are not paying their way —just hitch-hiking along the highway of Organized Medicine.

RE-PRINTS OF ARTICLES

There seems to be some confusion as to when reprints of articles published in the Journal can be acquired.

When an author is furnished with proof of his article there is always a slip enclosed for ordering reprints, with prices indicated. If the author wishes reprints they must be ordered at this time, because the forms are torn down almost immediately after publication of the current issue of the Journal. Late orders, consequently, cannot be filled unless the author would wish to go to the expense of having the article re-set.

Report of Committee on Study and Control of Tuberculosis

In view of the fact that less than 20 per cent of tuberculosis cases are discovered, or admitted to sanatoria, in an early stage of the disease, it is apparent that physicians need to be more alert to early diagnosis. Certainly prospects for success-

ful home care is greatest the sooner the disease is found.

A factor now favorable to the family physician is widespread public education about tuberculosis, thereby increasing the willingness of patients to accept a decision in early diagnosis. Another factor bringing the tuberculosis problem into the hands of the family physician is that the people are learning that infection in children may be discovered in advance of disease, and that such children need supervision and care to prevent active tuberculosis.

With the situation in regard to tuberculosis as herein outlined, encouraging a back-to-the-physician movement, the family doctor may logically play a more prominent part in its control. Therefore, we urge physicians to use routinely all modern diagnostic methods for the discovery of tuberculosis in the early stages. Also, at regular intervals checking known cases and contact cases in the home to determine progress and whether or not other members of the household have become infected. Furthermore, with our citizenship recognizing tuberculosis as still a national and local problem, the medical profession will gain in public esteem in taking a more active part in meeting it.

Carl Puckett, Chairman.
Will C. Wait.
L. J. Moorman.

Editorial Notes—Personal and General

DR. LEE K. EMENHISER announces the opening of his office at 1106 Medical Arts Bldg., Oklahoma City, having completed a two-year house service in Ear, Nose and Throat at Barnes Hospital, St. Louis. He was former head of the Department of Anatomy of the School of Medicine, University of Oklahoma.

DRS. FRED G. DORWART and HALSELL FITE, Muskogee, were the guests of the Pittsburg County Medical Society, June 17th. Their subjects were "Diuretics—Statistical Studies of" and "Urology in Children," respectively.

DR. and MRS. H. A. LILE, Cherokee, have returned from a vacation trip into the Rockies.

DR. and MRS. H. E. HUSTON and daughter, C h e r o k e e, are visiting relatives in Wenatchee, Washington.

DR. and MRS. ELTON LEHEW and children, Pawnee, are visiting in Galveston, going from there by boat to New York City.

DR. and MRS. JOHN F. PARK and children, McAlester, spent two weeks in June in Galveston.

Practice-Equipment For Sale

The practice, office equipment, and the office of the late Doctor H. L. Hille of Collinsville, Oklahoma, is for sale. In Collinsville and for an area of approximately 50 square miles around there, there is no other physician. This should be a good opportunity for some young physician.

The practice, office equipment, and the office of the late Doctor J. E. Adams, Cushing, Oklahoma, is for sale. This is an excellent opportunity for some young physician. If interested address Mrs. J. E. Adams, Box 507, Cushing.

OBITUARIES

Dr. C. M. Bloss, of Okemah, died at Okmulgee Hospital, Okmulgee, June 14th. He was born May 24th, 1878, at Clay Center, Kansas, and attended grade and high schools there, and the University of Oklahoma at Norman. On May 30th, 1908, he graduated in Medicine from the University of Texas Medical School. He practiced medicine in Okemah for 25 years and was a most useful citizen. A member of the First Presbyterian church, and an Elder in his church; a member of the Masonic fraternity; a member of the Oklahoma Medical Association for many years and at the time of his death he was secretary of the Okfuskee County Medical Society. He also held membership in the American Medical Association, Southern Medical Association, Okemah Chamber of Commerce, American Legion (Okemah Chapter), and Kiwanis Club.

Notice of Recent Deaths

(Insufficient data for obituary)

Adams, J. E., Cushing, Oklahoma, May 31, 1938.

Hille, H. L., Collinsville, Oklahoma, May 31, 1938.

Beg Your Pardon

OKMULGEE-OKFUSKEE County Medical Societies were reported, in a recent issue of the Journal, as having as their guests Drs. J. C. Brogden and E. G. Hyatt, of Oklahoma City. These doctors are from Tulsa, Oklahoma.

Need of Redetermining Schick Negativeness in School Children

A. B. Schwartz and F. R. Janney, Milwaukee (Journal A. M. A., May 21, 1938), state that during the last year or two there has been an apparent increase in the incidence of diphtheria among supposedly Schick negative children. These occurrences warrant serious consideration of the present status of Schick immunity in the present large school population. As it is now the practice to immunize against diphtheria at about nine months of age and to perform a Schick test within the following several months, many school children have had an interval of five years or more following the immunization procedure by the time they enter school. The importance of a Schick test following the immunization procedure has been repeatedly emphasized, but, once a negative Schick test has been obtained, the immunity has been generally assumed to be permanent. Whatever materials or method of immunization is followed, the immunity of the school child to diphtheria should be insured by either a routine Schick testing on all children entering school or by the administration of a routine dose of 1 cc. toxoid at the time of entering school, as suggested by Fraser and Brandon. In order to maintain the low incidence of diphtheria in the United States, one of these two measures should be made a routine part of preventive medicine.

Noise and its Effect on Human Beings: Noise Control as a By-Product of Air Conditioning

In their dissertation on noise and its effect on human beings Carey P. McCord, Detroit; Edwin E. Teal, Ann Arbor, Mich., and William N. Witheridge, Detroit (Journal A. M. A., May 7, 1938), conclude by saying that the American Medical Association's Committee on Air Conditioning recognizes that proper air conditioning is one factor tending to diminish the ill effects of noise of some types. The procurement of closed windows, doors and other sound barriers commonly associated with artificial climates in public buildings, office buildings, department stores, theaters and so on may eliminate as much as 75 per cent of the noises of extraneous origin. In industry, air conditioning offers little promise of protection against noise for workers employed near the origin of noise. Vibration in ranges below audibility has a prominent role in the production of injuries arbitrarily classed as noise diseases. Although inaudible vibrations may involve occupied areas that may be air conditioned, obviously no protection can be secured from such vibrations by air conditioning. The compilation of material making up this report presents extensive evidence that genuine injury is widespread as a result of noise action and that noise deafness is the chief of these dysfunctions in terms of both frequency and severity.

Multiple Primary Malignant Tumors

J. S. Eisenstaedt, Chicago (Journal A. M. A., June 18, 1938), reports the case of a man who died in 1936 and who had been operated on 21 years before for adenocarcinoma of the kidney. Later two other primary cancers developed in distinct and separate organs (prostate and sigmoid colon), one of which, that of the prostate, produced metastases to the lungs and lymph nodes. All three cancers were diagnosed clinically. It is the author's belief, after a rather complete survey of the literature, that: 1. Multiple primary cancers are more frequent than are reported. 2. They occur more frequently than chance alone would explain. 3. More percentage of multiple primary malignant tumors to be reported in the future will be higher than that recorded in the past, because: (a) More people are reaching advanced years, a period in which the incidence of cancer is generally high. (b) Since the inauguration of cancer clinics and commissions throughout the world, cancer patients have been more concentrated and more thoroughly studied. (c) Better results are being obtained in the treatment of cancer than heretofore. (d) As a result of longer survival after treatment for a single primary tumor, time is afforded for the development of subsequent primary cancers. (e) Autopsies are more widely done and with greater thoroughness than in the past. 4. Some factor, as yet unknown, possibly hereditary or hormonal in nature, plays an important part in susceptibility to malignant disease and the varied responses to environment in different individuals depends on this unknown element.

Cystic Hygroma of the Neck

Since hygromas of the neck rarely develop in adults Bruce L. Fleming, Philadelphia (Journal A. M. A., June 4, 1938), reports two adult cases that have been treated for this condition in the Jefferson Hospital since 1908 and in summary states that hygromas of the neck are thin-walled cystic tumors linew with endothelium and containing lymph. They grow from lymph sacs or buds that appear, in embryologic development near the junction of the internal jugular and subclavian veins. The endothelial cells lining these tumors are structurally different from and thicker than those lining lymphatic capillaries. They are structurally the same as blood capillary endothelial cells, which they resemble functionally, for they apparently produce the contained lymph. Evidence of phagocytic power is negligible. The treatment is complete surgical excision or partial excision and packing.

ABSTRACTS : REVIEWS : COMMENTS
and CORRESPONDENCE

SURGERY AND GYNECOLOGY
Abstracts, Reviews and Comments from
LeRoy Long Clinic
714 Medical Arts Building, Oklahoma City

The Treatment of Suppurative Cutaneous Wounds and Ulcerations with Cod Liver Oil and Allantoin; Salzmann and Goldstein; American Journal of Surgery; June, 1938; Page 523.

The use of living maggots and insects in the treatment of osteomyelitis, abscesses and non-healing wound infections dates back to antiquity. However, it is hardly likely that the medical men of old recognized the therapeutic value inherent in the maggot.

Allantoin, in the form of living maggots and extract of maggots, has been employed with remarkable success in the treatment of chronic cutaneous ulcerations, chronic osteomyelitis, severe burns and various dermatologic conditions.

Considerable evidence is available attesting to the beneficial effects of cod liver oil in the treatment of chronic non-healing wounds and chronic ulcerative affections.

The successful therapeutic use of cod liver oil and allantoin suggested a combination of these substances to obtain a double therapeutic action greater than the effect produced by either alone. It was found that such a combination with the addition of phenol was extremely effective in stimulating granulation tissue and encouraging healing in chronic ulcerative affections.

The ointment employed in this study contained 45 per cent cod liver oil, 2 per cent allantoin in a lanolin base with 0.5 per cent phenol.

Deep indolent ulcerative conditions and various cutaneous inflammatory affections respond promptly to applications of cod liver oil-allantoin ointment. The therapeutic procedure is simple and may be applied without any discomfort to the patient. It is tolerated better by the patient than the use of the actual maggots.

The preparation of cod liver oil-allantoin employed in this study is known as codalltoin and was made available through the courtesy of the Amfre Drug Company, New York.

LeRoy D. Long.

Mandelic Acid Therapy in the Treatment of Urinary Tract Infections; George H. Ewell; Editorial in Wisconsin Medical Journal; December, 1936.

"The introduction of a new drug in the therapy of urinary tract infections is always received with great enthusiasm in most quarters since the treatment of these infections is generally so disconcerting and the results generally unsatisfactory. Most of the drugs introduced are sponsored and advocated by the firms manufacturing them and must be accepted by the profession until their clinical value is established.

"The introduction of mandelic acid by Rosen-heim, in the treatment of urinary tract infections, which came about in his efforts to overcome certain objections to the ketogenic diet is a recognized therapeutic procedure, and, as has been pointed out, its efficacy depends upon the production of and the presence in the urine of a sufficient concentration of betaoxybutyric acid with the urine at a certain degree of acidity, the action of the acid being bactericidal and bacteriostatic. Sufficient concentration of this acid cannot always be obtained by dietary means, and efforts to supplement it by its administration were not satisfactory, since under normal metabolic conditions it is completely and rapidly oxidized in the body.

"Rosenheim employed several of the acids of this series attempting to find one which was not so easily oxidized, was non-toxic in adequate dosage, and would be excreted in the urine unchanged. Mandelic acid was the one chosen, and he employed the sodium salt for administration. The clinical results were very satisfactory.

"Again it is necessary for the urine to be acid to a certain degree. In some cases the drug will produce this degree of acidity, in others it is necessary to administer other acidifying agents such as ammonium chloride and nitrate; the acidity must be checked by a suitable indicator, and the common litmus paper is not satisfactory. Unless the proper acidity is obtained, satisfactory results cannot be expected.

"The majority of urinary tract infections are due to the organisms of the colon bacillus group. The members of this group are definitely sensitive to its action, exceptions being made for the Proteus and areogenes strains which are resistant.

"Impairment of kidney function may follow its administration; also gastro-intestinal disturbances. Its employment, therefore, must be supervised. The sodium and ammonium salts are the most commonly used and obtainable through the regular drug channels.

"The drug is expensive but not more so than the various dyes that have been introduced, and from the available clinical reports the results are much superior. The clinical reports are so 'encouraging as to warrant continued clinical trial."—G.H.E.

LeRoy D. Long.

The Postoperative Treatment of Exophthalmic Goiter; Lindon Seed; Clinical Medicine and Surgery; June, 1938; Page 258.

Immediately after an operation for exophthalmic goiter the patient needs: (1) fluids; (2) sugar; (3) morphine; and (4) iodine. The administration of these four substances constitutes 90 per cent of the postoperative treatment. Since, after this is carried out, there is very little else that one can do, it is imperative that it be carried out well.

Fluids: The fluid requirement after a thyroidectomy for exophthalmic goiter is larger than that after almost any other operative procedure. Three thousand (3,000) cubic centimeters of fluid in the first 24 hours is probably the minimum; 4,000 cc. is better; and 5,000 cc. is needed under many circumstances. The ease with which fluids can be given by the intravenous or the subcutaneous route often leads to disregard of the more effective administration by the oral route. In addition to the fact that no one as yet has devised a better way of giving fluids than by mouth, it seems that a glass of water, taken into the stomach, is more useful to the organism than twice that quantity injected under the skin or into a vein. Since after a thyroidectomy the gastro-intestinal tract is intact and uninjured, little caution need be exercised in the oral administration of fluids. A persistent effort will usually overcome the two obstacles to administration by this route—difficulty in swallowing, and vomiting.

The difficulty in swallowing begins soon after the operation and reaches its maximum in about 24 hours. Consequently the administration of fluids should be begun as soon after the operation as possible, for the effort to swallow will be more successful within the first 12 hours than in the second 12 hours. The tendency for the liquid to enter the larynx, causing a paroxysm of coughing, is greater when the patient is in a semi-reclining position than when she is in an erect position. The distress is only a little greater on boldly and quickly swallowing a large quantity of water than on sipping a few drops at frequent intervals. If the patient is instructed to sit up in bed, take a glass of water in her hand and drink it, distressing though it may be, she will usually succeed in drinking half a glassful. If a fit of coughing starts some bleeding, the surgeon will automatically be more careful of the hemostasis in future operations.

Vomiting, the second hindrance, is due in part to anesthesia, in part to the disease itself, and occasionally to morphine. Withholding of fluids by mouth does not lessen the vomiting; on the contrary, the patient will feel happier if she has something in the stomach to vomit, and the resulting involuntary lavage may stop the vomiting. A change of liquids is helpful; one of the carbonated beverages, especially ginger ale, may be satisfactory.

If the vomiting persists, one must turn to one or more of the three remaining methods of administering fluids. Of these methods, proctoclysis is the most inaccurate, but has the virtue of being the least distressing. If a proctoclysis is continued intermittently for 24 hours, the patient will nearly always absorb at least one liter. Physiologic saline solution is better than plain water, for it will counteract the hypochlorhydria not uncommonly resulting from the loss of chlorides due to excessive sweating. Venoclysis is, in many ways, preferable to hypodermoclysis, but it has one serious drawback in that, when the patient is extremely ill (when one most earnestly wishes to use the intravenous method), she is so restless that the needle cannot be maintained in the vein.

Sugar: Sugars are most effectively given by mouth. If the nurse will shift from grape juice to orange juice, to lemonade, or to ginger ale, the amount of sugar that will be taken in will be surprising. If vomiting prohibits oral feedings, the sugar must be given parenterally. The absorption of dextrose administered by proctoclysis is very uncertain. A five per cent solution of dextrose in physiologic saline solution is readily absorbed when given by hypodermoclysis; 2,000 cc., administered in the first 24 hours, will usually be adequate. If it is given intravenously, the sugar may easily appear in the urine when the rate of administration is too fast. To increase the nourishment, the intake of food is increased as rapidly as possible, and everything that the patient will eat is included.

Morphine: Morphine is essential for rest. Hypo-

dermic injections of 1/6 grain (0.01 Gm.) should be used freely. If the patient has an idiosyncrasy and becomes restless or vomits, a grain (0.06 Gm.) of codeine forms an excellent substitute.

Iodine: The administration of iodine should be continued for at least a week following the operation. Its withdrawal is not a calamitous blunder, but it can be followed by a sharp exacerbation of the symptoms several days later. The iodine can be conveniently given on the first day in the form of Lugol's solution (100 drops) in the proctoclysis, or as sodium iodide, 15 grains (0.9 Gm.) in the hypodermoclysis or venoclysis. On the second day, Lugol's solution can again be given by mouth. It is continued as long as the physician sees fit — as long as there is any doubt in his mind as to whether the thyrotoxicosis is completely controlled. The drug can do no harm and may be of some benefit. If it seems advisable to give it over a long period of time, the dose should be reduced to five drops once or twice daily.

Following the operation the patient is placed in bed in a semi-sitting position. If the position is comfortable, it is maintained; if not, there is no reason why it cannot be altered. The peak of the postoperative reaction is usually reached on the second night. On the third day the patient's comfort will be enhanced and recovery hastened if she is allowed to be out of bed. At this time neuralgic pains about the occiput, in the front of the chest, or in the teeth may be very troublesome. A standing order for one grain (0.06 Gm.) of codeine sulphate and 10 grains (0.6 Gm.) of acetylsalicylic acid, either or both or any part of either or both, whenever necessary, will be found very comforting to both the patient and the physician.

Comments: This is a commendable dissertation on the average routine care of postoperative toxic goiter patients in so far as the administration of these four important substances is concerned.

Personally we will never use glucose solution in any percentage under the skin. It is probable that five per cent solution of glucose in physiologic saline solution will not cause sloughing, but we have seen sloughing when glucose was used by others and we see no good reason for administration of glucose under the skin in the average case.

I am also prejudiced against the use of salicylate with these patients.

The author covers other phases of the postoperative care of exophthalmic goiter patients in his article such as crisis, hemorrhage, obstructive dyspnoea, and tetany. In general his ideas conform to those generally accepted.

LeRoy D. Long.

Trichomonas Vaginalis Vaginitis, A Comparative Study of Treatment and Incidence; Paul Peterson; American Journal of Obstetrics and Gynecology; June, 1938; Page 1004.

This report was made with a threefold purpose: (1) To present the figures of occurrence of true pathogenic cases, and of incidental cases discovered by routine examination for trichomonas vaginalis; (2) to review the treatment of trichomonas vaginalis vaginitis; and, (3) to report a case of trichomonas vaginalis proctitis.

Routine search was made for trichomonas vaginalis in all patients visiting the Obstetrical and Gynecological Clinic of the United States Naval Hospital, San Diego, California, with a total of 5,712 obstetric and gynecological patients being examined routinely.

It was found that 24.6 per cent of all patients examined had positive smears for trichomonas vaginalis whereas only 15 per cent of these patients

(3.69 per cent of the total number) had clinical symptoms.

On the basis of these findings the author is led to believe that the pathogenicity of the trichomonad is generally exaggerated.

In post-partum cases the incidence was 33 per cent as compared to 20.3 per cent in the ante-partum cases which is at slight variance with the general belief about the incidence of this type of infestation.

Some patients had a left lower quadrant pain and painful coitus with no other findings to account for it and the author speculates as to the possibility of patients with such symptoms having infestation of the rectum and sigmoid as in a particularly virulent type of proctitis described and reported in this article.

"Routine examination accounted for 64 per cent of the cases being found; 15 per cent were recognized clinical entities; 0.21 per cent occurred with a pathogenic abundance of Doderlein bacilli; 12.455 per cent were associated with gonorrheal endocervicitis; 8.26 per cent had a nonspecific endocervicitis; and 0.075 per cent occurred with monilia infection."

The treatment of 1,405 patients is reviewed. Three types of treatment were employed designated as carbarsone, vioform, and silver picrate methods. All these methods are given in detail. The author prefers the silver picrate method because he feels it is simple, effective and time saving and was employed in his series in 695 patients with no failures. In this group 80 per cent were cured with one course, 20 per cent required two courses and there were no failures.

In the carbarsone group 73 per cent were cured with one course, 25 per cent required two courses and 1.3 per cent were not cured after two courses and were considered failures.

With the vioform treatment 76 per cent were cured with one course, 23 per cent required two courses before remaining negative and 0.2 per cent were considered failures.

They considered an average course of treatment about 42 days and smears were taken following each of three menstrual periods.

Comments: By far the most interesting fact contained in this article is in relation to the pathogenicity of trichomonas vaginalis with the surprisingly large number of patients having positive smears with no symptoms and discovered only by routine examination.

The discussion and results concerning treatment are also of importance in several directions. In the first place, the treatment of trichomonas vaginalis vaginitis is more clearly defining itself and becoming crystalized in recent years. In the second place, one must agree with this author that the simplest possible means of treatment is probably more often applied correctly and, therefore, is superior.

The three methods of treatment outlined in this article closely parallel each other in results though the figures indicate a slight advantage in the use of silver picrate method. However, the manner of employing the carbarsone treatment in their clinic was a rather elaborate one and may not have given as satisfactory results if more simplified.

For a number of years I have depended upon the parasitocidal action of carbarsone as the primary factory in treatment and have studiously avoided any washing or trauma of the vagina in treatment of instances of trichomonas vaginitis. Such patients have been instructed about the introduction of carbarsone vaginal suppositories one each night before retiring for 12 nights. Following the use of such suppositories, with negative vaginal smears, floraquin tablets have been used one each night for 12 nights and usually one every other night for an additional 24 days, principally to maintain an increased acidity within the vagina. The results have been far more satisfactory in my hands than any former procedure employing local treatment and consequent inevitable vaginal trauma. The employment of the floraquin tablets has practically eliminated recurrences and the carbarsone vaginal suppositories alone have usually controlled symptoms within three to four days. Douches have been employed only for symptomatic purposes and if used, are employed in the evening before the carbarsone suppository is inserted.

Wendell Long.

A Comparison of the Three Types of Hysterectomy; Curtis H. Tyrone, New Orleans, La.; Annals of Surgery; May, 1938; Page 836.

This is a report based upon 764 consecutive operations performed by the late Dr. C. Jeff Miller and the author during a six-year period, 1931 to 1936, including ward and private patients.

The indications for hysterectomy are briefly reviewed and the pathological conditions found in operation in this series are tabulated with uterine fibroids and uterine fibrosis and chronic metritis composing the greatest incidence with 382 and 238 instances respectively.

Of the 764 hysterectomies 316 were supravaginal hysterectomies, 137 complete abdominal hysterectomies and 311 vaginal hysterectomies.

The mortality for the different types was: supravaginal, 1.9 per cent; complete abdominal, 2.2 per cent; and vaginal, 0.64 per cent. The mortality for the entire series was 1.4 per cent. The relatively large number of vaginal hysterectomies in this series is interesting as is also the fact that upon the basis of these statistics vaginal hysterectomy yielded lower morbidity and mortality and would, therefore, seem the operation of choice whenever it can be performed and is indicated.

However, the author is very emphatic that the patients for vaginal hysterectomy must be carefully and properly selected and the operation must never be used when extensive adnexal disease is present.

It is also an interesting fact that in more than half of the fatal cases peritonitis was the cause of death. In all of these patients there was extensive adnexal and parametral infection present at time of operation and the author emphasizes the danger of hysterectomy in the presence of such infection.

Comment: Such statistical reports relative to the employment of the various means of performing hysterectomy are of some importance in indicating the trend of surgical thought and approach. However, the use of the different surgical approaches for hysterectomy depends upon a number of factors and the choice of procedure as well as the indication for operation, must in the last analysis depend upon the individual circumstances of the patient's condition, the experience of the surgeon, and the associated lesions which are to be corrected at the time of operation.

The importance of proper preparation of all patients before surgical procedures, including hysterectomy, cannot be too emphatically recalled, if one is to expect a low mortality as well as good postoperative results. In this article the author has called attention to the careful preoperative control of pelvic inflammation as far as possible before operation is attempted. Equal importance can be assigned to the proper supportive measures pre-operatively such as replacement of blood loss and improvement of the patient's general condition wherever this is possible before a major surgical operation is undertaken.

Wendell Long.

---o---

EYE, EAR, NOSE AND THROAT
Edited by Marvin D. Henley, M.D.
911 Medical Arts Building, Tulsa

Rehabilitation of the Deaf Child. Dr. Max A. Goldstein, St. Louis. The Laryngoscope, April, 1937.

A general survey of the 50,000,000 children of school age in the United States showed:

- 40,000 Blind.
- 60,000 Totally deaf.
- 80,000 Partial-sighted.
- 300,000 Crippled.
- 3,000,000 Hard-of-hearing.
- 4,000,000 Defective in speech.

Or a total of 7,480,000 or nearly 15 per cent physically defective; mental defectives and other subnormal groups were not included in the survey.

The training of the deaf child is much more difficult than that of helping the hard-of-hearing child. The latter has acquired speech although it may be imperfect. Making contacts in and out of school presents the greatest problem due to the impaired hearing. Lip-reading and speech conversation are of paramount interest to this type of patient. Hearing aids are also useful.

The author tells of a class reunion of pupils from his Central Institute for the Deaf. The class was made up of 45 young men and women. Talking movies were made of the group as evidence of a successful rehabilitation.

The article re-emphasizes the fact that an Otologist has not completed his duty to his patient until he has successfully interested him in the technique of carrying on his life even though he is gradually becoming more hard of hearing or is totally deaf.

Treatment of Chronic Catarrhal Deafness With the Eustachian Heat Bougie. Emanuel Simon, M.D., Albany, N. Y. Archives of Otolaryngology, May, 1938.

The author presented a paper three years ago on this subject. He continues and reports the further development of this technique in his present article. The only way to tell whether or not this treatment will improve the patient's hearing or diminish the tinnitus is by trial. The article is very interesting and leaves the reader with the impression that the author is firmly convinced that his procedure is sound. The author's own summary is as follows:

1. Use of the heat bougie will open the eustachian tube for longer intervals than any other procedure. Opening up the eustachian tube helps only those patients who have no scar tissue in the middle ear restricting movement of the ossicular chain.

2. Chronic hyerplastic sinusitis is an extremely prevalent disease. Chronic nonpurulent otitis media is very common and is probably dependent on chronic nasal infection or chronic sinus infection (with its occasional acute flare-ups) for its source. These inflammatory processes are present in varying degree in most adults; they may exhibit no symptoms, slight symptoms or marked symptoms.

3. Chronic so-called catarrhal deafness may be helped by improving the rhinosinal mucosa and by direct treatment of the eustachian tube. Unfortunately, there is at present no known specific way to cure chronic sinusitis. One can, by various empiric methods, improve the condition of the mucosa in the nose and in the sinus to some degree, in most cases for a limited time, and thereby alleviate or temporarily stop the inflammatory process in the ear.

4. Direct treatment of the eustachian tube, particularly with the heat bougie, is of value in many cases of chronic catarrhal otitis media, but not in all, since it does not remove ossicular restriction. Aeration of the middle ear does help some patients, even if only temporarily; it seems to tide others over acute tubotympanic catarrh, leaving the ears apparently well thereafter. In some cases the condition gets worse regardless of all treatments. This is because one is unable to halt the course of hyperplastic sinusitis which is the source and cause of chronic progressive otitis media.

Naso-Pharynx Pathology After the Adenoid Period. C. C. Reid, M.D., Denver, Colo. The Eye, Ear, Nose and Throat Monthly, June, 1938.

The "adenoid age" is designated at from two to 14 years. By this the author means the time in life when the adenoids do the most harm to the body and also when they are most often surgically removed. He suggests that this period might well be extended from the time of birth to 30 years of age.

The author's opinion is that adenoids are frequently incompletely removed. If the LaForce instrument is used in their removal, then a wise procedure would be to follow with a Stubb's curette and lastly an inspection and completion of the operation with the operator's finger. If completely done the results are apt to be permanent.

Remnants of the adenoids probably cause pathology over a long period of years evidenced by infections, fevers, rheumatism, catarrh, sinus disease, deafness, heart disease, nephritis, diabetes, inefficiency and other complications. The pathology may be found in the naso-pharynx and throat. Repeated cold may produce a hyperplasia of the lymphoid tissue which in turn becomes and remains infected. The Fossa of Rosenmuller may become almost completely filled and extend down the sides of the throat to occupy the lower part of the fossa of the faucial tonsil, even after complete removal of the tonsils. Infected nodules often occur on the posterior wall of the pharynx. Absorption and trouble equal to that of a diseased tonsil not infrequently is the result. Adhesions may form between the turbinates and the septum. Synechia in region of the Fossa of Rosenmuller may cause the drainage to accumulate in the naso-pharynx. The formation of a plastic exudate may cause the lips of the Eustachian tube to adhere. Turgescence, hypertrophy and lymphoid hyperplasia may cause partial or total, continuous or intermittent, closure of the Eustachian tubes. So may be produced after a number of years a chronic progressive deafness due to obstruction.

The symptoms produced depend largely on the amount of pathology present. Mouth breathing may be produced by pathology in the naso-pharynx but it may also be produced by such nasal conditions as deformity or hypertrophy.

According to the author the word "catarrh" means "flowing down." Literally a running nose or a dropping into the throat. Unhygienic living, errors of diet, constipation, etc., in addition to a pathological condition in the naso-pharynx will produce this. Because there is not free drainage and ventilation present, a chronic rhinitis many times persists. Frequent colds complicated by sinus infections are not uncommon. The temperature may persist, day after day, for several weeks. The patient will often complain of a feeling of obstruction in the nose. Deafness is one of the later symptoms. Polypoid degeneration is another late evidence of the condition.

The treatment is cleaning up the naso-pharynx. A general anaesthetic is recommended. The author stresses what he terms "finger surgery."

Mycotic infections in Otolaryngology. William D. Gill, M.D., San Antonio, Texas. Southern Medical Journal, June, 1938.

The history of the bacteriology of mycology and the microscopic forms of vegetable life is briefly reviewed.

Pathogenic or non-pathogenic fungus may occur on the surfaces of the oral, pharyngeal and nasal mucous membranes as well as in the larynx, trachea and bronchi. Extension into the lung tissue is not uncommon. Varieties of importance to the otlaryngologist are the Actinomyces, the Blastomyces with their subdivisions, the Torulae, Oidia, Monilia and Saccharomyces, as are also the Aspergilli, Penicillia, Sporotrichi, Leptothrices and the Mucoraceal.

It seems some persons have an immunity to mycotic infections while others are especially susceptible to them.

The Oidia type of infection is probably the most c o m m o n l y seen, occuring usually in infacts (Thrush). Various pathogenic fungi infecting the skin of the external auditory canal has been designated as an otomycosis. It is of frequent occurrence. The presence of cereumen usually exerts a restraining influence against the invasion of fungi. However instances have been recorded where the fungi seemed to be actually flourishing on and in a ceruminous plug.

The prognosis is good if the initial focus is given early and vigorous treatment. The greatest danger is the extension from the focus of infection to deeper organs such as lungs and sometimes the central nervous system. Reinfections are prone to occur, especially those involving the ear. "In certain regions it is almost axiomatic to say that the reopening of swimming pools is a harbinger of the mycotic ear infections of the warmer months."

The treatment is essentially iodine or iodides and some form radiant energy such as X-ray. Particularly is this true of the infection in the air passages. Not such good results have been obtained in treating leptothricosis of the tonsil.

Torulosis, moniliasis and coccidiosis respond with varying degrees of success to vaccine and filtrates, autogenous. The author likes to use these as an adjunct with other forms of treatment. Usually when the general involvement is seen late, any treatment is ineffective.

Various treatments and drugs are discussed. In the author's experience, in order of clinical effectiveness, he recommends the following: (1) metacresylacetate or cresatin, (2) tricresol in glycerine, (3) Castellani's solution, (4) iodine in petrolatum or boric acid powder, (5) phenyl mercuric nitrate 1/3,000 alcoholic solution, (6) copper salts, such as copper sulfate, chloride, and oleate.

Essential points in treatment of otomycosis: (1) control of pain, (2) the control of the mycotic infection, (3) the prevention of reinfection. The use of the wick in the external auditory canal is preferable, moistened with the solution. After 24 hours, the canal is cleansed of debris. If water is used this must be carefully removed.

A long bibliography is appended to the article.

PLASTIC SURGERY
Edited by
GEO. H. KIMBALL, M.D., F.A.C.S.
404 Medical Arts Building, Oklahoma City

Reconstruction of Deformed Chin and Its Relationship to Rhinoplasty; Dermal Graft—Procedure of Choice. Jacques W. Maliniac, M.D., New York City. American Journal of Surgery, June, 1938.

The author points out that reconstructive rhinoplasty has come to be a common surgical procedure. With this popularity, however, attention is being focused on concomitant abnormalities of other components of the face and their relationship to the nose. The author points out that the chin should harmonize with the nose and profile.

Causative Factors: Under development of chin, trauma, scar formation, malocclusion, factors involving the jaw bone, teeth or temporomandibular joint.

Procedures in Use: (1) Ivory implant. (2) Bone graft. (3) Cartilage graft. (4) Fat graft. (5) Dermal graft.

The author points out the objection to ivory implant; principally that it is too hard, and second, that it is less suitable than auto-plastic grafts. Also he states that bone or cartilage gives an abnormal hardness, especially to touch about the chin. He favors, above all, the dermal graft for the reconstruction of the receding type of cnin and the cartilaginous graft for the under-developed chin.

Comment: The dermal graft should be kept in mind for filling out subcutaneous defects, especially about the scalp and forehead, face, chin, and any other part of the body that is exposed. The graft must be placed accurately and fixed to secure a good result.

———————o———————

INTERNAL MEDICINE
Edited by Hugh Jeter, M.D., 1200 North Walker, Oklahoma City

Protamine-Zinc-Insulin in Diabetes. By E. Perry McCullagh, M.D., Cleveland, Ohio. (Annals of Internal Medicine, May, 1938, Vol. 11, No. 11).

In this the author draws several practical conclusions which appear to be in line with the reported experiences of most present day students of diabetes mellitus. Some of the conclusions are as follows: "It is a remarkable fact that with the use of protamine and protamine-zinc-insulin, the blood sugar level may reach 40 mg. per hundred cubic centimeters or below without reactions. Reactions do occur, however, but for the most part they tend to be mild and gradual in their onset, thus allowing more time for treatment."

Protamine-zinc-insulin in common dosage appears to be active for 50 to 65 hours after injection, but the maximum effect is ordinarily from 12 to 18 hours. In some mild cases a dose of protamine-zince-insulin every second or third day may be sufficient to control fasting sugar levels.

The most obvious advantage of protamine-zinc-insulin is the reduction in the number of doses necessary.

Editorial by H.M.T., Jr., Protamine Insulin and Diet in Diabetes Mellitus. (Annals of Internal Medicine, May, 1938, Vol. 11, No. 11).

In this the recent trend in theory and practice in connection with the treatment of diabetes are nicely discussed. Some of the more critical physicians interested in diabetes mellitus say they have never seen a patient "regulated" on one daily dose of protamine-zinc-insulin.

Doubt as to the correctness of Mosenthols belief that the damage done to the patient with diabetes mellitus occurs not from the abnormally high level of blood sugar, but rather from the long continuous effects of glycosuria with its attendant polyuria, is questioned. It is impossible to say at present whether hyperglycemia and glycosuria are harmful if in other respects the sugar metabolism in the body is essentially normal. We can say that severe insulin shocks and possibly repeated mild attacks of hypoglycemia are harmful and in the face of arteriosclerotic coronary or cerebral arteries are actually dangerous.

The high protein diets as used in various clinics are discussed. Dietary adjustment and exercise are considered important factors in the satisfactory management of the diabetic.

"Moderate variations in blood sugar levels are unimportant and extreme ones make themselves evident to the watchful patient in a way that enables him to change his single dose of insulin or his diet to suit the situation. It has been shown that excellent regulation with protamine insulin can be obtained by proper dietary adjustment of an adequately high carbohydrate intake. The patient not only is happier and feels much better on this than on any other regimen but also the metabolic processes more nearly approach normal."

---o---

ORTHOPAEDIC SURGERY
Edited by Earl D. McBride, M.D., F.A.C.S.
717 North Robinson Street, Oklahoma City

Stenosing Tendovaginitis at the Radial Styloid Process, Harold Brown Keyes, Annals of Surg., April, 1938, Vol. 107, No. 4.

Stenosing tendovaginitis at the radial styloid, or DeQuervain's disease, is a condition which is not of infrequent occurrence and is not universally recognized, although it was first described in 1895. The author has seen two such cases within six months. Upon reviewing the literature he found relatively few cases described. DeQuervain describes it as follows: "It is a condition affecting the tendon sheath of the abductor pollicis longus, and the extensor pollicis brevis. It has definite symptoms and signs. The condition may affect other extensor tendons at the wrist."

It is known that the tendons of the abductor longus pollicis, and the extensor brevis pollicis, pass through a groove in the outer aspect of the styloid of the radius, and are contained in a separate compartment of the annular ligaments. A tendon sheath surrounds them, about an inch above, and below, the carpal ligament. This sheath is filled with synovial fluid.

The etiologic factors include (1) chronic injury, which is the most common type, and (2) a few cases of acute injury. Chronic injury is described as being of a type where one is required to work constantly repeating motion at the wrist, especially in ulnar abduction, with the thumb fixed on some object. The muscles become taut as they pass over the styloid process of the radius, and press on the tendon sheath. This also stretches the entire tendon sheath, with this motion.

The pathology consists chiefly of a fibrosis of the common sheath with a definite thickness. Sometimes it develops even to a cartilagenous-like consistency.

The characteristic findings consist of pain, which is usually directly over the styloid process of the radius, and is continuous, accentuated by motion, and radiates up the arm. It may even interfere with sleep. The anatomical "snuffbox" on the distal end of the forearm gradually disappears and eventually the area around the base of the thumb suggests atrophy of disuse. There may be a bulbous swelling in the region of the styloid of the radius. Point pressure directly over the styloid invariably causes the patient to wince. On grasping the hand and quickly adducting the thumb, a sharp pain occurs referred to the styloid process of the radius.

This condition must be differentiated from tuberculous tendovaginitis, tuberculous osteitis, tendovaginitis crepitans, periostitis, neuritis, arthritis of either gouty, rheumatic, gonorrheal or syphilitic origin, or fracture of the navicular bone.

Treatment is divided into conservative and operative methods. Conservative method consists of immobilization in the form of plaster cast holding the thumb at rest, or heat, massage and diathermy. This is not considered the ideal treatment, except possibly acute cases. The treatment of choice is that of operation, in which a small incision is made over the styloid of the radius and the tendon sheath is divided longitudinally, to permit the constricted tendon to expand to normal shape and to permit the tendon to slide back and forth normally. It is said to be remarkable how soon the pain disappears and the patient can resume normal function of the thumb.

Internal Fixation for Recent Fractures of the Neck of the Femur. Melvin S. Henderson. Annals of Surg. VCII, 132, January, 1938.

In a rather complete review of the subject, the author states that experience at the Mayo Clinic has showed that the risk of operative treatment is no greater than that of conservative treatment, provided operation is performed ten days or longer after injury.

Operative treatment promises a better chance for a good result than conservative treatment.

The author applies traction to the extremity immediately after the injury as preliminary treatment before operation. Pain is controlled by traction and by administration of opiates.

The operative treatment eliminates the need of prolonged confinement in a plaster spica and obviates the sequelae of stiff knees and hips.

The author reviews the various methods of internal fixation, the development of the cannulated nail and leg screw, and points out the technical difficulties of the operation and the importance of roentgenographic control with anteroposterior and lateral views. He describes in considerable detail the lag screw developed at the Mayo Clinic and compares its relative merits with the Smith-Petersen nail.

Fourteen days after the operation, motion of the hip and knee can be safely started. This is carried out by means of an overhead suspension apparatus which can be operated by the patient. Union cannot be expected under 90 days. Weight-bearing must be delayed for at least six months.

Henderson next discusses the results in 14 cases operated on more than a year ago in which the condition of the patients is known. Bony union and excellent function were obtained in 86 per cent of the cases. No serious infection occurred. Drainage followed late in two cases. There were no deaths from operation, and convalescence was much more satisfactory than by the conservative method.

---o---

UROLOGY

Edited by D. W. Branham, M.D.
514 Medical Arts Building, Oklahoma City

"I Was Rejuvenated," Liberty Magazine, June 18, 1938.

The only reason for comment on this article is that thousands of gullible people will read it and accept the information given as based on scientific facts. The article details the marvelous physical, mental and sexual invigoration noted by a senile individual following a vasectomy. No medical men believe now, that vasectomy, or the Steinach operation, is followed by anything more than permanent sterility, and that such improvement in general well-being that is noted is due to nothing more than suggestive therapy in a susceptible individual.

Quackery and charlantism will make profitable capital of such publicity with the ultimate result only of disappointment to the patients exploited.

"Observation on Impotence and Sterility Following Prostatectomy," Wilbur H. Haines, B.S., M.D. The Urologic and Cutaneous Review, May, 1938.

The author studied 75 patients who had undergone prostatectomy for prostatic hypertrophy in an attempt to determine whether the operation was followed by impotence or whether sterility results.

His conclusions were: 1. If potency exists prior to operation, its preservation following an otherwise successful operation may be assured 100 per cent. In some instances it may appear to be actually restored. Frequently it appears reinforced. 2. Fertility may be but seldom is preserved due largely to impairment of the mechanics of ejaculation, resulting in a blank. 3. The ecstatic climax is always present and occasionally prolonged.

"Lesions of the Urinary Tract Producing the Symptoms of Intra-Abdominal Disease." Richard Chute and Sylvester B. Kelley. Journal of Urology, May, 1938.

This article was prompted by the fact that various diseases of the urinary tract may masquerade as an intra-peritoneal lesion and unless the urinary tract is specifically studied an error in diagnosis will result.

The authors cite the report of Cecil where he found 19 per cent of calculus in the urinary tract and 30 per cent of hydronephroses had undergone abdominal operation for something else such as appendix or gall bladder, without relief of symptoms.

They state that ureteral calculus is the most frequent condition simulating intraperitoneal lesions, however, tumors, horseshoe kidney, duplication of the ureter with infection, and hydronephrosis will produce abdominal signs and symptoms. Case histories illustrating are presented.

In their conclusion they emphasize that the urinary tract should be continually kept in mind when the surgeon is confronted with a case presenting abdominal symptoms. Even an urinalysis and X-ray is not sufficient to clarify the diagnosis as often these are negative. They recommend the use of intravenous urography and even further urological study where puzzling abdominal symptoms are met with.

Comment: Mistakes in diagnosis which result in ill advised surgical procedures are not as common now as a few years past. Doubtless this is due to the technical aids which the careful surgeon will utilize when he doubts his diagnosis. Because a complete investigation and especially a urological examination is relatively expensive we are prone in those patients who, financially, are not well situated to omit such an examination, however, it must be continually borne in mind on the part of both the patient and doctor that a useless surgical procedure far outweighs the trivial cost of a complete diagnosis. No patient in the hope of saving a bit of money should run the serious risk of an unnecessary surgical procedure as also the surgeon should not hazard a blow to his professional prestige by performing an ill advised operation.

---o---

Thrombosis of Axillary Vein: Report of Five Cases With Comments on Etiology, Pathology and Diagnosis

Theodore Kaplan, New York (Journal A. M. A., June 18, 1938), cites five cases of thrombosis of the axillary vein in males. At the time that this process developed the patients were in good health and showed no pathologic defects to account for such a condition. The diagnosis of primary axillary thrombosis is made on the following symptoms and signs: (1) swelling of the arm and cyanosis within several hours or days after the accident, injury by strain or, occasionally, without any cause, (2) the absence of a rise in body temperature and absence of signs of local active inflammation, (3) the presence of dilated superficial veins on the affected arm and over the anterior part of the chest and also in the axilla, (4) the delay or absence in the collapse of the superficial veins of the upper extremity when the latter is raised above the level of the heart, (5) the presence of a cord in the axilla, (6) the increase of the venous pressure in the affected extremity, (7) prolongation of the circulation time in the affected arm, (8) X-ray visualization of new collateral formation, enlargement and dilatation of the veins, evidence of stasis on injection of radiopaque dyes into the veins of the affected arm and the failure of the axillary vein to be visualized and (9) the presence of numerous superficial veins on the affected side as shown by photography with the infra-red technic. Prognosis as to life is good. The duration of the disability is variable. Recurrences are occasionally noted following exertion. In the acute stage the treatment consists of rest, elevation and hot moist packs locally. If there is residual edema, an elastic bandage may be applied spirally, beginning at the hand an dextending upward to the shoulder. Diathermy is of value in reducing the swelling. Excision of the thrombus or the entire segment of the thrombosed vein has been recommended. However, such procedures are questionable, since after removal of the thrombus recurrence is likely, and if the venous segment is resected the chance for canalization of the organized thrombus is lost.

OFFICERS OKLAHOMA STATE MEDICAL ASSOCIATION

President, Dr. H. K. Speed, Sayre.

President-Elect, Dr. W. A. Howard, Chelsea.

Secretary-Treasurer-Editor, Dr. L. S. Willour, McAlester.

Speaker, House of Delegates, Dr. J. D. Osborn, Jr., Frederick.

Vice Speaker, House of Delegates, Dr. P. P. Nesbitt, Medical Arts Building, Tulsa.

Delegates to the A. M. A., Dr. W. Albert Cook, Medical Arts Building, Tulsa, 1938-39; Dr. McLain Rogers, Clinton, 1937-1938.

Meeting Place, Oklahoma City, 1939.

SPECIAL COMMITTEES 1938-39

Annual Meeting: Dr. H. K. Speed, Sayre; Dr. W. A. Howard, Chelsea; Dr. L. S. Willour, McAlester.

Conservation of Hearing: Dr. H. F. Vandever, Chairman, Enid; Dr. J. B. Hollis, Mangum; Dr. Chester McHenry, Oklahoma City.

Conservation of Vision: Dr. W. M. Galiaher, Chairman, Shawnee; Dr. Frank R. Vieregg, Clinton; Dr. Pauline Barker, Guthrie.

Crippled Children: Dr. Earl McBride, Chairman, Oklahoma City; Dr. Roy L. Fisher, Frederick; Dr. M. B. Glismann, Okmulgee.

Industrial Service and Traumatic Surgery: Dr. Marvin E. Stout, Chairman, Oklahoma City; Dr. Cyril E. Clymer, Oklahoma City; Dr. J. A. Rutledge, Ada.

Maternity and Infancy: Dr. George R. Osborn, Chairman, Tulsa; Dr. P. J. DeVanney, Sayre; Dr. Leila E. Andrews, Oklahoma City.

Necrology: Dr. G. H. Stagner, Chairman, Erick; Dr. James L. Shuler, Durant; Dr. S. D. Neely, Muskogee.

Post Graduate Medical Teaching: Dr. Henry H. Turner, Chairman, Oklahoma City; Dr. H. C. Weber, Bartlesville; Dr. Ned R. Smith, Tulsa.

Study and Control of Cancer: Dr. Wendell Long, Chairman, Oklahoma City; Dr. Paul B. Champlin, Enid; Dr. Ralph McGill, Tulsa.

Study and Control of Tuberculosis: Dr. Carl Puckett, Chairman, Oklahoma City; Dr. W. C. Tisdal, Clinton; Dr. F. P. Baker, Talihina.

ADVISORY COUNCIL FOR AUXILIARY

Dr. H. K. Speed, Chairman..Sayre

Dr. C. J. Fishman...Oklahoma City

Dr. W. S. Larrabee...Tulsa

Dr. J. M. Watson...Enid

Dr. T. H. McCarley..McAlester

STANDING COMMITTEES 1938-39

Medical Defense: Dr. O. E. Templin, Chairman, Alva; Dr. L. C. Kuyrkendall, McAlester; Dr. E. Albert Aisenstadt, Picher.

Medical Economics: Dr. Marvin E. Stout, Chairman. Oklahoma City; Dr. J. L. Patterson, Duncan; Dr. W. M. Browning, Waurika.

Medical Education and Hospital: Dr. V. C. Tisdal, Chairman, Elk City; Dr. Robert U. Patterson, Oklahoma City; Dr. H. M. McClure, Chickasha.

Public Policy and Legislation: Dr. Finis W. Ewing, Chairman, Muskogee; Dr. W. P. Neilson, Enid; Dr. C. P. Bondurant, Oklahoma City.

(The above committee co-ordinated by the following, selected from each councilor district.)

District No. 1.—O. C. Newman, Sr., Shattuck.

District No. 2.—McLain Rogers, Clinton.

District No. 3.—Thomas McElroy, Ponca City.

District No. 4.—L. H. Ritzhaupt, Guthrie.

District No. 5.—P. V. Annadown, Sulphur.

District No. 6.—R. M. Shepard, Tulsa.

District No. 7.—Sam A. McKeel, Ada.

District No. 8.—J. A. Morrow, Sallisaw.

District No. 9.—W. A. Tolleson, Eufaula.

District No. 10.—J. L. Holland, Madill.

Scientific Exhibits: Dr. E. Rankin Denny, Chairman, Tulsa; Dr. Robert H. Akin, Oklahoma City; Dr. R. C. Pigford, Tulsa.

Scientific Work: Dr. W. G. Husband, Chairman, Hollis; Dr. J. S. Rollins, Prague; Dr. J. L. Day, Supply.

Public Health:

Chairman—Dr. G. S. Baxter, Shawnee.

District No. 1.—C. W. Tedrowe, Woodward.

District No. 2.—E. W. Mabry, Altus.

District No. 3.—L. A. Mitchell, Stillwater.

District No. 4.—J. J. Gable, Norman.

District No. 5.—Geo. S. Barber, Lawton.

District No. 6.—C. E. Bradley, Tulsa.

District No. 7.—G. S. Baxter, Shawnee.

District No. 8.—M. M. De Arman, Miami.

District No. 9.—T. H. McCarley, McAlester.

District No. 10.—J. B. Clark, Coalgate.

SCIENTIFIC SECTIONS

General Surgery: Dr. F. L. Flack, Chairman, Nat'l Bank of Tulsa Bldg., Tulsa; Dr. John E. McDonald, Vice-Chairman, Medical Arts Bldg., Tulsa; Dr. John F. Burton, Secretary, Osler Building, Oklahoma City.

General Medicine: Dr. Frank Nelson, Chairman, 603 Medical Arts Bldg., Tulsa; Dr. E. R. Musick, Vice-Chairman, Medical Arts Bldg., Oklahoma City; Dr. Milam McKinney, Medical Arts Bldg., Oklahoma City.

Eye, Ear, Nose & Throat: Dr. E. H. Coachman, Chairman, Manhattan Bldg., Muskogee; Dr. F. M. Cooper, Vice-President, Medical Arts Bldg., Oklahoma City; Dr. James R. Reed, Secretary, Medical Arts Bldg., Oklahoma City.

Obstetrics and Pediatrics: Dr. C. W. Arrendell, Chairman, Ponca City; Dr. Carl F. Simpson, Vice-Chairman, Medical Arts Bldg., Tulsa; Dr. Ben H. Nicholson, Secretary, 300 West Twelfth Street, Oklahoma City.

Genito-Urinary Diseases and Syphilology: Dr. Elijah Sullivan, Chairman, Medical Arts Bldg., Oklahoma City; Dr. Henry Browne, Vice-Chairman, Medical Arts Bldg., Tulsa; Dr. Robert Akin, Secretary, 400 West Tenth, Oklahoma City.

Dermatology and Radiology: Dr. W. A. Showman, Chairman, Medical Arts Bldg., Tulsa; Dr. E. D. Greenberger, Vice-Chairman, McAlester; Dr. Hervey A. Foerster, Secretary, Medical Arts Bldg., Oklahoma City.

STATE BOARD OF MEDICAL EXAMINERS

Dr. Thos. McElroy, Ponca City, President; Dr. C. E. Bradley, Tulsa, Vice-President; Dr. J. D. Osborn, Jr., Frederick, Secretary; Dr. L. E. Emanuel, Chickasha; Dr. W. T. Ray, Gould; Dr. G. L. Johnson, Pauls Valley; Dr. W. W. Osgood, Muskogee.

STATE COMMISSIONER OF HEALTH

Dr. Chas. M. Pearce, Oklahoma City.

COUNCILORS AND THEIR COUNTIES

District No. 1: Texas, Beaver, Cimarron, Harper, Ellis, Woods, Woodward, Alfalfa, Major, Dewey—Dr. O. E. Templin, Alva. (Term expires 1940.)

District No. 2: Roger Mills, Beckham, Greer, Harmon, Washita, Kiowa, Custer, Jackson, Tillman—Dr. V. C. Tisdal, Elk City. (Term expires 1939.)

District No. 3: Grant, Kay, Garfield, Noble, Payne, Pawnee—Dr. A. S. Risser, Blackwell. (Term expires 1938.)

District No. 4: Blaine, Kingfisher, Canadian, Logan, Oklahoma, Cleveland—Dr. Philip M. McNeill, Oklahoma City. (Term expires 1938.)

District No. 5: Caddo, Comanche, Cotton, Grady, Love, Stephens, Jefferson, Carter, Murray—Dr. W. H. Livermore, Chickasha. (Term expires 1938.)

District No. 6: Osage, Creek, Washington, Nowata, Rogers, Tulsa—Dr. James Stevenson, Medical Arts Bldg., Tulsa. (Term expires 1938.)

District No. 7: Lincoln, Pontotoc, Pottawatomie, Okfuskee, Seminole, McClain, Garvin, Hughes—Dr. J. A. Walker, Shawnee. (Term expires 1939.)

District No. 8: Craig, Ottawa, Mayes, Delaware, Wagoner, Adair, Cherokee, Sequoyah, Okmulgee, Muskogee—Dr. E. A. Aisenstadt, Picher. (Term expires 1939.)

District No. 9: Pittsburg, Haskell, Latimer, LeFlore, McIntosh—Dr. L. C. Kuyrkendall, McAlester. (Term expires 1939.)

District No. 10: Johnson, Marshall, Coal, Atoka, Bryan, Choctaw, Pushmataha, McCurtain—Dr. J. S. Fulton, Atoka. (Term expires 1939.)

OFFICERS OF COUNTY SOCIETIES, 1938

COUNTY	PRESIDENT	SECRETARY
Adair		
Alfalfa	F. K. Slaton, Helena	L. T. Lancaster, Cherokee
Atoka-Coal	J. S. Fulton, Atoka	J. B. Clark, Coalgate
Beckham	R. C. McCreery, Erick	P. J. DeVanney, Sayre
Blaine	J. S. Barnett, Hitchcock	W. F. Griffin, Watonga
Bryan	P. L. Cain, Albany	Jas. L. Shuler, Durant
Caddo	J. Worrell Henry, Anadarko	P. H. Anderson, Anadarko
Canadian	A. L. Johnson, El Reno	G. D. Funk, El Reno
Carter	T. J. Jackson, Ardmore	Emma Jean Cantrell, Wilson
Cherokee	P. H. Medearis, Tahlequah	H. A. Masters, Tahlequah
Choctaw	G. E. Harris, Hugo	F. L. Waters, Hugo
Cleveland	O. E. Howell, Norman	J. L. Haddock, Jr., Norman
Coal	(See Atoka)	
Comanche	E. B. Dunlap, Lawton	Reber M. Van Matre, Lawton
Cotton	W. W. Cotton, Walters	G. W. Baker, Walters
Craig	W. R. Marks, Vinita	F. T. Gastineau, Vinita
Creek	C. R. McDonald, Mannford	J. F. Curry, Sapulpa
Custer	Ross Deputy, Clinton	Harry Cushman, Clinton
Garfield	E. J. Wolfe, Waukomis	John R. Walker, Enid
Garvin	G. L. Johnson, Pauls Valley	John R. Callaway, Pauls Valley
Grady	L. E. Wood, Chickasha	R. E. Baze, Chickasha
Grant	I. V. Hardy, Medford	E. E. Lawson, Medford
Greer	Leb B. Pearson, Mangum	J. B. Hollis, Mangum
Harmon	W. G. Husband, Hollis	R. H. Lynch, Hollis
Haskell	A. T. Hill, Stigler	N. K. Williams, McCurtain
Hughes	W. L. Taylor, Holdenville	Imogene Mayfield, Holdenville
Jackson	Jas. E. Ensey, Altus.	J. M. Allgood, Altus
Jefferson	C. S. Maupin, Waurika	C. M. Maupin, Waurika
Kay		R. G. Obermiller, Ponca City
Kingfisher	John R. Taylor, Kingfisher	F. C. Lattimore, Kingfisher
Kiowa	J. M. Bonham, Hobart	J. Wm. Finch, Hobart
Latimer	R. L. Rich, Red Oak	E. B. Hamilton, Wilburton
LeFlore	E. M. Woodson, Poteau	W. L. Shippey, Poteau
Lincoln	E. F. Hurlbut, Meeker	Ned Burleson, Prague
Logan	F. R. First, Crescent	E. O. Barker, Guthrie
Marshall	J. H. Logan, Lebanon	J. F. York, Madill
Mayes	S. C. Rutherford, Locust Grove	E. H. Werling, Pryor
McClain	J. E. Cochran, Byars	R. L. Royster, Purcell
McCurtain	R. D. Williams, Idabel	R. H. Sherrill, Broken Bow
McIntosh	D. E. Little, Eufaula	Wm. A. Tolleson, Eufaula
Murray	P. V. Annadown, Sulphur	Richard M. Burke, Sulphur
Muskogee	Finis W. Ewing, Muskogee	S. D. Neely, Muskogee
Noble	J. W. Francis, Perry	T. F. Renfrow, Billings
Nowata	M. B. Scott, Delaware	H. M. Prentiss, Nowata
Okfuskee	L. J. Spickard, Okemah	C. M. Bloss, Okemah
Oklahoma	C. J. Fishman, Oklahoma City	John F. Burton, Oklahoma City
Okmulgee	V. M. Wallace, Morris	M. B. Glismann, Okmulgee
Osage	R. O. Smith, Hominy	Geo. Hemphill, Pawhuska
Ottawa	Benj. W. Ralston, Commerce	W. Jackson Sayles, Miami
Pawnee	R. E. Jones, Pawnee	M. L. Saddoris, Cleveland.
Payne	E. M. Harris, Cushing	John W. Martin, Cushing
Pittsburg	A. R. Russell, McAlester	Ed. D. Greenberger, McAlester
Pontotoc	W. F. Dean, Ada	June Yates, Ada
Pottawatomie	E. Eugene Rice, Shawnee	F. Clinton Gallaher, Shawnee
Pushmataha	E. S. Patterson, Antlers	D. W. Connally, Antlers
Rogers	F. A. Anderson, Claremore	W. A. Howard, Chelsea
Seminole	A. N. Deaton, Wewoka	Claude B. Knight, Wewoka
Stephens	W. T. Salmon, Duncan	Fred T. Hargrove, Duncan
Texas		R. B. Hayes, Guymon
Tillman	J. E. Childers, Frederick	O. G. Bacon, Frederick
Tulsa	M. J. Searle, Tulsa	Roy L. Smith, Tulsa
Wagoner	S. R. Bates, Wagoner	Francis S. Crane, Wagoner
Washington	J. E. Crawford, Bartlesville	J. V. Athey, Bartlesville
Washita	J. Paul Jones, Dill	Gordon Livingston, Cordell
Woods	Arthur E. Hale, Alva	Oscar E. Templin, Alva
Woodward	C. W. Tedrowe, Woodward	V. M. Rutherford, Woodward

NOTE—Corrections and additions to the above list will be cheerfully accepted.

THE JOURNAL
OF THE
OKLAHOMA STATE MEDICAL ASSOCIATION

| VOLUME XXXI | McALESTER, OKLAHOMA, AUGUST, 1938 | Number 8 |

Acute Coronary Occlusion*

WILLIAM S. MIDDLETON, M.D.
MADISON, WISCONSIN

The first intravitam diagnosis of acute coronary occlusion (May 4, 1876), is attributed to Adam Hammer.[1] A German by birth, Hammer sought refuge in the United States at the time of the political disturbance of 1848. Settling in St. Louis he was one of the group to organize and operate the Humboldt Institut for medical instruction in the German language. Upon the occasion of his return to Europe he was called in consultation by Dr. Wichmann to see a patient in sharp collapse with a progressive myocardial incompetency. When Hammer suggested a thrombotic occlusion of a coronary artery in explanation of the striking clinical picture, Wichmann exclaimed, "I have never heard of such a diagnosis in my whole life." To which Hammer rejoined, "Nor I also." The accuracy of this explanation was established by necropsy; but singularly the occlusion had resulted from a large thrombus over small vegetations on the aortic cusp, which extended into the right sinus of Valsalva and effectively prevented the flow of blood into the right coronary artery. Twenty years elapsed before Dock[2] wrote the first American description of this condition, and even then the subject aroused no general interest.

The inertia of the medical profession may be explained in a measure by the lack of sound anatomic and physiologic knowledge of the coronary circulation. For ex-

ample in 1880 Weigert[3] had advanced evidence that capillary anastomoses between branches of the coronary arteries might become functional in event of occlusion. Cohnheim[4] maintained that these vessels were end-arteries and that occlusion resulted in death. Not until 1907 did Hirsch and Spalteholz[5] finally establish the existence of intercoronary anastomoses. In splended monographs Gross[6] and Spalteholz[7] independently afforded exact information relative to the distribution of the coronary arteries.

Returning to the matter of the anastomoses of the coronary arterial system it is interesting to observe that both Weigert[3] and Dock[2] predicted an extension of intercoronary capillary connections to functional proportions in impending occlusion. Gross[6] held a similar position and Oberhelman and Le Count[8] proved conclusively that adequate anastomoses occurred only in the presence of antecedent sclerosis. In the absence of such vascular change there was either little or no collateral communication between the coronary branches. The tiny arterae telae adiposae, especially abundant about the pulmonary veins, may afford some nutritional support through anastomoses with branches of the internal mammary arteries and of the aorta; but more interesting are the vessels of Thebesius. Wearn and his fellows[9-10] have attributed a peculiar shunt function to this system of vessels. In event of venous hypertension they may drain coronary blood directly into the chambers of the

*Read before the General Scientific Section, Annual Meeting, Oklahoma State Medical Association, Muskogee, Oklahoma, May 10, 1938. (From the University of Wisconsin Medical School).

heart and in the presence of coronary arterial interference they may serve a nutrient function. Such a collateral arterial supply alone would explain the survival of patients in whom occlusion of both major coronary arteries of long standing is established at necropsy. Thorel[11] suggested a fourth source of nutritional support to the myocardium, namely through pericardial adhesions. Injection studies[12] have confirmed this position by the demonstration of extensive anastomoses with the internal mammary arteries and anterior branches of the aorta through such adhesions. Upon this basis Beck[13] and others have opened an interesting field of surgical approach to the problem by suturing the omentum or the pectoral muscle to the heart after denuding the epicardium to favor granulations.

With this information it becomes apparent that coronary occlusion may result in varying degrees of myocardial injury. Three circumstances influence this end, namely the size and importance of the involved vessel, preexistent collateral channels and the time afforded to render such anastomoses effective. It is conceivable that a coronary vessel may be occluded without gross myocardial change, provided it be small enough and that adequate nutrition be supplied through collateral blood flow. Recanalization of the thrombus may restore a fair measure of circulation. Short of this advantageous outcome coronary occlusion may result in any degree of physiologic handicap and pathologic change. Its background is important. Spasm of the coronary arteries may give temporary ischemia and the clinical picture of angina pectoris. Vessels, the seat of atherosclerosis, are much more susceptible, and only by hardening less responsive to the stimuli that lead to spasm atherosclerosis is the common cause of gradual coronary occlusion; but in the present relation it is even more important as the virtually constant basis for coronary thrombosis. Embolism is so rare a cause of acute coronary occlusion as to merit scant attention.

Von Leyden[14] divided the pathologic changes incident to coronary occlusion, as follows:

1. Sclerosis, without myocardial change,

presupposing an intact nutrition until sudden occlusion.

2. Infarction with myomalacia cordis.

3. Slower occlusion with myofibrosis, diffuse or patchy, at times resulting in aneurysm of the heart.

4. Combinations of these types.

The area of myocardial infarction is essentially a foreign body. Reactive to the same are the fibrinous pericarditis and the mural thrombosis. The former may be succeeded by an effusion and synechiae; the latter, by remote embolism. Myocardial abscess is a rare occurrence, the consequence of septic embolism. From a clinical standpoint Levine's summarization of the pathologic sequences incident to acute coronary occlusion[15] is most valuable. Anemia, edema and hemorrhage mark the first three or four days; then necrosis takes precedence to the end of the third week; lastly, repair which has begun early, does not become adequate until after five weeks. Occasional calcium deposits may suggest the effort of nature to reinforce the scar of infarction.

The clinical picture of acute coronary occlusion should perforce include the less well defined symptomatology of coronary sclerosis, since the latter so regularly anticipates the former. Angina pectoris is the best recognized of symptoms dependent upon sclerosis of the coronary arteries, but it does not always have this background. Vague indigestion upon effort after eating is a singularly common story in patients who later develop acute coronary occlusion from thrombosis. By this token it should receive due attention in constructing the clinical picture of coronary sclerosis. Dyspnoea, at some time removed from physical effort and particularly at night, may mark this condition. Paroxysmal nocturnal dyspnoea may thus be explained in certain subjects. A sense of substernal oppression is an occasional manifestation. The myocardial insufficiency resultant from coronary interference may find its expression in remote circulatory symptoms and signs or there may occur an arrhythmia. More difficult to understand is the singular physical weakness from which certain of these patients with coronary sclerosis suffer.

Since a number of individuals showing

extreme atherosclerosis of the coronary arteries at necropsy had escaped serious subjective discomfort or physical handicap during life, certain workers have assumed that the importance of this lesion has been over-emphasized. The analysis of Willius and Brown[16] establishing the p e c u l i a r threat of coronary sclerosis to health and life, has been confirmed on every hand. In the present relation coronary sclerosis occupies a strategic position as the essential basis for the overwhelming majority of the cases of coronary thrombosis. In its classical form the clinical picture of coronary thrombosis lends itself regularly to the subdivisions suggested by Obratzow and Strachesko[17]:

1. Status anginosus.
2. Status dyspnoeicus.
3. Status gastralgicus.

In event of the occlusion of a branch of the coronary artery sufficient to induce pathologic changes a certain sequence of clinical symptoms and signs may be anticipated; but it must be borne in mind that if the branch be small enough and collateral blood supply adequate, the accident may occur without subjective cognizance or c l i n i c a l recognition. Then, too, the growing clinical variants jeopardize too sharp generalizations. Classically, pain initiates the kaleidoscopic expressions of coronary occlusion. It is agonizing in intensity and tends to be localized beneath the lower sternum or in the epigastrium. Its duration may extend over hours and days. It is resistant to the common vasodilators so useful in true angina. Even morphine may be ineffectual in its relief. The subsidence of the pain with gaseous eructations, vomiting or the voiding of large quantities of urine has added to the diagnostic confusion. Dyspnoea is marked and in many instances it partakes of a singular subjective quality far exceeding its objective evidence. The mental anxiety is extreme and in all save exceptional patients the appreciation remains clear. Delirium or coma may supervene. Drenching sweats accompany the marked asthenia. Diarrhoea is a common symptom. Embolism may lead to a variety of manifestations incident to their particular lodgment.

To physical examination the deep concern is written in the facial expression.

The skin is cool and l e a k y. Not infrequently the color is leaden. At times jaundice becomes a confusing detail. The pulse is rapid, small and easily compressible. The blood pressure is sharply depressed. In a word the picture is usually one of marked shock. The dyspnoea has been remarked. Marginal emphysema is noted and congestive rales are uniformly present in the bases. The cardiac dullness may be widened. A singular weakness of cardiac sounds is the rule. Embryocardia prevails and an arrhythmia may occur. After the first 18 hours a fine pericardial friction may be heard in those instances where the infarction has occurred in the anterior wall of the left ventricle. Interestingly this friction rub has a very evanescent character. Riesman[18] noted the absence of dorsalis pedis pulse in two patients with coronary thrombosis, a detail of inferential importance. A febrile reaction of one to three or more degrees Fahrenheit may be predicted on the second day in a majority of these subjects. Hydrothorax, anasarca and the complete picture of congestive failure appear in a minority. Hematuria, albuminuria and urinary suppression are occasional sequels. The physical evidences of embolism may be remote and widespread.

Among the laboratory data the most constant change is f o u n d in the leucocytes. Within a few hours leucocytoses of 15,000 to 30,000 with 80 per cent or more neutrophiles may be expected. The speed of sedimentation of the erythrocytes is commonly greatly increased. Both of these changes may be expressions of myocardial necrosis or reactions incident to the same. More d i r e c t l y the electrocardiographic studies reflect these changes in the myocardium. Isolated electrocardiograms may be diagnostic, but as a rule greater profit is derived from progress studies in this direction. Aside from the alterations in conduction t h a t constitute the common arrhythmias, diagnostic values have been assigned to certain deviations in the component waves. The work of Parkinson and Bedford[19], and Barnes and Whitten[20] in fixing the diagnostic importance of S-T segment deviations for the localization of the zone of infarction has been generally accepted. To this has been added an established place for the so-called body leads in patients where no typical change appears in the conventional leads.

The prognosis of coronary occlusion is influenced by many factors[21]. In general although age and sclerosis definitely en- -hance the adequacy of collateral b l o o d supply, the more advanced the years the less the chance for survival. Levine's figures[15] give 54.7 years as the average age of surviving patients and 61 years for those succumbing. Sex apparently bears no influence nor does the antecedent infectious or metabolic background except as it may establish the degree or grade of sclerosis. The cardinal symptom of pain might be expected to influence the prognosis. As a rule the more severe and the more protracted the pain, the greater will be the degree of myocardial injury and the less the chance of survival. Exceptions to this rule are so numerous as to render it very doubtful. One circumstance is particularly conspicuous. With weakening of the myocardium the same stimulus to pain may evoke "sinking spells" or dyspnoea with coincident fall in the blood pressure in the failing subject. Such equivalents of pain are especially o m i n o u s from a prognostic standpoint. The immediate shock levels are less significant than their duration. Maintained tachycardia w i t h persistent hypotension bodes ill. It should be remembered that the blood pressure of patients with prior arterial hypertension may not assume shock proportions. Yet the maintenance of new low levels is a poor prognostic sign. Decompensation carries with it an increased hazard. Of the evidences of disturbed conduction, alternans, auricular fibrillation, f l u t t e r and the various forms of heart block have the most serious prognosis. The presence and the extent of the pericardial friction have little bearing upon the prospect. Embolism carries with it the knowledge of mural thrombosis and the threat of further showers of a similar order. The constitutional response of fever gives little clue as to the extent or the outlook of a given myocardial infarct. The curve of the neutrophilic leukocytosis is an indirect index of the extent and the course of the infarction. More accurate than the leukocyte curve is the sedimentation rate. Its increased speed will be continued for some time after other evidences, including

the leucocyte count, have resumed normal levels. The roentgen ray may occasionally afford evidences of the extent and configuration of the myocardial infarction. Lastly, the electrocardiogram offers valuable prognostic information. Parkinson and Bedford[19] concluded that a movement of the distorted complexes toward, or a resumption of, previous conformations was a good sign. More specific were Barnes' observations[22]. In his studies a b e t t e r prognosis attended t h o s e subjects with typical T-1 and T-3 formulae. Atypical electrocardiographic findings w e r e commonly dependent upon multiple or complicated infarcts. Low voltage in the ventricular complexes occurred twice as commonly in the fatal group of his series as in those surviving. Hence these circumstances carry a poor prognosis.

Figures for the immediate mortality from acute coronary occlusion vary from 16.2 per cent[23] to 53 per cent[15]. Without exact information as to the type of practice of the recorder it is difficult to reconcile such a divergent spread; but in general it is recognized that many victims of this vascular accident die without medical attendance. This group falls into the category of fatalities from the lay diagnosis of "acute indigestion." In many of these patients digestive symptoms have dominated the picture, but death is determined by a gross disturbance of the cardiac rhythm, such as auricular fibrillation, ventricular tachycardia or fibrillation. Surviving the immediate shock of coronary occlusion, a second g r o u p of these patients dies between the fourth and the fifteenth day as the result of myocardial rupture or remote embolism. Still a third group of fatalities arises from deferred myocardial failure. Next to the immediate f a t a l i t i e s from grossly disordered rhythm the last group accounts for the largest number of deaths from coronary occlusion.

Surviving the a c u t e episode and convalescing satisfactorily by all clinical criteria, White and Bland[24] found an average expectancy of 2.4 years in 200 patients with coronary thrombosis. Cooksey's recent report[25] afforded an encouraging note in the complete rehabilitation of 78.1 per cent of 32 survivors from this vascular accident. In general a sharp curtailment of physical and mental activities may be predicted for the patients who weather the storm. An approximation to the life before the coronary thrombosis w i t h complete comfort should be counted the exception rather than the rule.

Certain clear indications d i c t a t e the treatment of a c u t e coronary occlusion. Rest, physical and psychic, is imperative. A p e r i o d of bedfastness of at least six weeks should be arranged. During the early phase of inequilibrium morphine in full therapeutic doses should be administered, in the interest of mental rest, even though pain be not well controlled by this drug. Detachment from the cares of home and business must be sought by the interdiction of visiting and the instruction of the family and attendants in their responsibility for the peace of mind of the patient. Mild sedation is urged for the control of restlessness and insomnia. Oxygen is remarkably effective in controlling the pain[26] and the anoxemia. While its effects are prompt and its need most evident in the first few days after the attack, it is logical to continue its use for two or three weeks. An atmosphere of 40 to 60 volumes per cent oxygen will usually afford the best results. Glucose is essential to muscular function and in the presence of such a serious disturbance of myocardial nutrition as acute coronary occlusion it should be s u p p l i e d regularly and in adequate amounts. If the patient be nauseated and absorption uncertain, glucose may be given intravenously to the extent of three injections of 500 cc. each of a five per cent solution a day. The isotonicity and slow injection of the glucose solution will prevent right heart overload. After the acute danger is past, five small rather than three average meals should be the rule. Theophyllin ethylendediamin[27] in doses of 1½ to 3 grains three times a day will appreciably decrease the precordial distress and l i m i t the frequency of anginal attacks. Acute cardiac failure may be met by venesection or a rapidly acting stimulant such as caffein, epinephrine or strophanthin. Quinidine should be reserved for the unusual occurrence of auricular fibrillation or ventricular tachycardia. Epinephrine and ephedrine are useful in the treatment of heart block. Digitalis is indicated when

signs of congestive failure make their appearance. It should not be used routinely in these patients. The special management of underlying conditions, such as syphilis and diabetes mellitus, requires detailed consideration beyond the scope of the present discussion. Coffee and alcohol may be permitted in moderation if the patient has used them previously. Tobacco is strictly forbidden.

The transition period from the shocking experience of coronary occlusion to a resumption of a measure of normal existence is a trying one not only to the patient but also to the family and the medical attendant. Anticipating the patient's n a t u r a l restiveness the physician must take him more or less completely into his confidence, explain the gravity of the situation and enlist his cooperation in outlining a regimen of rehabilitation. Probably no other extraneous factor so influences the outcome as does the patient's attitude in this respect. In just so many words he must be told that it is impossible to measure his cardiac reserve without effort, that in so far as possible this effort must be kept below a level that excites breathlessness, cardiac consciousness and fatigue[28], and that having exceeded this limit the steps must be retraced to insure a maximum of restoration of the cardiac reserve. Having enlisted the patient's complete confidence such a program of advancing physical effort by trial and error will not jeopardize his prospect by too serious psychic setbacks when evidences of myocardial limitation lead to a temporary or permanent retrenchment. In the last analysis the patient with a full understanding of the possible consequences should be the final arbiter in the decision that involves serious strictures upon his physical activities. If after a full review of the situation it becomes apparent that a measure of circulatory comfort may be assured only by comparative invalidism, then the patient may in all justice decide whether he prefers such an existence or a return to a more complete life at the cost of earlier myocardial incompetence.

REFERENCES

1. Major, R. H.: Classic descriptions of disease, Springfield, 1932.
2. Dock, G. L.: Some notes on the coronary arteries, M. and S. Reporter, 75; (1), 1, 1896.
3. Weigert, C.: Ueber die pathologischen Gerinnungsvor-

gange, Arch. f. Path. Anat. u. Phys. u. f. klin. Med., 79:87, 1880.

4. Cohnheim, J., and von Schulthess-Rechberg, A.: Ueber die Folgen der Kranzarterienverschliessung fur das Herz, Virchow's Arch f. Path. Anat., 85:503, 1881.

5. Hirsch, C., and Spalteholz, W.: Coronararterien und Herzmuskel (Anatomische und experimentelle Untersuchungen), Deutsch. Med. Wchnschr., 20:790, 1907

6. Gross, L.: The blood supply to the heart, New York, 1921.

7. Spalteholz, W.: Die Arterien der Herzwand, Leipzig, 1924.

8. Oberhelman, H. A., and Le Count, E. R.: Variations in the anastomoses of the coronary arteries and their sequences, Jour. A.M.A., 82:1321, 1924.

9. Wearn, J. T.: Role of the Thebesian vessels in the circulation of the heart, J. Exp. Med. 47:293, 1928.

10. Wearn, J. T.: Mettier, S. R., Klumpf, T. G. and Zschiesche, L. J.: The nature of the vascular communications between the coronary arteries and the chambers of the heart, Am. Heart J., 9:143, 1933.

11. Thorel, C.: Pathologie des Kreislauforgane, Ergebn. Allg. Path. u. path. anat., 9, pt. 1; 673, 1903.

12. Moritz, A. R., Hudson, C. L. and Orgain, E. S.: Augmentation of the extra-cardiac anastomoses of the coronary arteries through pericardial adhesions, J. Exp. Med., 56; 927, 1932.

13. Feil, H., and Beck, C. S.: The treatment of coronary sclerosis and angina pectoris by producing a new blood supply to the heart, Jour. A.M.A., 169; 1781, 1937.

14. von Leyden, E.: Ueber die Sclerose der Coronararterien und die davon abhangigen Krankheitzuzustand, Ztechr. f. klin Med. 7:459, 1884.

15. Levine, S. A.: Coronary thrombosis, its various clinical features, Baltimore, 1929.

16. Willius, F. A., and Brown, G. E.: Coronary sclerosis. An analysis of 86 necropsies, Am. J. Med. Sc. 168:165, 1924.

17. Obratzow, W. P., and Strachesko, N D.: Zur kenntnis der thrombose der konorararterien des herzens, Ztschr. f. Klin. Med., 71:116, 1910.

18. Riesman, D.: Coronary thrombosis, with an account of the disease in two brothers, Med. Clin. N. Amer., 6:861, 1923.

19. Parkinson, J., and Bedford, D. E.: Successive changes in the electrocardiogram after cardiac infarction (coronary thrombosis), Heart, 14:195, 1927.

20. Barnes, A. R., and Whitten, M. B.: Study of the R-T interval in myocardial infarction, Am. Heart J., 5:142, 1929.

21. Middleton, W. S.: The prognosis and treatment of coronary occlusion, Minn. Med., 18:710, 1935.

22. Barnes, A. R.: Electrocardiogram in myocardial infarction, Arch. Int. Med., 55:457, 1935.

23. Conner, L. A., and Holt, E.: The subsequent course and prognosis in coronary thrombosis, Am. Heart J., 1:129, 1930.

24. White, P. D., and Bland, E. F.: A further report on the prognosis of angina pectoris and of coronary thrombosis, Am. Heart J., 7:1, 1931.

25. Cooksey, W. B.: Coronary thrombosis, follow-up studies with especial reference to prognosis, Jour. A.M.A., 104:2063, 1935.

26. Rizer, R. I.: Oxygen in the treatment of coronary occlusion, Minn. Med. 12:506, 1929.

27. Smith, F. M.: Miller, G. H., and Graber, V. C.: The effect of caffein sodio-benzoate, theobromin sodio-salicylate, theophyllin and euphyllin on the coronary flow and cardiac action of the rabbit, J. Clin. Investig., 2:157, 1925.

28. Mackenzie, J.: Disease of the heart, New York, 1910.

———————————O———————————

Reconstruction Operation for Old Ununited Fracture of the Femoral Neck*

PAUL C. COLONNA, M.D.
From the Department of Orthopedic Surgery
Oklahoma University School of Medicine
OKLAHOMA CITY

In a discussion regarding non-union in the neck of the femur, the age period in which the fracture usually occurs and the severe disability arising from non-union at this site are the outstanding factors. On account of the pain and instability, these p a t i e n t s are usually u n a b l e to bear weight without the aid of crutches. In the consideration therefore of a reconstruction operation for this condition, it must be stressed at the beginning that to be effective, the operation should adequately reconstruct the joint mechanics. In other words, the patient must feel that the end has justified the means.

Necessarily upon the elderly type of patient, a very careful consideration of the general physical condition is of the first importance, for in certain cases, it must be

admitted that non-operative t r e a t m e n t only is justified. H a v i n g determined, however, that the individual is a satisfactory surgical risk, we are then faced with the decision as to the type of operation advisable. It should be remembered that in many of these old ununited fractures of the femur we have roentgenographic evidence of a necrotic head fragment, and that any attempt at bone grafting or fixation with metal nails or pins will almost always result in failure. A study of the roentgenogram will disclose complete or incomplete absorption of the neck, upward riding of the greater trochanter above its normal position with accompanying shortening of the limb, and often definite evidence of circulatory changes in the loose head fragment. Santos, Walcott, and others have c a l l e d attention to this increased opaqueness of the femoral head, pointing

*Read as invited guest before the New York State Medical Society, New York City, N. Y., May 11, 1938.

out that it indicates an aseptic necrosis. Therefore, an attempt to preserve a necrotic femoral head with the hope of its becoming revascularized following some type of pegging operation is hardly justified. It is in this type of non-union that the reconstruction operation to be described later is particularly suited.

Fig. I

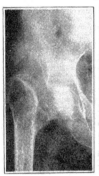 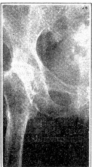

BEFORE   AFTER

A typical type of case for this reconstruction operation, showing complete absorption of neck and aseptic necrosis of the loose head fragment. With this type of reconstruction operation the line of force is a direct thrust downward from acetabulum to shaft, resulting in a mechanically stable articulation, because the shaft of the femur receives the body weight directly.

A more detailed study of the roentgenogram may give us other helpful data, and may also point to some of the *contra-indications* for the procedure under discussion. In some of these old ununited cases, not only necrosis of the head, but impairment of the acetabulum may be observed. There may be present a very shallow acetabulum or a destructive type of arthritis involving the hip joint may be present, producing an irregularity of outline in the acetabular floor. Again we may have a narrowed joint space indicating erosion of the cartilage covering the head fragment or acetabulum. As free mobility following this type of reconstruction operation is in large part dependent upon the integrity of the acetabular floor it follows that, if the acetabulum is not of sufficient depth, or if it presents any acquired deformation through disease or erosion, the opportunity for se-

curity or for free movement will be impaired.

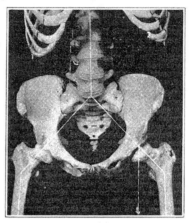

Fig. II

On the anatomical specimen shown there are illustrated lines of force which are transmitted normally from the acetabulum through the head and neck of the femur to the shaft. The position of the shaft following this type of reconstruction operation is shown by dotted line.

Any operative procedure should preferably be along simple mechanical lines. (Figure 2). Normal motion must not be expected from any type of reconstruction operation, but a certain degree of painless movement is greatly to be desired. The stability that the patient should possess in a reconstructed hip is necessarily of the first consideration. While a stiff hip may be a useful one, there can hardly be any question that from the patient's standpoint, loss of movement is never a desirable feature. If, therefore, the reconstructed hip can present an arc of motion from full extension to almost a right angle, it will permit the patient to sit comfortably in an ordinary chair, to climb stairs, or to walk on a flat surface with a good deal of facility. A satisfactory degree of abduction is also essential in order that equilibrium may be maintained while walking over rough surfaces or standing in a swinging vehicle.

Case 1—Ritterhof, New York City—In April, 1931, we had under our care on the orthopedic service in Bellevue Hospital, a woman of 55 in good general condition, who had been treated in an abduction plaster spica, and had received a satisfactory closed reduction following a recent fracture of the neck of the right femur. In spite of this excellent care, the neck had slowly undergone absorption with upward riding of the greater trochanter. The patient was first seen on the service six months after fracture, and was able to walk only short distances, and then only with the aid of two crutches, complaining of pain on any attempt at weight bearing. She presented a painful, unstable, shortened extremity. In an attempt to assure stability, preserve motion, and lengthen the already shortened extremity, a reconstruction operation was done as follows:

Under anesthesia, a curved incision was made over the lateral aspect of the right hip, and after dividing the fascia, the muscles attached to the greater trochanter were identified and sectioned close to the underlying bone, care being taken not to remove any osseous tissue. The capsule was then opened, and the necrotic head removed, and after completely freeing the upper extremity of the femur of its attached muscle tissue, it was placed deeply within the acetabulum. It was noted that the cartilage of the acetabulum was of normal color, shining, and showed no evidence of erosion. Before placing the greater trochanter region of the femur into the acetabulum, care had been taken to remove any small spicules so that the inner surface at the base of the neck region was smooth and flush with the inner border of the shaft of the femur and covered over with soft tissue.

A groove was made over the lateral surface of the shaft of the femur as far downward as the abductor muscles would reach, and after having replaced the greater trochanter into the acetabulum, these muscles were inserted into this bony trough and held in place by kangaroo tendon. This new insertion was reinforced by having the split vastus lateralis muscle sutured to the transplanted gluteus medius muscle at its new insertion. The wound was closed in layers, and a plaster of Paris spica was applied from the toes to the axilla, holding the limb in about 20 degrees abduction. Four weeks after operation the plaster was removed, and a long posterior shell made. With the limb suspended about an inch from the surface of the firm mattress, active and passive movement was instituted. Care was taken to place a pillow between the legs for the first few weeks in order that the reconstructed hip would not be suddenly pulled over into the adducted attitude. After this swinging apparatus had been used for two weeks, the patient was allowed out of bed and encouraged to use a walker, and shortly after this, graduated to crutches. Physiotherapy may or may not be necessary at this stage, but every effort is made to encourage the patient to discard all forms of support as early as possible. This patient made an uneventful recovery, and at present, seven years after operation, is doing her own housework. She presents a range of motion from 180 degrees to 90 degrees, complete extension, and a wide range of abduction with a gain of one and one-half inch in the length of the extremity.

Case 2—Alexander, 62, white, female. In December, 1936, this patient fell, sustaining a fracture of the left hip. She was in bed without support for seven weeks, and then allowed up on crutches. She was seen in the Department of Orthopedic Surgery of the Oklahoma University School of Medicine in November, 1937, presenting severe disability from the old fracture of the left hip, and was unable to walk except with the aid of crutches. A roentgenogram disclosed upward riding of the greater trochanter with almost complete absorption of the neck of the femur and definite non-union. Any movement of the hip caused pain. Patient was unable to stand on the affected limb without support. R.A. 33½", L.A. 32".

Patient was admitted to the University Hospital on January 20, 1938, and skin traction of 12 pounds was applied for the following two weeks. On February 3, 1938, a reconstruction operation of the type described was done, and her hospital convalescence was perfectly uneventful. The highest temperature after operation was 100.2, and on the fourteenth day after operation the plaster was removed from the posterior aspect of the foot and leg, and active movement of the knee begun. The entire plaster spica was removed two weeks later, and overhead suspension swinging apparatus used. Forty-nine days after operation, the patient was allowed out of bed, and cautious weight bearing with crutches started. One week later she was able to walk about the ward with only one crutch, and was discharged from the hospital about two months after operation, walking well, presenting no pain in the hip, and showing a gain of 1¼" in the length of the left lower extremity. On discharge she had a range of movement from 180 to 90 degrees, and a full range of abduction. The pre and post operative roentgenograms are shown.

Fig. III

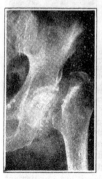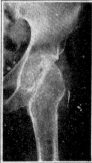

CASE 32

BEFORE   AFTER

This procedure since 1931 has been personally done in over 30 patients, and it is felt therefore that the procedure can be recommended as a safe and satisfactory one for the type of case under discussion.

BIBLIOGRAPHY

1. Colonna, Paul C.: A New Type of Reconstruction Operation for Old Ununited Fracture of the Neck of the Femur. J. Bone and Joint Surg., XVII, 110, January, 1935.

2. Colona, Paul C.: The Problem of Non-Union in Fracture of the Neck of the Femur. Virginal Medical Monthly, May, 1937.

3. Colonna, Paul C.: A Reconstruction Operation for Old Ununited Fracture of the Femoral Neck. J. Bone and Joint Surg., XIX, 945, October, 1937.

Carcinoma of the Prostate

HENRY S. BROWNE, M.D.
TULSA, OKLAHOMA

The mass of statistical data proves that about 15 to 20 per cent of all c a s e s of prostatic obstruction are due to carcinoma. In my experience this has run considerably lower for in 260 cases of prostatic enlargement operated on by me in the past four years only 30 have proved to be malignant. Seventy-one per cent of all cases occur b e t w e e n the ages of 60 and 79. Adeno-carcinomas make up the great majority and according to Baringer only 4½ per cent are confined to the prostate. A total of 7½ per cent are completely palpable while 88 per cent are extensive. Eighty to 90 per cent are slow in growth and radio resistant while the remainder are of rapid growth and radio sensitive.

As emphasized by Hugh Young most carcinomas originate in the posterior lobe of the gland. It is very unfortunate that the story of cancer every where is repeated here for three-fourths of the patients have metastases already when first seen and about half will have metastases a year after the symptoms first a p p e a r. The symptoms can scarcely be differentiated from those of benign obstruction. The burning and pain on urination are perhaps more severe. There is frequency, nocturia, difficulty and at times dribbling. Pain in the back, perineum and hips are suspicious of metastases. The patient has usually had symptoms for a year or more before examination and few live l o n g e r than three years after their onset. Early detection depends on rectal examination so it is not amiss to repeat that old saying that no physical examination is complete without a digital rectal exploration. This is especially true in men past 50. I am chagrined at my inability to diagnose early carcinoma of the prostate for in a number of cases of clinical benign hypertrophy resected by me the pathological r e p o rt has shown malignancy. This led me to believe that malignant nodules in an otherwise adeno-

matous gland are more frequent than the literature w o u l d indicate. The typical stony hardness with fixation to surrounding tissues is unmistakable. However, one should be suspicious of undue induration, hard nodules, and the obliteration of the median sulcus between the lateral lobes. On cystoscopy the congestion and fixation of the urethral m u c o u s membrane and veru montanum are an aid in diagnosis. X-ray of the pelvis and lower spine will show the snowflake appearing metastases when present. As the great majority are discovered too late the treatment is generally not satisfactory.

In the early cases the radical operation in which the prostate, seminal vesicles and neck of the bladder are removed en masse has been carried out by Hugh Young, Gilbert Smith, and Hinman with enough success for them to recommend it in v e r y carefully selected cases. Reports f r o m other men are notable for their absence. In other words, they do not perform it. An important thing is the relief of obstruction. This can be accomplished by a supra-pubic cystotomy and this was the accepted method until transurethral resection came into vogue. On this one point concerning resection all urologists are agreed—it will relieve the obstruction of carcinoma and allow the patient to void in comfort the rest of his days. It is not usually necessary to repeat the operation as carcinoma tends to grow outward and not to re-encroach on the urethra.

As stated before, I confess that I am unable to diagnose malignancy of the prostate by rectal palpation with any degree of regularity. It is possible that in these apparently early cases with no metastases the cancer cells may be few and isolated in one of the lobes. So in three recent cases where the diagnosis was made microscopically I have deliberately reoperated within a w e e k and removed all of the hypertrophied tissue down to the capsule, in the hope that by so doing I might be able to remove the cancer before it has spread through the capsule and invaded the surrounding tissues. This removal is not unusually difficult as there is only a thin shell of prostatic tissue left after the first resection and the concave, circular fibers of the capsule are easily differentiated from the firm, while irregular appearing hypertrophic tissue. The capsular bed was then lightly fulgurated with a roller electrode. I give you this idea for whatever you may think it worth. ·

Now, we come to radiation therapy. Radium can be applied by tubes through the urethra, or more readily, quickly and accurately by the implantation of s e e d s through the perineum. Up to the recent development of the very high voltage X-ray, deep therapy had little effect on the prostate itself. There is a well grounded belief that the super-voltage machines will have a more favorable effect on the gland.

Deep therapy is a distinct help in alleviating the pain caused by bone metastases, makes the patient more comfortable and probably prolongs life.

Cancer of the prostate occurs in men at the twilight of life. The great majority do not seek aid until metastases are present and they do not live usually over three years. If the diagnosis is made early the radical operation for cure is so extensive and so difficult that few are endowed with the ability to perform it so that the end results justify doing it. Transurethral resection offers the patient a chance to be comfortable for his remaining days. In the early cases, diagnosed microscopically following resection, a second resection, removing all of the prostatic tissue down to the capsule with fulguration of the capsular bed, may possibly remove all of the malignant tissue. X-ray and radium so far have proved only palliative but have undoubtedly prolonged life and made living more bearable.

Treatment of Infections of the Prostate

BASIL A. HAYES, M.D.
OKLAHOMA CITY, OKLAHOMA

As time goes on more and more urologists are learning that in some conditions treatment may be worse than the disease. Notably is this true of many cases of prostatitis where over enthusiastic massage or passage of instruments may bring on rheumatism or epididymitis. For the past ten years writers have been calling attention more and more forcibly to the dangers of traumatism and of o v e r treatment. In spite of this, however, it is my conviction that we are still having too many men attempt to cure infections of the prostate and seminal vesicles by r a d i c a l means. Twice during the past year I h a v e seen such cases brought into University Hospital with an acute bladder r e t e n t i o n which had to be relieved by catheterization because of intense swelling of the prostate gland. More than once have I seen an

acute gonorrheal rheumatism develop immediately after a prostatic massage. I have often seen gonorrheal proctitis and occasionally rectal fistulae develop following the same maneuver. These statements are made merely to emphasize the fact that massaging t h e prostate, particularly an acute one, is more or less dangerous and should not be done if at all possible of avoidance.

In looking over the literature and in discussing this matter with other urologists, it is surprising how few of them mention any treatment except the ordinary routine urethral injections, vaccines, or massage. The purpose of this paper is to summarize the various weapons with which we can attack this infection and to point out that practically every case can be cured if approached in the right manner. The remedial measures which may be utilized are as follows:

1. Constitutional measures.
   a. General tonics such as rest in bed, intravenous mercurochrome or neosalvarsan.
2. Specific medication.
   a. Sulfanilamide.
   b. Mandelic acid.
   c. Vaccines.
3. Urethral injections or irrigations.
   a. Argyrol, rivanol, potassium permanganate, etc.
4. Massage.
5. Heat locally applied.
6. Passage of sounds or meatotomy.
7. Vasotomy or injection of prostate.
8. Surgical drainage through the perineum.

Infections of the prostate and seminal vesicles logically divide themselves into acute and chronic stages. It is well known that acute infections u s u a l l y arise in younger men and in the course of a gonorrheal urethritis or following such an infection. It has been my observation that prostatitis usually develops about the third week of a gonorrheal a t t a c k and many times immediately follows some indiscretion on the part of the patient, such as drinking or intercourse; or some traumatism on the part of the attending physician, such as the injection of a strong solution into the urethra, or the passage of a sound or catheter. Following this event the patient will develop pain in the region of the prostate, straining on urination, pus in the second glass of urine, and in m a n y instances will have fever and will be forced to go to bed. Even in this stage of the disease there are three distinct types: First, the ordinary mild periurethral involvement of the shorter ducts of the prostate gland which in most instances will subside spontaneously within a week or ten days if all local treatment is stopped and the patient merely continued along on systemic tonics, vaccines, or sulfanilamide. A second type is more severe, involving the entire parenchyma of the prostate gland and causing an intense swelling which in many instances will block off the urethra as mentioned above. In some such cases the patient must be catheterized although I have

never had to do this in any case where I was in complete charge of the patient. As a rule he can squeeze out enough urine to keep him reasonably free from pain if he will sit in a tub of hot water and try to pass his urine. Meanwhile he can be given an intravenous injection of three ccs of one per cent mercurochrome and within eight to 12 hours the swelling of the gland will be down enough that he can void comfortably. At the same time he may be given hot rectal irrigations twice a day, sulfanilamide by mouth, calcium in the vein, or any other drugs which may appeal to the urologist's ideas. The one essential thing which I wish to call attention to is that an intravenous injection of mercurochrome will relieve the swelling and the acute pain in 90 per cent of the cases. I have been treating such patients this way for the past 12 years, and it is my happy experience that in no case have I failed to see an immediate improvement. The response to this drug is better than it is to any vaccine I have ever used. It is better than any heat treatment I have ever seen used. It absolutely avoids all local irritation or trauma and certainly builds up the systemic resistance of the patient against a gonorrheal infection. It is completely harmless, acts as a sedative, relieves the swelling of the gland so that the patient can urinate, and in nine times out of ten within one week the patient will be up and able to attend to his ordinary duties. In some cases the infection will continue to improve until it spontaneously disappears, while in others the process will drop into a chronic stage and must be dealt with in accordance with the principles which will be enunciated later in this paper.

In the third sub-group of acute prostatitis there is formed a definite abscess. This is manifested by swelling, leukocytosis, fever, i n t e n s e pain, and more or less urethral discharge. In any case of acute prostatitis or vesiculitis which does not respond to the previously mentioned routine of treatment and in which the patient suffers an unusual amount of pain, I suspect the formation of an abscess. Such a situation calls for the simplest and safest procedure of all, which is to open and drain it through the perineum. It goes against all surgical principles to rupture such an abscess through the rectal wall or through the urethral wall yet I have seen both procedures advocated by good men. When an organ is as easily approached as is the prostate through the perineum, it seems to me the unquestionable duty of the practitioner to open it in this manner, thus avoiding any danger of contamination from other sources or of fistula, or any other disagreeable sequel which may follow intraurethral or intrarectal procedures. Relief from such an operation is immediate and recovery is swift. The only danger involved is that which would come from cutting the urethra or the rectum, and a knowledge of the anatomy of the perineum would prevent such an accident. Even if it does happen, the damage can easily be remedied.

So much for the acute types of prostatitis; now for the chronic. These compose a vast majority of cases which come to the average urologist. They are not suffering from swelling, they have little or no pain, they simply have pus in the urine, an uneasy feeling about the neck of the bladder, rheumatic pains over the body, backache, i t c h i n g and crawling sensations in the urethra, and a general depression based upon the fact that they know they are sick and feel that they ought to be well. As a rule their infection is derived from a posterior urethritis due to gonorrhea. During the meeting of the American Urological Association in Minneapolis last summer, there was presented a symposium on pyogenic prostatitis and the essayists almost unanimously agreed that the prostatitis in the majority of cases was not due to the gonococcus. It seems to me that such a statement is completely erroneous and misleading. While it might be correct bacteriologically, it is certainly a m i s t a k e clinically because practically e v e r y one who has ever come under my observation knows himself that his infection started with an a t t a c k of gonorrhea. The fact that we can isolate B Coli, streptococci, or staphylococci in such c a s e s in no wise negates the fact that gonococci are also present. The only cases which I have seen which were not dependent upon a preceding gonorrheal infection were in elderly men where there was prostatic hypertrophy, carcinoma, or o t h e r attendant

pathology which blocked off drainage and brought about a necessity for instrumentation or lowered the resistance of the tissues to the point that infection could spontaneously develop either from other foci or from the urinary tract itself. I have no objection to eliminating focal infections anywhere in the body, but I do feel that urologists should keep their eyes upon the main point in prostatic infection and that is that the infection arose within the urinary tract and must be treated in that location. Whether or not we can isolate or culture gonococci from a chronically infected prostate is beside the point. The clinical fact is as we all know that if such men marry, they immediately infect their wives with gonorrhea even though we have been unable to demonstrate gonococci in the smear. Last year I read a report in the literature of a case where gonococci were isolated in a prostate and had apparently been present for as long as 30 years. It seems to me, therefore, that we should proceed upon the assumption that gonococci are present with or without secondary invaders and treat the patient accordingly plus any other specific medication which we may give to take care of the secondary bacteria. The plan of procedure which I have followed in the treatment of chronic prostatis and seminal vesiculitis is as follows: First, I attempt to determine the extent of involvement by a two glass test and a prostatic smear with a laboratory test to find out what organisms are involved. In the ordinary case there is a mild urethritis as shown by pus in both the first and second glasses, and there is a prostatitis as shown by numerous pus cells in the smear. Second, I attempt to build up the patient's resistance as much as possible by general hygienic measures and systemic drugs. He is instructed to avoid all sexual excitement, all alcohol, all loss of sleep, or heavy exertion or exposure of any kind. He is instructed to drink plenty of water and to avoid strong cathartics. He is ordered to come to the office every other day, at which time he is given an intravenous injection of three cubic centimeters of one per cent mercurochrome and after two or three such treatments, the anterior urethra is investigated to d e t e r m i n e whether there is a stricture or whether or not a meatotomy is needed. If the urethra is wide open and there is no stricture as demonstrated by passing a sound about three or four inches into the urethra, well and good; otherwise this passage is opened. Along with this the patient receives each time he comes to the office an anteroposterior injection of seven to ten ccs of five per cent argyrol or 1:1000 rivanol injected into the urinary meatus with a blunt nosed syringe and gently forced back into the bladder. If gonococci are isolated or if it seems plainly evident that the patient is suffering from this infection, he is given a course of sulfanilamide tablets. This is continued for about a week. If they produce results, well and good; otherwise no harm has been done and they are discontinued. If B Coli are present, he is given Mandelic Acid therapy, pushing it the full eight days as outlined by its originators. If the patient is suffering f r o m marked rheumatic symptoms, no massage is given; but if he is not, twice each week a gentle prostatic massage is given, catching the expressed secretion on a slide and examining it immediately. By this means I am able to keep up more or less roughly with the progress of the treatment and to determine the increase or decrease of pus cells in the prostatic field. In those cases where sulfanilamide s e e m to be of no value, after it is thoroughly out of the patient's system, I give one injection of .6 grams neosalvarsan each w e e k, substituting it for an injection of mercurochrome on that particular day. By following out such a conservative course the majority of cases of chronic prostatitis will respond in four to eight weeks, then the patient can be discharged. At the end of this time if the patient has failed to respond properly or is becoming dissatisfied or in my judgment is not making any progress, I suggest a bilateral vasotomy. This is a minor operation and can be done by going to the hospital for one day or can even be done in any well organized office where there is plenty of help. It consists of isolating the vas deferens on each side, lifting it up, splitting it, inserting a blunt needle, and injecting ten ccs of five per cent collargol or one per cent mercurochrome into the vas. I have only had to resort to it a few

times and in those cases it was the final step which brought about a cure. Another procedure along the same line which seems to be entirely harmless and which in all probability will cure many cases is injection of the prostate gland with one per cent mercurochrome by the m e t h o d of Granville Haynes. I have had no occasion to use this method but after hearing Dr. Haynes and others discuss it, I am completely convinced that it is without harm and that in many instances it will be of marked benefit to the patient. It can be done under Evipal anesthesia or under a s p i n a l or sacral block and according to those who have done many c a s e s, it is without pain or untoward consequences.

Finally, there remain those cases where we have tried the conservative treatment without avail, where we have done a vasotomy or injected the prostate, and still the patient has pus in the prostatic smear or pain about the bladder neck or rheumatic symptoms. What shall we do with him? Some 15 or 20 years ago Morrissey of New York reported brilliant results in a series of severe arthritic patients by removing the seminal vesicles through the perineum. Cunningham of Boston has reported similar results and has reported much benefit from mere incision and drainage of the prostate and seminal vesicles. The operation is simple, being done exactly according to the perineal incision as outlined by Hugh Young for his prostatectomy. The dissection is carried down t h r o u g h the prostate, both layers of the fascia of Denonvillier are opened, the prostate is incised, the seminal vesicles are located and opened, and a drainage tube is left in for a week or ten days. The treatment is adequately d e s c r i b e d by Cunningham in Lewis' Surgery and needs no further elaboration h e r e. It is completely surgical, gives perfect drainage, and will result in an absolute cure of infection of the vesicles and prostate in any case where it is needed.

Summarizing this paper, I would say that infections of the prostate and seminal vesicles, whether acute or chronic, should be treated by conservative measures and without t r a u m a. If, after a reasonable length of time, they do not respond properly or show that further measures are needed ,the prostate should be injected by the Haynes' method or a bilateral vasotomy should be done. If this fails to cure the patient, a perineal section should be done and true surgical drainage instituted.

-------------O-------------

Acute Nephritis and Nephrosis*

E. R. MUSICK, M.D.
Associate in Medicine, University of Oklahoma
OKLAHOMA CITY, OKLAHOMA

There has been much confusion during the last several years on the subject of nephritis. The old classification has been based on the pathology found at autopsy, which the clinician could not correlate with the clinical findings. Consequently, the clinician had one classification, and the pathologist another. Several years ago the term "nephrosis" was coined, which has not simplified the problem, but has added to the confusion. So at the present time most of us are still confused over the "nephritis problem."

There are several clinical classifications used, but probably the most simple to understand and a good one generally accepted is Christian's classification. It is clinically workable and is sufficient to cover the whole problem.

Whether you wish to class nephrosis as a distinct entity or as a grade or process in the nephritic state is open to controversy, and is unimportant so far as this discussion is concerned. This paper will deal only with acute nephritis with edema and with nephrosis. Focal nephritis, in which a small area of kidney is involved due to embolism, and the chronic forms of kidney disease will not be discussed.

The treatment of nephritis is well standardized, and all of us have treated our cases by this standard. It might be of interest to understand the reasons why we use these treatments. This is partially demonstrated on the slide prepared, which correlates some of the clinical and chemical occurrences in these two conditions.

*Read before the Medical Section at the Annual Meeting of the Oklahoma State Medical Association, Muskogee, Oklahoma, May 11, 1938.

The heavy solid line which you notice in the upper part of the diagram represents graphically the amount and degree of edema. You will observe that the immediate happening in the acute nephritic is an elevation of the blood urea nitrogen. It elevates abruptly. However, about 13 pounds of fluid must be present in the body tissues before an edema is demonstrable by pitting. Also, with equally as abrupt a rise is the albuminuria, shown by the heavy solid line at the lower part of the slide. You will also notice that the blood proteins—the serum albumin and serum globulin—show very little change except late when there may be a slight decrease in the total amount, but they remain in the normal ratio—4 to 4.5 milligrams of serum albumin to 2 of serum globulin. The blood cholesterol remains normal.

Pathologically, acute nephritis with edema is known to cause a swelling of all the glomerular cells. It is also known that in the edema of nephritis the sodium and chlorine ions together, in conjunction with water, are necessary to the formation of this edema. The cause is thought to be the raising of the kidney threshold for salt.

The treatment then of the acute nephritic is to rest the glomeruli as much as possible. This is accomplished by bed rest in order to place the kidney function at its lowest. Added warmth to the body surface is also useful. Second, the sodium and chlorine ions in combination as common salt should be entirely eliminated from the diet. If it is necessary to supply chlorides the potassium or calcium chloride, which are commercially available for table use, may be substituted. They have no deleterious effect on the edema. Third, use the amount of fluid intake necessary for body needs—2,000 to 3,000 cc. daily; because of the wasting of tissue which will occur if the body is dehydrated. This can safely be done in the absence of sodium chloride, unless the complication of a cerebral edema develops, when of course, the fluid intake should be restricted. Fourth, the b o d y caloric needs should be kept up, preferably in the form of concentrated carbohydrate. Proteins must be limited because of the retention of nitrogenous products, but not for too long a period because protein starvation brings equally as pernicious effects because of the eliminated albuminous material. Fats are not contraindicated since the b l o o d cholesterol remains normal. Fifth, diuretics are contra-indicated. This point deserves special emphasis. It has been p r o v e n experimentally on animals that diuretics not only do not help, but also that those diuresed died sooner than those in which no diuretics were used. This seems logical when we remember that all the cells of the glomeruli are swollen. To attempt overstimulation w o u l d have the same effect on the inflammed cells of the kidney as overwork on any inflammed organs. The first principle of surgery and medicine is rest to an inflammed part.

In some severe cases it may be necessary to place the patient on a milk diet for a few days. If the patient is vomiting, intravenous 5 or 10 per cent glucose solution, one or two litres daily should be used, and in addition chlorides other than the sodium should be given in order to combat the loss of chloride due to the vomiting. Since there is no anemia during the acute stage there is no indication for the use of iron.

With this type of treatment the patient will usually recover unless an intercurrent infection results. If this occurs, or if the acute case has been improperly handled, there is likely to be a recurrence of the edema—more marked than at the onset— and the p a t i e n t passes into the second s t a g e of nephritis—the nephrotic stage. Here we find an entirely different trend of findings. It must be mentioned here that by far the greater number will recover and will have no residual nephritis. This is demonstrated on the slide as this middle

area. The edema as a rule is shown by the weight curve, is much greater. The urea nitrogen is falling or is n o r m a l, which shows a return to normal of nitrogen metabolism—much in opposition to the happenings in the a c u t e nephritic. The blood cholesterol is beginning to rise, and most important there is a beginning change in the blood serum proteins: there is an inversion of the albumin-globulin ratio as shown by the two lowest curves, with of course a lowering of the total blood proteins. It is known that when the total proteins fall below four milligrams, edema will occur. The serum albumin seems to be the factor that holds the fluid in the blood stream, and prevents its escape into the body tissues. A nephrosis practically always runs a low metabolism.

The treatment of the nephrotic is first, rest and warmth for the reasons before mentioned. S e c o n d, elimination of the salt, and substitution of other than the sodium salt. Third, the s u p p l y of fluids necessary for body needs. Fourth, a high protein diet in order to replace the serum proteins in the blood so they may hold the fluids, and to replace the albumin lost. They are also not contraindicated because the urea nitrogen is normal. Carbohydrates should be used to give caloric value to the diet. Fat should be restricted, because of its p o s s i b l e bearing on the increasing cholesterol. Thyroid extract is sometimes used in order to increase the lowered metabolism and in order to utilize the cholesterol found.

Acute nephritis with edema involves primarily the glomeruli of the kidney, although there is also some tubular damage. The primary purpose of the glomeruli is to filter fluid from the b l o o d into the tubules. Nephrosis, on the other hand, is primarily an involvement of the tubular structure. Probably their most important function is the diffusion of fluids and materials in suspension which pass through the glomeruli back into the tissue spaces and then into the blood stream, so that the body can utilize the salts and materials needed in body function. During nephrosis the tubular action is badly damaged or destroyed. Organs such as the liver, spleen, and others may be swollen from the edema, and the body cavities may become filled with fluid. So really nephrosis becomes more than a kidney problem, it becomes a generalized metabolic disturbance.

All this work is investigative work, and the clinician usually does not have the facilities of utilizing t h e s e procedures to make the diagnosis. We can deduct our method of treatment in a great many cases f r o m understanding the happenings in these cases of nephritis. At times, however, it is absolutely impossible to make a diagnosis without the use of the laboratory. Massive edemas seen are usually, especially in young individuals, either an acute nephritis or a nephrosis. The amount of the edema is of no diagnostic value. Acute nephritis follows an acute infection, about 7 to 14 days, most often a streptococcic infection from the throat, tonsils, respiratory tract, middle ear, or gastro-intestinal tract. It is easily diagnosed. There is one condition that should be mentioned, for when it occurs in the presence of an acute nephritis, it demands a different treatment. That condition is cerebral edema. Any elevation of blood pressure over 160 systolic should cause immediate concern, and beginning dehydration treatment should be instituted. If it is allowed to progress, convulsions and death may result when the p r e s s u r e rises to 180 or 200. It is amenable to dehydration therapy of oral or intramuscular magnesium sulphate, intravenous hypertonic glucose, and limitation of fluids until reduction of blood pressure results. It is not a uremia, and must not be confused with uremia. With the presence of heavy albumin in the urine, blood in varying quantities, granular casts, and edema, with the history of a previous infection, acute nephritis with edema is easily diagnosed—*if this is the first attack of an edema.* If a urea nitrogen test can be made it will prove or disprove the diagnosis.

If, however, a case of acute nephritis which is apparently recovering develops an acute infection especially an u p p e r respiratory, and the edema becomes worse, it is nearly certain that this patient has developed a nephrosis. A check of the serum albumin-globulin ratio will reveal an inversion or beginning inversion of that ratio. If there is a history of a previous edema within two years, with an intercurrent infection of the upper respiratory tract, followed by a massive edema—that usually will also be found to be a nephrosis.

Both these types mentioned may give similar urine findings, and the blood pressure may or may not be elevated in either.

The question might arise as to why kidney function tests are not used to help in making the diagnoses in these types of cases. If we review the pathology that occurs it becomes clear. In the acute nephritis, as before stated, there is a generalized e d e m a t o u s involvement of all the glomeruli. The filtration through them is damaged because of the edema. There are 150,000 to 250,000 cc. of fluid that normally passes through the glomeruli daily. This fluid passes to the tubular structure, where there is reabsorption back into the body tissues. The remaining waste of approximately 1,500 cc. passes into the bladder and is excreted. Only one-tenth of the glomeruli of a normal kidney are active at any one time; the remaining nine-tenths are in the resting state. There are millions of glomeruli in the kidneys. There are 35 or 40 loops of blood vessels in the glomerulus, and only three to five of these loops are active at one time. The remainder are resting. The average output of day urine is 1,200 cc.; of night urine, 300 cc. The edema fluid of nephritis and nephrosis is a fixed fluid, and it can not be utilized for body needs. The needed intake of fluid daily is between 2,000 and 3,000 cc., since some fluid is lost in the perspiration, from the lungs, and in the intestinal tract.

By these facts it can be seen that it is only in the later stages of nephritis that functional tests can be of advantage in the diagnosis. They are worthless in the acute nephritis and nephrosis states. But the examination of the urinary sediment is v e r y important, and some writers have gone so far as to state that the coarse granular casts are indicative of acuteness, fine granular casts as showing the subacute stage, and the waxy casts as indicative of chronic progression of the disease. Microscopic examination may show the type of cellular structure that is diseased and that is consequently thrown off in the urine. It has also been s t a t e d that the presence of a few red blood cells persisting in the urine of a clinically improving case is not necessarily a bad sign; for it may signify that some blood is being supplied to the loops in the capsule and means that the loop is not entirely necrosed.

BIBLIOGRAPHY

Kerkhof, Arthur C.: Plasmapheresis Experiments upon Influence of Colloid Osmotic Pressure, Water and Salt in Edema Formation, Annals of Internal Medicine, February, 1938, Page 1407.

Leporte, Michael J.: Acacia Therapy in Neophrotic Edema, Annals of Internal Medicine, August, 1937, page 285.

Ziegler, Edwin E., and Brice, Arthur T.: Reaction and Specific Gravity of Urine in Relation to Nephritis (a Study of 10,000 Analyses), Annals of Internal Medicine, November, 1937, Page 768.

Stone, Willard J.: Bright's Disease and Hypertension, Text Book, 1936 Edition.

McCann, W. S.: Bright's Disease—Review of Recent Literature, Archives of Internal Medicine, March, 1938.

---O---

The Use of Cautery and Escharotics in the Nose

O. ALTON WATSON, M.D.
OKLAHOMA CITY, OKLAHOMA

It is not my purpose to delve deeply into the subject of physical therapy as applied to the nose and sinuses. I intend merely to discuss *two conditions*, very different in nature, that are greatly benefitted or relieved by cauterization either with heated applicators or some of the caustic agents such as Trichloracetic acid, chromic acid bead, strong solutions of silver nitrate, or the various drugs used in ionization of the nasal mucosa. In passing, I should like to state that in my opinion, the results obtained by ionization are no different from those obtained by the use of trichloracetic acid thoroughly applied. What I consider a proper technique of application will be described a little later.

The first condition to be discussed is *Hypertrophic Rhinitis*, which is described as a chronic inflammatory thickening of the nasal mucous membrane with an increase in connective tissue, especially on the inferior turbinate. Etiology of this disease is not specific—any condition which produces repeated attacks of irritation and inflammation of the nasal mucous membrane will cause hypertrophy—

1. Repeated attacks acute rhinitis.
2. Exposure to dust and chemical irritants.
3. Gas fumes.
4. Climatic conditions.
5. Improper diet.
6. Anemia.

All are listed as causes in different individuals.

Pathology is an increased blood supply with increase of connective tissue so that contractile power of the turbinate tissue is impaired or lost. The inferior turbinate is the most commonly involved.

Symptoms.

1. Nasal obstruction.
   a. Alternating.
   b. On lying down.
2. Sticky post-nasal secretion.
3. Headache—if drainage of sinuses is obstructed by pressure of middle turbinate.

Diagnosis is made on:

1. Dusky red color.
2. Increased size of turbinates.
3. Swelling is resistant to probe and depressions fill in slowly.
4. Symptoms.

If elimination of causative factors is not effective and other causes of nasal obstruction such as nasal polyps—deviated septum, etc., are ruled out—cauterization of the inferior turbinate will usually give relief: The electrode should be a narrow one to lessen the amount of tissue destruction. After the n o s e is properly anesthetized with 10 per cent cocaine solution, the electrode is heated to a cherry red color and beginning at the posterior tip of the inferior turbinate is drawn forward slowly, allowing enough time for the heat to coagulate the tissue entirely through the mucosa and periosteum—so that the resulting scar will be attached to the bone. Otherwise in a short time, a few weeks or months, the swelling is as great as ever. When the procedure is finished, there should be a line or eschar along the entire length of the inferior turbinate. What is the result? Temporarily there is increased swelling and for a few days the patient should use some oily medicant; the nose should be examined every two or three days to be sure there are no adhesions between the burned surface of the inferior turbinate and the septum which may have been accidentally burned in some area. Within a week or ten days, the swelling is subsiding and by the end of two weeks the mucosa is usually healed. Best results regarding breathing space are not obtained for about six to eight weeks. By this time there is adequate breathing space and consequently proper aeration of the nasal mucous membrane with decreased infection of the membrane, and less secretion formed. The normal secretions are dried out in a normal manner so that there is no excess to accumulate in the naso pharynx. In properly selected cases, this is one of the most satisfactory operations that the nasal surgeon may do.

The second condition of which I shall speak is vasomotor rhinitis, or hyper aesthetic rhinitis. It seems to me that the latter term offers a better description of the disease—since that is really what is present—an over sensitiveness to any irritant, whether dust, changes of temperature or from internal factors such as foods, drugs, etc.

The symptoms are:

1. Nasal blocking.
2. Sneezing.
3. Watery discharge.

Examination: There is a pale, edematous mucous membrane—throughout—which is more pronounced on inferior and middle turbinate. This may lead, in long continued cases, to the formation of mucous polyps either in the sinuses or in the nose, or to the formation of a polypoid middle turbinate.

X-ray or transillumination usually reveals sinuses all clear with the exception of each antrum which usually is slightly cloudy or quite cloudy depending on the amount of edema involving the mucous membrane lining of the sinus. These sinuses will become clear in a few minutes if an adrenalin or ephedrine tampon is used in the nose. Antrum puncture will be negative to pus unless secondarily infected. Eosinophiles are found to be numerous in any case. This type of patient has the same symptoms as seasonal hay fever except the eyes are usually not involved as much, if any, and the condition is not seasonal. There is a great variation in severity of the disease, some patients only sneezing a few times on arising and being normal throughout the day, while others have severe symptoms all day. Many of these patients later or coincidentally develop asthma, which points to the fact that the condition is not a local one but of constitutional scope.

I would like to state that in my opinion, many of these patients have been erroneously treated for sinusitis—and have run the gauntlet of treatment from Argarol tampons to sinus exenteration. I wish to make a plea for proper diagnosis with definite information to the patient that he or she is not suffering from sinusitis as ordinarily considered, but that they have a constitutional predisposition and will probably always have some tendency for recurrence of their symptoms as different factors arise in spite of any treatment that may be instituted. Regarding local treatment of this malady, I have a few suggestions that may be of benefit. There should be a minimum of surgery. The sinuses should not be opened unless there are definite indications of infection. A deviated septum or mucous polyps may be surgically handled with improvement of the local condition but even these operations are better done when the symptoms of vasomotor rhinitis are not at the most acute stage.

The use of trichloracetic acid (25-50 strength) as a coating for the entire mucous membrane of the nose is often of great value in lessening the symptoms and restoring the membrane to a more normal color and tone. This should be preceded by thorough anesthesia with 10 per cent cocaine and followed by an oily spray regularly for several days afterward. The acid should be applied sparingly with a fairly dry applicator, being careful that it is not allowed to run. If the nose is examined regularly for a few days, it is easy to prevent the formation of any adhesions.

I wish to say that I am not advocating this treatment in every case of vasomotor rhinitis—and that not more than 50 per cent of the patients are benefitted even temporarily. Many get more relief by an allergic review with elimination of specific reactors—food, dust, animal dander, etc., but for the mild cases, or those who have not obtained relief from the allergist, and for those who prefer to give this simple form of treatment a trial first—it is worth while. It may be repeated as found necessary if the patient has been given relief.

---o---

The Summer-Time Use of Mead's Oleum Percomorphum

During the hot weather, when fat tolerance is lowest, many physicians have found it a successful practice to transfer cod liver oil patients to Mead's Oleum Percomorphum.

Due to its negligible oil content and its small dosage, this product does not upset the digestion, so that even the most squeamish patient can "stomach" it without protest.

There are at least two facts that strongly indicate the reasonableness of the above suggestion: (1) In prematures, to whom cod liver oil cannot be given in sufficient dosage without serious digestive upset, Mead's Oleum Percomorphum is the antirachitic agent of choice. (2) In Florida, Arizona and New Mexico, where an unusually high percentage of sunshine prevails at all seasons, Mead's Oleum Percomorphum continues increasingly in demand, as physicians realize that sunshine alone does not always prevent or cure rickets.

Mead Johnson & Company, Evansville, Indiana, invite you to send for samples of Mead's Oleum Percomorphum for clinical use during the summer months to replace cod liver oil.

---o---

Summer Diarrhea In Babies

Casec (calcium caseinate), which is almost wholly a combination of protein and calcium, offers a quickly effective method of treating all types of diarrhea, both in bottle-fed and breast-fed infants. For the former, the carbohydrate is temporarily omitted from the 24-hour formula and replaced with eight level tablespoonfuls of Casec. Within a day or two the diarrhea will usually be arrested, and carbohydrate in the form of Dextri-Maltose may safely be added to the formula and the Casec gradually eliminated. Three to six teaspoonfuls of a thin paste of Casec and water, given before each nursing, is well indicated for loose stools in breast-fed babies. Please send for samples to Mead Johnson & Company, Evansville, Indiana.

DISEASES OF THE SKIN FOR PRACTITIONERS AND STUDENTS: By George Clinton Andrews, A.B., M.D., Associate Professor of Dermatology, College of Physicians and Surgeons, Columbia University; Chief of Clinic, Department of Dermatology, Vanderbilt Clinic; Fellow of the American Medical Association, of the American College of Physicians, and of the New York Academy of Medicine. Second Edition, Entirely Reset. 899 pages with 938 illustrations. Philadelphia and London: W. B. Saunders Company, 1938. Cloth, $10.00 net.

In this second edition of Andrews' book over 75 new diseases have been added, and there are new chapters on dermatoses due to filterable viruses, vitamin deficiencies, and cutaneous infiltrations with products of metabolism. Furthermore, several hundred additions have been made in subject matter, including remedies and prescriptions, discussions of allergy, sensitization tests, desensitization, and dermatologic surgery. Photographs in the first edition received much favorable comment and in this edition have been augmented and improved by substitutions and additions of over 200 pictures. There are many histological drawings and microphotographs have been added. Special prominence has been given to the more common skin diseases, making the text simple, easy to use and practical.

This will be a very acceptable work to students, and general practitioners.

---o---

Cutaneous Absorption of Sex Hormones

Carl R. Moore, Jule K. Lamar and Naomi Beck, Chicago (Journal A.M.A., July 2, 1938), applied testosterone or testosterone propionate to the skin of rats and guinea pigs as an ointment. It is readily absorbed and either maintains the accessory reproductive organs of castrate male animals in a normal reproductive state or stimulates their development precociously in the young or decidedly above the normal levels in adult animals. These androgens, so administered, exert effects similar to those obtained following subcutaneous injections. They (1) maintain reproductive accessories in castrate males at all ages, (2) reconstitute castrated guinea pigs within seven days of treatment to a state of producing coagulable ejaculates on electrical stimulation of the head, and (3) produce injuries to testes of normal growing young male rats. Face cream (stated to contain estradiol) sold commercially and recommended for the removal of wrinkles from normal women has decided internal effects when applied daily on the skin of experimental animals. Such treatments stimulate mammary development on normal male guinea pigs, induce cornified vaginal estrous smears in spayed female rats, maintain or increase normal growth of the uterus in young or mature spayed rats and reduce the weight of the testes by 80 per cent and the weight of seminal vesicles by 90 per cent in young male rats in comparison with normal litter mates. These results both emphasize the efficiency of applying hormones in a skin ointment and at the same time suggest caution in the use by normal persons of articles containing these active principles.

---o---

NOTICE

L. E. Gleeck, former State Factory Representative of H. G. Fischer & Co., is convalescing from an attack of Coronary Thrombosis and will be calling on his customers in September, for F. A. Davis Company, Philadelphia.

THE JOURNAL
OF THE
Oklahoma State Medical Association

Issued Monthly at McAlester, Oklahoma, under direction of the Council.

Copyright, 1938, by Oklahoma State Medical Association, McAlester, Oklahoma.

Vol. XXXI	AUGUST	Number 8

DR. L. S. WILLOUR..................................Editor-in-Chief
McAlester, Oklahoma

DR. T. H. McCARLEY..................................Associate Editor
McAlester, Oklahoma

Entered at the Post Office at McAlester, Oklahoma, as second-class matter under the act of March 3rd, 1879.

This is the official Journal of the Oklahoma State Medical Association. All communications should be addressed to The Journal of the Oklahoma State Medical Association, McAlester Clinic, McAlester, Oklahoma. $4.00 per year; 40c per copy.

The editorial department is not responsible for the opinions expressed in the original articles of contributors.

Reprints of original articles will be supplied at actual cost provided request for them is attached to manuscripts or made in sufficient time before publication.

Articles sent this Journal for publication and all those read at the annual meetings of the State Association are the sole property of this Journal. The Journal relies on each individual contributor's strict adherence to this well-known rule of medical journalism. In the event an article sent this Journal for publication is published before appearance in The Journal the manuscript will be returned to the writer.

Failure to receive The Journal should call for immediate notification of the Editor, McAlester Clinic, McAlester, Oklahoma.

Local news of possible interest to the medical profession, notes on removals, changes of addresses, births, deaths and weddings will be gratefully received.

Advertising of articles, drugs or compounds unapproved by the Council on Pharmacy of the A. M. A., will not be accepted.

Advertising rates will be supplied on application.

It is suggested that wherever possible members of the State Association should patronize our advertisers in preference to others as a matter of fair reciprocity.

Printed by News-Capital Company, McAlester.

EDITORIAL

PRACTICAL RECIPROCITY

It is again time to bring to the attention of our membership the matter of giving every consideration to our advertisers, not only that we may use Council approved products but to practice reciprocity with the firms who purchase advertising space in the Journal and exhibit space at our Annual meeting.

We are visited every day by detail men who bring to our attention both new and old preparations. Some firms depend entirely upon these detail men to place their products on the market and they are educated to try to teach us how to practice medicine. How many of us stop to inquire as to whether or not the products are Council Approved? There are a few pharmaceutical houses that carry on scientific research work and are sure before the detail man visits you that their claims are well founded and the product submitted to the Council for investigation. Again there are inferior houses who take advantage of this situation, add a little something that will not hinder the action and effect, change the name and claim a superior preparation. Perhaps they may even cut the price a little, for they have had no expense in carrying on the research work, which has been necessary to prove the effectiveness of the product.

The firms that do not use the ethical Journals in advertising in many instances have nothing to offer that your Journal will accept, as we will publish the advertising of no product that is not Council Approved. The service of this Council is offered to us without cost and we should be smart enough to take advantage of it. We can help to make the seal of this Council mean even more than it does now by insisting upon it being an important part of the recommendation of any product.

When an advertisement appears in this Journal you can be sure that after thorough investigation we have found it to be reliable and you can also be equally sure if the detail men can show you Council approval.

MORE SUB-STANDARD WORK

When the Public Welfare Commission agreed to spend its Crippled Children's money through the channels already established under the Crippled Children's law, it reserved the right to approve hospitals in addition to the list of accredited hospitals passed upon by the Board of Standardization.

At a meeting about a month ago, Major Kerr (and this is the same Kerr, who by his action on the Board of Regents destroyed our Post Graduate Program) secured approval of a Muskogee Hospital, and this hospital had never applied for approval from the Committee on Standardization. Following this Mr. Hyde secured approval of a hospital in Elk City, which institution has never been approved by the Board of Standardization.

Our Crippled Children's Law was modeled so as to protect the crippled child against inferior care and made it necessary for every hospital, as well as the Staff, to meet certain requirements, and it would be a sad misfortune indeed if this standard were lowered or in any way manipulated by politicians. This appears to be some more of the sub-standard work of the Public Welfare Commission as was evident in their management of the Pension matter.

The crippled child must be protected and assured the best professional care and there must be some way to accomplish this in an orderly manner.

------------o------------

SAN FRANCISCO MEETING OF THE AMERICAN MEDICAL ASSOCIATION

The 1938 session of the American Medical Association was the fifth one to meet in San Francisco, the last session held there being in 1923. The registration at the 1923 session was 3,726 while over 6,000 Fellows registered at the 1938 session. The membership of the Association in 1923 was 88,-159; today it is 109,435, the largest number ever recorded in the history of the organization.

At the opening session practically every delegate was present, and when the reference committee appointments were announced, you will be pleased to learn that your two delegates each had an appointment on an important committee, before which several important matters were presented and acted upon. At this meeting all alternate delegates, a l s o all presidents, secretarys and editors of State Medical Associations were invited to attend all sessions of the House of Delegates, including the executive session.

A resolution known as the Indiana Plan, "An Antidote for State Medicine," was approved in principle. This plan is similar to the recommendations submitted by the Missouri State Medical Association Committee on Postgraduate Course. The Indiana Plan follows:

AN ANTIDOTE FOR STATE MEDICINE

Frequently today the physician finds articles in the press questioning his efficiency and his methods of practice. Such articles accuse him of ignoring preventive medicine in his daily work. He is bewildered and defensive in his attitude for he feels that he is doing his job well. Even superficial observation will disclose the marked drop in death rate as a result of measures instituted by the medical profession in controlling tuberculosis, malaria, typhoid, diarrhea, yellow fever, puerperal sepsis and other infectious diseases. Preventive medicine is now being practiced by all physicians as private practitioners to some degree. In many parts of the state, county medical units have a definite program. The time is ripe to correlate these scattered activities, survey our local situations and acquaint the public with the extent of this phase of work.

Many phases of preventive medicine have advanced by stimulation from outside groups. Drives have been sponsored with much misunderstanding. Preventive medicine has now reached its maturity and should be utilized to the fullest by organized medicine and by the individual doctor. It is futile for one county or state to try to promote this alone. Disease and disaster are not aware of state borders. A national policy on the part of organized medicine is needed now.

Too long have we kept our light under a bushel. It is time to take the offensive. The amount of preventive medicine can be increased by the private practioner with definite benefit to his community and to himself, and the public will be made to realize that American medicine is pliable enough to continue as an individualistic enterprise.

Throughout the ages, medicine has adapted itself to social changes. We are now in one of those states of changing social customs and aspirations. The American public looks to organized medicine forleadership. Prevention of disease, early recognition of defects and diseases, reduction of hazards and prolongation of life are the important functions of a physician.

In Indiana we have visualized preventive medicine as a wheel with each spoke representing some important phase. Each phase is featured as a "Topic of the Month" in the Journal of the Indiana State Medical Association and is announced or discussed in each county medical society the month the subject is featured. The topic of the month is given support in the press and is discussed by speakers before medical and lay groups.

PURPOSE

To promote aggressive leadership by organized medicine in prevention of disease and early detection of defects.

To incorporate preventive medicine as an important phase of private practice and of county medical activity.

To promote a national health program with emphasis on prevention of disease sponsored by American Medical Association with due regard for local situations.

DIVIDEND OR RESULTS

1. Create good will and public approval.
2. Raise general standard of medical practice.
3. Prevent many deaths and much suffering.
4. Give longer ordered life for the doctor.
5. Give a steadier income for the doctor.
6. Intelligent defense against disease is our best defense against government encroachment.

The film "The Birth of a Baby" was endorsed for its educational value with the recommendation that its showing be limited to adults in counties where the county medical society approves the picture.

A resolution proposing the creation of a Council on Medical Care was not approved with the explanation that the Board of Trustees is considering the appointment of a special committee under the same name.

The Association voted to oppose all legislation which would restrict animal experimentation and urged all state associations to assist in an educational campaign emphasizing the humane use of animal experimentation in research and saving human life. The resolution was referred to the Board of Trustees.

The House of Delegates requested the Council on Foods to re-establish its rules on butter and dairy products.

The house approved in principle the establishment of the Rockefeller C a n c e r Control Fund on condition that a majority of the members of the advisory council be members of the American Medical Association.

A resolution requesting the establishment of a policy outlining the ethical and unethical features of fee schedules was referred to the Bureau of Medical Economics for study and report at the next Annual Session.

The name of the Bureau of Health and Public Instruction was changed to the Bureau of Health Education.

The resolution was adopted to the effect that no alien be granted a license to practice medicine in the United States unless he first became a naturalized citizen.

The report of the Judicial Council concerning physicians and cultists was adopted and the secretary was instructed to bring the r e p o r t to the attention of all State Associations to the effect that the American Medical Association does not approve of its members meeting in consultation with cultists or occupy joint reception rooms with them as it tends to lower the standing of the physician and has a tendency to elevate the cultists. Lecturing or teaching or appearing on the programs of osteopaths, chiropracters, optometrists or chiropidists was frowned upon.

The report of the Committee to Study Contraceptive Practices and Related Problems was endorsed as follows:

It is not the function of the American Medical Association to tell physicians what therapeutic advice they shall offer patients. However, it has been its policy to investigate various procedures, devices and drugs, and to publish the results of such studies in its official publications for the information of the profession.

The instructions to the Council on Pharmacy and Chemistry and the Council on Physical Therapy to investigate further the materials, devices and procedures used for the purpose of contraception do not indicate any change in the usual policy of the Association, nor do they constitute an endorsement by the Association of contraceptive practices.

Rigid visual standards for granting automobile drivers' licenses were recommended for adoption by the several states by the Section on Ophthalmology, which was adopted.

A resolution requesting that the Association establish standards for testing alcoholic intoxication was r e f e r r e d to the Board of Trustees for study and report at the next Annual Session.

A resolution denoting the teaching by physicians in schools of chiropody as unethical was laid on the table with the explanation that further study of this complex problem was needed.

Resolutions requesting the employment of p u b l i c relations counsel and the appointment of a committee on public relations were not adopted with the explanation that these contacts are now . being maintained.

A resolution suggesting legislation to authorize the giving of contraceptive advice by physicians to patients by mail was referred to the Board of Trustees.

The Association reiterated its recommendation that a Federal Department of Health be established with *a medical practitioner at its head.*

The report of the Bureau of Medical Economics, was adopted including t w o proposals as a resolution to the problem of medical service in group hospitalization contracts, as follow: (1) Restrict the benefits of the contract exclusively to the use of hospital facilities such as bed and board, operating room, medicines, surgical dressings and general nursing care; and (2) PAY CASH BENEFITS DIRECTLY TO THE INSURED FOR ALL M E D I C A L SERVICES.

An address on "Work of the Interdepartmental Committee of Coordinate Health Welfare Activities of the Federal Government" prepared by Josephine Roche was presented. The address was referred to the Committee on Executive Session which reported as follows:

Your Committee emphatically agrees with the statement in the address which reads: "No one formula or program can possibly be found adequate to meet the varied needs of medical care."

Your Committee notes with satisfaction that a group of physicians have been invited to take part in the discussions of the forthcoming National Health Conference and that it includes some of the officers of the American Medical Association. This will make available a vast amount of information concerning the subject involved which has been accumulated over a period of years including the result of our survey of medical service. We are confident that our official representatives will be guided by the principles and opinions that have been repeatedly expressed by the House of Delegates.

The report was unanimously approved by the House of Delegates.

Dr. J. H. J. Upham, Columbus, presided at all the Sessions, and Dr. Irvin Abell, Louisville, was installed as President to serve at the 1939 Session. Dr. Rock Sleyster, Wauwatosa, Kisconsin, was elected President-elect. Vice President, Dr. Howard Morrow, San Francisco.

Other officers elected were: Secretary, Dr. Olin West, C h i c a g o, (re-elected); Speaker of the House of Delegates, Dr. Harrison H. Shoulders, Nashville; V i c e Speaker, Dr. Roy W. Fouts, Omaha; Treasurer, Dr. Herman L. Kretschmer, Chicago, (re-elected).

Drs. Austin A. Hayden, Chicago, and Charles B. Wright, Minneapolis, were re-elected Trustees.

As meeting places for the next three annual sessions of the Association, the House of Delegates chose:

For 1939, St. Louis.

For 1940, New York.

For 1941, Cleveland.

Dr. Rudolph Matas, New Orleans, was chosen by the House of Delegates as the first recipient of the distinguished service medal for "meritorious services in the science and art of medicine" created by the Association in 1937.

We were very much interested in getting next years meeting to St. Louis and gave them our assistance and support, so that a large number of our members would have the opportunity of attending. We hope that at least half of our members will be able to attend the '39 meeting; but we consider the attendance of 56 at the San Francisco Meeting very good, when the distance is taken into consideration.

Your Delegates,
McCLAIN ROGERS.
W. ALBERT COOK.

---o---

Editorial Notes—Personal and General

DR. G. R. Booth, and family, LeFlore, have returned from a vacation trip to California.

DR. AND MRS. C. E. WILLIAMS, Woodward, spent the month of August in Colorado, where Dr. Williams took post graduate work at Denver.

DR. AND MRS. DAVID PAULUS, and children, have returned from a vacation spent on Square G Ranch, Jenny Lake, Wyoming.

DR. AND MRS. LEA A. RIELY, Oklahoma City, have returned from Honolulu and San Francisco where they spent some time.

DR. C. M. BLOSS, JR., Okemah, has taken over the office and practice of his father, the late Dr. C. M. Bloss. Dr. Bloss is a graduate of the University of Oklahoma Medical School.

DR. R. Q. ATCHLEY, Tulsa, spent the summer months at the Lahey Clinic at Boston.

DR. AND MRS. JOHN S. ROLLINS, and son, John Gordon, of Prague, attended the graduation of their daughter, Miss Mabel Geraldine, at Ward-Belmont, Nashville, Tenn., and spent their vacation in Washington, D. C., New York City, Niagara Falls, Toronto, Canada and Detroit.

The Valley View Hospital at Ada was dedicated with appropriate ceremony, Sunday, July 24th. This is a beautiful institution erected and equipped through the cooperation of contributors of Ada and the Commonwealth Fund of New York. It has the most modern equipment and facilities to well serve this particular community. The cooperation of the Commonwealth Fund insures an institution of high standard.

New X-ray equipment, costing $7,500, is being installed in the Western Oklahoma Charity Hospital, Dr. H. K. Speed, Jr., superintendent stated. The equipment includes an X-ray, a fluoroscope and a portable X-ray machine.

DR. J. L. DAY, superintendent of the Western Oklahoma Hospital, Woodward, and Mrs. Day were hosts to the doctors of the Northwestern district and their wives, June 28th, at their regular meeting. Dr. C. W. Tedrowe, president, presided and introduced Dr. C. P. Bondurant, Oklahoma City, who gave the principal address of the evening, "Some Common Skin Diseases."

The 23rd annual meeting of the American Association of Railway Surgeons will be held at the Palmer House, Chicago, September 19-23, 1938.

This Association includes members in practically every railroad company in the United States. An extremely interesting and highly profitable program has been arranged and all physicians and surgeons are invited to attend the sessions of this meeting as guests of the organization. There will be no rgistration fee to M.D. non-member guests. Complete program and information regarding the meeting may be secured by addressing Mr. A. G. Park, Convention Manager, Palmer House, Chicago.

ABSTRACTS : REVIEWS : COMMENTS
and CORRESPONDENCE

SURGERY AND GYNECOLOGY
Abstracts, Reviews and Comments from
LeRoy Long Clinic
714 Medical Arts Building, Oklahoma City

The Causes of Vaginal Bleeding and the Histology of the Endometrium after the Menopause; Howard C. Taylor, Jr., and Robert Millen; The American Journal of Obstetrics and Gynecology, July, 1938.

During the period 1921 to 1935, 12,350 patients were admitted to the Gynecologic Service of the Roosevelt Hospital and of these 4,362 had some form of abnormal vaginal bleeding.

There were 406 patients with postmenopausal bleeding. There was some type of malignant tumor present in 63 per cent of these.

"Benign tumors of the uterus and ovary were the lesions chiefly responsible for the symptom in 17 per cent of the cases. Of special interest was the association of hyperplasia of the endometrium with typical cystic pseudomucinous tumors of the ovary in two instances.

"Inflammatory lesions, usually in the cervix or vagina, were the apparent cause of bleeding in 11 per cent.

"In the remainder, or about eight per cent, no gross lesion to explain the bleeding was present in the pelvis. Several of this group showed evidence of a late ovarian effect on the endometrium or of an endometrial hyperplasia due to this or other causes. These instances of hyperplastic changes in the postmenopausal endometrium are important as possible pre-cancerous lesions."

The authors feel, however, that attention should be drawn to the fact that these statistics are based upon hospital patients and that consequently the incidence of major lesions is naturally higher than the average office practice. For this purpose, 291 patients with similar symptoms but seen in office practice gave an incidence of malignant disease of only 38 per cent. They feel that this figure is probably higher than the incidence of malignancy in the cases of postmenopausal bleeding which come originally to the family physician, because the office figures were taken from a gynecologist's practice and there were probably an unusual number of referred cancer cases to continue the emphasis upon cancer. It is felt that the incidence in an unsorted group in patients of postmenopausal bleeding would still range in the neighborhood of 20 to 25 per cent.

There is an extremely interesting discussion as to cause of bleeding after the menopause where there is no malignant tumor present and the endometrium shows very few changes, except endometritis. They have also discussed 34 patients in their group where there was no gross inflammatory or neoplastic lesion in the pelvis.

An attempt is made to explain the presence of typical hyperplastic endometrium after the menopause and there is an interesting discussion as to the possible correlation of this disease with malignancy of endometrial tissue.

Included in the article is a preliminary classification of their 4,362 patients with abnormal vaginal bleeding upon the basis of incidence of the disease causing such bleeding before the menopause. It shows that the relative frequency of functional and unexplained causes of bleeding remains about the same in any decade before the menopause. Bleeding due to some complication of pregnancy has its principal incidence in the twenties and even earlier, as does inflammatory disease. On the other hand benign tumors show both their greatest absolute and relative frequency as causes of bleeding shortly before the menopause due to the well-known age incidence of fibroids.

Comments: This is a valuable article for two principal reasons.

It contains statistical evidence as to the frequency of pathological lesions causing vaginal bleeding after the menopause. In this direction it is interesting that the incidence of malignant disease is about that shown by many series of figures which have demonstrated the presence of cancer in about two-thirds of the patients admitted to hospital services with postmenopausal bleeding.

In the second place, this article contains valuable information and discussion of the non-malignant endometrial changes found after the menopause which are at the present time causing so much concern as to the etiological factors involved and the significance of such endometrial changes as hyperplasia.

There has long been an attempt to establish a relationship between so-called hyperplastic endometrium and adenocarcinoma of the corpus uteri. It is the continuation of such studies as this one which will lead us to a proper evaluation in determining this relationship and consequently determining the proper therapeutic procedures to be employed in instances were hyperplastic endometrium is found.

Wendell Long.

An Evaluation of the Anterior Pituitary-Like Substance Intradermal Test for Pregnancy, With a Study of the Possible Relation of this Test to Prolan Content; Friedman and Fink; The American Journal of Obstetrics and Gynecology; July, 1938.

The following summary is an excellent condensation of the work done by these authors and their conclusions.

"1. The intradermal administration of anterior pituitary-like substance of pregnancy urine as a diagnostic test for pregnancy shows the following deviations from expected results on proved cases:

a. Of expected results in 88 pregnant women there were eight who gave negative results.

b. Of expected negative results in 40 non-pregnant women, only 13 gave a negative pregnancy reading, 27 were positive for pregnancy.

c. Of expected negative results in 33 men, eight showed the expected result, 25 showed positive pregnancy tests.

"2. Prolan studies done on 10 non-pregnant women who gave a definitely positive pregnancy reading were negative.

"3. Prolan studies done on six men who gave a definitely positive pregnancy reading were negative in five and positive in one.

"4. Of seven non-pregnant women with a positive prolan, five gave a positive pregnancy test and two a negative test.

"5. The results are in substantial agreement with other recent critical analyses of this diagnostic procedure."

Comments: An abstract of this article is submitted because there are still a good many physicians who have placed some confidence in this test for pregnancy whereas the numerous controlled studies show it to be entirely unreliable.

Wendell Long.

Vaginectomy; Masson and Knepper; The American Journal of Obstetrics and Gynecology; July, 1938, page 94.

There is a brief review of the history of this operative procedure and a discussion of the merit and indications for both total and subtotal vaginectomy.

The t e c h n i q u e of total vaginectomy is well described.

The authors report 23 cases in which complete vaginectomy was performed in the Mayo Clinic from 1910 to 1937. Of these 19 patients were traced and found to be cured without any incidence of recurrence of the prolapse or hernia. In their series they had no instance of the Le Fort partial vaginectomy. They expressed a preference for the complete operation over the subtotal operation of Le Fort.

The following conclusions well express the feeling of the authors:

"1. In gynecologic hernias, the selection of the operation best suited to the individual case is important.

"2. In the more difficult hernias which affect elderly patients some type of vaginectomy is justifiable.

"3. Comparatively few cases of either partial or complete vaginectomy are recorded in American literature.

"4. There is no doubt in our minds that a partial vaginectomy with removal of more or less of the upper part of the vagina is a rather common practice associated with a vaginal hysterectomy but that it is not reported.

"5. The Le Fort operation with preservation of the uterus is a safe and satisfactory operation.

"6. Complete vaginectomy with removal of the uterus is the operation of choice in many cases in which elderly women have procidentia of high degree and also is often indicated in cases in which vaginal hernia follows a previous hysterectomy."

Comments: The first conclusion of these authors that "In gynecologic hernias, the selection of the operation best suited to the individual case is important" is fundamental in the proper correction of this pathological condition.

To properly repair gynecological hernias, one must be familiar with and able to perform satisfactorily a relatively large list of operations in order to adapt the most ideal procedure to the various different lesions which occur together with complications of the primary hernia such as disease of the uterus itself.

In those where complete cessation of sexual relations is not objectionable, both the subtotal and total vaginectomy or colpectomy have a distinct place in the treatment of very advanced herniation especially in the aged, in those in poor general

condition, and in instances where there is a vaginal herniation following either a subtotal or total hysterectomy.

Both the Le Fort and complete colpectomy have been extremely useful to me in selected patients and the results have been quite satisfactory. These operations are also desirable when patients are in poor general condition, as they can be done quite satisfactorily under local infiltration anesthesia with much less consequent risk.

Wendell Long.

The Differential Diagnosis of Jaundice; Laboratory Tests Useful in the Distinction Between Surgical and Nonsurgical Conditions; Kyran E. Hynes and Clyde R. Jensen; western Journal of Surgery, Obstetrics and Gynecology; July, 1938, page 371.

In a critical review of cases of jaundice, it was found that errors are frequent in the differential diagnosis between various common causes of jaundice. The authors believe that many such errors are unnecessary, and that it is possible to differentiate with a high percentage of accuracy not only between surgical (mechanically obstructive) and nonsurgical (hepatocellular) jaundice, but also between various forms of mechanical obstruction, such as common duct stones and neoplastic obstruction of bile duct.

They point out that jaundice is not an emergency state and that haste is, therefore, unnecessary in its diagnosis.

In an attempt to attain this improvement in diagnostic efficiency they offer: (1) a discussion of the pathologic physiology of jaundice, with a simple classification of jaundice based primarily upon clinical needs; (2) a table of a few selected laboratory tests arranged so that results of these tests, if correctly interpreted, will fit readily into simple diagnostic patterns. The clinician must determine which of the tests are indicated in a given case and must interpret results with the realization that individual findings or details of the test may shift with the varying stages of each disease process, although the general pattern remains.

The tests which they mention may be enumerated as follows: (a) Tests of excretory phases; under this heading (1) serum bilirubin, (2) blood cholesterol and cholesterol esters, (3) bilirubinuria and urobilinogenuria, (4) excretion of dyes, and (5) d u o d e n a l drainage; (b) Tests of intracellular phases; (1) Carbohydrate tests of liver function, (2) tests of nitrogenous metabolism; (c) Miscellaneous laboratory tests; (1) blood Wassermann, (2) blood picture, and (3) X-ray.

All these tests are discussed in detail and must be read in the original in order to obtain a complete understanding of the authors' ideas.

LeRoy D. Long.

Modern Trends in the Treatment of Cancer of the Rectum and Rectosigmoid; Fred W. Rankin; Journal of the American Medical Association; November 20, 1937.

The author has operated on 578 patients for cancer of the rectum and rectosigmoid since 1927. This group on whom many different types of operation have been done (radical, exploratory and palliative) serves as a background for the following conclusions he has made as to the merits of different surgical procedures and their accompanying mortality, morbidity and applicability. As he points out experience shows that many methods are useless, many useful and a few essential. Radiation and surgical diathermy are discussed as palliative, not curative methods.

His conclusions which are of extreme interest and of great value to anyone interested in the handling of these serious cases are as follows:

"1. Acceptance of the principle that the most radical type of operation should be applied in all cases in which judgment indicates that such a procedure may be done with a reasonable hospital death list.

"2. The exertion of every effort to increase the scope of operability to the point of taking in all borderline cases. Other things being equal, I think that only hepatic metastasis and immovable fixation to the parietes or adjacent viscera should eliminate attempts at extirpation. This rule should be modified further in a certain percentage of cases by acceptance for palliative resection of a small group of movable tumors which have already metastasized to the liver.

"3. Abandonment of spinal anesthesia.

"4. Employment as a routine of postoperative transfusions and, in cases in which anemia and great dibility exist, preoperative transfusions as well.

"5. Extension of the preliminary preparatory period to at least seven days and insistence that decompression be complete whether it is accomplished by medical measures or by surgical procedure. If on exploration the preliminary measures are found not to have been successful in reducing the obstruction and eliminating a great deal of local infection, it is desirable to do immediately a graded operation, the first step of which usually is a cecostomy.

"6. The abandonment of the preoperative intraperitoneal vaccination. I do this regretfully, but a study of my private cases the last five years, in which vaccination was not done, in comparison with those which I reported for a previous six-year period, makes it impossible for me to escape the conclusion that vaccination is not the large factor in reducing mortality that I thought it to be.

"7. The employment of presacral neurectomy as a routine in the hope of lessening complications in the bladder. However, it must be admitted that this procedure has failed to achieve as brilliant results as were hoped for.

"A statistical study of end results, particularly of the more radical procedures, warrants the assertion that according to the present state of knowledge the choice of treatment for rectal cancer is operation. With an increasing operability curve and a lower mortality rate, this treatment of rectal and rectosigmoid cancer is rewarded by as favorable a prognosis as that for cancer of the same intensity elsewhere in the body."

LeRoy D. Long.

Common Duct Obstruction; Willard S. Sargent; American Journal of Surgery; May, 1938, page 396.

This is an excellent article which covers most of the phases of this important surgical condition. I personally do not use spinal anesthesia because I believe it carries an additional risk for these upper abdominal patients who are already seriously ill. I have, I admit, abandoned its use with considerable regret because the complete relaxation obtained certainly aids the surgeon.

The author apparently is also in favor of the use of prostigmin for the care of postoperative distention. I am convinced that the routine use of this drug may be frequently harmful.

A summary of the article follows:

"1. No one symptom of obstruction is diagnostic.

Since two conditions may be present, local pathology may show and general affections may be missed.

"2. A marked jaundice with clay-colored stools is usually significant of common duct obstruction, most likely due to cancer of the pancreas or bile ducts, chronic pancreatitis, gallstones or catarrhal jaundice. Transient jaundice, in the young, is usually catarrhal.

"3. A large liver, with jaundice, most often shows common duct obstruction, lues, cancer, abscess, cirrhosis or poisoning.

"4. Any jaundice should be relieved by palliative means as much as possible before surgery is done, inasmuch as the more nearly complete the obstruction is, the more the danger of cholemia. Early thorough treatment spares the liver, pancreas and kidneys. A slow pulse, in jaundice, is usually not present unless chronic pancreatitis occurs. If, with the jaundice, findings point to an essentially complete obstruction, the likely causes are tumors of the ducts or pancreas, stricture, or an accidentally ligated duct.

"5. Fever may be present with the attacks due to an infected gall-bladder, but when the hepatic ducts are infected, a continuous fever may result. Charcot's fever means cholangitis as a rule, although jaundice, fever and rigors can follow pylephlebitis and hepatic abscess; malaria and sepsis might give a similar picture.

"6. Biliary stones are often found post mortem. Icterus neonatorum has been caused by stones. Females who have been pregnant or had typhoid often have stones form in the gall-bladder and 20 per cent of them have common duct stone also, which usually gives a small gall-bladder with colic and jaundice. There may be no pain or jaundice, however, and the gall-bladder may be enlarged, especially if the cystic duct is blocked.

"Stones may accompany tumor or stricture. If jaundice follows right upper quadrant pain, it most likely is due to common duct stone. Recurring jaundice in a middle-aged woman, with or without colic, is almost pathognomonic of the same; chronic pancreatitis alone may confuse. Should pain occur without jaundice after cholecystectomy, it calls for duodenal drainage and examination of the bile for crystals of cholesterol and calcium bilirubinate.

"7. Tumors of the pancreas and biliary ducts usually give a painless jaundice with an enlarged gall-bladder, although pain, Charcot's fever, or a small gall-bladder may be present. Early diagnosis and treatment are imperative, because benign lesions may become malignant, and all malignant growths of the duct metastasize slowly. Carcinoma is more frequent in males, while stones form more frequently in females. Recurrences of jaundice for years is against malignancy, but on the other hand, a middle-aged person with loss of weight, having a history of short duration, together with a deep persistent jaundice without colic, and an enlarged gall-bladder, is almost surely suffering from carcinoma of the pancreas or the bile ducts.

"8. Pylephlebitis and cholangitic abscesses cause death, and diabetes is a very serious complication. Vocal cord paralysis may be dependent upon Ewald's node which might be the first sign of abdominal malignancy.

"9. Spinal anesthesia spares the liver, while ether, chloroform and avertin may further injure it. A fall in blood pressure is met by the Tredelenburg position combined, if necessary, with adrenalin or ephedrine by hypodermic, 50 c.c. of 50 per cent glucose by vein, a few whiffs of ether combined with artificial respiration, and even massage of the heart and adrenals through the abdominal wound.

"10. In the operative work the gallbladder should always be left in until it is made sure that the duct is all right. The duct should be explored in all suspicious cases, after needling it to be sure the portal vein is not entered; a stone may not be palpable if the duct is thick. It should be opened if there is or has been jaundice, and probed with a uterine sound. Suction should be used if necessary. Then the duct should be wiped out with gauze, and drainage inserted.

"Fistula of the duct into the gut calls for operation in most cases.

"The duodenum should be opened, if necessary, and if a condition is found which prohibits further surgery, the gall-bladder can be anastamosed to the duodenal wound. A stone in the ampulla may require transduodenal removal, if it cannot be removed through the duct above the duodenum. Tumors of the ampulla may be removed transduodenally and the duct reimplanted into the duodenum.

"11. Postoperative hemorrhage may be lessened by the use of blood transfusions before operation in conjunction with parathormone hypodermically, calcium chloride by vein, and duodenal drainage. Bile pigment is said to fix the calcium of the blood. Purpuric spots and increased sedimentation rates are indications for blood transfusions before operation.

"Prostigmin has recently been added to the armamentarium for the care of postoperative distention.

"Atelectasis after operation is more frequent following biliary surgery than any other type except gastric, and its incidence can be reduced by rebreathing of carbon dioxide and oxygen, deep breathing exercises, and frequent changing of position. Slapping the back sharply will often help loosen a plug of mucus from the bronchus.

"After release of obstruction, the bile for a few days shows absence of bile salts, increased calcium, and decreased sodium chloride content. If dehydration and loss of weight occur from loss of bile, the latter can be re-fed to the patient in grape-juice or given by rectum.

"Lipiodal through the drainage tube may be used to reveal the state of patency of the ducts, in cases not progressing normally."

LeRoy D. Long.

EYE, EAR, NOSE AND THROAT
Edited by Marvin D. Henley, M.D.
911 Medical Arts Building, Tulsa

Induced Hyperexia in Ophthalmology. Webb W. Weeks, M.D., New York, and Samuel A. Morris, M.D., Marysville, California. American Journal of Ophthalmology, June, 1938.

A series of 16 cases are reported that have the usual local therapeutic measures but in addition are treated by general hyperpyrexia.

Preparation includes complete physical examination, urinalysis, blood count, hemoglobin, Wasserman, blood nonprotein nitrogen, sugar, chlorides, X-ray study of chest, high caloric diet, 4,000 c.c. of six per cent saline by mouth the day before, exclusion of breakfast the day of, soap suds enema, sedative and explanation of the procedure to the patient.

Pulse, respirations and rectal temperature is taken every five minutes during the treatment. If the temperature fluctuates irregularly or pulse goes over 160, or if respirations go over 45 per minute,

treatment is discontinued. Treatment is given in an ordinary hospital bed.

Contraindications: old age, organic lesions of heart or kidney, thyrotoxicosis, anemia and marked emotional and nervous instability.

The 16 cases included: three cases of gonorrheal ophthalmia; four cases of iritis of probable gonococcal origin; three cases of iritis of unknown etiology; one case of superficial punctate keratitis; one case of scleritis and iritis; one case of uveitis; one case of trachoma with a secondary purulent staphylococcus conjunctivitis; and two cases of interstitial keratitis.

The results seemed to show that this treatment was of little value in cases of trachoma, luetic uveitis, and interstitial keratitis. In the other cases it seemed to be a valuable aid and the best results were obtained in the cases of iritis. It appeared to help greatly in quickly eliminating the gross exudate.

Meningitis of Otitic Origin. Oram R. Cline, M.D., Camden, N. J. Archives of Otolaryngology, June, 1938.

Meningitis is a dreaded complication of temporal bone suppuration, with a high mortality in the past. The author reports two cases of otitic meningitis with recovery. The article is short, interesting and to the point; his conclusions are:

"The recovery of more than 100 patients with hemolytic streptococcic meningitis following the use of sulfanilamide and its derivatives known as prontosil has been reported during the past year, whereas the mortality of patients with this disease was probably more than 95 per cent before these drugs were available.

Early symptoms of meningeal irritation demand an immediate mastoidectomy, with exposure of the dura.

In the presence of meningitis, after the focus of infection has been eradicated, a supportive and conservative method of treatment is followed.

Two cases of meningitis occurring as a complication of mastoiditis are reported. In each case the spinal fluid yielded a pure culture of Str. haemolyticus.

In the first case meningitis developed nine days after mastoidectomy. The infection was comparatively mild, as there was prompt improvement after one transfusion of convalescent blood.

In the second case meningeal symptoms were present from the onset of earache, the infection probably following the line of a former fracture. Bacteria in the spinal fluid were so numerous at the time of operation that the prognosis was considered hopeless; however, complete recovery occurred after the use of sulfanilamide and prontosil (the disodium salt of 4-sulfamidophenyl-2'-azo-7'-acetylamino-1'-hydroxynaphthalene-3',6'-disulfonic acid)."

Problems in Diagnosis and Treatment of Hyperplastic Sinusitis and Allergy. E. Ross Faulkner, M.D., New York. Annals of Otology, Rhinology and Laryngology, March, 1938.

The article opens with a general discussion of specialities and their interlocking interests with special reference to allergy.

Seasonal hay fever and an engrafted sinus infection present a picture in which the allergist and the rhinologist must cooperate, both in diagnosis and treatment.

Cases simulating acute nasal allergy that occur at any season of the year sometimes are quite difficult to differentiate. If symptoms occur following a coryza, there may be retention of pus in the ethmoid cells, which shrinkage and suction irrigation will correct. A careful nasal examination should be made.

A tickling sensation in the nose may be caused by contact between the middle turbinate and spurs or a deviated septum. Sudden change of temperature, an overloaded intestine, alcohol and other factors may cause swelling enough of the turbinate to touch some abnormally placed structure and so precipitate an attack. Removal of a part of the middle turbinate or a submucous resection or both, many times gives relief.

The most common causes of true allergic coryza are foods and drugs and inhalants such as house or occupational dusts, orris root, animal amanations and feathers. History and skin or mucous membrane tests help to discover the offender. Normal (apparently) persons may give positive reactions. and some allergic cases do not show positive so they cannot always be depended upon.

The hereditary factor is most important. Family groups show 25 to 30 per cent manifestations of allergy in some form. History should include incidence of asthma, hives, eczema, hay fever, angioneurotic edema, migraine, gastro-intestinal disturbances and allergic rhinitis, nasal smears should be taken. "Kahn and Stout consider that a nasal smear with 10 to 90 per cent eosinophils is positively diagnostic of nasal allergy." If the process is infectious there is an abundance of morphonuclear leucocytes.

In a patient subject to frequent coryza attacks, with sneezing and a free watery discharge, the author advises only palliative measures until the nature of the allergy is determined, which will guide the treatment.

The case that is more chronic in nature with enlarged turbinates and very little discharge, many times gives such a satisfactory result from a submucous and cauterization or scarification that one may well doubt if they were ever allergic.

Next there is a condition where there are no active manifestations of allergic phenomena but there is a positive history as well as positive skin tests, a hyperplastic type with polyp formation. The allergic factor must be treated as well as the polyps removed. After care is essential to take care of recurring polyps. The association of polyps with an allergic condition is a much discussed question. Cooke thinks hyperplastic conditions with or without polyp formation is due to an infection and that the allergy is a sensitization to the infection. These cases give usually a history of an acute infection at the beginning of their trouble, many times occurring only on one side. The nasal smear shows an abundance of polymorphonuclear cells. The author recalls cases where there has been no recurrence in 10 to 15 years following surgery on the polypoid type of case.

If the infection and the allergic condition are both present, before any surgery is attempted, it is best that the allergist do what he can. In bacterial allergy, vaccines have been found to be of questionable benefit.

The association of asthma with any of the discussed types is next reviewed. The average allergist holds to the opinion that intranasal polyp formation is an association that may occur with asthma rather than it being a condition that may have to do with cause and effect. Consequently they condemn attempts to cure asthma by intranasal surgery. Rhinologists themselves do not agree as to results obtained. This may be due in part to the variance in the skill of the operator. The author's experience shows always improvement and occasional cures of asthma following radical surgery in a nose with polypoid degeneration.

Ionization is next discussed. Alden and Tobey

have reported favorable results from their first cases. McMahon has shown it to be a destructive process. Dean's conclusion is "that it produces such deleterious results on the mucous membrane that the ill effect outweighs the good." Five to ten per cent silver nitrate applied often gives satisfactory results. Diathermy is not recommended.

Headaches may also be caused from migraine, local swellings or cerebral edema. Polypi within the cells of the ethmoids and sphenoids can exercise enough pressure to cause pain, while the nasal cavity may be filled with polyps without pain. X-ray before any intranasal medication helps in the diagnosis. Thorough exeneration of the ethmoids and making large openings into the sphenoids may be necessary." Incomplete operations may do more harm than good and merely stir up an infectious process without removing it.

Motor Disorders of the Central Nervous System and Their Significance for Speech. Part II. Clinical Forms of Motor Defects (The "Spastic Child"). Dr. Paul J. Zentay, St. Louis. The Laryngoscope, June, 1937.

"Spastic child" is a term generally applied to a number of conditions, such as athetosis, cerebellar lesions and even mental defects and all forms of motor disorders. The author suggests that to clear the present existing confusion, that the term "spastic child" be eliminated entirely and that in its place we have the term "motor defective child" or "motor deficiency." The classification would then be more clear and convenient.

This paper is limited to "motor defects that are due to antenatal or natal factors and consequently are present at the time of birth." These have to do with the acquisition of motor functions and the development of speech.

Central nervous system development may be impaired by: 1. Some fault in the anlage or due to some mechanical cause. 2. Intrauterine infection (causing fetal encephalitis). The author says: "Antenatal factors, as a rule, will lead to more decisive defects the earlier in fetal development they become operative."

The most important natal factor is accident at time of birth. During the molding of the head at the time of birth, there may occur an intracranial hemorrhage with subsequent destruction of tissue. The site and the extent of the lesion indicate the disability to be expected. Of paramount importance is whether or not the general intelligence of the individual has been damaged.

The pyramidal lesions include those known as birth palsy, Little's disease, etc. It is in this condition that there is a delay in the development of the motor functions. Spasticity may or may not be present. If absent, instead of the "scissors gait" and walking on tip toes, you then have circumduction of the leg and dragging of the foot when walking. Paraplegia will be accompanied by speech involvement less frequently than monoplegias with the dominant upper extremity or hemiplegias of the dominant side.

Motor and speech development result from the growth and development of the C. N. S. If the ganglion cells are destroyed, these do not regenerate. This lost function of the pyramidal ganglia cannot be taken over by other parts of the hemisphere. In this type patient the best that can be done is to bring the residues to their highest potential development.

Extrapyramidal and cerebellar lesions are discussed. The author's conclusions are:

Any motor defect must be looked upon as the problem of the whole person.

Motor defect in any one of the three central

motor systems disturbs tonus and balance also of the other two systems.

Any motor defect interferes with the total function of the central nervous system.

Any defect is irreparable and compensation for it depends on residual functions.

Improvement of functions largely depends on maturation.

Any form of training must have its limitations in the potentialities of the residues.

The teacher of speech must think realistically on this problem and avoid false hopes and unfounded optimism.

Cooperation with the neurologist, physiotherapist, psychologist is essential for best results.

The total personality of the child must be evaluated.

Methods of teaching and training have to be adapted not only to the nature of the motor defect, but also to the individual needs of the child.

---o---

PLASTIC SURGERY
Edited by
GEO. H. KIMBALL, M.D., F.A.C.S.
404 Medical Arts Building, Oklahoma City

Skin Graft for the Ambulatory Patient. Frederick L. Smith, M.D., Rochester, Minn. American Journal of Surgery, July, 1938.

The author points out that ulcers of the lower extremities present an economic problem, for the majority of the afflicted are laborers or indigent persons. He lists the causes of ulcers as follows:

1. Varicosities of the superficial venous system.
   A. Heredity.
   B. Thrombophlebitis.
   C. Injury.
   D. Intra-abdominal obstruction.
   E. Cellulitis.
   F. Over weight.

Technique: To begin with the patient is put to bed until the ulcer is clean or until the edema has subsided. The next step consists of applying small grafts under local anesthesia.

The dressing consists of silkloid sheet, double layer of sterile gauze, roller bandage, and finally the entire leg is encased in an elastoplast bandage.

After the operation the patient is allowed to be up and about. First dressing is done in ten days.

Comment: The author describes in detail a method for grafting ulcers of the lower extremities which allows the patient to be ambulatory after the operation. The technique is similar to that employed by most surgeons in such cases. I have not personally allowed patients to walk about after skin grafts on the leg. I recall one case that developed cellulitis and lost about one-third of the skin of the entire leg following application of an elastoplast bandage for an ulcer. I believe that the author's method is in general a good one. It certainly is inexpensive.

The Use of Fascia and Ribbon Catgut in the Repair of Cleft Palate and Hairlip. Addison G. Brenizer, M.D., Charlotte, N. C. Annals of Surgery, May, 1938.

The author points out that most cases of clefts in lips, palates, and alveolar processes are deficient only in hard palate and not in bony, muscular, and fibrous tissue, which can be used to close them. He states that most cases can be success-

fully repaired by the use of the so-called Langenbeck operation and its modifications, particularly those of Veau and Dorrance.

Certain cases, however, are extremely difficult to repair surgically:

1. Narrow flaps, not yielding.
2. Previously operated unsuccessfully.
3. Narrow flaps or double clefts where the model of the operation must be altered.
4. Simple cases showing failure, with scar thickened and unyielding flaps.

In such cases the author has for over 20 years used a rectangular strip of fascia as a means of support to the flaps, and relieved the tension in the stitch line from the hard palate, accompanied by a fascial tie at the musculature of the velum.

The author found that fascia so introduced apparently lived and bone cells grew across the defect.

Lately the author has employed ribbon catgut, instead of fascia. It is, of course, easier to obtain and seems to do as well.

The author points out that preliminary closure of the lip accomplishes much in bringing the cleft of the alveolus together.

There are a few cases of double harelip with projecting premaxilla in which the author employs ribbon catgut embedded between the mucosa and muscularis.

The article is accompanied by clear cut diagrams and illustrations explaining the technique used.

The article is discussed by very able physicians, who seem to understand considerable about this type of surgery.

Comment: The author has successfully used fascia in certain cases of cleft lip and cleft palate. I believe it would be very difficult for some men to use this technique. Personally, I have never used fascia in this type of surgery. So far, the sutures employed by myself are chromic catgut, horse hair, with an occasional silk worm gut, in older children especially. I, personally, do not feel the need of fascia in repair of the lip. It seems to me that one of the principle means of bringing about closure of a palate is to first close the nasal mucosa, then as the flaps of the aponeurosis are completely liberated from bony attachments, union will occur in most cases.

---o---

ORTHOPAEDIC SURGERY
Edited by Earl D. McBride, M.D., F.A.C.S.
717 North Robinson Street, Oklahoma City

*A Comparative Study of the Treatment of Oblique Fractures of the Shaft of the Tibia by Osteosynthesis, Osteotraction or only Reduction and Plaster. Oskar Liden. Acta Chirurgica Scandinavica, LXXX, 365, 1938.**

Follow-up examinations of some 250 cases of fracture of the shaft of the tibia furnish the material for 151 case summaries and the detailed tabulation of etiological data and end results. Errors from economic differences were minimal because all patients were from the same hospital and each method of treatment was used without selection of cases for a well defined period of time (1908 to 1932). Internal fixation was by means of a screw in all but one case. Skeletal traction was used for from three to six weeks and then removed for the application of plaster in all but two cases in which the cast was applied immediately. Throughout the period simple immobilization in plaster with or without reduction was employed whenever possible, but only the cases since 1919 are included in this report.

The writer found that skeletal traction frequently allowed shortening and angulation. He characterized this form of treatment as troublesome and uncomfortable. Open reduction and fixation with a screw gave better end results and shorter healing periods. When done immediately, open reduction and internal fixation showed better results in oblique fractures than did closed reduction and the application of a cast, in spite of the fact that the latter form of treatment was used chiefly in the simpler cases. Among the cases operated upon, however, there was one case of tetanus, and one thigh amputation was necessary because of infection. It is stipulated that open reductions should be done only by experienced surgeons and under reliable aseptic conditions.

Some Theoretical Considerations in the Construction of Active Scoliosis Braces. Josef Wolf. Amer. Jr. of Surg., XXXIX, 557, March, 1938.

The author reviews the literature in regard to the types of so-called active scoliosis braces, referring especially to apparatus worn during the day, with attempt to correct the deformity by mechanical means. He divides the components of the curve into: (1) curvature of the spine itself; (2) overhang on one side of the pelvis; (3) torsion and hump formation; (4) diminution of the height of the body.

The difficulty of bringing mechanical forces to play upon the spine itself is reviewed. This can only be done effectively through the ribs, with the correcting force applied below the apex of the curve and the line of pressure being directed obliquely in conformity with the position of the rib.

A design is suggested for the axillary crutch which would avoid undue pressure upon the anterior and posterior muscles of the chest. The author stresses the importance of a well-fitting rigid pelvic support, upon which the levering mechanism is dependent in the correction of the elements of the curve. He also emphasizes the futility of lifting the shoulder girdle in attempting to correct the thoracic deformity.

---o---

UROLOGY

Edited by D. W. Branham, M.D.
514 Medical Arts Building, Oklahoma City

Management of Pyelitis of Pregnancy, by H. K. Turley, M.D., Memphis, Tennessee; Journal of the Southern Medical Association; July, 1938, Page 729.

The author discusses the mechanism and etiology of pyelitis of pregnancy. He is of the impression that a combination of circumstances predispose to the production of this condition. The atony effect of an hormone in conjunction with the pressure effect of the enlarging uterus producing stasis, all of which favor the infection of the tract by organisms.

As far as treatment is concerned he is prone to be conservative in his therapy when the patient is in the first trimester. In this period he forces fluids and produces alkalinization of the urine. If no relief is obtained within 24 to 36 hours ureteral catheterization is performed leaving the catheters in for several days. Following this the patient is placed on urinary antisepsis using mandelic acid, urotropin, etc. Pelvic lavage is then carried out if necessary if the pyuria fails to respond to such antisepsis.

Patients with pyelitis after the fifth month are treated similar with ureteral catheterization but no intensive effort is made with antisepsis to eradicate the infection. As he states, treatment is not aimed at cure but to control the infection. As an adjunct to treatment posture often is a successful measure in favoring drainage of the kidney. He instructs the patient to sleep on a firm mattress with the foot of the bed elevated 12 to 14 inches. This position tends to stretch out the tortuous ureter and help drainage.

In cases that do not respond to treatment and especially if sepsis continues he is not against terminating the pregnancy. He suggests urologic examination of the patient three months after pregnancy to determine whether the urinary tract has returned to normal.

Comment: A practical article that details admirably the present day management of pyelitis of pregnancy. I feel that it should be stressed among obstetricians the importance of urological consultation in this rather common complication of pregnancy. This disease is basically an obstructive condition and one should have no more hesitancy in drainage of the pelvis by catheter than he should passing a catheter for acute retention of the bladder. In most of the cases the relief obtained is immediate and spectacular. A fear is wide spread that ureteral catheterization is conducive to abortion. This is certainly false and I personally feel the risk of abortion because of the continued sepsis far outweighs the trivial stimulus to the ureter that accompanies the passage of a small catheter.

The Lateral Pyelogram as a Diagnostic Aid in Perinephric Abscess; By John G. Menville, M.D., New Orleans; Journal of the American Medical Association; Page 231; July 16, 1938.

Perinephric abscess is an age old condition recognized as a clinical entity for many years but it remains undiagnosed in a large percentage of cases.

As an adjunct to accurate diagnosis lateral pyelography is performed in suspected instances. The procedure is simple in that the patient lies on the affected side perpendicular to the film. The developed plates show in instances where fluid has accumulated the kidney and ureter displaced anteriorly in an arc-like manner. The larger the quantity of material is present the more this displacement is accentuated.

Three cases with illustrations are presented to show this diagnostic sign.

Comment: Perinephric abscess is a condition that usually responds to treatment when surgery is instituted relatively early. The only mortality encountered is in those cases where rupture of the abscess has occurred into the peritoneal cavity, pleural cavity or a viscus, in which event is favored by neglect to recognize the condition for a length of time. Occasionally instances of suspected abscess do not show the typical spinal curvature with psoas obliteration on the X-ray; neither does aspiration reveal anything. I feel that the use of the lateral pyelogram will be of great diagnostic importance in such cases. Such a procedure should also be useful in the diagnosis of extra renal retroperitineal tumors.

Similarity of Interstitial Cystitis (Hunner Ulcer) to Lupus Erythematosus; By George M. Fisher; Journal of Urology, July, 1938; page 37.

The author points out the similarity of the two diseases by a study of the symptomatology, etiology and histopathology. He is somewhat convinced that the two disorders are possibly two phases of the same disease, one occurring in the bladder wall and the other in the skin.

A case report of a female patient with interstitial cystitis, who showed marked improvement with the administration of gold sodium thiosulfate, is presented. They feel that treatment of the disease with gold or bismuth salts is justified in view of the favorable experience with such treatment in lupus erythematosus.

Comment: I found great interest in reading this article as it presented a new approach to the problem of this most distressful and rebellious disease. I have tried a number of therapeutic procedures with only passable results as to the permanent cure. Undoubtedly fulgeration of the lesion is the best method of palliation with an occasional permanent cure achieved. The administration of bismuth to such cases offers an adjunct that may be of some therapeutic benefit.

---o---

The Care and Treatment of Cerebral Palsies

Winthrop Morgan Phelps, Baltimore (Journal A.M.A., July 2, 1938), states that the care of cerebral spastic paralysis is a general problem in which the orthopedic aspect is the biggest single factor, but orthopedic measures alone will not in many instances accomplish the desired results. The problem deals with a deviation from the normal which has existed since birth in most instances. The general care of the spastic and of the atnetoid patient and of the patient with any other type of cerebral palsy is complicated. There must be a program correlated by the orthopedist, the pediatrician, the neurologist, the physical therapist and the speech expert for the motor side and by teachers acustomed to handling the problems of the handicapped on the educational side, and psychologic aid is necessary in adjusting these children and their behavior to the world at large. Physical therapy in the primary stages of the condition should be followed by occupational therapy when the primary motions can be performed and grouped. This should give way to vocational training when the patient is old enough to determine the line in which he is to be trained. The program constitutes an effort to parallel the mental education of the normal child with a program for physical reeducation which for the normal child is to a great extent automatic.

---o---

Typhoid In The Large Cities of The United States In 1937: Twenty-Sixth Annual Report

As in the preceding annual reviews, data for the twenty-sixth annual report on typhoid (Journal A. M. A., July 30, 1938), have been obtained from the same 93 cities for which the annual statistical tabulations have been made. A communication addressed to the health officer of each city requested not only the total number of deaths from typhoid during the year 1937 but also a statement as to how many of these were among nonresidents. Furthermore, a comment was invited on any special outbreak of typhoid or any unusual protective measures taken to guard against this disease. The 14 New England cities as a whole (population 2,-640,933) again report the lowest rate for any group. Their rate of 0.45 is not quite as low as that of 1936 (0.42). There were recorded 12 deaths in 1937 (but 11 deaths in 1936). The Middle Atlantic states (18) have a group rate which is but slightly less than for the preceding two years (0.51 in 1937, 0.56 in 1936). The record for the nine South Atlantic cities is not as good as for 1936 but continues to show a marked improvement over the rate for 1935 (1.96 in 1937, 1.55 in 1936, 2.58 in 1935). The 18 cities in the East North Central states continue to remain in third place, first place being maintained by the New England group and second place by

the Middle Atlantic. The six cities in the East South Central group show a marked lowering in the death rate (3.35 in 1936, 2.1 in 1937). The West North Central group (nine cities) again report substantially the same number of deaths as have occurred during the past two years (21 in 1937, 22 in 1936, 23 in 1935). The eight cities in the West South Central group show a marked improvement over the rates for preceding years (2.34 in 1937, 3.99 in 1936, 3.82 in 1935). The 11 cities in the Mountain and Pacific states show a continued reduction in the rate (0.68 in 1937, 0.8 in 1936). The number of cities with no death from typhoid has increased to 27. In 1936 there were but 18 such cities. For the 78 cities for which complete data are available since 1910 there occurred 280 deaths from typhoid in 1937, which is the lowest record (336 in 1936).

---o---

Industrial Medicine of Tomorrow: Chairman's Address

Robert T. Legge, Berkeley, Calif. (Journal A. M. A., July 23, 1938), points out that the old-time factory doctor treated many symptoms, such as dyspnea, numbness, nausea or headache, as conditions arising from some functional or bacterial origin, while the modern well trained industrial physician recognizes that these are frequently the prodromal signs of a toxic element due to environmental labor conditions in which a special chemical is used. These call for preventive measures, the substitution of nontoxic agents, removal of workers from the atmosphere, introduction of forced ventilation, and so on. Industrial physicians recognized these early and late occupational diseases at their respective industries, and with the cooperation of chemists, engineers and the industrialists themselves, occupational diseases are being studied and controlled, while absenteeism and compensations are being minimized. The American Medical Association took a rather conservative or possibly badly advised attitude toward early recognition of the importance of industrial medicine. The Association, through its new Council of Industrial Health, now has its greatest opportunity to be a benefactor to American industrial medicine; to promote by research and uplift by education and mutual cooperation the humanizing of industry by preventive medicine. Its aim should be not only a whole hearted program in the study and prevention of occupational diseases but also to strengthen a loyal cooperative spirit to support medical practitioners who are so engaged. It must stimulate the consciousness of all industrialists to the need for the application of modern industrial medicine entailing the service of competent physicians and the development of standardized health services in which preventive medicine and surgery will be scientifically practiced. The new Council on Health must not fail in the new order of medicine. It has the opportunity to forestall a political form of medicine which the organized profession is not in sympathy with. It can, besides educating employers to the necessity of medical supervision of their plants, promote a standardized system of industrial medicine suitable for both small and great plants, stress ideal plants, and certificate such plants as conform to the requirements. It can do much to popularize the idea of how profitable to both employer and employee is the maintenance of an efficient health service in their plants in promoting efficiency and the reduction of absenteeism due to illness and accidents, and in the establishment of periodic physical examinations with scientific first aid medicine and surgery. Industry and organized labor have pointed the way and will look to the American Medical Association to cooperate in advancing industrial medicine.

The Menopausal Syndrome: One Thousand Consecutive Patients Treated With Estrogen

L. F. Hawkinson, Brainerd, Minn. (Journal A. M. A., July 30, 1938), points out that owing to the advances made in endocrine therapy, the physician's point of view regarding the treatment of the menopausal syndrome is changing. Tne tradition that they must be borne is unsound, for the administration of estrogenic preparations is rational and relieves the symptoms in a great majority of cases. Involutional melancholia, pruritus vulvae, senile vaginitis and menopausal hypertension are also frequently relieved by estrogens. The age limits for the syndrome are wide. The symptoms may begin months or years previous to the cessation of menstruation and often persist for years. Treatment should be instituted as soon as symptoms appear. Dosage must be adequate and treatment should be continued until the patient remains free from symptoms without therapy. Higher doses are usually required in patients with artificial menopause. Failure to obtain relief from the majority of the subjective symptoms in uncomplicated menopause is usually due to inadequate dosage. The results of the author's series of 1,000 consecutive patients presenting menopausal symptoms treated with estrogenic substances show that 691 were relieved of the majority of all symptoms, 149 were improved, 109 were doubtful and 51 obtained no relief. Results were evaluated by the disappearance of symptoms and by changes in the vaginal smears. The relief of symptoms is usually gradual. Flushes and chills, excitability, irritability, depression and crying, palpitation and insomnia usually disappeared after the seventh or eighth injection of 10,000 international units of estrogen in oil or after from two to three weeks of adequate oral treatment. Sweating, fatigue, lassitude and headaches responded after further administration of estrogenic preparations. Occipitocervical aching, a symptom complained of by 403 patients, proved very amenable to therapy. Migraine is often completely relieved by adequate estrogenic therapy. The administration of estrogen had little effect on the obesity that was present in some patients. Co-called menopausal arthritis seldom responds to estrogenic preparations. It is doubtful whether it should be included in a menopausal condition. If treatment is withdrawn after initial relief, symptoms are almost certain to recur within two to six weeks. This stresses the importance of continuous oral therapy with a gradual reduction of dosage until the patient is able to discontinue therapy and remain symptom free. Menopausal symptoms are often persistently troublesome and the average patient must remain on maintenance doses of estrogen for from two to three years. Patients at the menopause who are still menstruating may be more difficult to control, owing to the fact that symptoms are frequently intensified about a week prior to the menstrual period. Also, excessive bleeding may become a problem in these women, and large doses of estrogen may increase the already profuse flow. Oral therapy in the form of emmenin is best suited to these cases. No ill effects were seen in any patient even when doses up to 100,000 international units per week were given over a period of many weeks.

Clinical Aspects of Ultraviolet Therapy

Ethel M. Luce-Clausen, Rochester, N. Y. (Journal A. M. A., July 23, 1938), concludes that the value of ultraviolet radiation in the prevention and cure of rickets and tetany is an accepted fact and has been proved indisputably to be both safe and specific if given under accepted conditions. In the treatment of fractures of bone, experimental evidence points to radiation as being of little if of any value. In the treatment of tuberculosis, no claims for the specificity of ultraviolet radiation have yet been substantiated, though many authors still regard irradiation as a useful aid to other forms of treatment. In the treatment of diseases of the skin of bacterial origin ultraviolet radiation may be of value, provided the organisms lie within the range to which the rays penetrate and are killed or attenuated by doses safe for the host. In other diseases of the skin such as psoriasis, beneficial results might be due to the effect or radiation in producing hyperemia. Tumors of the skin have been produced in rats and mice with prolonged exposure to ultraviolet radiation, but the exposures needed are so far outside the range in general use by man, either in sun bathing or in the use of rays from artificial sources, that a warning of danger seems unnecessary. A caution, however, to avoid the abuse of radiation therapy, since its effects on the skin are imperfectly understood, is completely justified. More research is undoubtedly needed on the question of the photodynamic effect of radiation on the skin with special reference to the possible synthesis, in the skin, of the carcinogenic hydrocarbons.

Physical Aspects of Ultraviolet Therapy

W. W. Coblentz, Washington, D. C. (Journal A. M. A., July 30, 1938), emphasizes that the curative properties of a lamp are not necessarily measured by its power to generate an erythemia; also that the dosage, whether erythemal or suberythemal, should be left to the discretion of the physician. However, in order that a lamp may qualify as a therapeutic agent it should emit sufficient ultraviolet to produce an erythemia in a reasonable time of exposure (say 15 minutes or shorter) if the physician desires to give an erythemal dose. The physical aspects, the spectral range of antirachitic and erythemal reactions and the sources of radiation for use in ultraviolet light therapy are discussed.

Spontaneous Pneumothorax Complicating Pneumo-Thorax Therapy With Recovery After Pneumonolysis: Report of Three Cases

Since November, 1936, spontaneous pneumothorax has developed in three patients under the care of J. W. Cutler, Philadelphia (Journal A. M. A., July 30, 1938), following a therapeutic refill, which was the result of a tear in the visceral pleura at the base of an adhesion, with the adhesion remaining attached to the lung and preventing self closure of the perforation. In two, the spontaneous pneumothorax occurred two and 14 months respectively after pneumothorax therapy was instituted and successfully maintained. Both of these patients had a simultaneous bilateral artificial pneumothorax. In the third patient, with unilateral collapse, the spontaneous pneumothorax developed immediately after the first refill. The complication failed to respond to the usual therapeutic procedures, including continuous decompression. Closed intrapleural pneumonolysis was carried out to sever the plueral adhesions and was successful in permanently abolishing the spontaneous pneumothorax in each case.

OFFICERS OKLAHOMA STATE MEDICAL ASSOCIATION

President, Dr. H. K. Speed, Sayre.

President-Elect, Dr. W. A. Howard, Chelsea.

Secretary-Treasurer-Editor, Dr. L. S. Willour, McAlester.

Speaker, House of Delegates, Dr. J. D. Osborn, Jr., Frederick.

Vice Speaker, House of Delegates, Dr. P. P. Nesbitt, Medical Arts Building, Tulsa.

Delegates to the A. M. A., Dr. W. Albert Cook, Medical Arts Building, Tulsa, 1938-39; Dr. McLain Rogers, Clinton, 1937-1938.

Meeting Place, Oklahoma City, 1939.

SPECIAL COMMITTEES 1938-39

Annual Meeting: Dr. H. K. Speed, Sayre; Dr. W. A. Howard, Chelsea; Dr. L. S. Willour, McAlester.

Conservation of Hearing: Dr. H. F. Vandever, Chairman, Enid; Dr. J. B. Hollis, Mangum; Dr. Chester McHenry, Oklahoma City.

Conservation of Vision: Dr. W. M. Gallaher, Chairman, Shawnee; Dr. Frank R. Vieregg, Clinton; Dr. Pauline Barker, Guthrie.

Crippled Children: Dr. Earl McBride, Chairman, Oklahoma City; Dr. Roy L. Fisher, Frederick; Dr. M. B. Glismann, Okmulgee.

Industrial Service and Traumatic Surgery: Dr. Cyril C. Clymer, Medical Arts Bldg., Oklahoma City; Dr. J. Wm. Finch, Hobart; Dr. J. A. Rutledge, Ada.

Maternity and Infancy: Dr. George R. Osborn, Chairman, Tulsa; Dr. P. J. DeVanney, Sayre; Dr. Leila E. Andrews, Oklahoma City.

Necrology: Dr. G. H. Stagner, Chairman, Erick; Dr. James L. Shuler, Durant; Dr. S. D. Neely, Muskogee.

Post Graduate Medical Teaching: Dr. Henry H. Turner, Chairman, Oklahoma City; Dr. H. C. Weber, Bartlesville; Dr. Ned R. Smith, Tulsa.

Study and Control of Cancer: Dr. Wendell Long, Chairman, Oklahoma City; Dr. Paul B. Champlin, Enid; Dr. Ralph McGill, Tulsa.

Study and Control of Tuberculosis: Dr. Carl Puckett, Chairman, Oklahoma City; Dr. W. C. Tisdal, Clinton; Dr. F. P. Baker, Talihina.

ADVISORY COUNCIL FOR AUXILIARY

Dr. H. K. Speed, Chairman ....Sayre
Dr. C. J. Fishman..Oklahoma City
Dr. W. S. Larrabee..Tulsa
Dr. J. M. Watson..Enid
Dr. T. H. McCarley..McAlester

STANDING COMMITTEES 1938-39

Medical Defense: Dr. O. E. Templin, Chairman, Alva; Dr. L. C. Kuyrkendall, McAlester; Dr. E. Albert Aisenstadt, Picher.

Medical Economics: Dr. C. B. Sullivan, Cordell, Chairman; Dr. J. L. Patterson, Duncan; Dr. W. M. Browning, Waurika.

Medical Education and Hospital: Dr. V. C. Tisdal, Chairman, Elk City; Dr. Robert U. Patterson, Oklahoma City; Dr. H. M. McClure, Chickasha.

Public Policy and Legislation: Dr. Finis W. Ewing, Surety Bldg., Chairman, Muskogee; Dr. Tom Lowry, 1200 North Walker, Oklahoma City; Dr. O. C. Newman, Shattuck.

(The above committee co-ordinated by the following, selected from each councilor district.)

District No. 1.—O. C. Newman, Sr., Shattuck.
District No. 2.—McLain Rogers, Clinton.
District No. 3.—Thomas McElroy, Ponca City.
District No. 4.—L. H. Ritzhaupt, Guthrie.
District No. 5.—P. V. Annadown, Sulphur.
District No. 6.—R. M. Shepard, Tulsa.
District No. 7.—Sam A. McKeel, Ada.
District No. 8.—J. A. Morrow, Sallisaw.
District No. 9.—W. A. Tolleson, Eufaula.
District No. 10.—J. L. Holland, Madill.

Scientific Exhibits: Dr. E. Rankin Denny, Chairman, Tulsa; Dr. Robert H. Akin, Oklahoma City; Dr. R. C. Pigford, Tulsa.

Scientific Work: Dr. W. G. Husband, Chairman, Hollis; Dr. J. S. Rollins, Prague; Dr. J. L. Day, Supply.

Public Health:

Chairman—Dr. G. S. Baxter, Shawnee.

District No. 1.—C. W. Tedrowe, Woodward.
District No. 2.—E. W. Mabry, Altus.
District No. 3.—L. A. Mitchell, Stillwater.
District No. 4.—J. J. Gable, Norman.
District No. 5.—Geo. S. Barber, Lawton.
District No. 6.—C. E. Bradley, Tulsa.
District No. 7.—G. S. Baxter, Shawnee.
District No. 8.—M. M. De Arman, Miami.
District No. 9.—T. H. McCarley, McAlester.
District No. 10.—J. B. Clark, Coalgate.

SCIENTIFIC SECTIONS

General Surgery: Dr. F. L. Flack, Chairman, Nat'l Bank of Tulsa Bldg., Tulsa; Dr. John E. McDonald, Vice-Chairman, Medical Arts Bldg., Tulsa; Dr. John F. Burton, Secretary, Osler Building, Oklahoma City.

General Medicine: Dr. Frank Nelson, Chairman, 603 Medical Arts Bldg., Tulsa; Dr. E. R. Musick, Vice-Chairman, Medical Arts Bldg., Oklahoma City; Dr. Milam McKinney, Medical Arts Bldg., Oklahoma City.

Eye, Ear, Nose & Throat: Dr. E. H. Coachman, Chairman, Manhattan Bldg., Muskogee; Dr. F. M. Cooper, Vice-President, Medical Arts Bldg., Oklahoma City; Dr. James R. Reed, Secretary, Medical Arts Bldg., Oklahoma City.

Obstetrics and Pediatrics: Dr. C. W. Arrendell, Chairman, Ponca City; Dr. Carl F. Simpson, Vice-Chairman, Medical Arts Bldg., Tulsa; Dr. Ben H. Nicholson, Secretary, 300 West Twelfth Street, Oklahoma City.

Genito-Urinary Diseases and Syphilology: Dr. Elijah Sullivan, Chairman, Medical Arts Bldg., Oklahoma City; Dr. Henry Browne, Vice-Chairman, Medical Arts Bldg., Tulsa; Dr. Robert Akin, Secretary, 400 West Tenth, Oklahoma City.

Dermatology and Radiology: Dr. W. A. Showman, Chairman, Medical Arts Bldg., Tulsa; Dr. E. D. Greenberger, Vice-Chairman, McAlester; Dr. Hervey A. Foerster, Secretary, Medical Arts Bldg., Oklahoma City.

STATE BOARD OF MEDICAL EXAMINERS

Dr. Thos. McElroy, Ponca City, President; Dr. C. E. Bradley, Tulsa, Vice-President; Dr. J. D. Osborn, Jr., Frederick, Secretary; Dr. L. E. Emanuel, Chickasha; Dr. W. T. Ray, Gould; Dr. G. L. Johnson, Pauls Valley; Dr. W. W. Osgood, Muskogee.

STATE COMMISSIONER OF HEALTH

Dr. Chas. M. Pearce, Oklahoma City.

COUNCILORS AND THEIR COUNTIES

District No. 1: Texas, Beaver, Cimarron, Harper, Ellis, Woods, Woodward, Alfalfa, Major, Dewey—Dr. O. E. Templin, Alva. (Term expires 1940.)

District No. 2: Roger Mills, Beckham, Greer, Harmon, Washita, Kiowa, Custer, Jackson, Tillman—Dr. V. C. Tisdal, Elk City. (Term expires 1939.)

District No. 3: Grant, Kay, Garfield, Noble, Payne, Pawnee—Dr. A. S. Risser, Blackwell. (Term expires 1938.)

District No. 4: Blaine, Kingfisher, Canadian, Logan, Oklahoma, Cleveland—Dr. Philip M. McNeill, Oklahoma City. (Term expires 1938.)

District No. 5: Caddo, Comanche, Cotton, Grady, Love, Stephens, Jefferson, Carter, Murray—Dr. W. H. Livermore, Chickasha. (Term expires 1938.)

District No. 6: Osage, Creek, Washington, Nowata, Rogers, Tulsa—Dr. James Stevenson, Medical Arts Bldg., Tulsa. (Term expires 1938.)

District No. 7: Lincoln, Pontotoc, Pottawatomie, Okfuskee, Seminole, McClain, Garvin, Hughes—Dr. J. A. Walker, Shawnee. (Term expires 1939.)

District No. 8: Craig, Ottawa, Mayes, Delaware, Wagoner, Adair, Cherokee, Sequoyah, Okmulgee, Muskogee—Dr. E. A. Aisenstadt, Picher. (Term expires 1939.)

District No. 9: Pittsburg, Haskell, Latimer, LeFlore, McIntosh—Dr. L. C. Kuyrkendall, McAlester. (Term expires 1939.)

District No. 10: Johnson, Marshall, Coal, Atoka, Bryan, Choctaw, Pushmataha, McCurtain—Dr. J. S. Fulton, Atoka. (Term expires 1939.)

OFFICERS OF COUNTY SOCIETIES, 1938

COUNTY	PRESIDENT	SECRETARY
Adair		
Alfalfa	P. K. Slaton, Helena	L. T. Lancaster, Cherokee
Atoka-Coal	J. S. Fulton, Atoka	J. B. Clark, Coalgate
Beckham	R. C. McCreery, Erick	P. J. DeVanney, Sayre
Blaine	J. S. Barnett, Hitchcock	W. F. Griffin, Watonga
Bryan	P. L. Cain, Albany	Jas. L. Shuler, Durant
Caddo	J. Worrell Henry, Anadarko	P. H. Anderson, Anadarko
Canadian	A. L. Johnson, El Reno	G. D. Funk, El Reno
Carter	T. J. Jackson, Ardmore	Emma Jean Cantrell, Wilson
Cherokee	P. H. Medearis, Tahlequah	H. A. Masters, Tahlequah
Choctaw	G. E. Harris, Hugo	F. L. Waters, Hugo
Cleveland	O. E. Howell, Norman	J. L. Haddock, Jr., Norman
Coal	(See Atoka)	
Comanche	E. B. Dunlap, Lawton	Reber M. Van Matre, Lawton
Cotton	W. W. Cotton, Walters	G. W. Baker, Walters
Craig	W. R. Marks, Vinita	F. T. Gastineau, Vinita
Creek	C. R. McDonald, Mannford	J. F. Curry, Sapulpa
Custer	Ross Deputy, Clinton	Harry Cushman, Clinton
Garfield	E. J. Wolfe, Waukomis	John R. Walker, Enid
Garvin	G. L. Johnson, Pauls Valley	John R. Callaway, Pauls Valley
Grady	L. E. Wood, Chickasha	R. E. Baze, Chickasha
Grant	I. V. Hardy, Medford	E. E. Lawson, Medford
Greer	Leb B. Pearson, Mangum	J. B. Hollis, Mangum
Harmon	W. G. Husband, Hollis	R. H. Lynch, Hollis
Haskell	A. T. Hill, Stigler	N. K. Williams, McCurtain
Hughes	W. L. Taylor, Holdenville	Imogene Mayfield, Holdenville
Jackson	Jas. E. Ensey, Altus	J. M. Allgood, Altus
Jefferson	C. S. Maupin, Waurika	C. M. Maupin, Waurika
Kay		R. G. Obermiller, Ponca City
Kingfisher	John R. Taylor, Kingfisher	F. C. Lattimore, Kingfisher
Kiowa	J. M. Bonham, Hobart	J. Wm. Finch, Hobart
Latimer	R. L. Rich, Red Oak	E. B. Hamilton, Wilburton
LeFlore	E. M. Woodson, Poteau	W. L. Shippey, Poteau
Lincoln	E. F. Hurlbut, Meeker	Ned Burleson, Prague
Logan	F. R. First, Crescent	E. O. Barker, Guthrie
Marshall	J. H. Logan, Lebanon	J. F. York, Madill
Mayes	S. C. Rutherford, Locust Grove	E. H. Werling, Pryor
McClain	J. E. Cochran, Byars	R. L. Royster, Purcell
McCurtain	R. D. Williams, Idabel	R. H. Sherrill, Broken Bow
McIntosh	D. E. Little, Eufaula	Wm. A. Tolleson, Eufaula
Murray	P. V. Annadown, Sulphur	Richard M. Burke, Sulphur
Muskogee	Finis W. Ewing, Muskogee	S. D. Neely, Muskogee
Noble	J. W. Francis, Perry	T. F. Renfrow, Billings
Nowata	M. B. Scott, Delaware	H. M. Prentiss, Nowata
Okfuskee	L. J. Snickard, Okemah	C. M. Bloss, Okemah
Oklahoma	O. J. Fishman, Oklahoma City	John F. Burton, Oklahoma City
Okmulgee	V. M. Wallace, Morris	M. B. Glismann, Okmulgee
Osage	R. O. Smith, Hominy	Geo. Hemphill, Pawhuska
Ottawa	Benj. W. Ralston, Commerce	W. Jackson Sayles, Miami
Pawnee	R. E. Jones, Pawnee	M. L. Saddoris, Cleveland
Payne	E. M. Harris, Cushing	John W. Martin, Cushing
Pittsburg	A. R. Russell, McAlester	Ed. D. Greenberger, McAlester
Pontotoc	W. F. Dean, Ada	Glen W. McDonald, Ada
Pottawatomie	E. Eugene Rice, Shawnee	F. Clinton Gallaher, Shawnee
Pushmataha	E. S. Patterson, Antlers	D. W. Connally, Antlers
Rogers	F. A. Anderson, Claremore	W. A. Howard, Chelsea
Seminole	A. N. Deaton, Wewoka	Claude B. Knight, Wewoka
Stephens	W. T. Salmon, Duncan	Fred T. Hargrove, Duncan
Texas		R. B. Hayes, Guymon
Tillman	J. E. Childers, Tipton	O. G. Bacon, Frederick
Tulsa	M. J. Searle, Tulsa	Roy L. Smith, Tulsa
Wagoner	S. R. Bates, Wagoner	Francis S. Crane, Wagoner
Washington	J. E. Crawford, Bartlesville	J. V. Athey, Bartlesville
Washita	J. Paul Jones, Dill	Gordon Livingston, Cordell
Woods	Arthur E. Hale, Alva	Oscar E. Templin, Alva
Woodward	C. W. Tedrowe, Woodward	V. M. Rutherford, Woodward

NOTE—Corrections and additions to the above list will be cheerfully accepted.

THE JOURNAL
OF THE
OKLAHOMA STATE MEDICAL ASSOCIATION

| VOLUME XXXI | McALESTER, OKLAHOMA, SEPTEMBER, 1938 | Number 9 |

Mottled Enamel in Oklahoma Panhandle, and Its Possible Relations to Child Development

JOHNNY A. BLUE, B.A., M.D.
Director Panhandle District
Of Oklahoma State Health Department
GUYMON, OKLAHOMA

INTRODUCTION

The condition of chronic endemic dental fluorosis, commonly called "mottled enamel," is a defective formation of the enamel of the teeth whereby the enamel is streaked with defective areas of a chalky white color or brownish discoloration with areas of pitting according to the degree of mottling. This condition is prevalent in many areas of the United States, particularly in the Great Plains area, and is disfiguring as well as somewhat disabling to thousands of individuals.

It is an unpleasant and distasteful sight to see a strapping well built, apparently healthy, youngster bare a set of t e e t h which is the direct opposite to the "Smile of Beauty," and completely marring this individuals appearance. It must be more unpleasant and distasteful to this individual to have to brave a dentists chair for 10 to 20 fillings and in some cases extraction almost to complete adenture and the wearing of plates. Yet this condition is p r e s e n t in many communities and although considerable work has been done by the United States Public Health Service in locating the approximate areas where this condition is prevalent and in studying the causative factor in the production of this defective condition, little has been done to curb its development in the Oklahoma Panhandle. As a result c h i l d r e n continue to form their permanent defective teeth in their jaw bones by the time they are six to eight years old and parents are bewildered as to the cause of such unsightly teeth and many of the victims are accused of practicing poor oral hygiene.

It is not the purpose of this paper to criticize or to paint a picture that is darker than the condition really is, but merely to point out that the condition exists, to show the areas where it is prevalent, the source of the drinking water, the depth of the well from which this water is secured, the percentage of fluorine in the water, the element which is said to produce this condition, and to explain to the public what it is and what causes such a condition and to try and determine if there are any other physical defects accompanying this condition. To determine if possible, if there is any flaw or defective bone formations accompanying the mottled enamel, since both teeth and bone formations are related to the metabolism and assimilation of calciums, as well as to determine its possible relation to child development.

To say that the condition is present but to do nothing about it is to admit failure and if this article does nothing more than enlighten the public, the Medical and Dental professions and to stimulate thought and possibly some action to prevent this condition from developing in the generations to follow, since there is nothing that can be done as far as therapy is concerned after the permanent teeth are formed in the jaw bones, then it will have served its purpose.

DISCUSSION OF MOTTLED ENAMEL

Chronic dental fluorosis, enamel dystrophy or endemic hypoplasis of permanent teeth called mottled enamel is a water born disease associated with the ingestion of water termed rather high in an element called fluorine which produces a cumulative poisoning which is said to be carried in the blood stream to the tooth and thus interferes with the calcification of the tooth before it erupts, causing an excessive amount of calcium fluoride to be deposited thus changing the normal yellowish semi-translucent appearance of the tooth and g i v i n g it an appearance ranging from a chalky papery white to a corroded appearance with a tendency to chip, crumble and pit according to the degree of mottled enamel.

This condition was first reported by Edgar in 1901. The first investigation in the United States was done by Black and McKay in 1916.

Probably the most detailed and extensive study of this condition has been done by H. T. Dean, dental surgeon with the U. S. public health service who is at this time conducting further studies on this condition and who has already contributed several valuable papers to science treating on dental fluorosis, and locating endemic areas and mottled enamel index over the United States.

BASIS OF THIS STUDY IN OKLAHOMA PANHANDLE

Since this condition came to my attention it has been observed in the inhabitants of the Oklahoma Panhandle by numerous contacts with school children in particular while conducting school and immunization clinics. The presence of such a disfiguring condition in so many individuals here along with the complete ignorance of the cause of the condition by the laymen and by many professional men tempted the author to make a survey of the condition to study the degree of mottled enamel, the percentage of fluorine in the drinking water, the endemic areas and if possible to determine the mottled enamel i n d e x in the cities where there had been a continuous water supply for the past ten years and if possible to enlighten

the people of the prevalence of this condition, where the danger zones were located and try to stimulate methods of preventing such a condition developing in the endemic areas in future generations; as well as to ascertain if possible, the possible relations of this condition to child development and health, particularly to its association with r i c k e t s, orthopedic conditions and posture, since there has been little or no work done along the latter lines and since a pediatrician, Dr. Lemmon of Amarillo, Texas, has called to the attention of the medical profession that it was harder to prevent bowing of legs and rickets in children who lived in endemic areas although they received an adequate amount of the vitamines in their diets. Therefore, all of the schools in the four counties of the Oklahoma Panhandle were checked for mottled enamel and a physical examination done, a history taken of those who had the condition, and the finding recorded.

Approximately 400 school children were found to be afflicted with the condition in the endemic areas.

RELATION TO BONE FORMATION

It has not been so long ago that most people considered the teeth as something separate and distinct from the rest of the body. Today we know that the teeth are intimately connected with the body and derive their food from the blood stream and develop with the rest of the body and that conditions affecting the body as a whole will also affect the teeth. This can be illustrated by defects seen in teeth following long standing fevers and acute diseases of childhood.

Teeth are subjected to the same factors w h i c h influence the development and growth of the bones since both bone and t o o t h development is closely connected with the metabolism and assimilation of calcium. Mottled e n a m e l is the sign, manifested in defective e n a m e l of the teeth, of a disturbance of the calcification of the teeth.

There h a s b e e n considerable experimental work done on animals fed on a high fluorine diet. This w o r k showed that there was a derangement in bone formation along with the development of mottled enamel when the animal had a high content of fluorine in the diet.

An attempt was made to check this animal experimental work with children who had mottled enamel. Twenty-five students from an area where mottled enamel was endemic were chosen who had mottled enamel ranging from very mild to moderate. Blood calcium was run and X-rays of the bones taken.

The blood calcium was within normal range and the X-rays revealed no bony pathology or apparent bone changes over the normal that was detectable by X-ray films.

In the entire group of approximately 400 examined, who had mottled enamel, approximately 10 per cent gave a history of having experienced one or more fractured bones. This seems to be rather high when one considers that this is a plains area with practically no trees or hills for children to fall from. 15.30 per cent of this entire group showed definite signs of rickets by two or more detectable signs such as beading and flaring of the ribs, Harrisons groove, bowing of the legs, pigeon breast and prominent bosses, even though 76 per cent were breast fed and five per cent were breast and bottle babies combined. Whether this figure is high is purely a matter of opinion since the literature shows that signs of rickets in various groups of children ranges from 10 per cent to 90 per cent, however, when one considers that these individuals were practically all in fair economic circumstances and enjoyed fair dental and medical care up until three or four years ago and when one considers, too, that this country enjoys an abundance of sunshine 12 months out of the year one can assume, at least, that this rachitic index is above normal.

Forty-three per cent of the entire group were 10 per cent or more under weight, 20.25 per cent had poor postures.

Although there was no macroscopic pathology detected by X-ray and a single blood sample from 25 affected individuals showed a normal blood calcium. Taking all of the other points into consideration such as fractures, rickets, markedly high percentage of under weight, as well as to consider that bone and tooth formation are closely connected, it seems feasible that when one is affected the other is likewise affected and that there is a definite relation between mottled enamel and bony development.

RELATION OF MOTTLED ENAMEL TO OTHER ORAL CONDITIONS

Although no definite tabulations were done on the percentage or incidence of dental caries, gingivitis, malocclusions, pyorrhea and poor oral hygiene these conditions have been closely observed in frequent physical examinations of school children in the endemic areas in the Oklahoma Panhandle and from this observation I believe it can be truthfully stated that the incidence of caries is high especially in those cases which are beyond the questionable and very mild classifications of mottled enamel. Many of these individuals have malocclusions. A very high percentage of the cases which have pitting of the enamel have caries.

A very high percentage of these individuals, especially those who have the corroded appearing teeth and dark brownish staining have gingivitis and pyorrhea and poor oral hygiene. Whether there is some relation between dental fluorosis and gum infections cannot be said but it would seem more logical to assume that due to the inability of these individuals to improve the appearance of their teeth and remove the brownish stain by brushing and good oral hygiene, become discouraged and discontinue brushing the teeth and as a result of this poor oral hygiene gingivitis develops and then pyorrhea.

POSSIBLE RELATIONS OF FLUOROSIS AND CHILD DEVELOPMENT

The question of child development covers a wide field. There are many factors which must be weighed in this particular subject and many angles to be investigated. The viewpoint of the examiner determines the grade to a large extent because what is poor posture, etc., in the eyes of one examiner may not be so in the eyes of another. However, the author has tried to adhere to recognized standards to the letter and has approached this subject with an open mind.

In the relation of child development to chronic fluorosis it seems logical to assume that if this poisonous element is taken into the system in large enough quantities to affect the normal development of teeth that other protoplasmic substances and other parts of the body especially that which relies on the assimilation and metabolism of calcium would be affected in a like manner.

Laboring under this hypothesis t h o s e children who had signs of chronic fluorine poisoning manifested by signs of mottled enamel of the teeth were given a physical examination noting particularly defects in bodily development, posture and bony development. It should be stated here that the families of these children have all been in fair circumstances financially speaking until the past three or four years, all had fairly good medical and dental care. The larger per cent of which were breast fed and living in a country where there is an abundance of sunshine 12 months out of the year.

A total of 76.8 per cent of these students gave a history of being breast fed, only 10.3 per cent were artificially fed and 5.8 per cent were breast and bottle babies combined. Of the entire group 43 per cent were 10 per cent or more under weight measured according to Robert M. Woodbury, Bird T. B a l d w i n and Thomas D. Wood, chart of the American Child Health Association.

A total of 20.25 per cent had poor posture, 15.30 per cent had definite signs of rickets, 30.6 per cent had signs of chronically infected, hypertrophied and diseased tonsils, 3.60 per cent had systolic or dias-

tolic murmurs heard at the mitral area of the heart, 9.9 per cent gave a history of experiencing one or more fractured bones, 18.45 per cent of these students had brothers and sisters below six years old who were running the risk of developing chronic fluorine poisoning by consuming water from the same source of supply from which their afflicted brothers and sisters had partaken.

Weighing all of these figures and facts and assuming that children developing in an environment that is conducive to good development and in spite of this the examinations show that approximately 43 per cent are considerably under weight, 20 per cent have poor postures, and 15 per cent have definite signs of having had rickets and approximately 10 per cent having experienced broken bones and apparently more have malocclusions than in individuals with normal enamel. Knowing that fluorine is a protoplasmic poisoning and affected the assimilation of calcium, it would seem reasonable to think or assume and I think can safely be stated here that the above findings are ample proof that chronic fluorosis has a definite relation to child development and thus is a predisposition to rickets, poor posture and under w e i g h t and possibly a predisposition to fractures.

MAP OF OKLAHOMA PANHANDLE SHOWING ENDEMIC AREAS AND DEGREE OF MOTTLED ENAMEL
Colorado   Kansas

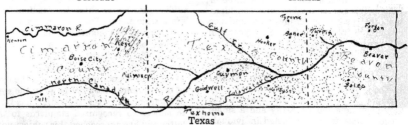

Texas

The above map shows the areas where mottled enamel is endemic in the Oklahoma Panhandle. The dotted area is the approximate boundary. The e x t r e m e north and w e s t e r n areas of Cimarron county and the extreme northwestern area of Texas county were not shaded because this area was not thoroughly checked due to a lack of schools and to sparseness of population.

The dotted area predominated in mottled enamel of the very mild class. The shaded area around Keyes was the area where the condition was more marked as to incidence and degree.

The following are graphic tabulations of the findings taken from the histories and physical examinations of those examined with mottled enamel.

TABLE I

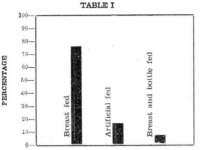

The above table shows 76.80% were breast fed, 10.35% were artificial fed and 5.85% were breast and bottle combination fed when infants. The remaining 7% could give no authentic history of infant feeding.

TABLE II

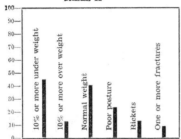

Table II shows 43% were found to be 10% or more under weight. 15% were 10% or more overweight. 42% ranged within normal weight. 20.25% had evidences of poor posture. 15.30% showed definite signs of rickets. 9.90% gave a history of experiencing one or more fractures of the bones.

TABLE III

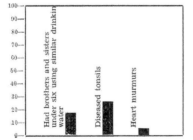

Table III shows some miscellaneous findings. 18.45% of those examined had brothers and sisters under six years old who were using similar drinking water and thus running the risk of becoming afflicted with mottled enamel. 30.60% had diseased tonsils. 3.60% had heart murmurs systolic in time, heard at the mitral area.

TABLE IV

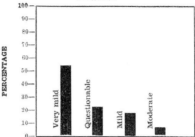

Degree of Mottled Enamel in percentage found on examination of approximately 400 school children in the areas in the Oklahoma panhandle.

The above graph is the degree of mottled enamel found in the endemic areas of the Oklahoma Panhandle.

The endemic areas were located by a survey of the s c h o o l s and by checking school physical examination records. When an endemic area was located the teeth of the children were checked, from the fifth grade up, and those having mottled enamel were classified as to the grade of mottled enamel using the H. T. Dean s y s t e m of grading, then a history was procured and a physical examination done.

TABLE V
MOTTLED ENAMEL INDEX

Guymon, Okla.	Texhoma, Okla.
Normal	
Mottled Enamel	

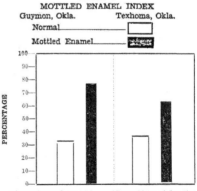

Mean fluoride (F) content in P.P.M. over six month period 1.45. Water supply two wells 150 feet apart depth 330 feet drilled 1928-1929.

Mean fluoride (F) content in P.P.M. over six month period 1.25. Water supply two wells depth 230 feet drilled 1924.

Only two places in the Oklahoma Panhandle have had a continuous water supply for ten years or more where enough children had consumed this water for the first six years of their life. Therefore this survey was restricted to these two areas as far as determining the mottled e n a m e l index.

In Guymon, Oklahoma, there has been a continuous water supply for ten years derived from two deep wells operated by the Oklahoma Electric and Water Company. These wells are 330 feet deep and showed a mean fluorine content, over a six month period, of 1.45 parts per million. Eighty-two children who had consumed this water all their lives were available for examination. Nineteen or 23 per cent of these had normal enamel. The remaining 63 or 77 per cent showed definite mottled enamel ranging from very mild to moderately severe, the greater per cent coming under the former classification.

Texhoma, Oklahoma, was the other community with a continuous water supply since 1924. They derive their city water from two wells 230 feet deep which are operated by the Cimarron Utility Company. The mean fluorine content of this supply was 1.25 parts per million over a six months period.

Thirty-three children were available for examination, who had used this s u p p l y continuously all of their lives or at least the first six years of their lives. Twelve of these, or 36 per cent, had normal enamel. The remaining 21, or 64 per cent, showed definite signs of mottled enamel ranging from very mild to moderately severe. The majority being very mild.

WATER SUPPLIES OF OKLAHOMA PANHANDLE

The entire w a t e r supply of the Oklahoma Panhandle is derived from wells. A rather thorough check of the municipal wells and s c h o o l wells in the endemic areas has been carried on over a six month period to determine the fluorine content of the water. These wells range from 132 to 330 feet in depth. The fluorine content ranges from 0.6 to 2.6 parts per million in the various wells.

Wells that were checked in areas where this condition was not e n d e m i c ranged around 0.6 p a r t s per million in fluorine content of the water.

A check was made of the few shallow wells ranging between 50 and 75 feet deep to determine the flourine content of this water. These wells were in creek and river bottoms and showed a flourine content of approximately 1. part per million.

Further investigation of the water supply both municipal, schools and private wells is being carried on but is rather slow due to the expense of the chemical analysis of the water.

POSSIBLE METHODS OF CONTROLLING
CHRONIC FLUORINE INTOXICATION

Since there is no cure of chronic fluorine poisoning once it has developed the chief aim is prevention. It has been suggested by some authorities investigating this condition that a low calcium intake hastens the onset and development of this chronic fluorine poisoning. In other words a high fluorine intake on a normal consumption of calcium in the diet will produce the condition as well as a comparatively normal intake of fluorine on a comparatively low calcium intake in the diet. In view of this evidence that a diet high in calcium tends to offset the effects of fluorine it would seem feasible that as a protective measure for children living in the endemic areas and questionable areas to partake of a diet relatively high in calcium content. Calcium salts do not dissolve in an alkaline medium but are soluble in an acid medium and can therefore be taken up by the blood stream and assimilated better. Fats react with calcium to form an insoluble soap. Thus a diet that is favorable to the increase in acidity of the intestines as well as one low in fat content may be considered even though some investigators have found that acid diets are conducive to carious teeth and that basic diets tend to arrest carious processes in four months time.

One cannot rely on the above too much for prevention however b e c a u s e there seems to be some difference of opinion of investigators as to the results of fluorine poisoning. Some state that there is a rarification of the calcium deposit while others state that there is an over abundance of calcium deposited.

At any rate the giving of calcium to correct teeth disorders as well as bone disorders has been over worked and calcium can be harmful as well as helpful.

It seems to be the concensus of opinion of the majority of those who have carried on investigations of this condition that the causative factor lies in the fluorine content of the water supply used for drinking and cooking purposes.

This being the case the safest thing as far as a preventive measure is concerned would be to seek a water supply for ingestion and consumption of c h i l d r e n in their formative years and years of greater development that will be below the danger level as to f l u o r i n e content. This may prove a troublesome task in an area where there are no cisterns, no s u r f a c e water supplies and where the majority of the people consume water from wells. However this task though great and expensive would seem well worth while when one views it from a public health angle and not from a financial view point.

SUMMARY AND CONCLUSIONS

1. Results of survey made in Oklahoma Panhandle on Chronic Fluorine Intoxication was stated, the endemic areas located, the mottled enamel i n d e x derived, the fluorine content of the water supply of the different areas given along with the depth of the wells, along with the findings on physical examinations of t h o s e afflicted with this condition.

2. That there is evidence which indicates that there is a definite relation between chronic fluorine poisoning as detected by mottling of the enamel and child development, particularly as to predisposition to developing underweight, p o o r posture, rickets and orthopedic conditions.

3. Possible methods of controlling and preventing this condition were suggested.

4. Dental c a r i e s, gingivitis, malocclusion, beginning phorrhea and poor oral hygiene incidence in mottled enamel is high.

ACKNOWLEDGMENT

I am indebted to, and wish to take this opportunity of thanking the following persons for their cooperation and help in carrying out this investigation. To Dr. Chas. M. Pearce, Oklahoma Health Commissioner, for his cooperation in making it possible for this investigation and for his reading and criticism of this script. To Drs. Collopy, Murhpy and Bell of the Child Welfare Department of Oklahoma Public Health Department for their assistance and suggestions. To Dr. Bertram and Kersey of the Dental Hygiene division of the Oklahoma State Health Department for their assistance, suggestions and grading of the cases of mottled teeth. To Drs. Lightner and Gruebbel of the dental profession in the endemic areas who offered valuable suggestions and criticisms; to the water superintendents and authorities of t h i s area for their cooperation, to the many school authorities and parents in the Oklahoma Panhandle without whose cooperation and assistance this investigation could not have been carried out. To Paul Thurber, sanitary engineer of this district for his handling of the investigation of the water supplies and to my office and nursing force for their assistance in the examinations and compiling the records.

BIBLIOGRAPHY

Further Studies In Mottled Enamel. Smith et. al., J.A.D.A., Vol. 22, May, 1935, Page 817.

Mottled Teeth. Isaac Schour & Smith, J.A.D.A., Vol. 22, May, 1935, Page 790.

The Occurrence of Mottled Enamel On Temporary Teeth. Margaret Cammack Smith & H. V. Smith, J.A.D.A., Vol. 22, May, 1935, Page 814.

Fluorine In Relation To Bone and Tooth Development. Floyd DeEds, J.A.D.A., Vol. 23, April, 1936, Page 568.

New Conception of the Development and Calcification of Teeth. E. C. McBeath, M.D., D.D.S., J.A.D.A., Vol. 23, April, 1936, Page 675.

Diet and Bone Development. Wm. J. Corcoran, M.D., J.A.D.A., April, 1934, Page 630, Vol. No. 21.

Relation of Rickets and Vitamin D to the Incidence of Dental Caries, Enamel Hypopasia and Malocclusion in Children. David H. Shilling, M.C., and George M. Anderson, D.D.S., J.A.S.A., Vol. 23, May, 1936, Page 840.

Relation of Diet and Dental Caries. Harold F. Hawkins, D.D.S., J.A.D.A., Vol. 21, April, 1934, Page 630.

The Cause of Mottled Enamel, a Defect of Human Teeth. Margaret Cammack Smith, Edith M. Lantz and H. V. Smith, Technical Bulletin No. 32, June 10, 1931, University of Arizona College of Agriculture.

Mottled Enamel in the Salt River Valley and the Fluorine Content of the Water Supplies. H. V. Smith, Margaret Cammack Smith, E. Osborn Foster, Technical Bulletin No. 61, May 15, 1936, University of Arizona College of Agriculture.

Chronic Endemic Dental Fluorosis. H. T. Dean, J.A.M.A., Oct. 17, 1936, Vol. 107, Page 1269-1272.

Summary of Mottled Enamel in Texas. H. T. Dean, D.D.S., U. S. Public Health Service, Texas Dental Journal, Vol 55 No. 3, Page 86.

Studies on the Minimal Threshold of the Dental Sign of Chronic Endemic Dental Fluorosis. H. T. Dean, Dental Surgeon, and Elias Elvove, Chemist U. S. Public Health Service. Public Health Reports, Vol. 50 No. 49, Dec. 6, 1935, Pages 1719-29.

Mottled Enamel in Texas. H. T. Dean, Dental Surgeon, U. S. Public Health Service, R. M. Dixon and Chester Cohen, Sanitary Engineer, Texas State Department of Health, Public Health Reports, Vol. 50 No. 13, March 29, 1935, Pages 424-45.

Studies On the Minimal Threshold of Dental Fluorosis. H. T. Dean, Dental Surgeon, and Elias Elvove, Chemist U. S. Public Health Service. Public Health Report, Vol. 52 No. 37, Sept. 10, 1937, Pages 1249.

Some Epidemiological Aspects of Chronic Endemic Dental Fluorosis. H. T. Dean, D.D.S., and Elias Elvove, P.H.D., American Public Health, Vol. 26 No. 6, June, 1936, Page 567.

Effects of Fluorine Upon Rate of Eruption of Rat Incisors and its Correlation With Bone Development and Body Growth. C. M. Smith, J. Dent. Research; 14-139-144, April, '34; Nelsons L. L. Living Medicine, Vol. III, PP. 127-133; Oxford Medicine, Vol. IV, Part I, PP. 229.

Bone Changes in Chronic Fluorine Intoxication. A. P. Bishop, American Journal Roentgenol, 35-577-585, May, '36.

Chronic Fluorine Intoxication (A Review). Medicine, Floyd DeEds, Ph.D., Vol. XII, No. 1, Page 1.

Rate of Apposition of Enamel and Dentine Measured by the Effects of Acute Fluorosis. I. Schour., D.D.S., Ph.D., Henry G. Poncher, M.D., American Journal of Diseases of Children. Vol. 45 No. 4, Oct., 1937.

Nutritional Influence on Teeth. Francis Krasnow. American Journal Public Health, Vol. 28 No. 3, March, 1938, Page 325.

Recurrent Iritis in Undulant Fever With Concurrent Rheumatic and/or Arthritic Disease*

JAMES R. REED, M.D.

E. GOLDFAIN, M.D.

OKLAHOMA CITY, OKLAHOMA

The diagnosis and treatment of arthritic diseases is a problem requiring the best that an internist can give to the patient. The patient needs to be considered as a whole and not only in respect to his joints. It therefore behooves the internist who is handling arthritic and rheumatic disease to ask for the assistance of specialists. In that way he may arrive at an opinion in respect to particular organs which can be correlated into the complex picture that makes up the rheumatoid syndrome.

While working with a number of cases having rheumatic or arthritic d i s e a s e symptoms a certain number that are quoted herewith had laboratory findings indicating the presence of undulant fever infection as well as eye symptoms. Curiosity having been aroused, and the problem requiring rather careful consideration from the eye standpoint, the ophthalmologist's help was enlisted in working out this rather unusual set of cases in which rheumatic disease symptoms, eye manifestations, and positive undulant fever skin and serological tests were present.

It is important to keep in mind that the collaborating ophthalmologist, co-author of this paper, does not positively and unequivocally hold that the chronic state of systemic brucellosis was the true and only cause of the ocular pathology. In view, however, of the fact that these cases had no definite foci of infection; that the Wassermann tests and urinalyses were negative; also no evidence of the presence of tuberculosis; it is justifiable to assume that chronic brucellosis was the etiologic factor. It is the desire of the ophthalmologist to stress the fact, in this paper, that in

proper geographical areas one should keep in mind that chronic brucellosis may be an etiologic factor in the causation of ocular disease, especially iritis. One should test for same properly and intelligently when the other more common causes of eye symptoms have been searched for and not found.

The cases reported herewith p r e s e n t rather similar history and findings in that each of them is suffering from either arthritis or has suffered from a rheumatic disease syndrome. Each case also had eye findings, some of which have been quite serious. Strongly positive skin tests when tested with the undulant fever organism were p r e s e n t. In addition to the very strongly positive skin tests, they yielded a positive opsonic index test for undulant fever, indicating a c t i v e infection when considered in connection with the s k i n test. Some of them also had positive agglutination tests. In accordance with the criteria of Huddleson a diagnosis of positive chronic undulant fever infection was established because of the fact that the opsonic index test revealed phagocytosis in mild, moderate or marked degree of less than 60 per cent and because of the presence of a positive skin test in all five cases, plus a positive agglutination test in four of the cases.

Tables I and II set forth below reveal the basis upon which a diagnosis of active undulant fever infection was arrived at in these cases.

*Read Before the Section on Eye, Ear, Nose and Throat, Annual Meeting, Oklahoma State Medical Association, Muskogee, Oklahoma, May 10, 1938.

TABLE I

Determination of phagocytosis activity as reported by Keller, Pharris and Gaub, and adapted from Huddleson, Johnson and Hamann. The opsonocytophagic activity of the blood.

Classification	Number of bacteria per polymorphonuclear cell
1. Negative	None
2. Slight	1 to 20
3. Moderate	21 to 40
4. Marked	41 or more

TABLE II

The diagnosis of undulant fever according to results of the skin, agglutination and opsonocytophagic tests as reported by Keller, Pharris and Gaub, and adapted from Huddleson, Johnson and Hamann.

Agglutination Test	Skin Test	Opsonocytophagic power of blood	Status toward Brucella
Negative	Negative	Cells negative to 20% slight phagocytosis	Susceptible
Negative	Positive	Cells negative to 40% marked phagocytosis	Infected
Positive	Positive	Cells negative to 40% marked phagocytosis	Infected
Negative	Positive	Cells 60% to 100% marked phagocytosis	Immune
Positive	Positive	Cells 60% to 100% marked phagocytosis	Immune

CASE 1, E. W. H., age 33: Recurrent iritis, both eyes. Eye symptoms began in 1926. He is now blind. They have consisted of redness and irritation of the eyes, attacks of iritis, and impairment of vision. He was treated by a number of good oculists, including the Mayo Clinic. He was told that he had iritis, detached retina, and scars of the retina and choroid, due to some type of infection. The trouble would come and go periodically. Tuberculin tests were made. The first was negative, the second tuberculin test was questionably positive. He received tuberculin treatment for one year. In spite of this treatment relapses continued to appear, at first only occasionally and mild in nature. He then noticed that his eyes became progressively worse until only light perception was present.

Laboratory tests for brucellosis revealed +4 agglutination in all dilutions including 1-200. Opsonic index test yielded 20 per cent moderate phagocytosis and 4 per cent marked phagocytosis. A very severe positive skin test with suppuration developing locally was present. Later skin tests with very small amounts of antigen continued to reveal strong positive reaction.

CASE 2, R. E. R., age 29: Recurrent iritis, left eye. This patient, who has a Marie Strumpell type of spondylitis, gives a history of reddening and irritation of the left eyeball occurring off and on since he began to have his serious symptoms of arthritis in the spine. March 1, 1937, he noticed redness present in the white part of his left eyeball, and photophobia. In June, 1937, pain in the left eyeball following a long drive appeared. Gradually loss of vision of the left eye began to appear in April, 1937, and became progressively worse until August, 1937, when only light perception was present. Tuberculin test was negative. Foci of infection were not found. Other commoner causes of iritis were not found. This patient experienced severe reactions to small doses of brucella bacterine. His tests for brucellosis revealed:

1. A +3 reaction on skin test.

2. Complete agglutination in all dilutions up to 1-200 on diagnostic examination.

3. Twelve per cent moderate phagocytosis on opsonic index test.

CASE 4, Dr. E. M., age 43: Recurrent ulcer, right cornea. Patient helped make antiserum Missouri State Farm, Agriculture Department, in 1911. In 1916 developed acute corneal ulcer right eye; also noticed general illness and cough. A tuberculosis specialist thought he had tuberculosis. This never could be definitely substantiated. In 1917 a rectal fistula developed. Later recurrent attacks of lumbago-like episodes occurred. Summer of 1928 had an influenza-like attack with recurrence of the old corneal ulcer in the old scar. At this time drank milk from a cow that had udder trouble but which tested negative for tuberculosis. In 1936 skin test for brucellosis revealed a severe positive test. Agglutination test was negative. The skin test caused his eye symptoms to flare up. It caused fever and general malaise and a flare-up of his back symptoms. Vaccine injections would cause severe reaction. While taking large dose injections of vaccine his eye trouble flared up in summer of 1937. Opsonic index test was strongly positive in 1937, after having taken vaccine treatment, however.

CASE 5, P. W. B., age 48: This patient some few years ago had a systemic infection which caused him to run fever with all of the associated signs of systemic infection, such as malaise, and muscle and joint aches. In addition at that time he had an iritis which according to his statement could not be explained on any definitely known basis. He was seen later by me with a subacute synovitis and swelling and discomfort of the left knee and left ankle. Medical management for his arthritic subacute symptoms resulted in a recession. No foci of infection were found. After the swelling disappeared the patient again developed trouble some seven months later. At this time there was swelling present in the right forefoot at the base of the toes. X-ray revealed demineralization of the head of the 2d, 3d, and 4th metatarsal bones.

Because of his recurrent symptoms serologic and skin tests for undulant fever were done. The agglutination test revealed complete agglutination in dilutions of 1-25 and 1-50, marked agglutination in dilutions of 1-100, and partial agglutination in dilutions of 1-200. The opsonic index test revealed 20 per cent marked phagocytosis, 70 per cent moderate phagocytosis, and 4 per cent slight phagocytosis. The skin tests revealed about a 2+ positive reaction for undulant fever. The patient was put on specific vaccine therapy. Disappearance of the arthritic symptoms again occurred.

CONCLUSION

This report is made for the purpose of calling attention to the following facts:

1. Ocular symptoms and signs may occur in an individual who has active chronic brucellosis.

2. Vaccine treatment may produce localizing reactions in the eye, as illustrated by Case 4.

3. While we cannot absolutely state that beyond all doubt the eye symptoms were caused by the chronic undulant fever infection in the quoted cases, we feel that it is quite probable that such is the case. The similarity of history and symptoms and of the presence of unmistakable serologic and immunologic skin tests for brucellosis are in favor of it.

4. We feel that in cases having ocular manifestations the factor of chronic brucellosis should be kept in mind and search-

ed for by proper laboratory and skin tests. This is especially true in cases in which a definite cause of the ocular manifestation cannot be adequately determined, such as syphilis, tuberculosis, or foci of infection.

5. Attacks of iritis in these cases were relatively free from pain.

REFERENCE

The Eye and its Diseases, edited by Conrad Berens, W. B. Saunders Company, 1936.

------------------o------------------

Undulant Fever
Correlation with Fatigue and Low Grade Fevers

ELEONORA L. SCHMIDT, M.D.
ELIZABETH DORSEY, M.D.
NORMAN, OKLAHOMA

Low-grade fevers have been found frequently among the women students of the University of Oklahoma. Too often they have been unexplained. They have always been a source of interest as well as concern. This past year we have had an additional staff member, so it has been possible to study and watch these students a little more carefully.

All women students who participate in any kind of physical education are given a complete physical examination before they may enter any activity. Since all freshmen and sophomore women are required to take some type of physical education this examination includes all the women in these two classes with the exception of those excused by their advisers or deans. The girls who were working were also required to have a complete examination. Because of this new ruling many juniors, seniors, and graduate students were seen. All upper classmen who had done their first or second year's work here had had an examination at that time. It was interesting to note that most of those students who had had unexplained elevated temperatures previously still registered above normal.

The Mantoux tuberculin test (O.T.) and the Wassermann test are included in these examinations. An effort was made to rule out early tuberculosis as a cause of the low-grade temperatures. All positive reactors to the tuberculin test had X-rays of their chests. In the doubtful cases they were referred to the specialist. Because of insufficient help in the laboratory a complete blood count and urinalysis were done only when indicated by family history, personal history, or findings at the time of examination.

One hundred cases of undulant fever are considered in this report. The ages ranged from 16 to 52. Each student had an intradermal test and a blood agglutination test. A suspension of killed organisms was used for the skin test. In reading the reaction edema less than 5 mm was considered negative. All the blood specimens were sent to the State Health Laboratory at Oklahoma City for an agglutination test at the same time that the skin test was given. This was done to prevent any possible error in the agglutination which might be due to the intradermal test. Those tests which were positive only in low dilutions are not considered in this report. The serum dilutions reported were 1:20, 1:40, 1:80, 1:160. We had no means of determining the opsonocytophagic index. This test could not be done in our laboratory and we had no way to get the citrated blood to the State Laboratory within the required time. Many of the tests were done on working students and they could not well afford the fee of a private laboratory.

Elevated temperatures were present in 87 per cent of the cases. The usual reading was from 99.4 to 99.8. The students of advanced standing who are included in this report are those who had had elevated temperatures recorded over a period of four to five years. Many had their temperatures taken at intervals, and some had as many as nine recorded temperatures above normal. There seems to be no special e l e v a t i o n in the afternoon, as the morning temperatures were frequently as high as those in the afternoon. Any temperature reading which might have been affected by an upper respiratory infection was discarded and the patient rechecked after the infection had subsided.

Fatigue was the almost universal complaint. One case seems to warrant special mention. A very normal-appearing girl returned to our office soon after classes began because of exhaustion w h e n she danced. We examined her chart and could see no reason for this, so we advised her to dance less strenuously for a while. A few weeks later she returned with the same complaint even though she danced l e s s strenuously. Her temperature was normal. Blood counts showed a white cell count around 10,000 each time. A test for undulant fever at this time showed a positive skin test and also a very positive agglutination test. Vaccine therapy proved very successful.

A s e c o n d girl complaining of fatigue provided an interesting study. She had fatigued easily for several y e a r s. Her mother and sister were diagnosed as having tuberculosis. She was under suspicion even though her tuberculin test had been negative five y e a r s prior to entry and again when taken here. An X-ray made three months before she entered school was read as being "suggestive." Her temperature taken at intervals was normal. Her systolic blood pressure was below 100. When tested for undulant fever her skin reaction was weakly positive, but the blood showed complete agglutination in all dilutions which are reported by the laboratory of the State Health Department.

Arthritis was a major complaint in 12 cases. The youngest girl was 17 years old, while the oldest was 52. A twin 21 years old consulted us because of arthritis. She gave a definitely positive s k i n reaction when tested, and her blood report showed complete agglutination in all dilutions. Her twin who had no complaints of any type was checked. Her skin reaction was negative and agglutination test two plus in the 1:20 dilution only. Seven years prior to this they had obtained milk from a neighbor whose cow had Bang's disease.

In this series of cases only one acute or semi-acute case is included. In November,

1937, while attending school in a neighboring state this girl became ill. The diagnosis was lobar pneumonia. Her temperature was 104, and she was irrational for several days. Her blood c o u n t showed 6,000 white blood cells. She never produced any sputum. After several weeks her temperature became normal, and she was brought to her home in Oklahoma by ambulance. One week later her temperature again rose to 105. Her chest was negative. This was in January, 1938. Gradually her temperature r e a c h e d the 99° level and remained there. On February 3 an undulant fever test was two plus in the lowest dilution. Fatigue and the low-grade fever continued. March 5 another specimen of blood was sent to the laboratory which reported complete agglutination in all dilutions. The skin test was slightly positive at that time.

In reviewing these 100 cases of undulant fever we find that the youngest was 16, the oldest 52. An attempt was made to determine the source of infection, but this was m o s t unsatisfactory. Even though they used pasteurized milk at present most of them had used raw milk for years. Then too, they had no idea of what type of milk was being used at their boarding houses or what had been used in previous years. A few came from homes where the cattle had been tested and some of the herd found to have Bang's disease.

Fifty-five per cent of the c a s e s gave both positive skin reactions and positive agglutination tests. Twenty-seven per cent gave only positive skin, while 18 per cent gave only positive agglutinations. Only two cases of this series had the opsono-cytophagic i n d e x determined, and they were both positive for infection. A most interesting observation in this relation to the tests was the fact that in all but one of our most positive skin reactors when the center sloughed the blood report came back absolutely negative or very weakly positive.

Complete blood counts were secured in only 60 per cent of the cases. Thirty-five per cent of these showed an anemia, the counts ranging from 3,180,000 to 4,000,000, while 65 per cent showed a c o u n t from 4,000,000 to 4,750,000. The hemoglobin varied from 65 per cent to 95 per cent Sahli. The white blood count seems to show a greater variation than the red blood count. The percentage of abnormal counts was greater than in the red blood count.

44% of cases had WBC of 3,700- 7,000
23% of cases had WBC of 7,000- 7,700
32% of cases had WBC of 7,700-11,500

The various counties represented in this group and the number from each county are given in the following list:

Cleveland	19%	Dewey	1%
Oklahoma	15%	Seminole	1%
McClain	6%	Cherokee	1%
Pottawatomie	5%	Johnston	1%
Tulsa	4%	Custer	1%
Carter	4%	Wagoner	1%
Major	3%	Kay	1%
Washington	3%	Jefferson	1%
Garfield	3%	Osage	1%
Choctaw	3%	Comanche	1%
Jackson	3%	Kiowa	1%
Grady	2%	Ottawa	1%
Logan	2%	Muskogee	1%
Caddo	2%	Rogers	1%
Stephens	2%	Okmulgee	1%
Garvin	1%	Out of state	7%
Kingfisher	1%		

It does not seem likely that these students acquired the disease while attending school in Norman since the greatest number of these cases were checked because of low-grade temperatures, and in almost all cases the initial temperature taken at the time of entering the university was elevated. Those complaining of fatigue had usually noticed it for a variable period of time prior to entry.

We believe that all persons who continue to have a low-grade temperature should be tested for undulant fever. Those persons who complain of fatigue, even though there may seem to be an adequate reason for this, should always be tested. We believe this is most important, especially so in younger people, since we think of youth as being symbolic of endless energy.

———o———

Chronic Gonorrhea

J. HOLLAND HOWE, M.D.
PONCA CITY, OKLAHOMA

Recent estimation made by public health officers showed that the population of the United States is heavily infected with venereal diseases. The greatest part of the infection is due to gonorrhea and its germ, the gonococcus. It was said that more than 80 per cent of the venereal diseases are caused by gonococci, and that about ten million men and women of this country are suffering from gonorrhea or its complications.

This great proportion of gonorrhea among the venereal diseases is due to the negligence of the patients who easily become used to a little discharge from the urethra or the vagina, and to the negligence of the doctors who still consider gonorrhea as an easily treated disease which can be cured with a few irrigations, instillations, and a couple of shots into the gluteal muscles.

Negligence of both the patient and the doctor is the main factor in pushing a gonorrheal infection into the chronic stage,

while the anatomical construction of the male genito-urinary apparatus is another. So it happens that gonorrhea persists, and there is little that we can do about it.

Preaching to the public the uselessness of quack remedies and the need of proper medical care does not help much alone if the medical profession in general does not change its attitude towards the disease, and does not treat the cases of gonorrhea more seriously.

It is improper to tell the patient that his discharge from the urethra does not amount to much; that it can be treated in a few weeks (or, as they have been led to believe by the newspapers, in a few days). Gonorrhea is a disease which is often more difficult to eradicate than syphilis. It is a disease which can destroy the happiness of family life more often than any other of the venereal diseases.

To make a diagnosis of chronic gonorrhea, it is not sufficient to rely upon the subjective symptoms and the local signs of the disease. Indeed, there are usually very few subjective complaints. The frequency of micturition is less marked than in the acute stage. There is no urgency in passing water, and the slight discharge, or morning drop, is often missing. The patient may have difficulties in his sex life which amount to a sexual neurasthenia. He may have pains vaguely localized to the perineum and the lumbar region or to some joints. Often, he is classified as a rheumatic p a t i e n t and treated as such with the innumerable remedies suggested lately for this affection.

No case of chronic gonorrhea can be diagnosed unless the doctor makes a routine inquiry as to the previous sex life of his patient. Of course, there are cases met by the specialist in which the presence of a chronic gonorrhea is evident, but I am speaking from the standpoint of the general practitioner, who acts as a sort of first casualty station for human suffering. He is the one who ought to have a specially sharp eye and become aware of the true nature of his patient's general ill health.

If chronic gonorrhea is suspected in a patient, the proper diagnosis is made by a series of tests:

1. The urine is examined by the four glass test (the fourth glass contains urine voided after a prostatic and vesicular massage) for the presence of pus and shreds.

2. The urinary sediment, the prostatic secretion expressed by massage, and, if there is any, the urethral discharge is examined microscopically for the presence of gonococci.

3. Cultures should be made on special media of the prostatic and vesicular secretions.

4. A complement fixation test made of the blood of the patient to show whether there are hidden metastatic foci of gonorrheal infection.

5. If all these tests are negative they are repeated after a provocative injection of gonococcal vaccine if the presence of gonorrheal infection is highly suspicious.

The value of these tests is very variable in certain cases. The four glass test may be negative today and positive a few days later. The microscopic examination and the staining of smears with the gram method may give doubtful results, especially when the number of gonococci is small. Russian physicians recently showed that often the gonococci remain gram positive, both in smears and in cultures. The complement fixation test is often negative; on the other hand, it may remain positive even after the cure of chronic gonorrhea has been established.

If both the clinical indications and the results of laboratory tests show that the patient has gonorrhea in the chronic form, the next step is to determine the focus of gonorrheal infection. As known from the anatomy of the male genito-urinary organs, there are m a n y side tracks, blind sacs, glands and ducts in the urethra where gonococci can easily hide themselves. Practically all these side tracks are inaccessible to l o c a l antiseptics and the usual methods of treatment by injection, irrigation, or instillation. Persistence of the gonorrhea is always due to a focus in these side tracts. Most of the hidden foci can be detected by means of palpation with bougies or by means of anterior or posterior urethroscopy.

The focus of a persistent gonorrhea may be in one or several of the following structures: 1. The paraurethral ducts. 2. Littre's glands and ducts and the lacunae of Morgagni. 3. Cowper's ducts and glands. 4. Prostatic ducts and the prostate gland. 5. The ejaculatory ducts and the seminal vesicles. 6. The vas deferens and the epididymes, and I have read but never have seen a case of lower ureteral infection.

Treatment of chronic gonorrhea is mainly a fight against an infection localized in one or several of the side tracts. Our aims s h o u l d be: 1. Establishment of proper drainage from these structures. 2. Efforts to reach the gonococcus with antiseptics. 3. Prevention of formation of fibrous tissue and stricture. The means are instrumental treatment, use of antiseptics of mild concentration, but sufficiently strong to kill the germs, massage, and the use of sulphanilamide in small doses.

If the paraurethral ducts are inflamed, they are obliterated best by an electric cautery.

Sometimes gonorrhea persists because the gonococci are stored in the subpreputial sac, and the ducts (Tyson's) at the base of the frenum, usually the instillation of a one per cent solution of picric acid is sufficient for the treatment and cleansing of the subpreputial sac. If there is an abscess of Tyson's duct it should be opened and the cavity cauterized.

One of the most frequent c a u s e s of chronic gonorrhea is a gonorrheal infection of Littre's glands and of Morgagni's lacunae. There may be a simple inflammation, or a purulent one, with occasional development of a periurethral abscess. The urine contains numerous pus shreds intermittently, and the urethroscopic examination will show which of the glands are involved. The treatment is irrigation followed by a straight bougie and massage of the u r e t h r a upon the bougie, followed again by irrigation. This treatment should be carried out once or twice a week. If only a single area in the urethra is affected, it can be cauterized in the urethroscope.

A periurethral abscess usually has to be opened and the abscess cavity cauterized with chemicals—one can do this with a knife through the skin. It is evident that the after treatment would include the use of sounds.

Suppurative cowperitis may occur. In that event put the patient to bed, use hot packs, and, if necessary, incise and drain.

The gonococcus has the ability to penetrate between the epithelial cells of the urethra into a subepithelial connective tissue which becomes hyperplastic. Such an event is shown by irregularity of the urethral surface felt on passing a bougie or a sound. Treatment is gradual dilatation of the urethra.

In a great majority of gonorrheal cases, a chronic prostatitis develops, mostly when the c a s e has not been properly treated. Here, besides the g e n e r a l symptoms of chronic gonorrhea, one finds the fourth glass of the four glass urine test with turbid fluid containing shreds. Rectal palpation shows irregularities of the prostatic surface, pain, and tenderness on pressure. The secretion expressed contains pus cells, occasionally also gonococci. If an old case, the inflammation is upheld by a mixed infection. Very often the ejaculatory ducts are also obliterated, and the seminal vesicles are a focus of infection. The chief measures of treatment are: 1. Massage. 2. Posterior irrigation, and 3. Dilatation with sounds;—some inject the gland transrectally.

The prostatic and the vesicular massage is the most important part of the treatment of c h r o n i c prostatitis. It is made twice a week for six or eight weeks followed by a week's rest, and repeated until the urine passed subsequent to massage is free from turbidity, the urine sediment and prostatic secretion is absolutely free from gonococci, its culture is sterile, and it does not contain more than five pus cells per high power field under the microscope. After each massage the urethra should be irrigated with an antiseptic solution, as potassium permanganate, silver nitrate, or mercury oxycyanide. The use of sounds is also important since they help drainage of the prostatic and ejaculatory ducts. If the condition does not quickly clear up by these measures, you can instill a one per cent solution of silver nitrate into the posterior urethra in order to cause a mild hyperemia and posterior urethritis. Sometimes the ejaculatory ducts have to be catheterized. It is only rarely that a vesiculitis does not clear up by this method of treatment so t h a t surgical intervention such as vasotomy, vasostomy, or vesiculectomy becomes necessary.

Epididymitis is usually known as an acute infection and complication of an acute gonorrhea, but it still exists in many cases after the violent, acute symptoms have subsided. The sterility of the male is due to c h r o n i c epididymitis, which mainly consists in fibrous tissue formation. Since a chronic epididymitis may any time exacerbate, and since the epithelial surfaces of the ducts are not accessible for local treatment, one has to use certain adjuvants. The use of adjuvants is indicated also for the reason that most of the chronic cases are due to a mixed infection.

Such adjuvants as: 1. Vaccines. 2. Foreign protein. 3. Chemicals. 4. Diathermic heat.

The use of chemicals has been recommended by many, and such substances as colloidal manganese, or dyes, as acriflavine, but I think they are more successful in the acute cases.

As a rare focus of gonorrhea may be mentioned the ureter. A case was shown by Friedman. His patient contracted gonorrhea in 1917, when 18 years of age, and in 1934, when he was 35, he still was suffering from gonorrhea. Cystoscopy showed that the orifice of the left ureter had a stricture. Intravenous pyelography revealed a dilatation of the lower third of that ureter. A ureter catheter was introduced, and a large amount of pus evacuated, in which gonococci were abundant. Here the oral use of sulphanilamide should work wonderfully.

We should also mention the joints, which perhaps is outside the field of the urologist—whether there are cases of chronic arthritis caused by a primary infection of the joints with gonococci. Tommasi mentions a case of a wife in whom gonorrheal arthritis developed without evident local signs of i n f e c t i o n of the genitals. The arthritis developed suddenly in s e v e r a l joints, and finally settled in the wrist joint.

One of the most difficult problems of chronic gonorrhea is to tell when a cure has b e e n established. Cessation of the clinical signs alone is not sufficient evidence of cure. The patient may remain a gonococcus carrier. Therefore, on stopping treatment, one should take smears and cultures daily for one week. If negative the examination is repeated once weekly for four weeks, and then once each month for three months. After six months a complement fixation test is made.

We can safely say that a cure has been established if: 1. There is no sign of urethral discharge for at least two weeks after treatment has been suspended. 2. There is no pus in the morning urine. 3. There are no gonococci in smears and cultures of urethral and prostatic secretion. 4. There is no sign of inflammation seen by means of the urethroscope. 5. The negativity of findings holds for six months.

---o---

Acute Gonorrhea

ROBERT H. AKIN, M.D., F.A.C.S.
OKLAHOMA CITY, OKLAHOMA

Due to the use of sulfanilamide the burden of acute gonorrhea has been greatly lightened during the past year. The question of the epidemiology and spread of the disease is still very important. The early amelioration of symptoms led to a caution by the original investigators that many new cases might develop. An effort was made to ascertain the incidence of new cases during the past three m o n t h s as compared to the same three months a year ago. In our own experience there was a reduction of about 50 per cent. This might be due to several factors, such as the drug counter sale of sulfanilamide, perhaps the g r e a t e r recognition of our competitors values, and the management of uncomplicated c a s e s by family physicians. The comments of several competent urologists indicate that the incidence is greater, while others indicate that it is less. At the present time, the question of spread of the disease is a very paramount one. In my own opinion m o s t physicians are cautiously watching their patients in this respect.

DIAGNOSIS

The diagnosis of active gonorrhea should not be made without confirmation by properly stained smears. In this connection, the use of the Gram stain is preferable. The typical Neisserian organisms, occurring in the urethral smears, are e a s i l y recognized, but the coffee-bean shaped, intracellular or extracellular diplococcus which is variable in its staining and has some tendency to pleomorphism, is more confusing. Such an organism, called a pseudo-gonococcus, has been described by Bolend[1]. The Gram negative diplobacillus (typical colon bacillus) should be very e a s i l y distinguished. These organisms seldom produce the characteristic purulent discharge.

A very confusing type of non-specific urethritis, presenting Gram positive lancet-shaped diplococci, has proven to be a very interesting problem in differential diagnosis so far as these discharges are concerned. The investigations of Moor and Brown[2], of the University of Oklahoma, proved that this organism was a pneumococcus; in most instances type 14, and that it occurred in one-third of a series of 400 cases having non-specific, subacute, chronic, and active urethritis. It has been found as an associated organism in several cases of acute gonorrhea.

CONTROL OF THE PATIENT

Just as important as the plan of treatment, is the problem of control of the patient. Patients presenting the symptoms of a c u t e gonorrhea, whether their discharge be specific or non-specific are never in a receptive mood on the first or second visit. They should return often enough to realize the seriousness of the infection, and the possibility of its transference to the patient's eyes or to other individuals. He should be taught to eat properly, secure adequate bed rest, and to avoid active emotional stimulation. He should also be informed of the joint legal obligations of patient and doctor to the United States Public Health Service in connection with case transfer, case holding and tests for cure.

SYMPTOMS AND PATHOLOGY

It has been shown by many investigators that the gonorrheal o r g a n i s m has passed beyond the basement membrane and is beyond the reach of local antiseptics when the symptoms have developed. Aside from this fact there are anatomical conditions which influence the course of acute gonorrhea. A tight foreskin or partial lymphatic obstruction in the coronal sulcus area may produce annoying meatal edema. The presence of a small urethral meatus indicates in m o s t instances the presence of excessive deep urethral crypts and sinuses along the entire penile urethra. Pelouze[3] calls attention to the variation in the structure of the posterior urethral mucosa as a cause for greater tendency to posterior extension. The r e d n e s s and edema of the urethral membrane gives a clinical estimate of the severity of the anterior urethritis. Suggestive symptoms of frequency, tenesmus, and difficult urination, indicate the development of posterior urethritis. Examinations of the first and second urine specimens still have great value as an o b j e c t i v e sign of posterior urethritis. The prostate and seminal vesicles should be examined only very gently

and then just to determine their involvement. When acute, no effort should be made to secure the secretion.

TREATMENT

The development of non-irritating, mild, mercurial and silver protein instillations have eliminated the necessity for overstimulation and destruction of the urethral membrane. However, mechanical injury can easily result from rapidly forced injections, pressure of the syringe in the meatus and the application of firm pressure with the thumb and forefinger. For the most part anterior injections should be only mild rinses. It is the author's impression that the prostate should receive practically no treatment during the active phase of acute gonorrhea. This applies with equal e m p h a s i s to the posterior urethra unless acute retention of urine develops as a result of acute prostatitis, then careful catheterization with a small catheter as needed for relief of the retention is indicated. When the active stage has subsided mild tonic massages may be instituted for microscopic study. Mild irrigations should follow the massage. Sounds should be left for treatment of chronic gonorrhea.

The Kettering type of hypotherm conditioned air cabinet seemed to reduce the period of involvement and the severity of symptoms in acute gonorrhea to about 50 per cent. This procedure was discontinued because it required five to seven hours for each application, with expensive equipment, to which was added the expense of constant medical attention, the employment of male and female nurses, and expenditures for hospital beds, laundry and electricity. In other words, such fever therapy is an institutional procedure and few patients with acute gonorrhea will submit to either the treatment or the expense, especially since the advent of sulfanilamide therapy. Most e v e r y physician has used sulfanilamide, in the treatment of gonorrhea. A summary of the facts established is, therefore, all that is necessary.

The administration of 60 to 80 grains a day for two or three days, will result in the disappearance of the discharge and the clearance of the urine in 70 to 80 per cent of the cases. The drug should be continued if well tolerated. The most desirable dosage seemed to be 10 grains every four hours, night and day. This dosage was considered most desirable as a result of the estimations of blood concentrations by Marshall, Eremson & Cutting[4]. They found that absorption from the intestinal tract was more than 99 per cent complete in four hours. The equilibrium between the amount ingested and the amount excreted in the urine was reached in two to three days and required about three days for elimination.

In cases with impaired renal function smaller doses raise the blood concentration and elimination requires a l o n g e r time. Practically the total amount of sulfanilamide taken by mouth can be recovered from the urine. Subcutaneous or intramuscular administration does not result in a higher blood concentration but excretion is slightly more rapid.

The water intake should not be limited. Normal water balance should certainly be maintained as an adequate concentration of the drug in the urine is easily obtained. Methods for determination of the free and conjugated sulfanilamide in the blood and urine are available to those using a colorimeter. Marshall, Emerson & Cutting[4].

The exact mode of action of sulfanila-. mide is not satisfactorily proven. The work of Helmholtz[5] and Farrell, Lyman . and Youman[6] indicates that it is bacteriocidal in the urine. That this is not its only mode of action is evident. Blood plasma has a greater concentration of sulfanilamide than does whole blood and evidently acts as a very efficient media for destroying the deep gonococci. Osgood and Brounlee[7] suggest that sulfanilamide did not kill streptococci in bone marrow cultures directly, but permitted greater efficiency of phagocytic action. This explanation is not satisfactory for gonorrhea b e c a u s e decreased phagocytic a c t i o n is present in cases responding to treatment.

It was unfortunate that great confusion resulted from fatalities occurring s o o n a f t e r the introduction of this excellent drug. Fortunately, the facilities and medical background existed and were placed into immediate action to accurately determine their cause, diethylene glyocol solvent[10].

The toxic manifestations may be divided into those associated with no important pathological changes and those with severe damage. Under the first group may be included such symptoms as headache, nervousness, mental confusion, nausea, anorexia, vertigo, weakness, precardial pain and abdominal discomfort. For the most part the drug need not be discontinued unless the symptoms are too severe to be tolerated but it is often wise to reduce the dosage, as a lower blood level will probably g i v e adequate therapeutic results. Cyanosis may indicate either sulphemoglobinemia or methemoglobinemia. The spectroscope is required to differentiate these. Marshall and Walzl[8] have not found any change in the oxygen-carrying capacity of a number of cases.

Skin rash on exposed surfaces indicates the production of a photosensitizing influence of the skin in some cases. Urticarial or exfoliative lesions sometimes occur but disappear in 48 to 72 hours, after discontinuing the drug.

The most dangerous toxic manifestations, well described in the literature, are changes in the blood picture, either hemolytic anemia or agranulocytosis. For this reason repeated studies of the blood picture are advisable and the drug immediately discontinued if a drop in the count occurs. The injury does not seem to be to the bone marrow but rather to the circulating cells so that blood transfusions, if given early, have usually resulted in rapid recovery. In such instances great fluid intake serves to avoid acid hematin crystalization in the renal tubules and alkalization is advisable. Vest, Harrell and Colston[9].

GONORRHEA IN THE FEMALE

Very little has been said about gonorrhea in the female, because we believe that the administration of sulfanilamide has about the same value in such cases as it does in the male. There are, however, more opportunities for the female to develop complications, due to her functional activities. She should have bed rest at the menstrual period, and only very careful nontraumatic local care.

Release of patients as cured should not be given under two and one-half to three months of repeated complete studies during which time the activities should be guarded to avoid exposure to others. I know of no new criteria of cure and time has to form one element in arriving at this conclusion. Sounds and sexual intercourse are uncertain tests for cure. Alcohol or beer will usually stimulate activity but may invite the production of a chronic carrier. Alas! I do not even know that another course of sulfanilamide is a positive test.

BIBLIOGRAPHY

1. Bolend, Rex—Journal Oklahoma State Medical Ass'n. 17:57, March, 1924.
2. Moor & Brown—J.A.M.A., June, 1937.
3. Pelouze—Gonorrhea in the Male.
4. Marshall, Emerson & Cutting—J.A.M.A., Vol. 108, No. 12, 953-957. March 20, 1937.
5. Helmholtz—Journal of Pediat. 2:243, 1937.
6. Farrell, Lyman & Youman—Vol. 110, No. 15, 1176. April 9, 1938.
7. Osgood and Brounlee—J.A.M.A., Vol. 110, page 349. January 29, 1938.
8. Marshall and Walzl—Bul. John Hopkins Hospital. 41: 14, 1937.
9. Vest, Harrell and Colston—Journal of Urology. 39 (2):198. February, 1938.
10. J.A.M.A., Vol. 109, No. 24, page 1985.

---o---

Necessity of Careful Eye Examinations*

D. M. K. THOMPSON

MUSKOGEE, OKLAHOMA

In the earlier days with primitive weapons there were wild beasts always waiting and hidden foes or savages ready to send an arrow or spear thrust and the ears and eyes were keen and sharp for preservation. These senses are just as essential today to cope with the wolves and foes of all kinds and the ever demand for speed, it is necessary that ones eyes should be kept keen and alert, not only for their protection but for the sake of other fellow men.

In this age of swift travel by plane and car we must be able in an instant to see clearly and accurately able to judge distance, not only speed, but with an active mind able to judge and act quickly and correctly. And, too, the machinery employed in all kinds of work while the hand must be skilled, yet the eye must be quicker and more accurate to help and guide the hand. So essential are good eyes that in practically all commercial enterprises a careful and accurate examination by a specialized physician is required and report is demanded before one will be employed, this for his own protection and of his fellow employees. In so doing the employer is many times saved compensation and law suits for injury and even those old in a service, who have rendered good and satisfactory service, have been dropped because of some physical defect.

*Read before the Section on Eye, Ear, Nose and Throat, Annual Meeting, Oklahoma State Medical Association, Muskogee, Oklahoma, May 10, 1938.

I will not undertake here to describe the various kinds of opthalmoscopes. Many advances in the styles and forms of these essential instruments with monocular, binoculars and many other varieties of suggestions and attachments, the red free attachments and the mechanisms for photographing and drawing to m e a s u r e distances and heights of the different changes taking place, the location and depth of opacities and a knowledge of kind and causes.

These more pretentious, expensive and electrically equipped machines, so handy and conveniently hooked up that the indirect method is not being used so much, although the image is reversed, yet we are given thus a very clear field and much magnified one and thus will reveal many points overlooked by the direct method and can be used to better advantage where pupil is contracted. So, in many ways, the better study can be made as in high myopia.

A normal fundus and medea we all try to recognize which ordinarily is not difficult to do, barring the anomalies of development, but when we have the patient coming apparently with symptoms pointing to some eye affection then with these means at our hands, we should, by making a careful examination, obtain a very perfect idea of existing changes, if any, not only the external eye structure and muscular inbalance the fields of vision and eye grounds for any anomalies of the vessels of the central artery, the retina, the choroid, lense, and change of vitreous.

Many of the patients come to you, referred by their physician, who wishes you to assist him in diagnosis and treatment of some obscure headache, neuritis and suspected brain lesion or some physical defect which may or may not be g i v i n g eye symptoms or any diminution of vision. By obtaining the history of the case, field of vision for white, for colors, blue, red and green, and careful fundus examination. Unfortunately many of these cases have been carelessly allowed to go to some ten cent store, drug store, or to some man who just fits glasses who knows nothing of the physiology or anatomy of the eye and what these symptoms mean and future bearing, not only on his vision or the delay in the necessary early treatment may mean the life of the individual when so much precious time may have been lost which, by a careful examination by a graduate of medicine who has specialized in the examination and treatment of eye diseases, and is able to diagnose systemic conditions with its relation to the eye.

The optic nerves come off as an elongated portion of the white matter of the brain, covered with the dura arachnoid and pia—being divided by spaces known as sub dural and arachuordal spaces, thus the spinal fluid circulates through this nerve, similarly to brain with the pia carrying many bundles of nerves so that we find a diseased condition or pressure acting on the brain will sooner or later, usually s o o n e r, be shown on the eye grounds. We may have a hyperemia, a congestion involving the disc and smaller vessels, due usually to some local infection or irritation. This usually clears up after removal of the local condition.

Optic neuritis or papillitis, c a u s i n g changes in the nerve head as to size, color and outline of nerve head, caused by severe and very deep p a i n s, usually affecting vision quickly, taking its toll according to s e v e r i t y, location and cause, always a symptom of some general disease or affection, frequently p r o d u c e d by brain lesions, meningitis, acute or chronic syphilis, usually secondary, are the more common chronic affections.

The acute infections may be brought about in many ways by febrile conditions of infectious diseases and their sequelae—in fact most any febrile disease may produce it. So, being a symptom, the offending cause may be found and treated, blood tests must be made, pus pockets, tonsils, teeth and sinuses, if possible found and eliminated, kidneys and urine checked.

Poisons, such as lead, arsenic, methyl alcohol, quinine and many other drugs affect the nerves and may bring about primary atrophy.

Pressure from tumors of the orbit and optic nerve may produce optic neuritis by pressure and blocking the spaces. Tumors of the brain, the pituitary body and other parts from pressure on the nerve fibers will cause an optic neuritis and result in an optic atrophy and blindness, depending upon location and amount of pressure.

Tumors of the choroid, most usually to be considered malignant, the sarcoma is the more common, and in this connection wish to relate one experience which came my way. Mr. Mac brought his wife, age a b o u t 60, for eye examination and for glasses, giving a history of flashes of light, like lightning at times, careful fundus examination revealed a very small tumor posteriorly, a d v i s e d enucleation as my opinion, asking consultation, the husband expressed a desire to take her to St. Louis, needless to say, they agreed with me and removed the eye, giving her only three years to live, vision was best in the affected eye. After .18 years she is living, in good health. Early diagnosis accounts for the prolonged life. I found the day before coming to me she had been examined by one of the best r e g a r d e d specialists in Kansas City and told she n e e d e d her glasses changed only.

Detachment of the r e t i n a, giving a blurred image of blind spots in the beginning, should be early recognized if any good results from treatment is expected.

Opacities of the vitreous brought about by changes in the circulation s y s t e m, hemorrhages and cause an amount of loss of vision proportionately due to the character of the density of such opacity. These may be seen by the examiner but may be remnants of embryonic life.

Injuries involving the optic nerve and

all or any part of the system leaves its mark and loss of function as to location and the severity of the i n j u r y, so frequently these penetrating injuries cause infections and suppuration. Naturally all penetrating wounds must be regarded as serious and the proper amount of care taken with early advise of removing the injured eye to avoid sympathetic ophthalmia if indicated. It behooves us to make a careful examination of any eye, even though so trivially injured, apparently as now since we have a corporation commission there are those claiming not only previous scars and diseases to have been recent so that we are called in court to be placed on the spot by these attorneys pro or con and even a small bruise may cause later a detachment of the retina as I have found from experience, after the case has been settled, patient apparently having no loss of vision for months afterward.

After this preamble I will endeavor to bring this paper up to date. In this day of mechanical devices doing so much of our work it is necessary that the eye be in as nearly perfect condition as possible. And to go a step farther there is the automobile, a necessity, trucks and cars going every where, moving rapidly so that any latent hyperopia or muscular unbalance must be corrected to avoid the strain and tired feeling produced by the long tedious drives, which in a flash, may cause a disastrous wreck and it should be only a short time until no driver will be permitted on the highway who does not have sufficient and stabilized vision for the safety of himself and others.

Examination of eyes for aviation has become increasingly important since flying has become more universal. Most nations have enormous air corps and since the speed of the airplane is now at the rate of 300 feet per second, in military operations, quick and a c c u r a t e eye sight is equally as important as in private or commercial f l y i n g from the standpoint of making safe take offs, landings, and in formation flying. In combat the "speck on the sun," as stated by one war ace may prove to be an enemy airplane necessitating a fight within the next few minutes.

Military operations may succeed or fail from no other cause than improper knowledge of terrain due to poor observation or inability to take proper pictures. Of course, in bombing quick and accurate eye sight is always very important.

In every day life the necessity for quick and accurate eye sight is especially important to all when you consider the rapid transportation by autos and airplanes and the careless driving which is seen daily on the highways.

While the exceptional pilot is sometimes found who can fly with one poor eye or with poor muscular balance, as for instance, Wiley Post, who never could receive a Department of Commerce license because of visual defect. Also a famous war ace who flies with one eye has a handicap in case of an accident to that eye.

Early in the World War, b e c a u s e air pilots were so few, the British army investigated the cause of many accidents and found that out of 100 crashes 90 were due to defective pilots, two to the enemy and eight to mechanical defects. After organizing a medical examining corps and elimination of epileptics, blind and mentally and physically inadept men from flying this mortality was cut to only 32 per 100 in the first year. Out of some million of military flyers in the United States air service in recent years there has only been one accident due to physical or mental defects of the pilot.

When the United States entered the war we had a medical aviation school of Eastern Specialists who, t h r o u g h extensive study of the pilots, both good and bad, devised the physical examination for aviators called 609. This has been largely used by practically every civilized nation in the world with very little change.

(Wilmer, Ike Jones, Col. Lester, Dr. Snyder, who worked out the physical defects of the air to know how the high and low altitudes affect the eyes.)

Limiting ourselves to the discussion of the eye the examination becomes important to eliminate all disease and major as well as minor defects. The examination goes further in search for latent tendencies which, under stress, strain and fatigue, will become aggravated and may be the cause of an accident. As, for instance, a man with apparent normal distance vision cannot receive a license in the army if he has normal muscular balance but is found under the prism test to have weak muscles which, under fatigue, may develop into diplopia which is a c o m m o n cause of crashes in making landings. Eye fatigue in recent years has become one of the important subjects of research for the air license because the pilot flying at 250 to 300 miles per hour has to be constantly on the alert for other people, for emergency landing fields, and has to be able to see clearly and quickly as many as 85 instruments or dials on his instrument panels. All applicants are examined under complete mydriatic to bring out all latent defects.

Since it is to the advantage of the air forces in time of war and to the commercial licensed pilot in time of peace to fly at a high altitude because of cross currents the effect on the pilot, his eye fatigue and general nervous instability, has become increasingly important.

Eye and nerve changes will d e v e l o p more rapidly under low oxygen at high altitude if the pilot is in any stage of fatigue or acidosis, or fatigue before starting. This exposure to the low oxygen accounts for an accident to pilots who have flown over the same course many times previously.

Muscular balance, depth perception or distance judgment is a necessity in all and any kind of flying.

It is very evident that the diseased eye or one with poor vision is a definite handicap to flying. This has been recognized by many states which require acute vision tests and good v i s i o n before issuing a driver's license for automobiles.

The stress and strain of flying, especially at low oxygen, in the high altitude on the normal eye is very difficult to overcome and practically impossible for one having diseased or weakened eyes of any kind.

In conclusion the necessity of eye examinations by the use of the opthalmoscope is recognized as a means of diagnosing by every recognized school of today. All students are required to become familiar with its use and now you will see the surgeon obstetrician, neurologist, general medicine and urologist examining for eye changes, looking for disease and changes which may be produced by certain drugs, such as arsenic, quinine or diseases of pregnancy, kidney troubles, tuberculosis, syphilis and the different variety of interocular tumors and pressures of tumors of the brain, systemic diseases and disturbance of the circulatory system, auto intoxication, drug poisonings and nervous symptoms, headaches, irritable s t o m a c h and system should be eliminated or proven by a careful eye examination. No eye should ever be tested for lenses without an opthalmoscopic examination.

––––––––o––––––––

Typhoid Pyelonephritis, Renal Typhoid Fever

Hobart A. Reimann, Philadelphia (Journal A. M. A., Aug. 20, 1938), cites a case of typhoid pyelonephritis presenting systemic symptoms and signs of typhoid lasting 47 days; the clinical features were remarkable in that no symptoms referable to the intestinal tract were observed. The main interest centered about the typhoid state with threatened uremia and evidence of retention of metabolites, typhoid bacilluria, pyuria, hematuria and pain in the right lumbar region, which were present as early as the eighth day of illness. The patient recovered, but pyuria, bacilluria and hematuria persisted. Typhoid bacilli disappeared from the urine after the administration of mandelic acid. Evidence of active renal disease ten months after the acute attack supports the growing mass of evidence that renal infections, particularly in childhood, must be looked on as a cause of subsequent kidney disease. Whether chronic nephritis and hypertension will eventually develop in this case can be determined only by future examination. It is important to establish etiologic diagnosis promptly in all cases of acute or chronic pyelonephritis, since there is no doubt that patients like the one described may serve as a dangerous source of infection to others if proper precautions are not taken to sterilize the urine before its disposal.

––––––––o––––––––

"Is This Product Council-Accepted?"

This is the first question many physicians ask the detail man, when a new product is presented.

If the detail man answers, "No," the doctor saves time by saying, "Come around again when the Council accepts your product."

If the detail man answers, "Yes," the doctor knows that the composition of the product has been carefully verified, and that members of the Council have scrutinized the label, weighed the evidence, checked the claims, and agreed that the product merits the confidence of the physicians. The doctor can ask his own questions, and make his own decision about using the product, but not only has he saved himself a vast amount of time but he has derived the benefit of a fearless, expert, fact-finding body whose sole function is to protect him and his patient.

No one physician, even if he were qualified, could afford to devote so much time and study to every new product. His Council renders this service for him, freely. Nowhere else in the world is there a group that performs the function so ably served by the Council on Pharmacy and Chemistry and the Council on Foods.

Mead Johnson & Company cooperates with both Councils, not because we have to but because we want to. Our detail men can always answer you, "Yes, this Mead Product is Council-Accepted."

Mead Johnson & Company, Evansville, Ind., U. S. A.

THE JOURNAL
OF THE
Oklahoma State Medical Association
Issued Monthly at McAlester, Oklahoma, under direction of the Council.

Copyright, 1938, by Oklahoma State Medical Association, McAlester, Oklahoma.

Vol XXXI	SEPTEMBER	Number 9

DR. L. S. WILLOUR..............................Editor-in-Chief
McAlester, Oklahoma

DR. T. H. McCARLEY..............................Associate Editor
McAlester, Oklahoma

Entered at the Post Office at McAlester, Oklahoma, as second-class matter under the act of March 3rd, 1879.

This is the official Journal of the Oklahoma State Medical Association. All communications should be addressed to The Journal of the Oklahoma State Medical Association, McAlester Clinic, McAlester, Oklahoma. $4.00 per year; 40c per copy.

The editorial department is not responsible for the opinions expressed in the original articles of contributors.

Reprints of original articles will be supplied at actual cost provided request for them is attached to manuscripts or made in sufficient time before publication.

Articles sent this Journal for publication and all those read at the annual meetings of the State Association are the sole property of this Journal. The Journal relies on each individual contributor's strict adherence to this well-known rule of medical journalism. In the event an article sent this Journal for publication is published before appearance in The Journal the manuscript will be returned to the writer.

Failure to receive The Journal should call for immediate notification of the Editor, McAlester Clinic, McAlester, Oklahoma.

Local news of possible interest to the medical profession, notes on removals, changes of addresses, births, deaths and weddings will be gratefully received.

Advertising of articles, drugs or compounds unapproved by the Council on Pharmacy of the A. M. A., will not be accepted.

Advertising rates will be supplied on application.

It is suggested that wherever possible members of the State Association should patronize our advertisers in preference to others as a matter of fair reciprocity.

Printed by News-Capital Company, McAlester.

EDITORIAL

BEWARE OF FALSE GODS!*

AN EDITORIAL FROM THE KANSAS CITY MEDICAL JOURNAL, AUGUST, 1938

If you are not familiar with the impending investigation of the A.M.A. at Washington, it is just that you have not read the recent issues of your own J.A.M.A. or you have not picked up the papers from the front lawn. The build-up of the government to dissipate and dilute the influence of the A.M.A. is showing progress in all directions. Members who have never participated in the o r g a n i z a t i o n and progress of the medical profession have

*From the Journal of the American Medical Association, August 20, 1938, Vol. III, No. 8.

been uncovered and minority groupings in different thought channels have been encouraged to display their antipathy. The barrage has been amplified by a t t a c k s from different bureaus and departments of the government. The scare and the threat of the law and the grand jury has not been overlooked.

The unfortunate part about the present situation is that while all of these attacks have some small elements of fact, when combined they tend to obscure the great values for the good of the whole people which organization in the profession has established. Enough wolves nipping at the heels and annoying a strong man will wear down any enthusiasm for existence.

One may declare a vacation for tradition for a period of time. One may wink at ethics for another period. One may argue that public policy demands a cessation of standards. Some may insist that it is not necessary to balance the science and the art of medicine. There is no doubt but that you can tear down the structure of better and honest medicine in America if the fitness of change in the house of medicine is not judged by the profession itself. It is notorious that laymen are not able to choose medical attention or rather health attention by any measure of their judgment.

Only as the medical profession, through organized medicine and the A.M.A., has erected standards of medical education, eliminated quackery, qualified specialists and criticized hospital methods, etc., has the quality of medical practice of America developed. There has never been any police power to the A.M.A. There have never been any laws conferring any measure of p e n a l t y or legal action by the A.M.A. There has never been any big boss such as o t h e r groupings in business and sports have devised.

All of the progress of American medicine has been through the better education of physicians, through the moral persuasion of the Councils of the A.M.A. and through the traditional application of ethical standards. Such means are bound always to have more weight than mere laws. Public opinion has supported these various items of progress and gradually the quackery and charlatanism of A m e r i c a has faded into disrepute.

Medical schools with their huge establishments may feel that they are peculiarly fitted to practice mass medicines with governmental subsidies. L a r g e non-profit metropolitan and even smaller hospitals may feel that they are ordained through the merit of their physical establishments to be the center for medical and health needs of their communities.

These modern factors of civilization and progress are prone to forget that it is really the personality and peerage of their medical staff that establishes their fame and their clientele. It is now apparent that even the physicians who staff such institutions sometimes arrogate to themselves an u n u s u a l ability to serve the people. Physicians in groups promptly believe that in their small union rests the local tenens of Aesculapian lore.

All these things may be true. But one must realize that only a small minority of all the people can take advantage of such institutions and such groupings. The great majority of p e o p l e scattered over the country must be taken care of by the physicians of their locality. The quality of such medical care can only be maintained by supporting the progressive type of physician who keep up with the times and who does not indulge in unethical methods or tamper with traditional items of good medical manners. It is further maintained by a better distribution of well educated physicians.

These factors of medical progress are maintained by the inherent good will and the promotion of better standards by the Councils of the A.M.A. and other national medical organizations. If you dissipate the influence behind these standards, you are cutting out the foundations that are responsible for better medicine for all the people in America. One should not listen to the sirens who will cheer on those who are willing to scuttle the ship. Hold fast to those things that are good! Beware of false gods!

—E. H. S.

HELPFUL POSTGRADUATE COURSES

Reports from the f i e l d on the Post-Graduate Program in Obstetrics are that the second circuit was completed in southeastern Oklahoma Friday night, August 26. The centers of this circuit were Poteau,

McAlester, D u r a n t, Hugo, and Idabel. Seventy-seven physicians in the s o u t h-eastern counties registered and completed the course. The number of practicing physicians in some of these counties is sparse, and we consider this a record enrollment.

In addition to the practical instruction being given .by Dr. Edward N. Smith, the Instructor, doctors are reporting that the private consultations are, from a teaching angle, some of the most valuable h e l p s they have received in any form of postgraduate study. Many state they regret seeing the course closed, and wish that it could go on indefinitely.

The next circuit will be confined to the mideastern section of the state, and will include Tulsa, Muskogee, Okmulgee, Shawnee, and Ada. The instruction will open in early September in these centers. The Course lasts ten weeks, and the fee is only $5.00. This is the most economical postgraduate study that doctors of Oklahoma will probably ever receive. Doctors may correspond or enroll in advance for the course, and the Committee solicits your cooperation.

All correspondonce should be addressed to Dr. Henry H. Turner, Chairman, Committee on Post-Graduate Medical Teaching, 304 Osler Building, Oklahoma City.

INVESTIGATE BEFORE YOU BUY

Apparently the doctors of Oklahoma are being swindled by a concern known as the Underwriters Service Bureau of Philadelphia. They have been investigated by the Merchants Protective Credit Association of Elk City, Oklahoma, and by reading the following telegrams you will be informed as to this swindle.

Better Business Bureau, Philadelphia Penn.: Can you recommend Underwriters Service Bureau Morris Building Philadelphia selling doctors listing service for twenty-five dollars as reliable? Telegraph immediately collect. Merchants Protective Credit Association, Elk City, Oklahoma.

Merchants Protective Credit Association, Elk City, Okla.: Have received many complaints against Underwriters Service Bureau. Understand they have recently moved without leaving forwarding address. The Better Business Bureau of Philadelphia, Inc.

HOUSE OF DELEGATES

A special meeting of the House of Delegates of the American Medical Association has been called to meet in Chicago at 10 a.m., September 16, 1938. The official call states the business to be transacted at this special session will be limited to consideration of the medical health problems submitted to the National Health Conference recently held in Washington and to such other matters as may be submitted to the House of Delegates by the Board of Trustees.

This will be a very important meeting and the membership of our State Association will be advised as to these transactions as soon as possible.

COUNTY POSTGRADUATE COURSES IN VENEREAL DISEASE

The Oklahoma State Health Department announces through Chas. M. Pearce, M.D., Commissioner of Health, that postgraduate courses in venereal disease will start Monday, October 3, in Rogers county, running every Monday through the month. Courses in Osage county start Tuesday, October 4, running every Tuesday up to November 1. Courses in Washington county start October 5, running every Wednesday through November 2. Courses in C r a i g county start October 6, running through every Thursday until November 3.

Lectures will be held in Rogers county at C l a r e m o r e, Craig county at Vinita, Washington county at Bartlesville, Ottawa county at Miami, Osage county at Pawhuska. These courses will be given without cost to the physicians and will be conducted by Dr. David V. Hudson.

U n d e r the LaFollette-Bulwinkle Bill each State receives its pro rata share of funds for venereal disease control according to population. A certain amount of these funds is to be spent for educational purposes; therefore, our setup consists of one consultant, Dr. David V. Hudson; one director, Dr. Vance F. Morgan; two epidemiologists, Dr. Louis Dakil, (one to be named); two publicity men, William Riddle and Jack Muller.

These courses will be given until the entire state is covered. The president and secretary of each county medical society will be notified in advance as to when lectures will be held and will be contacted by one of the men in this setup some several weeks before the course begins. These courses are limited to M.D.'s only.

As in the past, arsenicals will be furnished to all ethical practicing physicians in the state of Oklahoma for the care of indigent patients on requisition through the local county health superintendent. Indigent patients are classed as to the amount that can be paid by such patients. We want every physician to get what he can out of the patient for treatment, but we consider that a patient who can pay more than $1.00 for a treatment should not be classed as indigent.

LEGAL DEFINITION OF "DOCTOR"

The following is a copy of a letter from the State Board of Medical Examiners written by the Attorney General of the State of Oklahoma, g i v i n g his opinion relative to the law concerning the "Indian Herb Doctor," or any "herb doctor" or doctor who administers simple remedies. This opinion is published in full for your information and should it be applicable to anyone in your County you may know now how to proceed.

Dr. J. D. Osborn, Jr., Secretary
State Board of Medical Examiners
Frederick, Oklahoma.

Dear Sir:

The Attorney General acknowledges receipt of your letter dated August 10, 1938, wherein you ask:

1. If a person, commonly referred to as an "Indian herb doctor" or an "herb doctor" or a "doctor who administers simple remedies" who has never been licensed under the laws of this State to practice any branch of the healing art but who has been registered by the Basic Science Board under the last proviso of Section 19, Article 28, Chapter 24, Oklahoma Session Laws, 1936-37 (commonly called the Basic Science Law) has the right to treat disease, injury, or deformity of person by drugs of any kind, whether derived from herbs or otherwise, *for compensation?*

2. Would the Attorney General's answer to the above question be the same in the event said person makes no specific charge for his services but does charge for the medicine prescribed and furnished by him?

In reply to your *first question,* you are advised that the material part of Section 4635, Oklahoma Statutes 1931, (same being a part of Chapter 59, Oklahoma Session Laws 1923) is as follows:

"Every person shall be regarded as practicing medicine within the meaning and provisions of this Act, who shall append to his name the letters 'M.D.,' 'Doctor,' 'Professor,' 'Specialist,' 'P h y s i c i a n,' or any other title, letters or designation which represent that such person is a physician, *or who shall for a fee or compensation treat disease, injujry or deformity of persons by any drugs,* surgery, manual or mechanical treatment *whatsoever."*

Section 4634, Oklahoma Statutes 1931, is in part as follows:

"Every person b e f o r e practicing medicine and surgery or any of the b r a n c h e s or departments of such, within the meaning of this Act, (meaning as defined in Section 4635, supra) within the State of Oklahoma, must be in legal possession of the unrevoked license or certificate herein provided for, and any person so practicing in such manner within this State, who is not in such legal possession thereof, shall be guilty of a misdemeanor, and shall, upon conviction thereof, in any court having jurisdiction, be fined for the first offense in any sum not less than One Hundred ($100.00) Dollars, and not more than Five H u n d r e d ($500.00) Dollars, . . ."

In the case of Reeves v. State, 36 Okla. Cr. 186, 253 Pac. 510, the fourth paragraph of the syllabus is as follows:

"Section 12, c. 59, Session Laws 1923, which provides that every person shall be regarded as practicing medicine within the meaning and provision of that act who shall append to his name the letters, 'M.D.,' 'Doctor,' 'Professor,' 'Specialist,' 'Physician,' or any other title, l e t t e r s, or designation which represent that such person is a physician, is an expression of the legislative intent, broadening the meaning of the words, 'Practicing Medicine.' The acts forbidden, in a substantial sense, amount to a practice of medicine or an assuming to practice medicine. Such section is not invalid as creating a conclusive presumption or an unreasonable prima facie presumption."

In the case of Needham et al. v. State, 55 Okla. Cr. 430, 32 Pac. (2d) 92, it was held that when an unlicensed person assisted a licensed physician in treating diseases for compensation, both violated Sections 4634 and 4635, supra.

In the case of Holt v. State, 51 Okla. Cr. 263, 300 Pac. 430, the Criminal Court of Appeals held that the evidence in said case was sufficient to sustain conviction for practicing medicine without a license or certificate from the State Board of Medical Examiners. In this c o n n e c t i o n it should be noted that said evidence was summarized by the court as follows:

"The evidence of the state was that the defendant represented himself as superintendent of an institution known and designated as 'Utilitarian Vitality Unity, A Mutual Cooperative Health Society'; that he issued numerous advertisements of this institution, one of which was received by the prosecuting witness, Mrs. Mitchell; that she entered into a contract with the defendant, and paid him $100 cash, and took the treatments given her by defendant; that *defendant charged the prosecuting witness for medicine;* and that defendant possessed no license to practice medicine."

By an examination of the Basic Science Law, supra, referred to by you, it will be found that the purpose thereof is to require applicants for examination before the examining boards of the various branches of the healing art, to *first* take and pass an examination in the basic sciences before the Basic Science Board. After the applicant passes said preliminary examination he is given by said board "a certificate of ability" in the basic sciences, which, *if he is otherwise qualified,* when presented to the examining board of the branch of the healing art in which the applicant desires to obtain a license, will entitle him to be examined by said board, and, upon his successfully passing the examination thereof, to be issued a license to practice said branch of the healing art, thereby.

Section 19 of said Basic Science Law, after making c e r t a i n exceptions to the provisions of said law not material here, states:

"It is expressly provided that the provisions of this Act shall not apply to Indian Herb Doctors, Herb Doctors or Doctors who administer s i m p l e remedies who register with this Board within sixty (60) days after the passage of this Act and who have practiced in Oklahoma for two (2) years."

Under the above proviso, what is designated as an Indian herb doctor, an herb doctor, or a doctor who administers simple remedies and who has practiced as such in Oklahoma for at least two years, if he registers with the Basic Science Board within 60 days after the passage of the Basic Science Law, is made eligible, *if he is otherwise qualified*, to take an examination befor the examining board of any branch of the healing art (such as Medicine and Surgery, Chiropractice, and Osteopathy), without first securing a certificate of ability from the Basic Science Board. This is the only effect of said proviso.

It is therefore the opinion of the Attorney General that under the facts set forth in your first question a person such as is mentioned by you *does not now and never has had the right* to treat disease, injury or deformity by drugs of any kind, whether derived from herbs or otherwise, for compensation.

In answer to your *second question,* you are advised that in an opinion dated October 15, 1932, addressed to the Hon. Hiram A. Butler, County Attorney, Boise City, Oklahoma, the Attorney General held that a person is practicing medicine for compensation if he receives remuneration for his services "consisting of free-will offerings," and cited in support of said holding the case of Singh v. State, (Texas) 146 S. W. 891, the thirteenth paragraph of the syllabus thereof being as follows:

"Under Acts 30th Leg. c. 123, prohibiting any person from practicing medicine for compensation received, directly or indirectly, without a license, proof that defendant did not charge for his services directly, but told all who applied for treatment that he would receive from them 'free-will offerings,' and that he actually did receive pay from patients, was sufficient to show that he practiced medicine for compensation."

In the case of Harris v. State, 41 Okla. Cr. 221, 271 Pac. 263, it is stated:

"The prosecution is under the Medical Practice Art (chapter 59, Session Laws 1923). The information charges that defendant, without having a license or certificate to practice medicine and surgery, did treat and prescribe as physician and surgeon to Velma Weidman, and for compensation, certain drugs for an a l l e g e d tumor. . . .

"In enacting this law, the Legislature evidently intended to prevent persons not properly educated in the science of medicine and not properly licensed from acting or assuming to act as a physician or surgeon and to protect the public from quacks, humbugs, and charlatans who so often prey upon the public, pretending to have marvelous remedies or pretending to cure incurable diseases.

"By c r o s s - examination defendant sought to show that the charge of $125 was for the preparation of 'oil of radium' only; that defendant made no charge for any advice or examination. He argues that it is no violation of law for any person to sell medicine in his home, and that the evidence does not sustain the charge. This contention cannot be sustained. It is evident that the physical examination, the pretended diagnosis, and the imposing on the credulity of the patient by the sale of a worthless preparation for $125 constitutes but a single transaction, and while it is probably true that at the time defendant informed his patient he was charging the $125 for the two bottles of drugs and not for the examination and diagnosis, this does not alter the situation. The entire transaction is a practice of medicine within the definition of the Medical Practice Act. The fact that defendant informed his patient at the time that this charge was for the pretended m e d i c i n e is plainly but a subterfuge to avoid the provisions of the law."

In the case of Tucker et al. v. Williamson et al., 229 Fed. 201, the third paragraph of the syllabus is as follows:

"Under Gen. Code Ohio, 1286, a person who examines patients, diagnoses their diseases, and then prescribes and sells his own proprietary remedies is engaged in the practice of medicine, although his ostensible and apparent motive may be the sale of his medicines, and he is subject to the laws of the state regulating such practice."

Attention is called to the following cases which are in harmony with the cases last above cited, to-wit, State v. Van Doren (N. C.), 14 S. E. 32; Underwood v. Scott (Kansas), 23 Pac. 942, and Katsafaros v. Agathakas (Ohio), 3 N. E. (2d) 810.

Therefore, in answer to your second question, you are advised that under the authorities above set forth the Attorney General is of the opinion that the mere fact the person mentioned by you makes no specific charge for his services, but does charge for the medicine prescribed and furnished by him, does not prevent him from unlawfully practicing medicine for compensation within the meaning of Section 4643 and 4635, Oklahoma Statutes 1931. Your second question is, therefore, answered in the negative. You will also note from the Reeves case, supra, that if said person appends to his name the word "Doctor," such fact also constitutes a violation of said sections. Furthermore, if the person mentioned by you is not registered and licensed under the provisions of Sections 4696 and 4697, Oklahoma Statutes 1931, relating to the practice of pharmacy, he is subject to the penalties provided in the pharmacy law.

Yours very truly,

FOR THE ATTORNEY GENERAL
FRED HANSEN,
Assistant Attorney General.

Approved in Conference 8-17-38.

Editorial Notes—Personal and General

DR. AND MRS. JOHN S. PINE, Oklahoma City, have returned from Havana, Cuba, to Florida and will spend some time motoring there and in other southern states.

DR. AND MRS. JOSEPH W. KELSO have returned from Corydon, Iowa, where they visited Dr. Kelso's family.

DR. GERALD ROGERS, Oklahoma City, announces the removal of his office from 404 to 328 Osler Building. His practice is limited to obstetrics and gynecology.

DR. AND MRS. ALLEN R. RUSSELL, McAlester, and daughter, Betty Sue, spent two weeks in August in Little Rock, Hot Springs and Memphis.

DR. AND MRS. P. K. GRAENING and children, Oklahoma City, have moved to Waverly, Iowa, where they will establish their home.

DRS. E. H. SHULLER and L. S. WILLOUR and

their families, McAlester, spent a week in August at Roarin' River, Mo.

County Health Superintendent Appointments

Dr. James O. Hood, Norman, Cleveland County.

Dr. F. S. Hassler, Muskogee, Muskogee County.

Dr. Hood fills the place with the City-County Health Unit which was resigned by Dr. Guy H. Williams. Dr. Hassler was appointed director of the full-time City-County Health Unit which was organized July 1, 1938.

International Assembly

The twenty-third International Assembly of the Inter-State Postgraduate Medical Association of North America will be held in the public auditorium of Philadelphia, Pennsylvania, October 31, November 1, 2, 3 and 4, 1938. All scientific and clinical sessions will take place in the auditorium. Hotel headquarters will be the Benjamin Franklin Hotel.

The members of the medical profession of Philadelphia are correlating for the clinics, an abundance of hospital material representing various types of pathological conditions which will be discussed by the contributors to the program.

In the neighborhood of 80 distinguished teachers and clinicians will appear on the program, a tentative list of which may be found on page XIII of the advertising section of this Journal. The subjects and speakers have been selected to consider practically all the subjects of greatest interest to the medical profession in general.

A full program of scientific and clinical sessions will take place every day and evening of the Assembly starting each morning at 8 o'clock. On account of the fullness of the program, restaurant service will be available at the auditorium at moderate prices.

The members of the profession are urged to bring their ladies with them as a very excellent program is being arranged for their benefit by the ladies' committee. Philadelphia has many places of historic and other interests, which will make this year's program especially attractive to them.

Pre-assembly and post-assembly clinics will be held in the Philadelphia Hospitals on Saturday, October 29, and Saturday, November 5.

It is very important that you make your hotel reservations early by writing Mr. Thomas E. Willis, Chairman of the Hotel Committee, Chamber of Commerce Building, 12th and Walnut streets, Philadelphia, Pa.

The Association, through its officers and members of the program committee, extend a very hearty invitation to all members of the profession in good standing in their State and Provincial Societies to attend the Assembly. The registration fee is $5.00.

Dr. Elliott P. Joslin, President, Boston, Mass.

Dr. George W. Crile, Chairman Program Committee, Cleveland, Ohio.

Dr. William B. Peck, Managing-Director, Freeport, Illinois.

ADDITIONS TO ROSTER

Johnston County
CLARK, GUY L. ....Milburn

LeFlore County
BEVILLE, S. D. ....Poteau
LOWRY, R. W. ....Poteau
ROLLE, NEESON ....Poteau

Logan County
MEAD, W. W. ....Guthrie

Kay County
YEARY, G. H. ....Newkirk

Okfuskee County
BLOSS, JR., CLAUDE M. ....Okemah

Payne County
WRIGHT, J. M. ....Stillwater

OBITUARIES

DOCTOR FRANCIS BARTOW FITE

Dr. F. B. Fite, Muskogee, died at his home, August 13, 1938, after a long illness.

He was the second in three generations of physicians, coming to Indian Territory as a young man and almost alone sponsoring growth of the medical profession in this vast wilderness. He was founder of the first hospital in Muskogee; one of the founders of the Indian Territory Medical Association, being president in 1893.

Dr. Fite was born near Cartersville, Bartow County, Georgia, October 17, 1861. His father was Dr. Henderson W. Fite, who served as surgeon of the 40th Georgia regiment, Confederate army, during the Civil War. Dr. Fite's early education was received in the public and private schools near his boyhood home. He later entered Pine Log Academy at Pine Log, Georgia. At the age of 19 he began the study of medicine with his brother, Dr. R. L. Fite, and his half-brother, Dr. J. A. Thompson, at Tahlequah. In 1884 he returned to Georgia and entered the Southern Medical College at Atlanta. This institution is now Emory Medical College. He graduated in 1886 with high honors, receiving the class medal. In 1886 he returned to Tahlequah where he first began practicing with his brother, Dr. R. L. Fite, but in 1888 he went to New York where he took extensive post graduate work.

On November 1, 1889, he established his office in Muskogee, and in 1893, he formed a partnership with Dr. J. D. Blakemore and the late Claude A. Thompson.

The Fite Clinic was established in 1923 with his son, Dr. W. Pat Fite. Later another son, Halsell, joined the organization.

Dr. Fite was a member of the International Association of Railroad Surgeons; the Oklahoma State Medical Association; the American Medical Association; North Texas Medical Association and a Fellow of the American College of Surgeons. He was a member of the First Methodist Episcopal Church, South, and a charter member of St. Paul's M.E.S. Church. He was also a member of Muskogee Commandery of the Knights Templar; Independent Order of Odd Fellows, and the Benevolent and Protective Order of Elks.

Dr. Fite is survived by the widow, four sons, Drs. Wm. P. and Halsell Fite; Julian Fite, an attorney, all of Muskogee; Francis Bartow Fite, Jr., an attorney of Seattle, Washington, and a daughter, Mrs. Frances Fite Ambrister.

Funeral services were held at St. Paul's Methodist Church, with Dr. L. S. Barton officiating. Interment in Greenhill Cemetery.

This ends the career of one of the pioneer practitioners of Indian Territory, a man who has done much for his profession and the people of his state.

DOCTOR WALTER N. JOHN

Dr. W. N. John, born at Galveston, Texas, May 18, 1871, died August 15, 1938, following a long illness.

His early education was received at Nashville, Tenn., completing his high school education in that city. He then entered Texas University, graduating from the medical department, May 1, 1894. The following year he spent as an interne at the John Seely Hospital, Galveston, and in October, 1894, he located at Nelson, Indian Territory, as physician to the Choctaw School Spencer Academy. When this school burned in 1897, he remained at Nelson, doing private practice until 1902, moving to Antlers Jack Fort, now in Pushmataha County. In 1908 he moved to Hugo and became County Health officer and surgeon for the Frisco railroad.

Dr. John was a Royal Arch Mason, an Odd Fellow, a Pretorian and a Maccabee; a member of the Woodmen of the World and Modern Woodmen of America, and charter member of the Hugo Lions Club. He was a member of his County Medical Society, the State and National Medical Associations.

Dr. John is survived by his widow and four daughters.

Interment was in Mount Olivet Cemetery, Hugo.

DOCTOR FREDRICK L. SMITH

Dr. F. L. Smith, pioneer physician of McIntosh County, died August 22, 1938, at his home in Eufaula. He was born in Florida in 1867 and came to Oklahoma long before statehood. For many years he resided at Fame, a small town west of Eufaula, but was a resident of Eufaula for the past seven years. He was a member of the City Council and Eufaula Masonic Lodge No. 1. He was a member of his County, State and National Medical organizations.

Dr. Smith is survived by his widow and one son and daughter. Interment was in the Eufaula Cemetery.

---o---

Ruch, Walter A.: Analgesia During the First Stage of Labor. Am. J. of Obst. & Gyn., 35:830-834, (May) 1938.

In this series of 755 obstetric cases, Ruch has reported on the effects of a combination of Dilaudid 1/32 grain and scopolamine 1/130 grain used for first stage analgesia. Also, an analysis was made of the possible effect of ethylene, nitrous oxide, ether and other drugs used for second stage anesthesia on the condition of the baby.

By far, most of the mothers obtained good analgesia from the Dilaudid-scopolamine combination. Apnoea in the infants was of no great consequence in most cases, as they responded to minor resuscitation procedures, such as rubbing of the back, thumping of the feet, and began to breathe very quickly after mucous had been removed from the throat. The incidence of asphyxia was slightly greater when ether was used for second stage anesthesia. The only cases of deep asphyxia (three in all) which occurred followed the use of the latter anesthetic. There were three stillborn babies, one of which had an intracranial hemorrhage following a rapid second stage in a multipara; the other two were stillborn as a result of a prolonged period of "molding" in primiparae.

Several of the babies were X-rayed on the second day of life to determine whether or not they had an enlarged thymus gland. Some of these mothers had entered the hospital too late for semi-narcosis, but others were included in the series. In the 378 cases examined by X-ray, it is found that atelectasis was present in 24 of the babies, but only one of the babies showed any active symptoms. The lungs were completely expanded at the end of three to five days in all except four or five babies. Several of the babies who showed slight atelectasis in the X-ray picture from mothers who had no semi-narcosis during the first stage.

Ruch concludes his report: "In a series of 755 cases, 1/32 grain of Dilaudid and 1/130 grain of scopolamine proved to be a satisfactory combination for the production of semi-narcosis during the first stage of labor, providing a pleasing analgesia for the mother with little, if any, effect on the baby. In some cases a small dose of one of the barbiturates was administered in conjunction with Dilaudid-scopolamine analgesia. When ethylene or nitrous oxide was used for anesthesia in the second and third stages, apnoea occurred in only 4.2 per cent of the babies. With ether, respiratory difficulty was encountered more frequently."

ABSTRACTS : REVIEWS : COMMENTS
and CORRESPONDENCE

SURGERY AND GYNECOLOGY

Abstracts, Reviews and Comments from
LeRoy Long Clinic
714 Medical Arts Building, Oklahoma City

Modified Double Enterostomy (Mikulicz) in Radical Surgical Treatment of Intussusception in Children. By Barnes Woodhall, Durham, N. C. Archives of Surgery, June, 1938.

The author says that the procedure which he reports was previously advocated by Dr. Dean Lewis, Johns Hopkins Hospital, Baltimore, Lewis "stressing particularly the control of intestinal obstruction and the protection from extensive fluid loss gained by its use."

After referring to eight types of surgical operations proposed and done by as many different surgeons, the conclusion is that none has been as satisfactory as that advocated by Lewis. In discussing it he says, "The optimal surgical technic for the treatment of irreducible or gangrenous intussusception occuring in early life should insure the following essential points: (1) rapidity of execution; (2) complete removal of the irreducible or gangrenous bowel; (3) control of the concomitant intestinal obstruction; (4) control of the loss of fluid, and (5) restoration of the continuity of the intestinal canal."

There are two case reports. The first patient was a white male child 10 months of age. Illness had lasted about 72 hours and was characterized by vomiting and intermittent severe cramp-like abdominal pain. There had been much blood in the stool after an enema on second day. A physician prescribed castor oil, child became much worse— vomiting, massive bloody stools.

On admission to hospital about 72 hours after onset pulse 140, respiration 28, temperature 98, W.B.C. 12,000, Hgb. 96 per cent, well nourished but dehydrated. "The abdominal wall was soft and relaxed, with evidence of intraabdominal distention. There was a readily palpable mass extending from the right lower quadrant of the abdomen to the costal margin on the right side and thence across to the midepigastrium." It was not possible to feel the mass per rectum, but the examining finger was smeared with blood.

After consultation 150 cc. of 5 per cent dextrose solution was given intravenously, blood grouped and matched for a transfusion and patient sent to surgery for immediate operation.

"The operation consisted of resection of an irreducible and gangrenous intussusception and a double enterostomy with lateral anastomosis.

"After anesthesia had been induced with ether by the drop method, the child's abdomen was cleaned with a 3.5 per cent solution of iodine followed by 70 per cent alcohol and was draped in the usual fashion. A long midright rectus incision was made. When the peritoneum was opened, many dilated loops of small intestine presented. A mass could be felt in the right side of the abdominal cavity. With some difficulty, this was brought out into the operative wound for inspection. It consisted of an ileocecal intussusception extending to the middle of the transverse colon. The portion of the large bowel at the ring and the entering ileum were bluish black, dull and obviously gangrenous. Tentative attempts to reduce the intussusception manually by milking the distal end of the mass were futile. Resection was commenced by cutting across the ileum, with the actual cautery between crushing clamps ,at a point 3 cm. from the beginning of the intussusception. The mesentery of the ileum was divided between Kelly clamps. The cecum and the ascending colon were quite mobile, and after incision of the lateral peritoneum the mass was easily retracted mesially, exposing the mesentery of the large bowel. This was clamped and divided. Division of the transverse colon in its midportion completed the resection. The mesenteric vessels were ligated with No. 1 plain catgut sutures. The ends of the bowel, with clamps attached, were exteriorized in the upper angle of the incision, the colonic stoma being uppermost. At the suggestion of Dr. Dean Lewis, an ileocolic lateral anastomosis was performed at a point 8 cm. from the resected ends of the bowel, an outer layer of continuous fine black silk and an inner layer of No. 1 plain catgut being used. The upper peritoneal angle was closed about the exteriorized bowel with interrupted sutures of No. 1 plain catgut. The remainder of the peritoneum was closed with a continuous suture of similar material. Four stay sutures of braided silk were laid. The fascial sheath was closed with interrupted figure-of-eight sutures of No. 0 chromic catgut. The edges of the skin were approximated with interrupted sutures of fine black silk.

"Postoperative Course—The child was given a transfusion immediately after the operation of 100 cc. of citrated blood, and a continuous intravenous 'drip' of 5 per cent dextrose solution and 1.5 per cent saline solution was started. During the evening he vomited, and continuous gastric lavage was instituted. On the following day his condition rapidly improved, and the gastric siphonage was discontinued. On the third day after the operation water by mouth was given. This was followed by vomiting and by increasing abdominal distention, which became so alarming that the ileostomy was opened. Earlier in the day two stools had been passed by rectum. Relief from distention and from vomiting was immediate, and on the following day feeding by mouth was resumed. The parenteral intake of fluids was discontinued. During the next ten days the status quo was maintained, with drainage from the ileostomy and normal stools about equally divided in amount. The ends of the bowel could have been closed at any time, but this step was deferred because of the presence of an infection in the operative wound. Sixteen days after the operation bronchitis and bilateral otitis media developed. Loss of fluid through the ileostomy increased, the child's weight began to decrease, and his condition became progressively more critical. After 24 hours of parenteral intake of fluid the ends of the bowel were inverted with interrupted sutures of fine No. 1 catgut and the skin edges were approximated with silk sutures above the inverted bowel. The improvement after this procedure was dramatic, and the child was discharged on the twenty-eighth day after the operation.

"Pathologic Diagnosis:—The diagnosis was ileo-cecal intussusception with necrosis of bowel."

The second patient was a male child seven months of age, admitted to hospital after 30 hours during which time there had been vomiting, cramp-like pain, blood per rectum. Following is quotation from notes made at time:

"The adbomen is not distended, is soft and is not tender. Just below the umbilicus and slightly to the left of the mid-line a mass can be seen and felt. It is about the size of a peach, is fairly firm and is slightly movable. The baby does not seem to object to palpation. On rectal examination one can feel the mass very plainly, and also a de-pression in the center, which feels like a cervix. No blood is present on the examining finger."

At operation, after 150 c.c. 5 per cent dextrose solution intravenously, and after grouping and matching for transfusion, it was found that there was "a typical ileocecal intussusception, involving the entire large bowel to the rectosigmoid junc-tion." It was possible to do a partial manual re-duction by "milking" but when the last segment was reached it was necessary to incise the intus-suscipiens longitudinally in the manner advised by Brown, after which the mass was forcibly reduced exposing a gangrenous terminal ileum and partial gangrene of cecum and appendix. The operation was completed as in the case of the first patient and the post-operative treatment was practically the same. The ends of the bowel were inverted with interrupted No. 1 plain catgut sutures on the 10th day. There was healing per primam and the patient was discharged cured on the twenty-eighth day after admission.

The summary as written by the author is as fol-lows:

"Resection, or similar radical method, for the treatment of irreducible or gangrenous intussusep-tion occuring in early life has a mortality of 70 per cent. In the two most recent consecutive and suc-cessful resections in the Johns Hopkins Hospital, the usual Mikulicz procedure has been modified by the addition of a lateral anastomosis. In addi-tion to guaranteeing immediate continuity of the lumen of the bowel this technical modification has proved distinctly valuable in controlling the re-sultant intestinal obstruction and fluid loss."

LeRoy Long.

Premenstrual Tension; S. Leon Israel; Journal of the American Medical Association; May 21, 1938; page 1721.

This author treated seven patients with marked premenstrual tension by use of progesterone upon the basis that it was due to defective luteinization with subsequent progestin deficiency or relative hyperestrogenemia.

The seven patients were given one international unit of progesterone intramuscularly daily or every other day during the second half of each men-strual cycle for from two to three months. Five were entirely symptom free and the remaining two noted improvement, but in six of the patients the premenstrual tension returned with withdrawal of treatment. The remaining patient was symptom free as far as premenstrual tension was concerned for two years.

The recurrent instances were treated by roent-gen therapy with low dose irradiation of the pitui-tary gland and ovaries. In all the periodicity of the menstrual cycle was undisturbed and they re-ceived symptomatic relief with the premenstrual tension.

This author, naturally, strongly emphasizes the importance of the most careful application of the roentgen therapy for this symptom. He is unable to explain the functional alterations of the pitui-tary gland and ovaries produced by low dose X-ray.

Comments: Premenstrual tension is entirely sub-jective symptomatology. One would, therefore, feel that the patient suffering from this symptom would require the most careful general physical investi-gation and proper treatment prior to the use of progestin or X-ray for its relief. Also, the degree of debility or in other words the severity of the symptoms would naturally have to be rather mark-ed prior to the tedious, almost purely substitutional progestin therapy or to the rather questionable use of deep X-ray therapy for a symptom of this char-acter.

However, with the proper conscientious complete investigation of the individual and in the instances of very severe premenstrual tension, it is well to have the basis of this work in which substitutional relief can be obtained by the use of progestin dur-ing the last half of the menstrual cycle and that permanent relief was obtained in this series of pa-tients by the employment of properly administered roentgen therapy of the pituitary gland.

Wendell Long.

The Menopause and its Management; Emil Novak; Journal of the American Medical Association; February 26, 1938; page 619.

This is a most excellent article dealing with the management of the menopause which Dr. Novak thinks should be based almost entirely upon the particular woman's entire menopausal syndrome, making it an individual problem in her instance and employing glandular preparations as indicated as an adjunct to the remainder of her medical care. In other words, the simple use of organo-therapy routinely without the combined individual medical attention of the patient is certainly an improper approach to the care of the average woman in the menopause period.

"There are wide variations in character and de-gree of the symptoms presented by menopausal women, depending not only on the severity of the hormonal readjustment but also on such factors as the patient's psychic make-up, her social, in-tellectual and economic status, her family life and her general physical condition. The method of approach must therefore be adapted to the in-dividual case but should always be combined with sympathetic understanding and reassurance and a patient effort to discover, evaluate and adjust such factors as I have mentioned.

"The well known vasomotor group of symptoms are the only ones which seem clearly attributable to the hormonal readjustment of the menopause, though it is possible that others may at times be directly produced. However, the menopausal wo-man may present many other manifestations only indirectly of menopausal significance, and yet often constituting real problems in treatment, which must be along psychic and general rather than endocrine lines. Only a minority of menopausal women need medical treatment, and a much smaller proportion require organotherapy.

"While the mechanism of the vasomotor meno-pausal symptoms is not clear, the immediate factor is quite certainly the cessation of ovarian func-tion, and ovarian therapy with the now available effective preparations of estrogens is a rational procedure. The results are variable, rarely brilliant, but often satisfactory to both patient and physi-cian. Light irradiation of the hypophysis may be tried if organotherapy is unsuccessful, but its too promiscuous use should be decried."

As to the dosage, "In many instances rather small doses of estrogenic substance seem to suffice; in others much larger doses are required. If, for example, intramuscular injections of 2,500 or 5,000 international units of estrogenic substance in oil (such as theelin, amniotin, or progynon-B) do not give relief, the dosage may be increased to 10,000, 20,000 or rarely even 50,000 units.

"The duration of treatment is likewise to be adapted to individual indications. Menopausal symptoms are rarely persistently troublesome, and it is usually only during exacerbations that active hypodermic medication is necessary, and only a few injections may be required. In the intervals the patient may need no medication, or at most the administration of some simple sedative of the bromide or barbituric acid group.

"In other cases the oral administration of an active estrogenic preparation (amniotin, theelin, theelol, progynon-DH) may be necessary and, in fact, the milder forms of disturbance may require nothing more than oral treatment at any time."

Comment: It is evident that it is fallacious to attribute practically all symptoms which occur in women between the ages of 35 and 60 to the menopause and it is equally fallacious to treat practically all symptoms in women in this age group by routine estrogenic administration.

There is no question as to the advantage associated with the proper administration of estrogenic substances in elected patients in the menopause who have vasomotor symptoms and who have been carefully examined with proper treatment of any other physical defects.

The importance Dr. Novak places upon the individualization of examination and treatment of all women in the menopause cannot be too highly regarded if the results of therapy in individual hands of particular women is to be satisfactory.
Wendell Long.

A Consideration of Artificial Fever Therapy and Sulfanilamide Therapy in the Treatment of Gonorrheal Infections of Women. By Randall, Krusen and Bannick, Rochester, Minn. American Journal of Obstetrics and Gynecology, August, 1938.

A group of 37 patients were treated by fever therapy. Thirty-one of these received a single 10 hour session in the fever cabinet. Six were given multiple artificial fever treatments. Thirty-four of the 37 patients treated with fever therapy were found to have consistently negative cultures following treatment. In two cases having positive cultures after fever treatment sulfanilamide was employed and negative cultures were obtained.

Sixteen patients were treated by oral administration of sulfanilamide. Fifteen had consistently negative chocolate blood agar cultures after treatment. The average duration of treatment was 10½ days and the average amount of drug administered was 590 grains with average daily dose of more than 54 grains. The one failure of sulfanilamide treatment was given fever therapy and developed negative cultures.

From their experience these authors feel that gonorrheal infections of the female genital tract should first be treated by the administration of sulfanilamide and when the infections are intractable to this method of treatment, a combination with artificial fever therapy is desirable.

They feel that the greatest care should be employed in the administration of sulfanilamide and that it should be done under the constant supervision and direction of a physician.

They also feel that fever therapy, to be effective, must be most carefully controlled with a well trained team giving the patient constant supervision and careful attention to all details.

Comment: These are amazingly good results. There is no information contained in the article about the average age of the patients and their general physical condition, but it is taken that they were selected patients of reasonably early adult life in otherwise good general physical condition making good risks for strenuous treatment of this character.

My experience with sulfanilamide and fever therapy in the treatment of gonorrheal infections in women is small, but it is quite clear that every possible precaution should be taken in general examinations before sulfanilamide is employed and that the individual should be under constant care during the time that the drug is employed.

It is also my observation that fever therapy should be undertaken as a hospital treatment only and only where there is a trained personnel with a doctor familiar with the entire treatment in direct charge all of the time. The physical equipment is of course necessary but the most careful direction and management of the treatment is essential to avoid injury if not death of the patient.

It would therefore seem wise at this time to consider sulfanilamide in large effective dosages and fever therapy as agencies to employ in the resistant infections rather than in every instance of infection, many of which will respond to other means of treatment satisfactorily.
Wendell Long.

---○---

EYE, EAR, NOSE AND THROAT
Edited by Marvin D. Henley, M.D.
911 Medical Arts Building, Tulsa

Preoperative Management of Acute Streptococcic Mastoiditis. E. Miles Atkinson, M.D., F.R.C.S. (Eng.), New York. Archives of Otolaryngology, July, 1938.

Ambroise Pare is quoted as saying "that he dressed the wounds but God healed them." What immunity is, is hard to definitely state, but without this defense mechanism, whatever it is, surgery and medicine would be quite impotent.

Surgery is discussed from the time of and before Lister, when the localization of the infection was awaited before drainage was instigated. In the space of approximately 50 years, surgery has as the author expressed it become "superabundant." "Judgment gave way before dexterity." The right iliac fossa and the tonsillar region were the most popular areas of investigation. Subsequently an area of infection was opened earlier and earlier not awaiting localization. The defense mechanism or the pathology of the body apparently were more or less ignored. Surgical intervention in the early infections must insure entire removal of the infected area, as say an appendix. A streptococci infection of the finger was widely incised. When the infection occurs at a site that cannot be entirely removed then according to the author "the arguments in favor of early surgical intervention fall to the ground." This is applicable to the mastoid region. A virulent infection here is one of the most dangerous in the body. Operation before localization and walling off of avenues of extension, i.e. blood stream, petrous portion of the temporal bone and the mastoid bone itself, is most dangerous. The different types of mastoiditis are discussed.

The author's version is that a patient with mastoiditis is suffering from a bacteremia if not a septicemia. Rest is of paramount importance and to get this morphine is used freely. Transfusions are advisable. Sulfanilimide is valuable but should not be used indiscriminately. If shock therapy is used, it should be employed late.

Seven to ten days should show definite signs of localization, such as a lowering of temperature with a daily swing, leukoocytosis and localized tenderness over the mastoid.

There is a table of the author's patients operated early and late. The results show "that when the expectant treatment is adopted there are fewer complications, a lower mortality and a shorter period of hospitalization."

Sulphanilamide in Gonorrheal Ophthalmia. Luis J. Fernandez, M.D., and Ricardo F. Fernandez, M.D., San Juan, Puerto Rico. American Journal of Ophthalmology, July, 1938.

Fourteen cases were reported in December, 1936, which were treated with parenteral milk injections, frequent irrigations and local antiseptics. This series is made up of eight cases of gonorrheal ophthalmia where sulfanilamide was also used. Diagnosis was made with Gram's stain. The dosage is given. The patients were not hospitalized. The summary and conclusions are:

1. All patients who received sulfanilamide recovered in a spectacular manner and in a shorter period of time than that required by other accepted forms of treatment.

2. Cases of primary eye infection, where no pre-existing focus of gonorrheal infection could be demonstrated, responded as well as those of secondary eye infection. We must emphasize that these cases of primary infection of the eye failed, as a rule, to respond to any other type of treatment hitherto employed.

3. The results obtained in this series of cases warrant the judicious use of sulfanilamide in all cases of gonorrheal ophthalmia in adults, whenever there is no serious contraindication.

4. It is highly desirable that this method of treatment be tested by our colleagues to corroborate our findings.

5. The mode of action of this drug needs more thorough investigation. We have only checked our clinical findings by routine laboratory examinations (smears and cultures), but it is yet necessary to determine the minimal effective dose.

6. We have had no opportunity to treat ophthalmia neonatorum by this method, but see no reason why it should not be as effective as in adults.

7. Smaller doses and special precautions must be used for patients with renal insufficiency, because the excretion of sulfanilamide is slow, and in such patients would tend towards accumulation of the drug in the blood.

The Effects of Sulfanilamide as Determined in the Eyes of Rabbits. V. C. Rambo, M.D., Boston. American Journal of Ophthalmology, July, 1938.

The author's conclusions are:

The eye is an excellent organ in which to test the action of sulfanilamide. The rabbit stands sulfanilamide well. The injection of a saturated solution of sulfanilamide into the conjunctiva, or directly into the anterior chamber, produces no permanent observable damage to the eye. Injection of sulfanilamide into the vitreous produces moderate opacity of the vitreous, and after a few days a low-grade iritis of short duration, but has no observable effect on the retinal function.

Sulfanilamide by mouth in adequate, regularly repeated doses, markedly checks the growth of an observable culture of hemolytic streptococci in the vitreous of a rabbit. But even if the treatment is continued, the vitreous eventually becomes completely purulent.

When streptococcus hemolyticus is injected into the anterior chamber, sulfanilamide administered by mouth for only four or five days not only checks but permanently overcomes the infection.

Obviously, leucocytes can reach organisms in the center of the vitreous much less readily than they can reach organisms in the anterior chamber. Hence our experiments support the view that sulfanilamide alone inhibits streptococci, but that to destroy the organisms, leucocytes and possibly other factors are early required in addition.

Injection of streptococci into the anterior chamber with 0.20 gm. of sulfanilamide in water suspension, has protected three out of four eyes from infection as effectively as sulfanilamide by mouth. That the protection was not from the blood stream was proved by the fact that the other eyes of the same rabbits, injected with hemolytic streptococci and not treated, were lost from the infection. It is, therefore, evident that sulfanilamide is effective when used locally only. It is very important, however, that the sulfanilamide be kept at an effective concentration at the site of infection. This is difficult to accomplish because of the great diffusibility of the drug.

These experimental observations indicate that, properly administered, sulfanilamide will overcome certain intraocular infections. They do not indicate, however, that it will save the eye in a case of rapidly progressive purulent endophthalmitis such as may follow accidental or operative trauma. Sulfanilamide by mouth should be useful in treating less virulent infections already established in the anterior chamber, or even in the vitreous. Other treatment, however, such as the use of diphtheria antitoxin, should be employed in addition, especially when the vitreous is infected. Sulfanilamide in 0.5 per cent or saturated solution, as a powder, or as an ointment, may be used locally for infections of the conjunctiva or cornea. If the r e q u i r e m e n t of sufficient, constant, necessary strength of solution is fulfilled, and the organisms are susceptible to the drug, the results should be good. In recent wounds of the cornea or conjunctiva, sulfanilamide solution may be used as a cleansing agent, all needed surgery then done, and sulfanilamide powder dusted into the wound.

Our experiments c o n f i r m Jaeger's conclusion, based on clinical observations, that sulfanilamide is of service by local application. However, he was possibly over-enthusiastic concerning the number of conditions which he found benefited by the local use of sulfanilamide. Other methods of applying the drug locally than have been mentioned by Jaeger may prove successful in local infections which are not amenable to known treatment. However, the giving of sulfanilamide by mouth, in addition, should not be omitted unless contraindicated by the general condition of the patient or by special circumstances.

The local use of sulfanilamide ,even if of itself insufficient, may make the amount needed by mouth much smaller, and vice versa. In certain conditions, full local and general treatment may be needed—for instance sulfanilamide might be dusted into the conjunctival sac as well as given by mouth, in a case of pneumococcic ulceration of the cornea.

By injections of the drug into an organ such as the eye, a concentration far greater than that possible in the blood can be maintained. This greater concentration may make it possible to treat successfully local infections with organisms resistant to treatment with the drug administered by mouth.

Preliminary treatment with sulfanilamide before expected infection, as from a foreign body in the eye, or from an operation in a poor risk, should receive consideration. For this purpose, it is possible that the local use of sulfanilamide may be sufficient.

---o---

ORTHOPAEDIC SURGERY
Edited by Earl D. McBride, M.D., F.A.C.S.
717 North Robinson Street, Oklahoma City

Treatment of Fractures of the Shaft of the Femur. An analysis of One Hundred and Twenty Cases. Robert H. Kennedy. Annals of Surgery, CVII, 419, March, 1938.

One hundred and twenty consecutive cases of

recent fractures of the shaft of the femur treated by the staff of the Beekman Street Hospital from January, 1924, to March, 1932, are analyzed by the author. Patients are classified according to the location of the fracture and according to age.

Seventeen early deaths are reported in the series, including one patient who died after amputation was performed. Two other patients required amputations. This leaves 101 patients with severe multiple injuries.

Forty-eight of the patients analyzed were under 16 years of age. Forty-seven had fractures resulting from automobile accidents. There were but four compound fractures and 20 comminuted fractures in the series.

The primary hospital treatment in 43 cases was adhesive plaster traction with suspension in a Thomas splint; skeletal traction was used in 35 cases; overhead adhesive plaster traction in 11 cases; reduction and application of a plaster spica in 11 cases, and open reduction in one case.

The final treatment, except when complications occurred, was skeletal traction in 43 cases; adhesive plaster t r a c t i o n with suspension in a Thomas splint in 31 cases; reduction and application of a plaster spica in 12 cases; overhead adhesive plaster traction in 11 cases, and open reduction in four cases.

The initial treatment was unsatisfactory in 14 cases of adhesive plaster traction with suspension and in two cases treated by reduction and application of plaster spica.

Traction methods were employed in treating 87 per cent of these patients. The author prefers the Kirschner wire to tongs and Steinmann pins which were used in the earlier cases.

There were four open reductions, all in children. In three cases there were simple fractures and one was compound. In the compound-fracture case infection developed, followed by osteomyelitis, but solid union occurred. Three patients required late open reductions for complications. Four patients sustained refractures. In 84 patients solid bony union was known to have developed and in one non-union developed.

The conclusion of the author is that by traction methods bony union with relatively little shortening and good functional results may be obtained in a high percentage of cases. He does not feel that the results obtained in this series were good enough. Overhead adhesive traction was satisfactory in children under five years of age. Skin traction was unsatisfactory in children over five years of age from the point of view of recovering original length. Skeletal traction in adults gave too high an incidence of infection. He condemns closed reduction and application of a plaster spica.

In March, 1932, the surgeons changed to Russell traction in all of these groups. They are still not satisfied with their results and believe that they should perform more open reductions with internal fixation especially in transverse fractures of the middle and lower thirds of the femur.

Skeletal traction has been a marked improvement over reduction and application of a plaster spica or adhesive plaster traction with suspension in a Thomas splint. No single method is applicable to all cases and one should be ready to use each type of treatment according to the individual indications.

Injuries About the Shoulder Joint in Children, Exclusive of Fractures of the Clavicle. John E. Sullivan. Annals of Surgery, CVII, 594, April, 1938.

A study was made of the records of 61 children under 12 years of age, with injuries about the shoulder joint, exclusive of fractures of the clavicle, who had been admitted to the Children's Surgical

Service of Bellevue Hospital during the past ten years.

Fifty-five of these patients had fractures of the upper end of the humerus, four had fractures of the scapula, one had a subluxation of the head of the humerus, and one had an acromioclavicular separation. There were no instances of separation of the upper humeral epiphysis or of apparent injury to this epiphysis.

Most of the fractures were produced by a fall, and the author describes in detail the mechanics of the injury. Various methods of treatment did not give anatomical reductions but functional results were excellent and in many instances complete anatomical readjustment occurred in a few months.

There were three pathological fractures of the upper end of the humerus in the series. Fractures occurred more often in the left than in the right humerus. There were three cases of fractures of the body of the scapula which were all caused by severe trauma. The methods of treatment used were manipulations under anesthesia or traction.

The following reprints of articles of interest have come to my desk recently:

"Posterior Dislocation of the First Cervical Vertebra with Fracture of the Odontoid Process," Rudolph S. Reich, Surgery, Vol. 3, No. 3, p. 416-420, March, 1938.

"Treatment of Intercondylar Fractures of the Elbow by Means of Traction." Rudolph S. Reich, Jr. of Bone & Joint Surg., Vol. XVIII, No. 4, p. 997-1004, October, 1936.

"Extra-Articular Disabilities of the Shoulder Joint," Rudolph S. Reich, The Ohio St. Med. Jr., Vol. 32, October, 1936, No. 10.

"Treatment of Fractures of the Shaft of the Femur," Robert H. Kennedy, Annals of Surg., Vol. 107, No. 3, March, 1938.

"Osteomyelitis in Compound Fractures," Robert H. Kennedy, Amer. Jr. of Surg., New Series, Vol. XXXVIII, No. 2, p. 327-331, November, 1937.

"Amputations: General Considerations," Robert H. Kennedy, Surgical Clinics of N. A., April, 1938. New York Number.

"Treatment of Birth Fractures of the Femur," Wilton H. Robinson, Jr. of Bone & Joint Surg., Vol. XX, No. 3, p. 778-780, July, 1938.

---o---

INTERNAL MEDICINE
Edited by Hugh Jeter, M.D., 1200 North Walker, Oklahoma City

Blood, a Review of the Recent Literature. Frank H. Bethell, M.D., Raphael Isaacs, M.D., S. Milton Goldhamer, M.D., and Cyrus C. Sturgis, M.D., Ann Arbor, Mich. (Archives of Internal Medicine, Volume 61, No. 6, June, 1938).

This represents a remarkable review of blood dyscrasias and allied diseases covering 842 entirely different articles written on the subject.

Pernicious Anemia

Kahn studied case records of 840 persons with pernicious anemia and found none in which hydrochloric acid was secreted normally and incidentally none which had peptic ulcer. Other interesting observations relative to the intrinsic and extrinsic factors as related to pernicious anemia are recorded.

The problem of bioassay of preparations proposed for the treatment of pernicious anemia has attracted a number of investigators. It is generally concluded that animals do not satisfactorily supplant the human being as a basis for the assay of potency of liver extracts.

The Average Length of Maintenance

Moench studied the liver extract requirement in 32 patients. Therapy consisted of the intramuscular injection of an average monthly dose of the amount of commercially prepared concentrated liver extract derived from 300 grams of liver. This dosage maintained the red cells of 70 per cent of the patients above the minimum normal. Time factors are also recorded.

Sellers made the statement that prior to the introduction of liver in the treatment of pernicious anemia the average duration of life after the diagnosis was made was estimated at two to two and one-half years. Now it is generally agreed that with proper liver therapy the fatal termination may be postponed indefinitely in a majority of cases. He quoted Stocks as stating that since 1926, when liver treatment was introduced, there has been "an average lengthening of life of all persons affected with pernicious anemia in England and Wales of about three to three and one-half years."

Interesting reports of many other varieties of anemia and observations in connection with these are also reported. Interesting cases of polycythemia and purpura hemorrhagica are mentioned.

Hemophilia

Specific treatment seems to remain a mystery. Whole blood, citrated blood, human plasma, human and animal serum, defibrinated blood, hemostatic preparations, fibrinogen, cephalin, calcium, sodium citrate, protein shock, liver and its derivatives, whole ovary, ovarian extracts, histidine, estrogenic substance and even the use of maggot therapy have all been tried, but favorable results are doubtful.

Banti's Disease

The existence of this disease at present is questioned. The pathologic c h a n g e s, which were thought by Banti to be specific, have been shown by Thompson and his co-workers to be due to increased pressure in the splenic vein, with secondary effects in the spleen.

Infectious Mononucleosis

The etiology seems to remain unknown. Davidsohn as a result of a careful serological study of 30 cases has given important technical data relative to the agglutination of sheep cell test.

Agranulocytosis

Here again no single etiological factor can be established. Reports indicate a variety of factors, drug therapy, infections, allergic reactions and auto intoxication, play important roles in different cases. No new or more specific therapeutic measures have been suggested.

Sulfanilamide has been definitely included among the drugs capable of causing or playing an important role in the cause of agranulocytosis.

Myelogram

Many reports are made with observations on bone marrow and bone marrow biopsies. Sedimentation rates and methods are discussed.

---o---

PLASTIC SURGERY
Edited by
GEO. H. KIMBALL, M.D., F.A.C.S.
404 Medical Arts Building, Oklahoma City

Carcinoma Developing On Extensive Scars. The Inefficiency of Pinch Grafts as a Prophylactic Measure. Max Danziz, M.D., F.A.C.S., Milton Friedman, M.D., and Louis J. Levinson, M.D.

Carcinoma is encountered rather infrequently on old scars both following burns and trauma. Extensive, thick, dense scars, which are avascular and poorly nourished, do not tolerate mild injuries due to pressure, irritation of clothing, scratching, etc., as well as the normal skin. After a period of years, varying from 12 to 20, the incompletely developed and poorly nourished skin overlying the scar loses its capacity to repair these minor injuries, and a persistent ulceration develops, which may become malignant.

The authors point out that prophylactic treatment should be employed to avoid such scars. They believe that pinch grafts are useless in preventing the future development of carcinomata. As stated by Treves and Pack: "The Thiersch grafts do not simulate normal skin, since none of the skin accessories, such as hair follicles, sweat and oil glands, are present, and consequently the grafted area is dry, without oil, and subject to the same degenerations as scar tissue." Also, "Cancer has been known to originate on Thiersch-grafted regions."

The authors report two cases which illustrate the development of carcinoma at the site of an old scar. These lesions were originally covered by pinch grafts.

Comment: One sees not infrequently malignant transformation at the site of a scar. I have seen more malignant changes occur in scars left by burns than in those caused by trauma. Some of the cases have been seen where no grafts had been used but healing had been allowed to occur by a natural process. I have not yet seen a malignant change occur at the site of a skin graft.

I believe the authors somewhat exaggerate the possibilities of malignant changes following this type of graft. The changes as I have observed occur when no graft is used. It is true that a split graft or a full thickness graft gives a much better final result than a pinch graft. It is not always possible to obtain the type of graft that is ideal. It is common in children especially to encounter extensive burns where one is unable to secure any kind of graft except a small Thiersch graft.

One is extremely grateful to be able to cover or epithelialize an extensive raw surface by any means whatever. Many of the children survive and are apparently leading useful lives.

---o---

UROLOGY
Edited by D. W. Branham, M.D.
514 Medical Arts Building, Oklahoma City

The Antipyretic Action of Intravenous Administration of Mercurochrome in Acute Pyelonephritis, John L. Emmett, M.D., Journal of U r o l o g y, August, 1938.

Although mercurochrome given intravenously has been in use at the Mayo Clinic for a number of years, of late it has been administered more frequently as a therapeutic measure for shortening the acute manifestations of pyelonephritis. Sufficient favorable results have been obtained when it is given in smaller doses (less than 10 c.c. of a one per cent solution) without bad reactions to prompt the author to recommend its use. Statistical data is presented to reinforce his argument as to its value. The drug is given two or three times at daily intervals, however, if no improvement is noted after the first two doses it is discontinued.

It is emphasized that it is not a potent preparation for its bactercidal effect and other chemotherapeutic measures must be prescribed later to complete the cure.

Comment: Careful reading of this article failed to convince me that mercurochrome has any place in our therapeutic armanentarium as far as its use intravenously is concerned. One has only to remember the case reports presented a few years back detailing the severe reactions, with their irritative and degenerative effect on the kidney following its administration. It is true the dose given then was somewhat larger than that recommended in this article but nevertheless the danger is only slightly less. I do not believe any mercurial preparation has a place in modern medicine as far as its intravenous use is concerned due to its potential destructive effect on renal tissue. The profession in general had its day with mercurochrome intravenously and its judgment has found the drug unsafe and even dangerous. In this day of much more efficient drugs and therapeutic measures for the treatment of urologic infections, mercurochrome intravenously had best be left in the list of discarded remedies.

Vas Deferens Anastomosis, Successful Repair Four Years Subsequent to Bilateral Vasectomy, Elmer D. Twyman, M.D., and Charles S. Nelson, M.D., Kansas City, Missouri, The Urologic and Cutaneous Review, August, 1938.

A report that details the successful repair of a vas deferens following a vasectomy performed for the production of sterility four years previously. Not only were spermatozoa found in the seminal fluid, but the sexual partners later gave birth to a child.

The technique in repairing the strictured vas was essentially the removal of the strictured area and the two ends were brought together by a catgut suture threaded up the lumen of both portions and tied together forming a hammock loop—following which all layers were approximated.

Comment: In this day of mass vasectomies for the production of sterility it is a comforting bit of news to hear of a successful anastomosis after such a long duration of time. One must, however, remember chances are rather slight for such a fortunate outcome and for that reason both patient and doctor should think twice before allowing such a mutilating operation to be performed.

-----o-----

Human Requirement of Vitamin D

P. C. Jeans and Genevieve Stearns, Iowa City (Journal A.M.A., Aug 20, 1938), define the requirements of vitamin D as those amounts which, with ample intakes of calcium and phosphorus and a diet otherwise adequate, insure sufficient retention of calcium and phosphorus to permit normal growth and mineralization of the skeleton and teeth of infants and children, maintenance of bony and dental structures during adult life and a sufficient supply for mother and infant during pregnancy and lactation. Individual variation in ability to utilize the calcium and phosphorus of the diet without added vitamin D exists at all age periods. A high proportion of infants have poor retention and only a very few retain an ample amount without vitamin D. As the age increases persons in increased proportion are able to retain adequate amounts of these minerals without vitamin D, but at all age periods some persons are found who are not efficient. In defining a standard for the vitamin D requirement it seems desirable to state an amount which will be satisfactory for those who are less efficient. Vitamin D does not decrease the minimum requirement of calcium and phosphorus and this vitamin cannot produce a good retention in a person who is ingesting less than the requirement for these minerals. Vitamin D is not as well utilized on a unit for unit basis from the more concentrated preparations as from those preparations in which it is more widely dispersed. The most desirable concentration has not been determined, but apparently the concentration found in cod liver oil is as effective as any lesser concentration studied. The vitamin D requirement of the full term artificially fed baby is probably between 300 and 400 units a day. Vitamin D is necessary for many and useful for most breast-fed babies. It is tentatively considered that prematurely born babies may require twice as much vitamin D as full term babies during the early period of most rapid growth, after which time the requirement should be the same as for babies born at term. For children between infancy and adolescence a daily allowance of at least 750 cc. of milk together with from 300 to 400 units of vitamin D permits consistently ample retention of calcium and phosphorus. For adolescents a need for vitamin D exists, but insufficient data are available to permit an estimate of the quantity required. It seems probable that from 300 to 400 units a day would be satisfactory. For adults the optimal amount of vitamin D, if a need exists, remains to be determined. It appears strongly advisable to give vitamin D during pregnancy and lactation. The optimal amount is not known. During lactation the requirement may be greater than at any other period of life and a daily dosage of 800 units or more is suggested, together with an abundant intake of calcium and phosphorus.

-----o-----

Rabies: Report of Twelve Cases, With Discussion of Prophylaxis

Maurice L. Blatt, Samuel J. Hoffman and Maurice Schneider, Chicago (Journal A.M.A., Aug. 20, 1938), discuss the 12 cases of rabies admitted to the Cook County Hospital between 1929 and 1937. All proved fatal. The diagnosis in each case was confirmed by necropsy. The incubation period for the patients varied from two weeks to two months. The closer the site of the bite to the central nervous system the shorter was the incubation period. Wounds made by the bites of animals should immediately be cauterized with nitric acid. The Pasteur treatment or one of its modifications should be instituted in accordance with rules outlined and accepted. The 12 persons whose cases are reported died after suffering great agony and might have been saved if adequate prophylactic measures had been instituted immediately. They were admitted to the hospital after having been ill from two to seven days and anywhere from two weeks to two months after they had been bitten by dogs. Stringent enforcement of regulations governing ownership, licensure, muzzling and leashing of dogs would have prevented the bites. The extent of this problem is evidenced by the fact that in the state of Illinois alone 18,466 dog bites were reported to the state department of public health in 1936 and that there were ten deaths from rabies. A knowledge of similar facts would divulge a tremendous loss of time and of lives of human beings and animals in the United States from a preventable cause. When such knowledge becomes public it will be of inestimable educational value in the eradication of this dreadful malady.

-----o-----

Use of Serum in Treatment of Higher Types of Pneumonia

Pneumonia of the higher types is an important part of the pneumonia problem. In a collected series of 6,545 cases of pneumococcic pneumonia Norman Plummer, New York (Journal A.M.A., Aug. 20, 1938), finds that more than 50 per cent of the cases were of the higher types, 30 per cent being of types IV, V, VII, VIII and XIV. He and his associates used antipneumococcus serum in 111 cases, with a rather marked clinical response and an appreciable effect on the mortality rate for the combined series of cases of pneumonia of types IV, V, VII, VII and XIV. At present there are available refined and concentrated preparations of horse and of rabbit serum that are high in antibody content and almost entirely free from reaction-causing substance. With such products the prospects are excellent for obtaining increasingly better results in the treatment of all types of pneumococcic pneumonia. Nine patients with type III pneumonia were treated with concentrated antipneumococcus rabbit serum, the last six having had no untoward reactions. Of the nine, three died and six recovered. Of those who recovered, one had a positive blood culture when serum treatment was instituted. Three were treated very early in the course of the disease and showed prompt response to a large unitage of serum. Antipneumococcus rabbit serum has taken the focus of attention recently, but whether rabbit serum, unit for unit, is more effective than horse serum remains to be proved.

---o---

Vitamin B1: Methods of Assay and Food Sources

Hazel E. Munsell, Washington, D. C. (Journal A.M.A., September 3, 1938), states that the importance of vitamin B1 in physiologic and pathologic conditions has emphasized markedly the need of devising accurate methods for the quantitative determination of this substance in foods. Until recently the chemical identity of vitamin B1 was unknown, rendering it impossible to develop chemical methods of analysis, and accordingly recourse was had to biologic methods of assay using rats and pigeons as test animals. Much information regarding the vitamin B1 content of foods has been gained in this way, especially by the method in which the growth of rats was used as the measure

of potency. The technical aspects of various methods of bio-assay for vitamin B1 are presented from the point of view of quantitative interpretation of the results obtained and the chemical methods that are being developed are discussed. The article also evaluates foods as sources of the vitamin.

---o---

Gastroduodenostomy For Certain Duodenal Ulcers

Howard M. Clute and John S. Sprague, Boston (Journal A.M.A., September 3, 1938), urge that gastroduodenostomy be given more consideration when surgical treatment is necessary in the management of certain duodenal ulcers. Although opinions and experiences as to the occurrence of stomal ulcers after gastroduodenostomy differ widely, they have been unable to discover evidence of a high percentage of these postoperative complications. They believe that gastroduodenostomy results in a nearer approach to normal gastric physiology than other short-circuiting operations. They discuss the technic and present the results that they obtained following gastroduodenostomy in seven cases of pyloric stenosis, in two cases of persistent pain from duodenal ulcer in spite of long medical treatment, two cases of duodenal ulcer with serious hemorrhages, two cases of ulcer high on the lesser curvature of the stomach and two bleeding gastrojejunal ulcers.

Report of Licenses Granted to Practice Medicine

NAME	Year of Birth	Place of Birth	School of Graduation	Year of Graduation	Permanent or Present Address
Wiggins, Howell Ernest	1911	Hobart, Okla.	Oklahoma University	1936	Los Angeles, Calif.
Howard, Robert Bruce	1913	Oklahoma City, Okla.	Oklahoma University	1936	Los Angeles, Calif.
Morgan, Vance Fredrick	1909	Foster, Okla.	Oklahoma University	1934	Oklahoma City, Okla.
Evans, Logan I.	1868	........, Kansas.	Oklahoma University	1916	Oklahoma City, Okla
Shaver, S. Robert	1905	Quinton, Okla.	Oklahoma University	1937	Oklahoma City, Okla.
Lachmann, Ernst	1901	Glogau, Germany	University Breslau	1925	Oklahoma City, Okla.
Spencer, Walter Carlton Edw.	1808	Bradford, Pa.	University Texas	1931	Greenville, Miss.
Word, Lee Bailey	1904	Windom, Texas	University Arkansas	1936	Bartlesville, Okla.
Wilson, George Stewart	1895	Eaton, Kansas	Washington Univ.	1927	Enid, Okla.
Willis, James Asa	1904	Corsicana, Texas	University Texas	1929	Oklahoma City, Okla.
Whitney, Merle Lemuel	1905	Talmage, Kansas	University Kansas	1935	Oklahoma City, Okla.
Trent, Robert Irvine	1908	Goodwill, W. Va.	University Virginia	1933	Oklahoma City, Okla.
Oakes, Charles Gratton	1908	Batesville, Ark.	University Kansas	1934	Sapulpa & Tulsa, Ok.
Mantz, Earl Russell	1908	Elgin, Ill.	Univ. Wisconsin	1932	Ada, Okla.
Mitchell, Tom Hall	1900	Bessemer, Ala.	Med. Col. of Va.	1931	Tulsa, Okla.
McKenzie, Walten Holt	1909	Enid, Okla.	Washington Univ.	1934	Enid, Okla.
Lovett, Ivan Clair	1906	Lineville, Iowa.	Univ. of Iowa	1934	Tulsa, Okla.
Colonna, Paul Crenshaw	1892	Norfolk, Va.	Johns Hopkins Univ.	1920	Oklahoma City, Okla.
Shackelford, John William	1902	Carrollton, Miss.	Tulane University	1926	Greenville, Miss.
Newell, Waldo Bee, Jr.	1912	Hunter, Okla.	Vanderbilt Univ.	1937	Enid, Okla.
Cotton, Bert Hollis	1911	Sallisaw, Okla.	Oklahoma University	1937	Sallisaw, Okla.
Henke, Joseph Reid	1912	Hydro, Okla.	Oklahoma University	1937	Hydro, Okla.
Young, Andrew Merriman III	1913	Oklahoma City, Okla.	Oklahoma University	1937	Oklahoma City, Okla.
Mead, William Wesley	1913	Whitecloud, Kans.	Oklahoma University	1937	Guthrie, Okla.
Bohlmann, Wilbur F.	1912	Okarche, Okla.	Oklahoma University	1937	Okarche, Okla.
Blair, Claude M., Jr.	1910	Tecumseh, Okla.	Oklahoma University	1937	Okemah, Okla.
Fulton, W. R.	1867		Barnes Medical Col.	1902	Blackgum, Okla.
Grant, Verne V.	1882	Columbia City, Ind.	University Med. Col.	1907	Oklahoma City, Okla.
Epps, Curtis Howard	1911	Springfield, Mo.	Washington Univ.	1936	Oklahoma City, Okla.
Ryan, Robert O.	1902	Hickory, Okla.	Oklahoma University	1937	Canton, Okla.
Gallagher, Clarence Alfred	1911	Stillwater, Okla.	Oklahoma University	1937	Stillwater, Okla.
Clark, Ralph Otis	1908	Ravia, Okla.	Oklahoma University	1937	Roff, Okla.
Layton, Otto Earl	1906	Cleveland, Okla.	Oklahoma University	1937	Collinsville, Okla.
Talbott, George Albert	1902	McKinney, Texas	Oklahoma University	1936	Konawa, Okla.
Hoyt, Jonathan	1897	Fresno, Calif.	Oklahoma University	1937	Wayne, Okla.
O'Leary, Charles Marion	1909	........, Okla.	Oklahoma University	1934	Oklahoma City, Okla.
Brundage, Bert Truman	1913	........, Okla.	Oklahoma University	1936	Thomas, Okla.
Loy, William A.	1914	Enid, Okla.	Oklahoma University	1937	Guthrie, Okla.
Melnish, Robert Kerr, Jr.	1913	Bennington, Okla.	Oklahoma University	1937	Tahlequah, Okla.
Pugh, Robert Eugene	1910	Lawton, Okla.	Oklahoma University	1936	Haskell, Okla.
Murray, Forney Long	1906	........, Okla.	Oklahoma University	1937	Malta Bend, Mo.
Melness, James Thermon	1910	Carthage, N. C.	Oklahoma University	1937	Pampa, Texas.
Mahneel, Earl I.	1915	Oklahoma City, Okla.	Oklahoma University	1937	Oklahoma City, Okla.
Oglesbee, Corcos LeRoy	1906	New Canton, Ill.	Oklahoma University	1937	Trousdale, Okla.
Matthews, Newman Sanford	1904	Clarendon, Okla.	Oklahoma University	1937	Oklahoma City, Okla.
Gross, Francis Warren	1912	Orr, Okla.	Oklahoma University	1937	Erie, Pa.
Petway, Aileen (F)	1911	Eastman, Ga.	Oklahoma University	1937	Oklahoma City, Okla.
Ohl, Charles Wallis	1909	Vineland, N. J.	Hanemann Medical	1937	Chickasha, Okla.
Kersch, Clyde	1909	Gatewood, Mo.	Oklahoma University	1937	Oklahoma City, Okla.

OFFICERS OKLAHOMA STATE MEDICAL ASSOCIATION

President, Dr. H. K. Speed, Sayre.

President-Elect, Dr. W. A. Howard, Chelsea.

Secretary-Treasurer-Editor, Dr. L. S. Willour, McAlester.

Speaker, House of Delegates, Dr. J. D. Osborn, Jr., Frederick.

Vice Speaker, House of Delegates, Dr. P. P. Nesbitt, Medical Arts Building, Tulsa.

Delegates to the A. M. A., Dr. W. Albert Cook, Medical Arts Building, Tulsa, 1938-39; Dr. McLain Rogers, Clinton, 1937-1938.

Meeting Place, Oklahoma City, May, 1939.

SPECIAL COMMITTEES 1938-39

Annual Meeting: Dr. H. K. Speed, Sayre; Dr. W. A. Howard, Chelsea; Dr. L. S. Willour, McAlester.

Conservation of Hearing: Dr. H. F. Vandever, Chairman, Enid; Dr. J. B. Hollis, Mangum; Dr. Chester McHenry, Oklahoma City.

Conservation of Vision: Dr. W. M. Gallaher, Chairman, Shawnee; Dr. Frank R. Vieregg, Clinton; Dr. Pauline Barker, Guthrie.

Crippled Children: Dr. Earl McBride, Chairman, Oklahoma City; Dr. Roy L. Fisher, Frederick; Dr. M. B. Glismann, Okmulgee.

Industrial Service and Traumatic Surgery: Dr. Cyril C. Clymer, Medical Arts Bldg., Oklahoma City; Dr. J. Wm. Finch, Hobart; Dr. J. A. Rutledge, Ada.

Maternity and Infancy: Dr. George R. Osborn, Chairman, Tulsa; Dr. P. J. DeVanney, Sayre; Dr. Leila E. Andrews, Oklahoma City.

Necrology: Dr. G. H. Stagner, Chairman, Erick; Dr. James L. Shuler, Durant; Dr. S. D. Neely, Muskogee.

Post Graduate Medical Teaching: Dr. Henry H. Turner, Chairman, Oklahoma City; Dr. H. C. Weber, Bartlesville; Dr. Ned R. Smith, Tulsa.

Study and Control of Cancer: Dr. Wendell Long, Chairman, Oklahoma City; Dr. Paul B. Champlin, Enid; Dr. Ralph McGill, Tulsa.

Study and Control of Tuberculosis: Dr. Carl Puckett, Chairman, Oklahoma City; Dr. W. C. Tisdal, Clinton; Dr. F. P. Baker, Talihina.

ADVISORY COUNCIL FOR AUXILIARY

Dr. H. K. Speed, Chairman..Sayre
Dr. C. J. Fishman...Oklahoma City
Dr. W. S. Larrabee...Tulsa
Dr. J. M. Watson...Enid
Dr. T. H. McCarley...McAlester

STANDING COMMITTEES 1938-39

Medical Defense: Dr. O. E. Templin, Chairman, Alva; Dr. L. C. Kuyrkendall, McAlester; Dr. E. Albert Aisenstadt, Picher.

Medical Economics: Dr. C. B. Sullivan, Cordell, Chairman; Dr. J. L. Patterson, Duncan; Dr. W. M. Browning, Waurika.

Medical Education and Hospital: Dr. V. C. Tisdal, Chairman, Elk City; Dr. Robert U. Patterson, Oklahoma City; Dr. H. M. McClure, Chickasha.

Public Policy and Legislation: Dr. Finis W. Ewing, Surety Bldg., Chairman, Muskogee; Dr. Tom Lowry, 1200 North Walker, Oklahoma City; Dr. O. C. Newman, Shattuck.

(The above committee co-ordinated by the following, selected from each counsellor district.)

District No. 1.—Arthur E. Hale, Alva.
District No. 2.—McLain Rogers, Clinton.
District No. 3.—Thomas McElroy, Ponca City.
District No. 4.—L. H. Ritzhaupt, Guthrie.
District No. 5.—P. V. Annadown, Sulphur.
District No. 6.—R. M. Shepard, Tulsa.
District No. 7.—Sam A. McKeel, Ada.
District No. 8.—J. A. Morrow, Sallisaw.
District No. 9.—W. A. Tolleson, Eufaula.
District No. 10.—J. L. Holland, Madill.

Scientific Exhibits: Dr. E. Rankin Denny, Chairman, Tulsa; Dr. Robert H. Akin, Oklahoma City; Dr. R. C. Pigford, Tulsa.

Scientific Work: Dr. W. G. Husband, Chairman, Hollis; Dr. J. S. Rollins, Prague; Dr. J. L. Day, Supply.

Public Health:

Chairman—Dr. G. S. Baxter, Shawnee.
District No. 1.—C. W. Tedrowe, Woodward.
District No. 2.—E. W. Mabry, Altus.
District No. 3.—A. A. Mitchell, Stillwater.
District No. 4.—J. J. Gable, Norman.
District No. 5.—Geo. S. Barber, Lawton.
District No. 6.—C. E. Bradley, Tulsa.
District No. 7.—G. S. Baxter, Shawnee.
District No. 8.—M. M. De Arman, Miami.
District No. 9.—T. H. McCarley, McAlester.
District No. 10.—J. B. Clark, Coalgate.

SCIENTIFIC SECTIONS

General Surgery: Dr. F. L. Flack, Chairman, Nat'l Bank of Tulsa Bldg., Tulsa; Dr. John E. McDonald, Vice-Chairman, Medical Arts Bldg., Tulsa; Dr. John F. Burton, Secretary, Osler Bufilding, Oklahoma City.

General Medicine: Dr. Frank Nelson, Chairman, 603 Medical Arts Bldg., Tulsa; Dr. E. R. Musick, Vice-Chairman, Medical Arts Bldg., Oklahoma City; Dr. Milam McKinney, Medical Arts Bldg., Oklahoma City.

Eye, Ear, Nose & Throat: Dr. E. H. Coachman, Chairman, Manhattan Bldg., Muskogee; Dr. F. M. Cooper, Vice-President, Medical Arts Bldg., Oklahoma City; Dr. James R. Reed, Secretary, Medical Arts Bldg., Oklahoma City.

Obstetrics and Pediatrics: Dr. C. W. Arrendell, Chairman, Ponca City; Dr. Carl F. Simpson, Vice-Chairman, Medical Arts Bldg., Tulsa; Dr. Ben H. Nicholson, Secretary, 300 West Twelfth Street, Oklahoma City.

Genito-Urinary Diseases and Syphilology: Dr. Elijah Sullivan, Chairman, Medical Arts Bldg., Oklahoma City; Dr. Henry Browne, Vice-Chairman, Medical Arts Bldg., Tulsa; Dr. Robert Akin, Secretary, 400 West Tenth, Oklahoma City.

Dermatology and Radiology: Dr. W. A. Showman, Chairman, Medical Arts Bldg., Tulsa; Dr. E. D. Greenberger, Vice-Chairman, McAlester; Dr. Hervey A. Foerster, Secretary, Medical Arts Bldg., Oklahoma City.

STATE BOARD OF MEDICAL EXAMINERS

Dr. Thos. McElroy, Ponca City, President; Dr. C. E. Bradley, Tulsa, Vice-President; Dr. J. D. Osborn, Jr., Frederick, Secretary; Dr. L. E. Emanuel, Chickasha; Dr. W. T. Ray, Gould; Dr. G. L. Johnson, Pauls Valley; Dr. W. W. Osgood, Muskogee.

STATE COMMISSIONER OF HEALTH

Dr. Chas. M. Pearce, Oklahoma City.

COUNCILORS AND THEIR COUNTIES

District No. 1: Texas, Beaver, Cimarron, Harper, Ellis, Woods, Woodward, Alfalfa, Major, Dewey—Dr. O. E. Templin, Alva. (Term expires 1940.)

District No. 2: Roger Mills, Beckham, Greer, Harmon, Washita, Kiowa, Custer, Jackson, Tillman—Dr. V. C. Tisdal, Elk City. (Term expires 1939.)

District No. 3: Grant, Kay, Garfield, Noble, Payne, Pawnee—Dr. A. S. Risser, Blackwell. (Term expires 1938.)

District No. 4: Blaine, Kingfisher, Canadian, Logan, Oklahoma, Cleveland—Dr. Philip M. McNeill, Oklahoma City. (Term expires 1938.)

District No. 5: Caddo, Comanche, Cotton, Grady, Love, Stephens, Jefferson, Carter, Murray—Dr. W. H. Livermore, Chickasha. (Term expires 1938.)

District No. 6: Osage, Creek, Washington, Nowata, Rogers, Tulsa—Dr. James Stevenson, Medical Arts Bldg., Tulsa. (Term expires 1938.)

District No. 7: Lincoln, Pontotoc, Pottawatomie, Okfuskee, Seminole, McClain, Garvin, Hughes—Dr. J. A. Walker, Shawnee. (Term expires 1939.)

District No. 8: Craig, Ottawa, Mayes, Delaware, Wagoner, Adair, Cherokee, Sequoyah, Okmulgee, Muskogee—Dr. E. A. Aisenstadt, Picher. (Term expires 1939.)

District No. 9: Pittsburg, Haskell, Latimer, LeFlore, McIntosh—Dr. L. C. Kuyrkendall, McAlester. (Term expires 1939.)

District No. 10: Johnson, Marshall, Coal, Atoka, Bryan, Choctaw, Pushmataha, McCurtain—Dr. J. S. Fulton, Atoka. (Term expires 1939.)

OFFICERS OF COUNTY SOCIETIES, 1938

COUNTY	PRESIDENT	SECRETARY
Adair		
Alfalfa	F. K. Slaton, Helena	L. T. Lancaster, Cherokee
Atoka-Coal	J. S. Fulton, Atoka	J. B. Clark, Coalgate
Beckham	R. C. McCreery, Erick	P. J. DeVanney, Sayre
Blaine	J. S. Barnett, Hitchcock	W. F. Griffin, Watonga
Bryan	P. L. Cain, Albany	Jas. L. Shuler, Durant
Caddo	J. Worrell Henry, Anadarko	P. H. Anderson, Anadarko
Canadian	A. L. Johnson, El Reno	G. D. Funk, El Reno
Carter	T. J. Jackson, Ardmore	Emma Jean Cantrell, Wilson
Cherokee	P. H. Medearis, Tahlequah	H. A. Masters, Tahlequah
Choctaw	G. E. Harris, Hugo	F. L. Waters, Hugo
Cleveland	O. E. Howell, Norman	J. L. Haddock, Jr., Norman
Coal	(See Atoka)	
Comanche	E. B. Dunlap, Lawton	Reber M. Van Matre, Lawton
Cotton	W. W. Cotton, Walters	G. W. Baker, Walters
Craig	W. R. Marks, Vinita	F. T. Gastineau, Vinita
Creek	O. R. McDonald, Mannford	J. F. Curry, Sapulpa
Custer	Ross Deputy, Clinton	Harry Cushman, Clinton
Garfield	E. J. Wolfe, Waukomis	John R. Walker, Enid
Garvin	G. L. Johnson, Pauls Valley	John R. Callaway, Pauls Valley
Grady	L. E. Wood, Chickasha	R. E. Baze, Chickasha
Grant	I. V. Hardy, Medford	E. E. Lawson, Medford
Greer	Leb B. Pearson, Mangum	J. B. Hollis, Mangum
Harmon	W. G. Husband, Hollis	R. H. Lynch, Hollis
Haskell	A. T. Hill, Stigler	N. K. Williams, McCurtain
Hughes	W. L. Taylor, Holdenville	Imogene Mayfield, Holdenville
Jackson	Jas. E. Ensey, Altus	J. M. Allgood, Altus
Jefferson	C. S. Maupin, Waurika	C. M. Maupin, Waurika
Kay		R. G. Obermiller, Ponca City
Kingfisher	John R. Taylor, Kingfisher	F. C. Lattimore, Kingfisher
Kiowa	T. M. Bonham, Hobart	J. Wm. Finch, Hobart
Latimer	R. L. Rich, Red Oak	E. B. Hamilton, Wilburton
LeFlore	E. M. Woodson, Poteau	W. L. Shippey, Poteau
Lincoln	R. F. Hurlbut, Meeker	Ned Burleson, Prague
Logan	F. R. First, Crescent	E. O. Barker, Guthrie
Marshall	J. H. Logan, Lebanon	J. F. York, Madill
Mayes	S. C. Rutherford, Locust Grove	E. H. Werling, Pryor
McClain	J. E. Cochran, Byars	R. L. Royster, Purcell
McCurtain	R. D. Williams, Idabel	R. H. Sherrill, Broken Bow
McIntosh	D. E. Little, Eufaula	Wm. A. Tolleson, Eufaula
Murray	P. V. Annadown, Sulphur	Richard M. Burke, Sulphur
Muskogee	Finis W. Ewing, Muskogee	S. D. Neely, Muskogee
Noble	J. W. Francis, Perry	T. F. Renfrow, Billings
Nowata	M. B. Scott, Delaware	H. M. Prentiss, Nowata
Okfuskee	L. J. Snickard, Okemah	C. M. Bloss, Okemah
Oklahoma	O. J. Fishman, Oklahoma City	John F. Burton, Oklahoma City
Okmulgee	V. M. Wallace, Morris	M. B. Glismann, Okmulgee
Osage	R. O. Smith, Hominy	Geo. Hemphill, Pawhuska
Ottawa	Benj. W. Ralston, Commerce	W. Jackson Sayles, Miami
Pawnee	R. E. Jones, Pawnee	M. L. Saddoris, Cleveland.
Payne	E. M. Harris, Cushing	John W. Martin, Cushing
Pittsburg	A. R. Russell, McAlester	Ed. D. Greenberger, McAlester
Pontotoc	W. F. Dean, Ada	Glen W. McDonald, Ada
Pottawatomie	E. Eugene Rice, Shawnee	F. Clinton Gallaher, Shawnee
Pushmataha	E. S. Patterson, Antlers	D. W. Connally, Antlers
Rogers	F. A. Anderson, Claremore	W. A. Howard, Chelsea
Seminole	A. N. Deaton, Wewoka	Claude B. Knight, Wewoka
Stephens	W. T. Salmon, Duncan	Fred T. Hargrove, Duncan
Texas		R. B. Hayes, Guymon
Tillman	J. E. Childers, Tipton	O. G. Bacon, Frederick
Tulsa	M. J. Searle, Tulsa	Roy L. Smith, Tulsa
Wagoner	S. R. Bates, Wagoner	Francis S. Crane, Wagoner
Washington	J. E. Crawford, Bartlesville	J. V. Athey, Bartlesville
Washita	T. Paul Jones, Dill	Gordon Livingston, Cordell
Woods	Arthur E. Hale, Alva	Oscar E. Templin, Alva
Woodward	C. W. Tedrowe, Woodward	V. M. Rutherford, Woodward

NOTE—Corrections and additions to the above list will be cheerfully accepted.

THE JOURNAL
OF THE
OKLAHOMA STATE MEDICAL ASSOCIATION

VOLUME XXXI	McALESTER, OKLAHOMA, OCTOBER, 1938	Number 10

An Analysis of 1514 Inguinal Herniotomies*

W. PAT FITE, M.D., F.A.C.S.
MUSKOGEE, OKLAHOMA

The group of cases u n d e r discussion represents 1514 consecutive operative procedures for cure of indirect and direct inguinal herniae. It is confined to males of the age limits of veterans of the great war. These represent a social type somewhat diferent from that seen in the average private practice in that a far better check up is available and the individual tends in the case of a recurrence to return to the bureau for reoperation, something which is seen with far less frequency in the private practice of surgery.

ANESTHESIA

The first 371 procedures were done almost exclusively under local anaesthesia with an occasional ether anaesthesia. The last 1,143 were operated under spinal anaesthesia with an occasional local when the other was untra-indicated. We prefer spinal anaesthesia as it gives excellent relaxation, no oedema in the operative field —only a relatively low anaesthesia is necessary—and greatly facilitates the handling of successive cases on the same morning in the operating room.

MORTALITY RATE

There was one death in the series, that from cerebral hemorrhage in a man who had previously had a hemiplegia.

TERM OF HOSPITALIZATION

All cases are required to remain in bed a minimum of 21 days, in severe cases 28 days.

*Read Before the Surgical Section of the Oklahoma State Medical Association's Annual Meeting, May 10, 1938, Muskogee, Oklahoma.

PERCENTAGE OF DIFFERENT TYPES OF INGUINAL HERNIAE

		%
Indirect	1,072	70.8
Direct	297	19.6
Sliding (indirect)	5	.3
Strangulated (indirect)	2	.1
Recurrent	138	9.1

By this it is seen that by far the greatest number seen was of the indirect type. That we did not see more strangulated cases is no doubt due to' the fact that almost all cases have to come s o m e distance, and there were relatively few in the advanced age group, by far the largest number being between 35 and 50 years of age.

In this same period there were operated 87 ventral, 44 epigastric and 12 femoral herniae. These last are mentioned only to show their relative frequency in the same group of patients in the same period of time.

These 1,514 inguinal herniae represent 3.48 per cent of the 43,429 admissions during this period.

TYPES OF OPERATIVE PROCEDURES

The Bassini type of o p e r a t i o n with transplantation of the c o r d w a s u s e d throughout. Approximately 50 per cent of the operations were done by one man whose procedure differed from that used by the others only in that he inspected the posterior wall of the canal in all cases and repaired it whenever weak areas were f o u n d, removed all cremasteric muscle from the inguinal canal, imbricated the fascia of the external oblique and in most recurrent and all direct cases transplanted the cord to a subcutaneous position over the internal ring.

RECURRENCES

One hundred and thirty-eight recurrent inguinal herniae were operated, 24 were on individuals that had previously been operated in the institution as a part of the series under discussion, a known recurrence rate of 1.54 per cent plus. Twenty-one of these, 1.3 per cent, were operated by those not taking care to repair the posterior wall of the canal and follow the other procedure described above. Four, or .2 per cent, recurred in about 50 per cent of these cases that these procedures were used in.

DESCRIPTION OF PROCEDURES

Indirect Inguinal Hernia. The canal is exposed in the usual way by splitting the fascia of the external oblique. The cremasteric muscle is thus opened and all of this lying in the inguinal canal is removed. Next the sac is isolated, ligated high, removed, and the neck transplanted beneath the internal oblique muscle. All extra peritoneal fat, when present, is removed from the upper portion of the canal. Following this the posterior wall of the canal is examined and where any weak places are found in the transversalis fascia, this is dissected out and overlapped, care being taken to always reduce the internal ring to the smallest size to safely carry the cord elements. The b o r d e r of the internal oblique and the conjoined tendon is then sutured by interrupted sutures to Poupart's ligament behind the cord followed by overlapping of the fascia of the external oblique by a double row of interrupted s u t u r e s, the cord coming out t h r o u g h the reduced external inguinal ring.

Direct Inguinal Hernia. The repair of the direct type of inguinal hernia is carried out in the same way with the following variations. The fascial covering of the sac is carefully defined and dissected off the sac and the sac is invaginated by one or more purse string sutures. The borders of the dissected transversalis fascia are thus overlapped by a double row of interrupted sutures and the cord transplanted by being brought out the reconstructed internal ring where the fascia of the external oblique muscle has been imbricated medially, thus placing the cord

in a subcutaneous position. Then the external ring may be completely closed.

Recurrent Herniae. The same principle of disposing of the cord is used in these as in the management of direct herniae. Care is taken in all repairs to do away with abnormal relaxations, to refrain from injury to the ilio-inguinal and ilio-hypogastric nerves, and not to include them in any sutures. Occasionally there is too much tension of the fascia of the external oblique muscle and when this occurs we prefer to make a longitudinal incision through the fascia over the rectus medial to the repair.

We have not as yet had to have recourse to the Galli type of suture for the repair of any hernia, and have operated all cases unless right of domicile had been forfeited by the hernial contents of the general condition of the patient made operation inadvisable or too dangerous.

SUTURES

In this series c a t g u t has been used throughout.

LOCAL COMPLICATIONS .

There have been a few superficial wound infections, none have led to a recurrence.

In one case a cord and testicle became gangrenous and had to be removed but the hernial repair held.

Occasionally there has been oozing in the upper part of the s u t u r e s but this has never been a serious complication.

The bladder was injured in one case, immediately repaired, no sequellae.

UNDESCENDED TESTICLE

Now and then an undescended testicle is found complicating the hernia. These, if they appear normal, are usually placed within the abdomen and a tight closure made. If there is any question of neoplasm, the testicle is removed.

In this series there were found two malignant tumors in intra-abdominal testes. No case of epididymitis has been noted associated with an undescended testicle, nor have we ever seen one.

We have been particularly interested in operating recurrent inguinal herniae in trying to ascertain why that certain hernia recurred and we believe repair of the posterior wall, reduction in the size of the internal ring, removal of the cremasteric muscle, and in certain cases the transferring of the cord into a subcutaneous position over the internal ring in addition to the usual Bassini procedure, will greatly reduce recurrences. At least analysis of this series of cases tends to emphasize that possibility. It is not unusual to operate a recurrent hernia and find little evidence that the case had ever been operated before. Such cases we feel sure had little done other than removal of the sac and a simple closure.

When we realize that some 50 per cent of individuals have a preformed indirect hernial sac of some degree, it is little wonder that "rupture" or clinical inguinal hernia is so common as to be almost a social problem, especially as it is a disqualifying defect for employment. Heredity must play a part as it is not unusual to have h e r n i a in successive generations of the same family.

An individual is often turned down for employment because of enlarged external rings, on the grounds that he may have a potential hernia. This may be true so far as direct hernia is concerned. Our experience shows that with each decade the percentage of direct herniae increases. But we doubt seriously if the ordinary enlarged external ring alone has anything to do with the development of an indirect hernia as its occurrence depends upon a preformed sac, a large or relaxed internal ring and ample space in the inguinal canal.

In conclusion, let me suggest that in the repair of inguinal herniae, that in addition to the removal of the sac that each layer be made as intact as possible and all spaces be made as fibrotic as possible. If this last were not true the injection treatment would in no way succeed.

* * *

DISCUSSION

Dr. H. C. Weber, Bartlesville: Most of the hernias which I do are industrial hernias. Up in our part of the country we have not accepted spinal anesthesia. We do practically all under ether, local, or nitrous oxide. I think perhaps the cause of a lot of failures with local anesthesia that a great many people have is due to the fact that they don't inject their anesthetic deep enough. They get it into the fascia and expect that to hold from pain,

when the nerves are much deeper than that. I always try to get my anesthesia as deep as I can get it without going into the peritoneal cavity. Occasionally I find one who does not want a local, and those you can do under nitrous oxide.

So far we have had no deaths from simple hernia. I had a death a month or two ago in a case of strangulated hernia. A woman came to the hospital who had had this hernia out for four days; on the fourth d a y h e r f a m i l y put her in a car and brought her 300 miles from Kansas. The hernia was as large as your fist and it was becoming considerably inflamed. I operated her and it was necessary to resect about a foot or two of the ileum, and she did not get along very well, and on the third day she died of an embolus. The peculiar part of this case was that the hernia had been out that long, and this w o m a n was apparently not very sick. There was no rise in temperature and her p u l s e was good. She had no vomiting. You could hardly believe it to be as serious as it was.

About the length of time in the hospital, insurance companies don't want them to stay longer than they have to. I make it a rule to keep them two weeks and then let them go home. I would like to keep them all three weeks, but I can't do it.

As to sutures, I use continuous suture m o s t l y rather than interrupted. The most men use interrupted sutures, but I never knew of any of them giving way on that a c c o u n t. I think there are three points of importance—isolate the sac, ligate it high enough, and close the internal ring around the cord both above and below as tightly as you can get it without strangulation, and proper closure of the muscle to Poupart's ligament, and then I think you have accomplished all anybody can.

This thing Dr. Fite brought out about examination for employment is valuable to anybody who does a lot of examinations. Perhaps a large external ring is not a potential hernia, but in a good many cases where they have a large external ring, we find them coming in with hernia. It is a bad thing to have to turn them down, but you have to do it. I believe that is all I have to say.

Dr. F. L. Flack, Tulsa: Most of the recurrences of inguinal hernia that I have seen have been in the external ring or the subcutaneous layer, and I think that one point of value is to close the external ring. You can transplant the cord clear up on top of the fascia, but you can close the psoas inguinalis tightly down under the cord and there is no danger of compressing the cord, because of course the cord is on top. In regard to suturing the conjoin tendons or your Poupart's ligament so that there will be fibrosis of the sac, that requires about two weeks and 20-day chromic catgut will last 10 days or two weeks. The principal advantage in using Galli sutures or fascia sutures, would be the saving of the price of a tube of catgut. Another thing to look for is when you get the sac out and open it up is to see if you haven't a n o t h e r sac. You may have sometimes two sacs, and that accounts for some recurrences. The sutures must be tied tightly enough to produce some strangulation of the conjoin tendon to produce this myositis and make the thing hold.

Dr. A. Ray Wiley: I enjoyed this paper very much indeed for several r e a s o n s. Most of my work has been in the industrial field, the same as Dr. Fite's and Dr. Weber's. I have very little to add to what has been said. Dr. Fite has covered the field very well. A few points might be somewhat worthwhile. I b e l i e v e in what both Dr. Fite and Dr. Weber have said. Dr. W e b e r remarked that local anesthesia sometimes, not in his experience but in some cases, had not been sufficient. If you make your local injection correctly you will get a nice anesthetic clear down through to the peritoneum.

In closing the fascia, I have been very c a r e f u l where you have the congenital type of hernia extending into the tunica vaginalis not to close or tie off the lower sac. Excise your sac, but leave that opening into the tunica opening, otherwise you will almost certainly get a hydrocele.

I had a very interesting case recently. This patient was operated in Texas by a very good man. He had a recurrence. In the previous operation the interrupted sutures were of black silk so that every stitch showed distinctly. The hernia had not recurred in the line of suture, but to one side.

I think this subject has been very well covered.

Dr. Woolsey, St. Louis: Mr. Chairman, it looks like Wiley put me on the spot. I was unfortunate in being so far away from the kitchen that I was late with my lunch and did not get to hear the paper. I don't know why he mentioned my name. I am a guest, living up on the Mississippi river.

I have had something to do with hernias, and the most important thing I have to say is that a hernia is the result of a poster anatomical wall defect of the inguinal canal. You talk about lifting and other things, but you are not going to get an inguinal hernia unless you have direct violence to the point of hernia, and it will follow immediately. A lot of people have hernias for many years before they are aware of it, and they find it accidentally. As far as traumatic hernia is concerned, our state laws, our compensation laws, etc., the majority of them are wrong in figuring that lifting, etc., causes hernia. When you find the wrestler, the strong man in the circus, etc., without hernia you will know that the anatomical wall if properly made is greatly in excess of any exertion.

As far as the repair of the hernia, back in 1920 I became convinced that white meat would not grow to red meat, and I devised an operation of my own which I have followed since that time. I reported it in 1925 in Dallas, and just before I reported it, Major Selig of St. Louis, after having gotten my idea on fascia to muscle suture, made extensive investigations on rats, etc., and wrote an article for the American Surgical Society to the effect that the fascia would not grow to muscle. In my operation I put three layers of fascia under the cord. Bassini is responsible for the first really proper idea in hernia operation, and with these three layers I have been criticized on the grounds that there might be trauma to the cord, but one can readily see that your trauma to the cord would have to be over the pubes and that part of it hasn't been disturbed in this operation. The most important part in this operation is to carry your substitute suture line not only to the internal ring but above the internal ring, and if you carry it high enough and never put a suture in that first line of sutures above your internal ring, because you will get a constriction atropy and get into trouble. Your suture line should go a little above the internal ring.

In direct hernia the inguinal canal has nothing to do with direct hernia, and if it has nothing to do with it, there must be a weak posterior wall. Now with that so, and with the internal ring having the inguinal hernia appear through the internal ring is a weak canal wall too, so that all operations should be the same. The first thing to do is to properly repair the internal ring, the posterior canal wall. If that is properly done you will not get recurrences. In the old operations we had the most recurrences in the direct hernia. In the operation that I have used, I have not seen a recurrence in direct hernia. The only hernia that I have seen recur—and that had very few recurrences—is that of the internal ring and it is either because the posterior canal wall was not carried high enough or the top suture is broken by coughing, or the conjoin tied, or something of that kind. I use in my first line No. 1 20-day double catgut and I have the knots so that the knots are all outside the fascia. Since 1925 when I reported the operation I have had five recurrences in over 700 cases. In my particular work I am more apt to get the recurrences than the majority of surgeons. If a person is operated by a surgeon and gets a recurrence, he is pretty apt to go to some other surgeon to get repair. In my work, railroad work, I feel more apt to get the recurrences than the majority of surgeons.

* * * *

CONCLUSION

Dr..Fite: I think we are all agreed that one of the essential things in closure is repair of the posterior wall, and the comparative figures in this paper go to show that that is at least a significant thing, because one-half of these 1,500 cases were done without any particular attention to the posterior wall, the other half with a great deal, and there were seven times as many recurrences in the first group as in the second. In the first group there were 21, and in the second group three recurrences.

Like Dr. Woolsey we are able to follow our cases pretty well for the reason that they come back to get it done for nothing. That is one of the first things, and the bureau has a pretty good follow-up, so that we are fairly accurate in the number of recurrences that we have. No private cases were included in these cases at all, because we realized that we cannot follow these and we don't know how many recurrences we might have, and any figures we might get up would be wide of the mark.

But this subject of hernia in our present industrial life is made important, and it behooves us to see that we operate them and get good results. From the standpoint of insurance companies, if the hernia occurs during the time of employment, if it does not recur, the man can get a position. I haven't any figures to show on it, but the incidence of chronic hernia is about one in 15. I know it is pretty high. I do know at the average examination there is a preformed sac in at least 50 per cent of all individuals. If there is a preformed sac in 50 per cent, it is not strange that one in 15 should develop a hernia.

I appreciate the remarks you gentlemen have made. I believe we all know what we should do. If we can cut down our recurrences we have done something for the problem.

———————o———————

Corpus Luteum Hormone in Early Pregnancy: Report of Case in Which There Was Early Removal of Corpus Luteum

Using the gravimetric method of Venning, Howard W. Jones and Paul G. Weil, Baltimore (Journal A.M.A., August 6, 1938), studied the excretion of pregnanediol in a case of early pregnancy in which the corpus luteum of pregnancy was removed 58 days after the last menstrual period. Abortion did not take place. Following this operation, the daily urinary content of pregnanediol, an excretion product of progesterone, was determined. Progesterone is probably produced by the placenta, beginning, in this case at least, at about the end of the second month.

———————o———————

The Treatment of Addison's Disease

Edward H. Rynearson, Rochester, Minn. (Journal A.M.A., September 3, 1938), discusses the treatment of Addison's disease by presenting hypothetic case histories, which include the patient in a crisis of Addison's disease, the patient with Addison's disease who requires an operation, the patient with chronic Addison's disease and the patient suspected of having Addison's disease. Progress in the treatment of Addison's disease is being reported and it is believed that the best available treatment should consist in (1) the restriction of potassium in the diet, (2) the addition of sodium salts to the diet, (3) the use of an active extract of the adrenal cortex when it is needed, (4) the training of the physician and the patient in the details of treatment of the chronic state of the disease and (5) the early recognition of acute remissions and their energetic treatment.

Surgical Diseases of Gallbladder and Bile Ducts

D. L. GARRETT, M.D.

TULSA, OKLAHOMA

The biliary system attracts the attention of the surgeon largely because of inflammatory processes and the results of inflammation. Anomalies, t u m o r s, traumatic injuries, parasitic and other lesions are of much less importance to the clinical surgeon.

The symptoms are frequently of slow insidious onset, so that the patient is unable to fix an exact date for their beginning. A sensation of fullness and distension, vague epigastric discomfort and distress, eructation of gas, increase of discomfort to the point of actual epigastric or right upper quadrant pain often mark the course of the malady, until the patient finally seeks relief. Other cases present a sudden dramatic attack, usually after a period of years of milder distress. The attacks, the well k n o w n gallbladder or cystic duct syndrome, are said to begin suddenly, often at night, following the eating of a heavy meal. The pain is epigastric or in the right hypochondrium, radiating to the right scapular and interscapular region. Nausea and vomiting may occur. Localized tenderness over the gallbladder area, below the ninth costal cartilage becomes manifest. Murphy's first percussion sign may be elicited. There is little disturbance of the pulse or temperature early.

There are not to be found the agonizing pain of acute pancreatitis, the board-like rigidity of perforating ulcer, the posterior tenderness of acute kidney lesions, the fall in blood pressure of coronary thrombosis, the f e v e r and dyspnoea of pulmonary lesions. Early in an attack, acute appendicitis may mimic a gallbladder syndrome with considerable fidelity. Relief of the pain and spasm by use of an opiate terminates the attack and after a few days the patient resumes her customary routine.

If the inflammation becomes severe, seriously compromising the gallbladder wall with suppuration or gangrene, the story becomes prolonged. We have fever, prostration, anorexia and persistent pain and tenderness, with or without the development of a palpable mass. The process may then subside, be terminated by surgery or result in rupture of the gallbladder either into the peritoneal cavity or an adjacent viscus.

When a stone establishes its residence in the c o m m o n bile duct, a new train of symptoms develops. Intermittent f e v e r with chills and sepsis, with or without pain may be present. If the common duct is completely blocked jaundice becomes evident. This jaundice varies in intensity, develops r a p i d l y and subsides quickly. There may be more than one attack. Thus it differs from the jaundice of malignancy which is progressive, never fades and becomes deeper and darker as the weeks pass.

The diagnosis is to be made from consideration of history, elimination of other possible causes of epigastric and upper right abdominal pain by physical examination, X-ray examination, including the dye, electro-cardiograph when necessary, and the standard laboratory procedures. It is somewhat useful and interesting to have an icterus index and van den Bergh test made. The bleeding time is quite important in jaundiced cases.

In selecting cases for operation who present vague atypical symptoms, with few physical findings, we must be careful not to include the neuroses and the patients with functional digestive disorders. Certain neurologic cases may present deceptive findings. The interpretation of the films of the gallbladder must be made with care. When the findings are not distinct and positive, it is wise to wait awhile and repeat the tests.

The preparatory treatment for operation includes the administration of abundant fluids, citrus fruit juices, glucose intravenously and blood matching for donors. A bed rest period is useful for many patients. The frequent and judicious use of consultants is a distinct aid in lowering morbidity and perhaps mortality.

The choice of anesthesia depends upon circumstances and individual peculiarities of patient, surgeon and anesthetist. We frequently use spinal.

A transverse incision has been quite satisfactory to us, g i v i n g good exposure, closing easily, producing sound scars and few hernias. Technique of various procedures upon the gallbladder and ducts is too well k n o w n to consume your time describing it.

---o---

A Case of Actinomycosis in Man

Wm. H. Bailey, A.B., M.D.

WESLEY HOSPITAL LABORATORY

OKLAHOMA CITY, OKLAHOMA

Cases of actinomycosis in man, although not extremely rare, are not f r e q u e n t enough to make us very familiar with the clinical picture. We are very likely to overlook the diagnosis, if the condition is not suspected and special methods used in making the laboratory examination of pus. The diagnosis is confirmed by the finding of the "sulphur" granules, which float in the pus as small pinhead, or smaller size white or light yellow, particles and which h a v e, on microscopic examination, the characteristic ray-like fungus appearance. Although such a positive finding might be considered essential for a definite diagnosis, it must, as always, be considered only as one factor in the whole clinical picture of the case.

The other laboratory findings in the ordinary case are not especially distinctive and are what you might expect in any infection.

Blood: The white blood count runs from 13,000 to 17,000, with a tendency to the higher count if a severe secondary infection has t a k e n place. The differential count is from 80 per cent to 90 per cent polymorphonuclears. As the c o n d i t i o n progresses, a secondary anemia of more or less severity develops, the red cells dropping to 3,000,000 or below with a proportionate decrease in the hemoglobin.

Urine: No characteristic findings occur in the urine. If the case is quite acute with considerable fever and general toxemia, a slight amount of albumen, often with hyaline and granular casts, will be found.

Pus from lesion: It is the appearance of this pus and the discovery in it of the small, so-called "sulphur" granules that often first brings the thought of actinomycosis to one's mind. Microscopic examination of this pus and especially of the "sulphur" g r a n u l e s, if they show the ray fungus, confirms the diagnosis. The ray fungus, if examined properly, is quite distinctive, but can be easily overlooked. Too heavy crushing of the granules will destroy their typical ray-like form. We have found that just the w e i g h t of the cover-glass alone, or possibly with the very slightest pressure on it, is sufficient and makes the best preparations. Examination is made of wet preparations, unstained, u s i n g a subdued light. Stained preparations, both with simple stains and Gram's are made and add to the findings but are not entirely satisfactory by themselves.

The infection is a c h r o n i c condition which is due to the invasion and growth of the ray fungus (Actinomyces Bovis), a microscopic parasitic plant that c a u s e s "lumpy jaw" in cattle. It is considered that the infection usually enters the body through the mouth, from which location it is carried to other portions of the body, most frequently to the neck, intestines or lungs. These three most common sites for the spread of the infection give rise to the three clinical types of the disease that are recognized in man.

1. *Cervico-facial:* This probably is the most frequent type and carries a mortality of around 25 per cent. In it, the submaxillary region on one side of the throat becomes swollen, hard and indurated. The jaw soon becomes enlarged and tender. Later, multiple abscesses form and numerous sinuses discharge a thick, mucoid bloody pus, in which can be seen the small "sulphur" granules. There may be a slight septic type of fever in the more acute or extensively involved c a s e s. Often the other side of the jaw, as well as the tongue, may become involved.

2. *Abdominal:* This is the second most frequent type and gives a mortality of around 50 per cent. Any o r g a n in the abdomen may be affected, but some part of the gastro-intestinal tract is more often primarily involved. As would be expected, during the time the gastro-intestinal tract is the system primarily attacked, the symptoms will be those referable to it such as nausea, vomiting, diarrhea, etc. As soon as the infection gets outside of the digestive tract, the organs and structures then involved give the m o s t prominent symptoms. Sooner or later, the infection works its way through the abdominal wall and appears on the external surface of the body, first as a hard indurated painful swelling which soon breaks down and discharges, usually through multiple sinuses, a characteristic pus in which the "sulphur" granules can be seen. Even while this drainage is going on, the pus burrows its way in o t h e r directions and penetrates any structure that comes in its way. It may go through into the pleural cavity, or even through the vertebrae into the spinal canal. A frequent route for infection in the lower abdomen is down the ilio-psoas muscle into the thigh.

3. *Pulmonary:* This type is the l e a s t frequent, but it has the highest mortality, about 80 per cent or higher. The symptoms are those referable to a chronic infection of the lungs, cough, some fever, varying quantities of thick sputum, either purulent or muco-purulent, often bloody. The "sulphur" granules can usually be found in the sputum, but often the case goes on to an extension through the chest wall and the escape of pus through the skin, before a diagnosis is established.

We are permitted to report the following case through the courtesy of Dr. G. H. Kimball, Oklahoma City, under whose care he was while in the hospital, and at the time the diagnosis was made: Mr. B. F., age 36 years, white, male, married, oil field worker, was admitted to Wesley Hospital, 3-31-38, complaining of pain and tenderness in lower right rectus muscle, with some burning on urination and nocturnal frequency. He gave a history of having received a slight trauma to the front of his abdomen, 1-6-38, which was some four months previous to his entry into the hospital. He was working with a grader at the time and was pushed aside more than actually being struck by it. At least, it was not severe enough to cause him to stop work at the time. A few days later, however, he did stop work and was seen by his family physician who treated him a little and he soon returned to work. Then, after a short time, he was forced to stop work a second time. This was on or about 3-8-38, some three weeks before his admission to the hospital. On entering the hospital, his physical examination was essentially negative except for a tender area at the median edge of the right rectus muscle just above the pelvis, and a slight daily temperature. Laboratory findings: Blood, W.B.C., 13,300-16,800 per cu. mm. Diff. Ct.—80 per cent to 90 per cent polymorphonuclears. R.B.C.—4,100,000-3,300,-000 per cu. mm. Hb—54 per cent to 60 per cent. Wassermann and Kline—negative. Urine—Normal, except for a slight trace of albumen.

Several possible diagnoses w e r e discussed, chronic appendix, ruptured appendix, with walled-off abscess, incarcerated right inguinal hernia, infected hematoma of the right rectus muscle, acute myositis of right r e c t u s, even malingering was mentioned. On 4-8-38, the lesion was incised and dissected. A small amount of pus escaped from a small mass underneath the right rectus. The surrounding tissue was quite firm and fibrous. Microscopic examination of this tissue showed only chronic inflammation. There was no microscopic evidence of T.B., s y p h i l i s, or malignancy of the tissue. Actinomycosis was not suspected at this time and was not picked up.

At the time of the operation, a s m a l l sinus was found extending down towards the right psoas muscle, but it was not completely explored. On 4-16-38, the drainage material from the operative wound was described as very foul and fecal in character. His general condition seemed improved and the p a t i e n t was allowed to l e a v e the hospital on 4-22-38, with the wound draining freely. The wound did not heal, but continued to drain the fecal-like pus while at home. At this time also the pain and "drawing-up" of his right t h i g h increased, so that he had to use crutches to get around. He was re-admitted to the hospital on 5-21-38, X-ray examination of kidneys and colon gave no additional information as to the cause of the condition. The p a t i e n t had developed symptoms of a general sepsis with marked anemia. He was given two or more blood transfusions, which seemed to benefit him a great deal.

On 6-1-38, a second abdominal operation was done and the a p p e n d i x removed, which was r e p o r t e d as about normal length, but thick-walled with some adhesions to its surface. It was a chronic, rather than an acute appendix. There was not found any special amount of adhesions or walled-off abscess or abscess wall, so it was thought that the original condition could not have been a ruptured appendix, which was one of the possibilities discussed at first.

This second incision continued to drain and did not heal so that now there were two draining wounds. The right leg, by this time, was rather acutely drawn up and flexed at the hip and knee joints, and there was apparent danger of at least partial ankylosis, if not firm fixation, in this crippling position, so the leg was forcibly extended and put in a cast.

On 6-28-38, a third operation was performed, the two incisions being re-opened widely and·packed open and the right leg straightened and fixed in an extended position by a cast. On 7-6-38, some of the pus from the wound was sent to the laboratory for culture and microscopic examination, but only the ordinary pyogenic organisms found. Actinomycosis was still not thought of. After the sinuses had been partially occluded for a day or two with lessened drainage, on 7-25-38 a large amount of pus escaped when the dressing was changed, and Doctor Robert Choice, the interne on

the case, noticed many small yellowish-white granules floating in it. Smears of this pus were sent to the laboratory with the request to examine for Actinomyces, but only pus cells and the ordinary pyogenic bacteria were found in the stained preparations. Unstained preparations of the crushed "sulphur" granules d i d n o t show the ray fungus, for the reason, we believe, that too much pressure was put on the cover-glass and the typical arrangement of the rays destroyed. The next day, additional specimens were taken at the bedside, in the unstained preparations the cover-glass was allowed simply to settle down on the pus by its weight alone, and when examination in a subdued light, the characteristic rays, with bulbous ends and coccal and bacillary forms in the center of the granules were definitely identified.

As soon as the diagnosis was established, the patient was put on K.I. by mouth and sodium iodide intravenously. L a t e r, he was g i v e n thymol, also sulphanilimide. Although the patient s e e m s much improved physically, and is running v e r y little fever, on 8-25-38 a new abscess down below Poupart's ligament on the inner side of the upper part of the right thigh ruptured and drained. The two former sinuses seem to be healing slowly.

We are unable to give the final outcome of this case because the patient is still under treatment in the hospital. We can say, however, that he is much better, physically, and the prognosis seems much more favorable than at the time the diagnosis was established. The treatment instituted apparently has had a beneficial effect up to this time.

CONCLUSIONS

Here is a case of actinomycosis of the lower part of the abdominal wall in a man who gives the history of having had an injury to that part of the body some three or four months before. He was working for an oil company at the time, so there is the question of compensation in this case. The location of the lesion is at or near the site of the alleged injury, but at the same time, is in one of the three most frequent locations in which the disease is found, when the infection enters through the mouth. We also must remember that cases can develop through trauma, the infection being introduced through a wound with the entrance of a foreign body. Most authors do not consider the condition contagious. The finding of the fungus in the tonsillar crypts and in the cavities of decayed teeth has been reported in the literature. These must, therefore, be considered as possible foci for infection. In some cases, it will be most difficult and at times impossible to decide the exact route of infection. If the infection entered through the mouth and passed through the wall of the intestines before reaching the abdominal wall, there should be some extensive peritoneal adhesions, but none were reported as having been found at the time the appendix was removed.

SUMMARY

A case of actinomycosis in man is reported in which the diagnosis was not established until late in the course of the disease. The inadequacy of the ordinary routine methods of examining the pus from these cases in the laboratory is pointed out. The fact that the condition must be suspected, and special laboratory technique used in examination of the pus, is emphasized. The possible routes of invasion are discussed.

Thoracoplasty in the Treatment of Tuberculosis*

R. M. SHEPARD, M.D.
TULSA, OKLAHOMA

The purpose of this paper is to demonstrate by a case presentation selected from our files the place for thoracoplasty in the course of treatment and cure of tuberculosis. No one method used can usually be considered a cure within itself. It is a combination of methods, each being used as indicated and deemed advisable for a permanent cure.

In the treatment of tuberculosis every method of treatment and means of cure should be used to return a patient to a useful life, a permanent cure, and to prevent the spread of the disease as soon and as permanently as possible.

Tuberculosis is a local disease with systemic manifestations. The attack on the lungs by the infection causes a lowering of the red blood cells, hemoglobin and general resistance of all the organs of the body. Tuberculosis is not primarily a surgical disease, but often it is necessary to resort to surgery to r e d u c e the constitutional symptoms as well as to produce a permanent cure of the local infection.

No two clinics or clinicians use the same technique or method in arriving at their end results, so the phthisilogoist and surgeon should carefully weigh each case for the best method to pursue for the best results. Statistics will not give one the results and working knowledge that the study of each patient will give. Therefore, when thoracoplasty is decided upon as the surgical method indicated in any particular case to c o n t r o l the symptoms such as cough, expectoration, fever, and loss of weight, the patient must be prepared for the operation by a complete study of the blood and all the organs, their functions and reaction to the strain which will be thrown upon them by the operation. A study must also be made as to the extent of the lesion and its location to determine the number of stages of operation and the extent of the operation to be done.

Thoracoplasty is the only method whereby the lung is completely immobilized. In pneumothorax collapse of the lung there is some expansion of the lung tissue on inspiration regardless of the degree of collapse. This can easily be demonstrated by X-raying a patient with pneumothorax on deep inspiration and then again on deep expiration.

In performing the operation of thoracoplasty which we are discussing today, it must be so timed, judged and performed as to avoid any future complications.

*Read before the Medical Section, Annual Meeting, State Medical Association at Muskogee, Oklahoma, May 10, 1938.

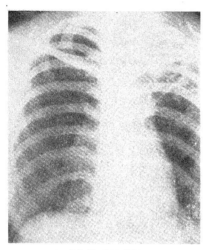

Cut Number One

This particular case p r e s e n t e d is a typical illustration of using the necessary methods of treatment when indicated and was so timed and completed for ideal results.

Female, 32 years old, appears for examination January 28, 1937, complaining of cough, expectoration, blood streaked sputum and fever over a few weeks' duration. Previous history recalls that the patient was examined and X-rayed in A u g u s t, 1931, which showed a tuberculous involvement in the upper lobe of the left lung. No treatment more than bed rest was advised and carried out. Then she was examined and X-rayed again in August, 1936, which still showed an a c t i v e process in the upper lobe of the left lung. When she appeared for examination in January, 1937, (See Cut No. 1) there was active tuberculosis in the upper lobe of her left lung with small cavitation. At this time she was put to absolute bed rest for observation to determine the method of treatment.

On February 22, 1937, this patient developed influenza and was sent to the hospital where she remained very sick for two weeks. After this the X-ray (See Cut No. 2) showed marked extension of the tuberculosis in the left lung. Pneumothorax was administered, 15 treatments b e i n g given, but because of massive adhesions only a partial c o l l a p s e was obtained.

Cough, expectoration and fever continued with positive s p u t u m. Pneumothorax was discontinued in July, 1937, (See Cut No. 3) and thoracoplasty recommended because at this time there was very little air space in the pleural cavity.

The first stage thoracoplasty was done July 22, 1937, the upper four ribs being removed from the vertebral junction to near the costa-cartilaginous junction. The second stage was done August 9th, the next six ribs being removed from the vertebral junction to n e a r the costa-cartilaginous junction.

This patient made an uneventful recovery and gained weight from 112 to a present weight of 150. Very little cough, expectoration and fever remained after the first stage of the operation and completely subsided after the last operation (See Cut No. 4). She has had no symptoms since.

I wish to emphasize at this point that a thoracoplasty should not be done as long as there is a large quantity of air in the pleural space because you realize the ribs will re-ossify in a few weeks' time and the air will continue to be absorbed, which will leave a portion of uncollapsed lung which may cause serious trouble in the future.

I also wish to emphasize the importance of removing as much of each rib as possible

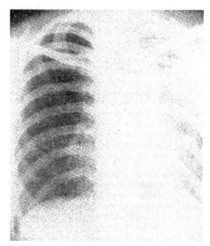

Cut Number Two

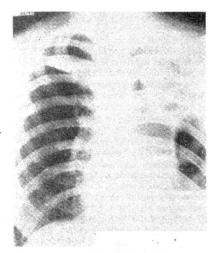

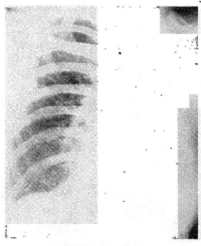

Cut Number Three

Cut Number Four

in order to collapse the entire lung. If much of the ribs is left near the vertebral body or near the sternum, there is some danger of having some uncollapsed lung area. Furthermore, these short pieces of para-vertebral rib remaining may cause pain by pressure on the inter-costal nerves and some immobilization of the shoulder, which in the future may develop diminished usefulness of the shoulder and arm. That also applies to the costa-cartilaginous portion of the ribs which may produce adhesions of the muscle which will also give limited functions.

The efficacy of the results of any method of treatment a n d particularly thoracoplasty is judged by the immediate abatement of symptoms such as fever, cough and expectoration together with a negative sputum.

When the operation is complete and the patient leaves the hospital, the cure is even yet not complete and there should be no let up in medical supervision and medical care to put the patient back to social and economic well being for all time to come.

---------------o---------------

Acute Infective Laryngotracheobronchitis*

CARROLL M. POUNDERS, M.D., F.A.C.P.
OKLAHOMA CITY, OKLAHOMA

I wish to deal here with a dangerous disease which occurs not uncommonly in small children. The fact that discussions and writings upon the subject are largely limited to those who are specializing in

*Read Before the Section on Obstetrics and Pediatrics, Annual Meeting, Oklahoma State Medical Association, Muskogee, Oklahoma, May 11, 1938.

otolaryngology leads one to fear that the pediatrician and family physician k n o w too little about it. And still it is we of the latter groups who first see such cases; and upon us rests the responsibility for recognizing the true condition and seeing that proper medical service is rendered. The symptoms, diagnosis and treatment will be briefly dealt with and an illustrative case report presented.

According to Chevalier Jackson[1], Blaud[2] first described the condition in 1823; but we are indebted to Jackson[3,4] himself, for much of our present day knowledge of it. Baum[5] discussed the endoscopic findings in 1924 and later reported 24 cases[6]. Gittins[7] reported 14 cases in 1926 and is the author of subsequent papers dealing with it[8,9]. Reference to several articles which have appeared in print during the past 15 years, will be found in the bibliography which follows[10,39].

It can be said of the disease that it is infectious and contagious and occurs sporadically and epidemically throughout most parts of the country during the c o l d e r months. While the most typical and severe form is seen in children under three, it can occur at any age. Davis[40] reports a fatal case in an adult and Gittens[8] had one that recovered. The onset is apt to be insidious and to appear in the guise of a common cold with a l a t e r development of hoarseness and croup. The fulminating type of case may come on more rapidly, accompanied by high fever and prostration with a quickly developing dyspnoea. I have seen two cases which followed the bronchoscopic removal of vegetable foreign bodies and Gittins[8] had three such instances in his series. The onset sometimes occurs in the middle of the night and simulates spasmodic c r o u p. When first seen most of these children have considerable dyspnoea, a croupy cough and are restless. The degree of temperature varies but may not be very high. One is often at a loss to r e c o n c i l e the rather striking symptoms with the few physical findings. The lungs are usually resonant but moist rales may be heard over the entire chest. The throat is congested and the ear drums may be reddened.

The d y s p n o e a grows progressively worse, the difficulty being largely inspiratory. Cyanosis may become apparent but instead of this, the more severe cases often have an ashen gray color. There is retraction at the suprasternal spaces and the epigastrium. Many cases develop a wheeze with stridor. Mucous plugs may occlude portions of the tracheobronchial tree and produce evidence of atelectasis over corresponding parts of the lung. Due to anox-

emia the fever may be low until a tracheotomy is done and then it may be greatly elevated. T h e progressively increasing dyspnoea is apt to become so marked as to rapidly exhaust what r e s e r v e strength there might be. In due time the inflammation extends well throughout the tracheobronchial tree. Some of the milder cases will go on to recovery in a few days without operative interference while the severe ones will succumb unless a tracheotomy is done without too much delay. The mortality in the severe type is generally about 50 per cent. Gittins t h i n k s that many cases of bronchiectasis seen in later life may be the result of fibrosis and dilatation of the bronchi following this disease.

On seeing such a case one is apt to experience considerable uneasiness b e f o r e making a final diagnosis. The possibility of (1) asthma, (2) foreign body aspiration, (3) bronchopneumonia, (4) enlarged thymus and (5) laryngeal diphtheria m u s t u s u a l l y be considered. Absence of the typical expiratory difficulty and the characteristic musical rales eliminates asthma. In the condition under discussion there is dificulty with both inspiration and expiration but it is usually greater with inspiration. Moist rales may be heard over the entire chest but not the peculiar musical variety belonging to asthma. Absence of a history of a sudden attack of coughing and strangling helps to rule out a foreign body. This, with the lack of characteristic physical findings, is usually sufficient but the aid of the roentgenogram may also be employed. It is my feeling that the condition is often erroneously d i a g n o s e d bronchopneumonia and more particularly when it occurs in young infants. We are helped by noting the fact that retraction of the supraclavicular and epigastric spaces is out of proportion to the chest findings and that the lungs are generally resonant throughout. Here, too, the roentgenogram may be of much assistance. It is entirely likely that many cases which live long enough do later develop pneumonia; but early in the course such a diagnosis is apt to be wrong. If one cannot satisfy himself otherwise as to the possibility of an enlarged thymus, he can readily do so with a chest picture. The condition has much in common with laryngeal diphtheria and one should not be too severely criticized for confusing the two. Certainly, the giving of antitoxin in doubtful cases is a logical procedure. The respiratory difficulty with retraction of the supraclavicular and epigastric spaces is common to both but there is not the s a m e type of hoarseness or aphonia here as in diphtheria. This is because most of the trouble is below the vocal cords and they are not covered by a membrane. There is more evidence of widespread involvement of the tracheobronchial tree than in diphtheria. Examination with the laryngoscope clears up the question quite readily and is an important procedure. The laryngeal mucosa appears red and swollen and may be covered with an exudate which, when wiped off, s h o w s no membrane or ulceration. Smears and cultures can thus be made directly from the larynx.

As yet, no specific organism has been found constantly present. It seems that the bacteria recovered correspond fairly well to what is found in routine throat cultures in ordinary upper respiratory infections w i t h different varieties predominating at different times. Pneumococci and staphylococci are often f o u n d and streptococci (both hemolyticus and viridans) are quite frequently reported. It has been suggested that a fliterable virus may some day be discovered as the primary cause.

As was previously stated, the disease is serious and, unless properly d e a l t with, carries a very high mortality rate. The patient's strength is not only exhausted by the dyspnoea but it is also impaired by the toxemia and anoxemia. Atelectasis of portions of one or both lungs may contribute to the bad outlook with added difficulty from the thick, tenaceous tracheobronchial secretions. At times, there is very little cough reflex. The cardiac muscle, weakened by the toxemia, may be completely exhausted and death ensue from circulatory failure. However, asphyxia is probably the greatest single lethal factor. The ordinary croup remedies are not effective and the oxygen tent is not sufficient to overcome the anoxemia.

Proper management of these cases demands the services of some one who can use a laryngoscope and perform a tracheotomy on a small child. It is often neces-

sary to employ the bronchoscope, as well. First of all, a laryngoscopic examination is necessary in order to make a diagnosis. Through this instrument it can be determined whether or not a diphtheritic membrane is present and the presence or absence of diphtheria can be further verified by smears and cultures taken directly from the larynx or trachea. The severe type of case will be saved only by maintaining the breathing s p a c e through a tracheotomy opening. Baum likes to try intubation first but most authorities favor tracheotomy instead. This should be done when marked signs of obstruction are present and should not be delayed until the child is so greatly exhausted or until such destructive changes have taken place in the respiratory center as to prevent recovery. And tracheotomy alone will save very few unless the air passages are kept open by proper after care. This is particularly important because the thick, tenacious secretions continue to accumulate and to form plugs and crusts which not only block the trachea but shut off portions of the lungs aerated by the smaller bronchi. A suction machine must be available at all times and a competent nurse in attendance. By means of a soft rubber catheter attached to the suction machine the secretions must be cleared out as often as they b e c o m e troublesome. It is sometimes necessary to first introduce a half dropperful of warm normal saline to soften the crusts. Young and Wautat[41] were successful in actually irrigating the tracheobronchial tree, with injections of from 5 to 10 cc of saline in a two-year-old child. Instillation of a few drops of a 1 to 1,000 solution of epinephrin into a trachea has often been found helpful. At times the bronchoscope may have to be introduced in order to remove obstructing plugs from the bronchi. Warm moist air from a vaporizer both b e f o r e and following the tracheotomy is very helpful in soothing the irritated mucosa and in helping to prevent the secretions from becoming dessicated. The oxygen tent is also useful where there is continued difficulty with aeration as evidenced by cyanosis. Since dry cold air is irritating and c a u s e s dessication, the temperature and humidity should be controlled. There is little indication for drugs. Opiates are dangerous because they depress the respirations, inhibit the cough reflex and cause retention of secretions. Atropine may contribute to a fatal ending by thickening the secretions. After seeing that the air passages are sufficiently clear for breathing one may quiet the child's restlessness by cautiously giving pheno-barbital. The iodides and other expec-torants do not seem to be of much prac-tical value and, since they are usually un-palatable, it is generally better to not dis-turb the child with them. Many of these children do not take liquids well and they all lose much moisture through the rapid respirations. Since dehydration leads to disturbed body chemistry and causes the secretions to be thicker, it is important to give plenty of fluids and electrolytes. In some cases these can be given by mouth but it will often be necessary to give nor-mal s a l i n e or Hartmanns solution sub-cutaneously or intraperitineally. While the child should be disturbed as little as possible, he should be given a thorough examination once daily to determine the condition of the heart and the possibility of such complications as otitis media and pneumonia. B e c a u s e of the prominent part so often p l a y e d by the hemolytic streptococcus the question of giving sulfan-ilamide naturally arises. It has seemed to help in some cases but I do not believe there has been sufficient opportunity to evaluate it.

CASE REPORT

J. K., a 26-month-old white female, was seen because of a croupy cough and diffi-cult breathing of 24 hours' duration. For two or three days preceding this she had had a cold with a moderate coryza and cough. Her twin sister and older brother were just recovering from colds with mod-erate hoarseness and cough. A cousin, one year of age, had shown symptoms which were similar to those of the patient and which necessitated a tracheotomy three days before. These children had all been in contact with each other. The patient had been troubled with eczema and asthma nearly all her life.

When seen the child was quite restless and had a moderate degree of retraction of the suprasternal, supraclavicular and epigastric spaces. The lungs were reso-nant throughout but numerous moist rales were heard. The throat was moderately injected. The rectal temperature was 103.

A blood count showed: hemoglobin 80 per cent, total erythrocytes 4,000,000, t o t a l leucocytes 11,600, polymorphonuclears 43 per cent. She was admitted to the hos-pital where Dr. J. C. McDonald did an im-mediate laryngoscopic examination. There was considerable swelling of the laryngeal. mucosa with some exudate but no mem-brane. Cultures taken were later reported as showing no diphtheria bacilli or strep-tococci. Steam inhalations were begun. She became more restless, the dyspnoea grew more marked and cyanosis devel-oped which was not relieved by oxygen. Finally an ashy gray color developed and the child looked very bad. Dr. McDonald did a tracheotomy under local anesthesia. A moderate amount of dark colored, tena-ceous e x u d a t e was expelled when the trachea was incised. The c o l o r imme-diately returned to normal and the patient looked quite well. During the next three days it was necessary to repeatedly remove the heavy mucus from the trachea by in-troducing the catheter attached to a suc-tion machine. The temperature gradually subsided, the breathing became normal and the tracheotomy tube was removed on the fourth day. She made a complete re-covery.

COMMENT

This case is fairly typical of the mod-erately severe type that will recover with prompt and efficient treatment. She came from a community where there had been other cases; this and the fact that she had been in contact with a relative who had the same condition illustrates the infec-tious and contagious nature of it.

SUMMARY

Acute infective laryngotracheobronchi-tis is a dangerous disease of early child-hood. The real diagnosis is probably often overlooked. It o c c u r s endemically and epidemically during the cooler months.

For proper treatment it is necessary to secure the services of some one who can use a laryngoscope, do a tracheotomy and, if possible, use a bronchoscope. Among the severer type of cases the mortality will be around 50 per cent.

BIBLIOGRAPHY

1. Jackson, Chevalier and Chevalier, L.: Acute Infective Laryngotracheobronchitis, Brennemanns Practice of Pedi-atrics, Vol. 2, Chap. 45.
2. Blaud, P.: Nouvelles Recherches Sur La Laryngo-

tracheite Connue sous le nom de Croup, Paris, 1823.

3. Jackson, Chevalier; Croupy Cough and Dyspnoea Simulating Diphtheria due to Infective Laryngotracheobronchitis, Med. Clin. North America, 5:648, 1921.

4. Jackson, Chevalier and Chevalier, L.: Acute Infective Laryngotracheobronchitis, J.A.M.A., 107:929-932, September 19, 1936.

5. Baum, H. L.: Some Endoscopic Observations on Laryngotracheobronchitis, Ann. Otol. Rhin. and Laryng., 33:728-788, September, 1924.

6. Baum, H. L.: Acute Laryngotracheitis, J.A.M.A., 91:1097-1102, October 13, 1928.

7. Gittins, T. R.: Membraneous Laryngitis and Tracheobronchitis (Non-Diphtheritic). Annals of Otol. Rhin. and Laryng., 35:1110-1129, December 26, 1926.

8. Gittins, T. R.: Laryngitis and Tracheobronchitis: Reference to Non-Diphtheritic Infections, Ann. Otol. Rhin. and Laryng., 97:1165-1174, December, 1936.

9. Gittins, T. R.: Laryngitis and Tracheobronchitis in Children, Special Reference to Non-Diphtheritic Infections, Annals of Otol. Rhin. and Laryng. 41:422, June, 1932.

10. Richards, Lyman: Fulminating Laryngotracheobronchitis, Ann. of Otol. Rhin. and Laryngol., 42:1014-1040, December, 1933.

11. Beare, Frank: A Series of Cases Resembling Laryngeal Diphtheria, The Med. J. of Australia, May 24, 1930.

12. Johnson, M. C.: Acute Laryngotracheobronchitis in Infants, Arch. Otolaryngol., 17:230-234, February, 1933.

13. Thembe, C. L.: Acute Non-Diphtheritic Obstruction, The New England J. of Medicine, 207:740, October 27, 1932.

14. Cultra, G. M. and Streit, A. J.: Non-Diphtheritic Infectious Laryngitis, Texas State J. of Med. 31:364-368, September, 1930.

15. Leigh, H.: Sudden Death from Acute Laryngeal Obstruction of Non-Diphtheritic Origin, Southwestern Med., 11:210-213, May, 1927.

16. Seitz, R. P.: Acute Streptococcic Laryngitis in Children, Calif. and Western Med., 30:259-260, April, 1929.

17. Kirkpatrick, S. and S. M.: Non-Diphtheritic Laryngotracheobronchitis, South. Med. J., 26:287, March, 1933.

18. Marks, S. B.: Acute Laryngotracheobronchitis in Children, Kentucky Med. J., 31:381-384, August, 1933.

19. Hyde, C. I., and Ruckman, J.: Acute Infectious Edematous Laryngitis in Which Recovery Followed Tracheotomy, Arch. of Ped., 48:124, February, 1931.

20. Strachan, J. G.: Acute Septic Tracheitis, The Can. Med. Assoc. J., 15:708-711, July, 1925.

21. Schenck, C. P.: Non-Diphtheritic Laryngotracheobronchitis, Texas State J. of Med., 27:493, November, 1931.

22. Peeler, C. N.: Acute Non-Diphtheritic Laryngitis in Children, Southern Med. and Surgery, 88:661, October, 1926.

23. Codd, A. N.: Obstructive Laryngeal Dyspnoea, Annals Otol., Rhin. and Laryng., 40:242, March, 1931.

24. Hart, V. K.: Streptococcic Laryngitis, Report of a Case With a Very Rare Complication, Annals of Otol., Rhin. and Laryng., 36:781, September, 1927.

25. Mathew, R. Y.: The Staphylococcus Aureus as the Possible Cause of a Fatal Disease Simulating Laryngeal Diphtheria, The Medical J. of Australia, January 11, 1930.

26. Bradford, W. L. and Leahy, A. D.: Acute Obstructive Laryngitis, Am. J. Dis. of Children, 40:298-304, August, 1930.

27. Champion, A. N.: Acute Stenotic Laryngitis of Infectious Origin, Texas State J. of Med., 23:669, February, 1928.

28. Simpson, W. Likely: Pheumothorax Complicating Tracheotomy in Fulminating Laryngotracheobronchitis, Arch. Otolaryng., 26:411-414, October, 1937.

29. Spearman, Maurice P. and Vandevere, W. E.: Acute Laryngotracheobronchitis (Case Report). Southwestern Med., 21:165-168, May, 1937.

30. Morris, M. E.: Laryngeal Stenosis as a Complication of Measles, N. Y. Med. J., 106:1125, December 15, 1917.

31. Mainzer, F. S.: Acute Laryngotracheobronchitis, Penn. Med. Jour., 33:24, October, 1929.

32. Spake, Laverne B: Acute Infective Laryngotracheobronchitis, Jour. Kans. Med. Soc., May, 1930.

33. Silverman, A. Clement: Acute Laryngotracheobronchitis, Arch. Ped., 51:257, April, 1934.

34. Smith, W. Jewell: Acute Laryngotracheobronchitis in Children, Arch. Otolaryng., 23:420, April, 1936.

35. Richards, Lyman: Can Fulminating Tracheobronchitis be Cured, N. Eng. J. of Med., 207: July 21, 1932.

36. Gatewood, E. Trible: Bronchoscopic Observation of Laryngotracheobronchitis in Children with Obstructive Dyspnoea, Virg. Med. Monthly, 63:600-601, January, 1937.

37. Brennemann, Joseph; Clifton, Willie Mae; Frank, Albert and Holinger, Paul: Acute Laryngotracheobronchitis, Am. J. of Dis. of Children, 55:667-695, April 1938.

38. Tolle, D. M.: Croup: Analysis of Three Hundred and Forty-Four Cases, Am. J. Dis. Children, 39:954-968, May, 1930.

39. Neffson, A. H., and Wishik, S. M.: Acute Infectious Croup: A General Study of Acute Obstructive Infections of the Larynx, Trachea and Bronchi with an Analysis of 727 Cases: II. Acute Non-Specific Group, J. Pediat., 5:617-641, November, 1934.

40. Davis, David: Acute Fulminating Laryngotracheobronchitis in an Adult, Arch. Otolaryngology, 23:686-690, June, 1936.

41. Young, Nelson A., and Woutat, Philip H.: Fulminating Laryngotracheobronchitis, The Journal Lancet, 57:287-289, July, 1937.

1200, North Walker street.

---o---

What Every Woman Doesn't Know—How To Give Cod Liver Oil

Some authorities recommend that cod liver oil be given in the morning and at bedtime when the stomach is empty, while others prefer to give it after meals in order not to retard gastric secretion. If the mother will place the very young baby on her lap and hold the child's mouth open by gently pressing the cheeks together between her thumb and fingers while she administers the oil, all of it will be taken. The infant soon becomes accustomed to taking the oil without having its mouth held open. It is most important that the mother administer the oil in a matter-of-fact manner, without apology or expression of sympathy.

If given cold, cod liver oil has little taste, for the cold tends to paralyze momentarily the gustatory nerves. As any "taste" is largely a metallic one from the silver or silverplated spoon (particularly if the plating is worn), a glass spoon has an advantage.

On account of its higher potency in Vitamins A and D, Mead's Cod Liver Oil Fortified With Percomorph Liver Oil may be given in one-third the ordinary cod liver oil dosage, and is particularly desirable in cases of fat intolerance.

---o---

Hodgkin's Disease: Sixty Cases in Which There Were Intrathoracic Lesions: Clinical Lecture at San Francisco Session

C. B. Wright, Minneapolis (Journal A.M.A., Oct. 1, 1938), has reviewed 60 cases of Hodgkin's disease, in all of which, during the period of observation, there were intrathoracic complications; all had been observed long enough so that there was a fairly good clinical history and a physical examination had been made. All the patients had roentgen treatment and were under observation for a considerable period. The patients did not all have intrathoracic lesions on first examination. Some had them then and the rest acquired them later. The intrathoracic lesions are of four varieties: (1) enlargement of the mediastinal glands, (2) involvement of the pulmonary parenchyma, (3) involvement of the pleura and (4) combinations of these regional types. In 57 cases enlarged mediastinal glands were demonstrated roentgenographically. Twenty-one patients had parenchymal involvement, and 18 of these had also enlarged mediastinal glands. Three of these patients had parenchymal lesions only. Seventeen patients had pleural effusion; all of these had mediastinal enlargements. Seven had pleural effusion and involvement of the mediastinal glands. Forty-five of the 60 patients observed were followed until their death. The average duration of life was 40 months. For the 13 patients now living, the average length of the disease is 50 months. Seven of these patients have had the disease 72 months. The majority are in fairly good health. Some are working, and others are in a condition of semi-invalidism. Two patients were lost track of. An attempt was made to estimate the length of life after the onset of intrathoracic complications. In some cases there were in addition other complications. In the 39 cases in which this estimate could be made, the average survival period was 23 months.

THE JOURNAL

OF THE

Oklahoma State Medical Association

Issued Monthly at McAlester, Oklahoma, under direction of the Council.

Copyright, 1938, by Oklahoma State Medical Association, McAlester, Oklahoma.

Vol. XXXI	OCTOBER	Number 10

DR. L. S. WILLOUR..Editor-in-Chief
McAlester, Oklahoma

DR. T. H. McCARLEY..Associate Editor
McAlester, Oklahoma

Entered at the Post Office at McAlester, Oklahoma, as second-class matter under the act of March 3rd, 1879.

This is the official Journal of the Oklahoma State Medical Association. All communications should be addressed to The Journal of the Oklahoma State Medical Association, McAlester Clinic, McAlester, Oklahoma. $4.00 per year; 40c per copy.

The editorial department is not responsible for the opinions expressed in the original articles of contributors.

Reprints of original articles will be supplied at actual cost provided request for them is attached to manuscripts or made in sufficient time before publication.

Articles sent this Journal for publication and all those read at the annual meetings of the State Association are the sole property of this Journal. The Journal relies on each individual contributor's strict adherence to this well-known rule of medical journalism. In the event an article sent this Journal for publication is published before appearance in The Journal the manuscript will be returned to the writer.

Failure to receive The Journal should call for immediate notification of the Editor, McAlester Clinic, McAlester, Oklahoma.

Local news of possible interest to the medical profession, notes on removals, changes of addresses, births, deaths and weddings will be gratefully received.

Advertising of articles, drugs or compounds unapproved by the Council on Pharmacy of the A. M. A., will not be accepted.

Advertising rates will be supplied on application.

It is suggested that wherever possible members of the State Association should patronize our advertisers in preference to others as a matter of fair reciprocity.

Printed by News-Capital Company, McAlester.

EDITORIAL

SOUTHERN MEDICAL ASSOCIATION

To ALL PHYSICIANS OF OKLAHOMA:

The Southern Medical Association, with a membership recruited from all over the South, will hold its thirty-second annual meeting in Oklahoma City on Tuesday, Wednesday, and Thursday, November 15 to 18, 1938. This Association is unique in that its scientific exhibits feature the work of individuals and not of institutions. In other words, the Southern Medical Association exists for the individual doctor and not for any group, faculty, department or association. Exhibits this year will consist of subjects demonstrated by means of p i c t u r e s, motion films, diagrams, and printed placards. The booths will be of uniform construction, and the entire group of exhibits will be well worth the effort of any physician who will take the necessary time to go through them.

The program of the meeting will be divided into 19 different sections covering every field of medicine, both in science and practice. Each section will have its complete program, making a total of more than 600 papers and discussions on various subjects. Meeting simultaneously with the Southern Medical Association will be four or five other national meetings on public health, tropical medicine, etc. The first day's program will consist of 86 papers, each lasting 15 minutes, given by members of the profession in Oklahoma City. All papers will be of a practical nature even when the subject matter is distinctly technical. Specialties covered in this program will include general surgery, eye, ear, nose and throat, traumatic surgery, urological surgery, obstetrics, and gynecology.

Oklahoma City feels distinctly honored to be the host city this year. Previous meetings since 1934 have been held in San Antonio, Texas, St. Louis, Missouri, Baltimore, Maryland, and New Orleans, Louisiana. Never before has it been held in a city as far northwest as Oklahoma City, and it will probably be many years again before such a meeting comes to us. Every physician of Oklahoma is urged to consider himself as a part of the entertainment committee since in reality the Southern Medical Association is the guest of all the physicians of this state. Every member of the State Association should make it his business to be present and do his part in assisting the visitors to find their way around and also to see that they are entertained in a manner fitting this great occasion. Let's do our part and show them that Oklahoma City is a leader among the southern states.

----o----

REPORT OF REFERENCE COMMITTEE ON CONSIDERATION OF THE NATIONAL HEALTH PROGRAM

(Adopted at Special Session, House of Delegates, A.M.A., Chicago, September 17, 1938)

(In this editorial you will find a report taken from the minutes of the called meeting of the House of Delegates of the American Medical Association. These conclusions were made after serious deliberation of a Committee of 25 and the report adopted as we hand it to you. We are giving you this information for two reasons: One, that you may inform the laity as to the cooperation of the medical profession in a plan to increase public health facilities and care for our sick citizenship. Second, that you may prepare to cooperate with this move made by organized medicine as 100 per cent cooperation will be necessary to make it effective.)

Since it is evident that the physicians of this nation,. as represented by the members of this House of Delegates convened in special session, favor definite and decisive action now, your committee submits the following for your approval:

1. Under Recommendation I on Expansion of Public Health Services: (1) Your committee recommends the establishment of a federal department of health with.a secretary who shall be a doctor of medicine and a member of the president's cabinet. (2) The general principles outlined by the Technical Committee for the expansion of public health and maternal and child health services are approved and the American Medical Association definitely seeks to cooperate in developing efficient and economical ways and means of putting into effect this recommendation. (3) Any expenditure ma'de for the expansion of public health and maternal and child health s e r v i c e s should not include the treatment of disease except in so far as this cannot be successfully accomplished through the private practitioner.

2. Under Recommendation II on Expansion of Hospital Facilities: Your committee f a v o r s the expansion of general hospital facilities where need exists. The hospital situation w o u l d indicate that there is at present greater need for the use of existing hospital facilities than for additional hospitals.

Your committee heartily recommends the approval of the recommendation of the technical committee stressing the use of existing hospital facilities. The stability and efficiency of many existing church and voluntary hospitals could be assured by the payment to them of the costs of the necessary hospitalization of the medically indigent.

3. Under Recommendation III on Medical Care for the Medically Needy: Your committee advocates recognition of the principle that the complete medical care of the indigent is a responsibility of the community, medical and allied professions, and that such care should be organized by

local governmental units and supported by tax funds.

Since the indigent now constitute a large group in the population, your committee recognizes that the necessity for state aid for medical care may arise in poorer communities and the federal government may need to provide funds when the state is unable to meet these emergencies.

Reports of the Bureau of the Census, of the U. S. Public Health Service and of life insurance companies s h o w that g r e a t progress has been made in the U n i t e d States in the reduction of morbidity and mortality among all classes of people. This reflects the good quality of medical care now provided. Your committee wishes to see continued and improved the methods and practices which have brought us to this present high plane.

Your committee wishes to see established well coordinated programs in the various states in the nation, for improvement of food, housing and the other environmental conditions which have the greatest influence on the health of our citizens. Your committee wishes also to see established a definite and far reaching public h e a l t h program for the education and information of all the people in order that they may take advantage of the present medical service available in this country.

In the face of the vanishing support of philanthropy, the medical profession as a whole will welcome the appropriation of funds to provide medical care for the medically needy, provided, first, that the public welfare administrative procedures are simplified and coordinated; and second, that the provision of medical services is arranged by responsible local public officials in cooperation with the local medical profession and its allied groups.

Your committee feels that in each state a system should be developed to meet the recommendation of the National Health Conference in conformity with its suggestion that "The role of the federal government should be principally that of giving financial and technical aid to the states in their development of s o u n d programs through procedures largely of their own choice."

4. Under Recommendation IV on a General Program of Medical Care: Your committee approves the principle of hospital

service insurance which is being widely adopted throughout the country. It is capable of great expansion along sound lines, and your committee particularly recommends it as a community project. Experience in the operation of hospital service insurance or group hospitalization plans has demonstrated that these plans should confine themselves to provision of hospital facilities and should not include any type of medical care.

Your committee recognizes that health needs and means to supply such needs vary throughout the United States. Studies indicate that health needs are not identical in different localities but that they usually depend on local conditions and therefore are primarily local problems. Your committee therefore encourages county or district medical societies, with the approval of the state medical society of which each is a component part, to d e v e l o p appropriate means to meet their local requirements.

In addition to insurance for hospitalization we believe it is practicable to develop cash indemnity insurance plans to cover, in whole or in part, the costs of emergency or prolonged illness. Agencies set up to provide such insurance should comply with state statutes and regulations to insure their soundness and financial responsibility and have the approval of the county and state medical societies under which they operate.

Your committee is not willing to foster any system of compulsory health insurance. Your committee is convinced that it is a complicated, bureaucratic system which has no place in a democratic state. It would undoubtedly set up a far reaching tax system with great increase in the cost of government. That it would lend itself to political control and manipulation there is no doubt.

Your committee recognizes the soundness of the principles of workmen's compensation laws and recommends the expansion of such legislation to provide for meeting the costs of illness sustained as a result of employment in industry.

Your committee repeats its conviction that voluntary indemnity insurance may assist many income groups to finance their sickness costs without subsidy. Further development of group hospitalization and

establishment of insurance plans on the indemnity principle to cover the cost of illness will assist in solution of these problems.

5. Under Recommendation V on Insurance Against Loss of Wages During Sickness: In essence the recommendation deals with compensation of loss of wages during sickness. Your committee unreservedly endorses this principle as it has distinct influence toward recovery and tends to reduce permanent disability. It is, however, in the interest of good medical care that the attending physician be relieved of the duty of certification of illness and of recovery, which function s h o u l d be performed by a qualified medical employee of the disbursing agency.

6. To facilitate the accomplishment of these objectives, your committee recommends that a committee of not more than s e v e n physicians representative of the practicing profession under the chairmanship of Dr. Irvin Abell, President of the American Medical Association, be appointed by the Speaker to confer and consult with the proper federal representatives relative to the proposed National Health Program.

———————o———————

The Post-Graduate Instruction Program in Obstetrics is now well into its sixth month. Two circuits of five teaching centers each have been completed, and a third circuit is just beginning. The first circuit included Claremore, Pawhuska, Bartlesville, Vinita, and Miami, with an enrollment of 75 physicians. The second circuit included Poteau, McAlester, Durant, Hugo, and Idabel, with an enrollment of 77 physicians. The third circuit just opened in Wewoka, Muskogee, Okmulgee, Ada, and Shawnee. At the present time, there is an enrollment of 92 physicians in this circuit. These figures show that 152 doctors in Oklahoma have c o m p l e t e d this postgraduate course in obstetrics, and that 92 more physicians are now attending the lectures in their respective centers. For the small fee of $5.00, it is the belief of the Committee that, with a few exceptions, every physician in Oklahoma should take advantage of this course.

The instructor, Dr. Edward N. Smith, has received many demands upon his time for free private consultations with class members. During the circuit in southeastern Oklahoma, the i n s t r u c t o r was called in on consultations over many and varied complicated malaria cases—malaria being a frequent complication with pregnancy.

It is contemplated that the next circuit will either include teaching centers in the north middle section of the state or in the extreme southwestern corner of Oklahoma. . This will be determined shortly. Prior to the meeting of the Southern Medical Association w h i c h convenes in Oklahoma City November 15, announcements will be mailed to the section where the course will function next. Doctors of that particular area may enroll at the booth which the post-graduate committee will establish at that meeting. Physicians of all sections of the state are invited and urged to call at this booth and see outlines of the course, becoming acquainted with the plans from maps which will indicate when the course will occur for the county where each and every doctor resides.

————————o————————

MEDICAL TECHNOLOGY; ITS VALUE TO OKLAHOMA DOCTORS

What is a Medical Technologist?

In 1928 the American Society of Clinical Pathologists established the Registry of Medical Technologists as a voluntary bureau for certifying laboratory technicians who had minimum qualifications for this important field, properly called medical technology. It was the clinical pathologists who were especially interested in seeing that the assistants in their private and hospital laboratories were competent in their work. They realized that many laboratory workers had received very poor or no laboratory training at all, or that they were the victims of unscrupulous and blatantly advertised commercial schools that gave them but a smattering of procedures and failed to instill in them a realization of the responsibility that they were assuming. The American Society of Clinical Pathologists desired to establish a standard for laboratory workers and some means of signifying to the medical profession that certain technicians were qualified. The Registry became the means to that end. It assumed the responsibility for instituting standards for training schools; it inaugurated systematic and timely examinations conducted bi-annually. The result of these efforts is the Medical Technologist, a laboratory worker certified by the Board of Registry and found competent to practice medical technology within the bounds of the Code of Ethics.

Code of Ethics

"Registered Medical Technologists shall agree to work at all times under the supervision of a qualified physician, and shall under no circumstances, on their own initiative, render written or oral diagnosis except so far as it is self-evident in the report. They shall not advise physicians or others in the treatment of disease or operate an independent laboratory, or when employed by a physician accept work outside of his own practice."

A.M.A. Acceptance of Medical Technologists

In 1936 the A.M.A. accepted the recommendations of the house of delegates to recognize the examination and certification of laboratory workers by the A.S.C.P., thus making the Registry of Medical Technologists the authoritative bureau for licensing and q u a l i f y i n g laboratory workers throughout the United States and Canada. Moreover the standards for training schools of the A.M.A. and the A.S.C.P. are the same. A list of approved schools for technicians appears in the J.A.M.A., March 26, 1938, Vol. 110, page 982.

The requirements for admission to the examination for registration in medical technology are graduation from high school and two years college work (in a college or university approved by the regional college associations) with special emphasis on basic science subjects; chemistry, biology, bacteriology, and physics. Ninety quarter hours must be completed before admission to an approved training school or to the registry examination for medical technologists is granted.*

Examination and Certification

The examination is divided into an oral and a written portion; the applicant is asked to carry out certain standard laboratory procedures under the eye of examiners appointed by the Board of Registry. All questions, written and oral, are formulated by the Board of Registry and submitted to the appointed examiners under seal by the Board of Registry. By this method, a uniform, fair, and impartial examination is conducted.

Organization of Oklahoma Society of Medical Technologists

In April, 1936, every medical technologist in Oklahoma was invited to meet in Oklahoma City for the purpose of forming the Oklahoma Society of Medical Technologists. A representative group gathered at the medical school, and the Society was created to further the cause of Medical Technology, to bring about a closer fellowship among medical technologists and a better understanding between the physicians and technologists. Officers were elected, committees appointed, and a program for growth in medical technology was formulated.

At the present time there are 66 registered technologists in Oklahoma, and two recognized training schools for technicians, namely; the University of Oklahoma Hospital, and St. Anthony's Hospital, both in Oklahoma City.

One of the chief objectives of the organization has been to further the cause of the Board of Registry. An official Board of Registry exhibit has been placed at nearly every medical or hospital meeting held in Oklahoma since the organization of the society. The purpose is to bring to the attention of every licensed physician the service that the Board of Registry is rendering all doctors, in their program of certification, standards for competency, and ethical practices in Medical Technology.

A.S.C.P. Accomplishments

The A.S.C.P. has rendered a service of inestimable value to doctors, patients, and medical technologists, for the establishment of the Board of Registry has brought about a stabilization of laboratory medicine in that it has:

1. Established a professional standing for laboratory workers.

2. Provided an adequate code of ethics to protect patients, hospitals, and doctors from deleterious practices.

3. Established standards of competency for the practice of medical technology.

————————

*A laboratory worker who does not come up to the requirements but who had received his or her training prior to January 1, 1933, and whose technical qualifications are vouched for by a clinical pathologist, may, by special action of the Board of Registry, be considered eligible for the examination.

4. Certified training schools for training Medical Technologists.

5. Standardized examinations for registration throughout the United States.

6. Provided a title and insignia for Medical Technologists.

7. Elevated the scientific, economic, and social status of registered laboratory workers.

8. Obtained the support of the A.M.A., American College of Surgeons, American Hospital Association, and the Catholic Hospital Association.

9. Safeguarded interest and promoted welfare of M.T.

10. Outlined a program of post-graduate study and organized post-graduate seminars for medical technologists as a means of keeping them abreast of present day Medical Technology.

The Oklahoma Society of Medical Technologists' November Meeting

It is the hope of medical technologists in Oklahoma to launch a precedent which will consist of annual post-graduate seminars for technologists to be held in various medical centers where inspiration and ideas for technical improvements in their profession may be gleaned. With this in mind the O.S.M.T. has invited the technicians of the South to meet for study and fellowship in Oklahoma City, November 17 and 18, where they will be able to enjoy some of the speakers of the Southern Medical Association. Among the outstanding men in laboratory medicine who will speak and give demonstrations to us are Dr. R. R. Kracke, Dr. Meyer Bodansky, and others.

There will be a $1.50 registration fee to help defray the expense of the seminar, and will include the banquet ticket. Trips to the oil fields, hospitals, and points of interest will be available. A banquet and informal get-acquainted reception are other features of interest in addition to a worthwhile program which will be published in the November issue of this Journal.

The O.S.M.T. Appeal to Oklahoma Doctors

We urge every doctor who attends the Southern Medical Association in Oklahoma City to bring his technician with him. Give your technician an opportunity to hear the guest speakers and to get acquainted with other Medical Technologists. Even though a technician is not registered, he will be welcome to join us in these meetings and if he is interested in becoming registered, Dr. R. R. Kracke, past president of the A.S.C.P. and member of the Board of Registry, who will be there with the official registry exhibit, will be very glad to give your technician sound and authentic advice.

Doctors, we appreciate your interest and cooperation. We depend upon you for leadership and inspiration to attain greater efficiency. We are striving for technical excellence, sincerely hoping that we will be able in our small way to assist you in your efforts to solve the problems of disease.

More detailed information regarding registration may be secured from Mrs. Anna Scott, Registrar of the American Society of Clinical Pathologists Board of Registry, 234 Metropolitan Building, Denver, Colorado.

Editorial Notes—Personal and General

DR. E. O. TEMPLIN and family of Alva spent a week in Colorado during September.

DR. W. E. SIMON of Alva is taking a three months' vacation and resting in Massillon, Ohio.

DR. C. A. ROYER, formerly of Kiowa, Kansas, has recently returned from a two years' post-graduate course and has located in Alva, being associated with Dr. A. E. Hale in the practice of eye, ear, nose, and throat.

DR. C. A. TRAVERSE returned September 5 from taking a 16-week post graduate course in Vanderbilt University.

DR. D. B. ENSOR returned August 28 from a month spent in eastern Tennessee and Kentucky.

DR. E. A. McGREW, Beaver, has returned from a meeting of the International Goitre Assembly at Washington, D. C.

DR. F. E. DARGATZ has been appointed as Director of the full time Health Unit, Ardmore, to fill the place resigned by Dr. R. M. Parish.

DR. REED WOLFE has been appointed as County Health Superintendent of Choctaw County.

DR. H. T. BALLANTINE, JR., Muskogee, and MISS ELIZABETH ELLIOTT MIXTER, daughter of Dr. and Mrs. William Jason Mixter of Brookline and Hardwick, Mass., were married in Boston September 24. They are at home at 77 Revere Street, Boston.

DR. AND MRS. JAMES L. PATTERSON and son, James, have returned from a vacation in Canada and down the west coast of the States to San Francisco.

News of the County Medical Societies

WOODS-ALFALFA County Medical Society held their regular meeting September 27 in Cherokee. Dr. J. W. Mercer and E. E. Talley, both of Enid, read papers on "Pre-Natal Disturbances, Symptoms and Treatment," and "The Thyroid," respectively. Dr. Talley's paper was discussed by Dr. E. A. McGrew, of Beaver. The next meeting of the joint Societies will be held in connection with a crippled children's clinic in December.

WESTERN Oklahoma Medical Society held its quarterly session at Hobart, September 13th. Following the dinner Dr. Carroll M. Pounders, Oklahoma City, read a paper on "Rheumatic Fever in Childhood." Dr. J. Wm. Finch, Hobart, read a paper on "The Etiology of Nausea and Vomiting of Pregnancy." Other Oklahoma County physicians visiting this meeting were Drs. C. P. Bondurant; J. Worth Gray; J. F. Kuhn, Sr.; Floyd Moorman, and Horace Reed.

APPOINTMENTS

Additions to the Faculty of the University of Oklahoma School of Medicine.

Dr. Donald B. McMullen, D. Sc., Johns Hopkins University, 1935, has been appointed Assistant Professor of Bacteriology (Division of Parasitology).

Dr. Rudolph F. Nunnemacher, Ph. D., Harvard, has been appointed Instructor in the Department of Histology.

The following men have been appointed Assistants in Medicine:

Dr. Allen G. Gibbs.

Dr. Vern H. Musick.

Dr. Ralph A. Smith.

Dr. Hubert E. Doudna has been appointed Lecturer in Anaesthesia and Head of the Department of Anaesthesia in the University and Crippled Children's Hospitals.

Rob't. U. Patterson, M.D.,
Dean and Superintendent.

OBITUARIES

DOCTOR WALTER P. HAILEY

Dr. Walter P. Hailey of Haileyville, Oklahoma, died at the Albert Pike Hospital, McAlester, September 12 as the result of a long illness.

He was born in McAlester in June, 1876, son of the late Dr. D. M. Hailey, who was a pioneer physician and coal operator in Pittsburg County. Dr. Walter Hailey practiced medicine in Pittsburg County during his entire professional career and was one of the participants in the development of organized medicine in Indian Territory. He attended Kemper Military Academy at Boonville, Mo., took a pre-medical course at Cornell University and graduated from Columbia, New York City, in Medicine. He was married to Miss Grace Moulten of Greenville, Texas, in 1899, who preceded him in death in February, 1935.

Dr. Hailey was a gracious gentleman, who never spoke ill of any fellow practitioner and gave his services freely both in a civic and professional way.

The last rites were held September 14 at the Haileyville home by the Rev. Charles F. Schwab, pastor of the First Christian Church, McAlester, with burial in McAlester.

Another pioneer medical man of Indian Territory has passed to his reward, leaving many close and intimate friends to mourn his demise.

DOCTOR GILES E. HARRIS

Dr. G. E. Harris, Hugo, pioneer physician of Choctaw County, died following an automobile accident September 14 in which his car overturned after striking another head-on.

Dr. Harris was born at Quitman, Texas, 58 years ago. He attended and graduated from the Louisville University at Louisville, Ky., after which he served his internship in St. Louis. In 1906 he moved to Boswell where he began the practice of medicine, living there until 1918, when he moved to Hugo, where he remained until the time of his death.

Dr. Harris was a member of his County Medical Society, State Association and the American Medical Association. He was a charter member of the Hugo Lions Club, a member of the Masonic fraternity, State Historical Society and the American Legion.

He is survived by his widow and two daughters. Burial was in Mount Olivet Cemetery, Hugo.

RESOLUTIONS

Report of Committee on Resolutions. Muskogee County Medical Society. August 17, 1938.

DR. F. B. FITE

WHEREAS, our esteemed co-worker, Dr. F. B. Fite, has been called by the Great Physician, and,

WHEREAS, for many years he was a prominent and active member of our society, and our profession, and,

WHEREAS, his professional attainments, and sterling qualities were known and admired both within and without the profession,

THEREFORE, be it resolved, by the Muskogee County Medical Society, that we record our sadness in his untimely passing, holding in memory his splendid skill and personality as a professional man, a loving and generous husband and father, an active civic leader, and, withal, kindly and generous, and,

BE IT FURTHER RESOLVED, that a copy of these resolutions be spread upon the minutes of the Muskogee County Medical Society, and that a copy be sent to the Journal of the Oklahoma State Medical Association, and the Journal of the American Medical Association.

Respectfully submitted,

J. Hutchings White, Chairman
L. S. McAlister, Member
J. T. Woodburn, Member.

Proctologic Tumors

During the last six years C. C. Tucker and C. A. Hellwig, Wichita, Kans. (Journal A.M.A., Oct. 1, 1938), studied by microscopic methods every specimen removed during anorectal operation. In the majority of cases nothing was detected by histologic study which changed the prognosis or treatment based on clinical examination. There are, on the other hand, so many cases in which the microscopic examination revealed conditions which were not suspected clinically that the routine histologic study of proctologic specimens seems well justified, in the interest of the patient. McCarty, basing his statistics on 150,000 surgical cases, found that routine microscopic examination revealed in 0.5 per cent of all operations a malignant condition which was not suspected by clinical methods or during operation. In the authors' 951 proctologic cases this percentage of clinically unrecognized cancer is almost four times higher, namely 1.9 per cent. The conclusion therefor eis justified that, more than in other regions, early malignant lesions of the anal and canal may closely resemble harmless conditions. Many of the malignant tumors in th ematerial were small and 18 of the 52 malignant tumors were discovered during routine histologic examination of what seemed clinically harmless anal lesions. Two adenocarcinomas and a basal cell carcinoma were completely removed by hemorrhoidectomy and in the specimen removed at the subsequent radical operation after the histologic diagnosis was established no trace of malignant tissue could be detected. In six of the 52 malignant cases, cancer developed in previously existing anal lesions. One adenocarcinoma was found originating in a fistulous tract, one squamous cell carcinoma in a fissure, three adenocarcinomas in hemorrhoid nodules and one basal cell carcinoma in an external hemorrhoid. The material of adenomatous polyps could be classified with one exception by histologic criteria as either benign or frankly malignant tumors. Only one polyp showed atypical glands in a small area, probably a transitional stage of a benign into a malignant growth. The fact that hypertrophic anal papillae are often confused with adenomatous polyps has been stressed in a recent paper by Tucker of San Antonio. In several cases the diagnosis of adenoma was made by an occasional proctoscopist, when the location in the dentate line and the whitish surface characterized these structures as enlarged papillae. The authors agree with Tucker that hypertrophic papillae do not carry a serious prognosis as compared with adenomas. Not infrequently, patients seek proctologic advice while their symptoms are caused by extra-anal conditions. The complex embryologic changes occurring in the sacral region explain the origin of chordoma (two cases), teratoma (one case) and dermoid cysts. Of pelvic tumors which produced symptoms calling for proctologic examination were one ovarian dermoid which became infected and perforated into the rectum and one adenomyoma of the recto-vaginal septum. A patient with a tumor of the cauda equina consulted a proctologist first because of anal discomfort. A sweat gland adenoma, a myxoma and a hemangioneruromyoma of the glomus type were observed in the perianal region.

ABSTRACTS : REVIEWS : COMMENTS
and CORRESPONDENCE

SURGERY AND GYNECOLOGY
Abstracts, Reviews and Comments from
LeRoy Long Clinic
714 Medical Arts Building, Oklahoma City

Conization of the Cervix; Miller and Todd; Surgery, Gynecology and Obstetrics; September, 1938; page 265.

This article is based upon 899 conizations performed in the University of Michigan Hospital during the past four years. While at first the procedure was carried out in the office as well as hospital, they now prefer to hospitalize every patient for three or four days. They state that it takes about six weeks for complete epithelization to occur following conization. To guard against stricture they place an iodoform wick in the cervical canal at the time of conization, remove it on the third day, have the patients take daily cleansing douches and report every two weeks for introduction of sterile sound into the canal.

They have come to the conclusion that extensive conization cannot be viewed as a substitute for simple cauterization, coagulation, or other valuable means of treating benign cervical disease. However, they feel that the benefits of extensive conization are real and should have a place in everyday gynecological surgery.

Though their indications have fluctuated somewhat, their present indications for using this method of treatment follow:

"1. As a means of correcting minor cervical disease and preventing remote complications of the cervix, **in patients for whom subtotal hysterectomy is planned.**

"2. As a means of eradicating deep s e a t e d, chronic infections of the cervical canal **in older women.**

"3. As a complete substitute for the Sturmdorf operation any condition of the cervix for which Sturmdorf operation is indicated.

"4. As a means of obtaining adequate biopsy material in cases in which original biopsy material presented cytological abnormalities strongly suggesting neoplastic change.

"5. As a substitute for older methods of trachelorrhaphy in most women but especially in elderly women.

"It is difficult not to become enthusiastic over the use of conization and we feel a word of caution is justified for the procedure is not without drawbacks. Extensive conization as here described is a hospital procedure and should be reserved for the more severe types of cervical lesions."

They had no serious immediate complications in their group of 899 conizations.

In their follow-up study the late results showed a stricture incidence of 8.97 per cent but they feel with the more recent greater care during the healing period the number of strictures has decreased. They state that the majority of strictures were mild and required only dilatation or the passage of a sterile sound or hemostat.

They note that the number of pregnancies subsequent to conization in this series was small, the trend certainly suggesting a harmful influence on subsequent pregnancies. "This tendency to early interruption of pregnancy is another drawback and suggests its use only in women past the childbearing period, and even then we do not consider it a substitute for the less radical office procedures in mild cervical disease."

Their concise evaluation, summary, and conclusions follow:

"Electrosurgical conization of the cervix appears to have a real place in gynecology. As a means of treating stubborn chronic cervicitis in women past the childbearing age, it far surpasses any other procedure known to us short of total hysterectomy. The excision of gland bearing tissue can be made complete although such extensive conization is probably not often necessary. We have found it a satisfactory substitute for the Sturmdorf operation and for most trachelorrhaphies.

"We believe that our experience with this operation justifies certain general conclusions:

"1. Conization of the cervix as here described is a valuable, safe, rapid, and eminently satisfactory way of treating the **more extensive benign lesions of the cervix in older women.**

"2. In general its use should be limited to women past the child-bearing age and even in this group should not be looked upon as a substitute for the less radical office procedures now in use in the treatment of simple cervical disease.

"3. Conization is many times faster, simpler, and a bloodless substitute for—and in our clinic has completely replaced—the Sturmdorf operation. The amount of tissue removed can be controlled and conization equals in efficiency any means of cervical gland reaming now available. Ultimate healing is but little slower than in the Sturmdorf procedure and the incidence of severe stricture probably no greater.

"4. Conization is a desirable, quick, and convenient method of treating the cervix prior to subtotal hysterectomy."

COMMENTS: This is an excellent article based on a fine piece of work done in a most practical field. It will do much in assisting the proper appraisal of this operative procedure upon the uterine cervix for the elimination of chronic irritations and chronic infections.

While it was originally indicated by Hyams of New York as an office procedure, it is quite evident that most men now consider it far better to hospitalize patients. It is also recognized that conization is a more formidable procedure than it was at first considered and that the proper selection of patients is of the utmost importance.

Wendell Long.

The Problem of Intra-Abdominal Injuries Due to External Trauma—Two Cases of Rupture of the Intestine. (Le Probleme du Traumatisme Ferme de l'Abdomen—Deux cas de Rupture Intestinale). By A. Bellerose—Notre-Dame Hospital, Montreal.

Translation of the French title is free because a reading of the article indicates that the author is discussing the question of intra-abdominal lesions due to external, non-penetrating injuries of the abdomen resulting from the sudden application of force, like blows upon the abdomen.

Attention is directed to the importance of systematic and uniform examination of the patient from hour to hour, particularly in those cases in which the situation is not at first perfectly clear.

The cases are divided into those where there is rupture of a solid organ, like the liver, for example, with hemorrhage; and those in which there is rupture of a hollow organ, like the gastro-intestinal tract or the urinary bladder.

When there is immediate severe hemorrhage, shock is pronounced, the clinical picture being characterized by great weakness, small and rapid pulse, cold and sweating skin, paleness, with, sometimes, dullness in the flanks. In such a situation the author advises immediate operation in order to stop the hemorrhage. (L'hemorragie reconnue, l'acte operatoire s'impose d'emblee sans qu'il soit tenu compte de l'etat general due malade; seule, une hemostase peut lui sauver la vie). I shall say something about this radical advice in the comments following the abstract.

When there is rupture of a hollow organ, most often the intestinal tract, without hemorrhage, there is frequently severe pain and temporary prostration, but the patient may apparently recover within a very short time, and be able to be up and about for a little while, this period of relief being followed by evidences of peritoneal irritation, such as rigid abdomen and the return of severe pain.

The cases of two patients are reported, there being a rupture of the intestine in each case.

In the first case a youth of 18 years was struck upon the abdomen by the knee of a companion while in play. There was immediate intense pain with partial loss of consciousness and a little later vomiting. Within a short time, however, he was apparently all right, and walked home, the distance not being indicated. Soon after that there was return of abdominal pain. A physician was called and he was sent to hospital. On admission to the hospital the pulse was 74, the temperature in the neighborhood of normal, blood pressure 124/80, respiration 24, s h a l l o w and distinctly thoracic in type. There was rigidity of the entire abdominal wall. The white blood count was 45,000. There was a diagnosis of a rupture of the intestinal tract. Laparotomy revealed some liquid in the abdomen having the gross characteristics of pus, but without odor (the article is not clear as to how long it had been after the accident, but probably about 24 hours). There was congestion of the peritoneum which was covered by diphtheroid membranes. ("Le peritoine visceral est congestionne, recouvert de membranes dithteroides"). A perforation of the small intestine about 60 centimeters from the duodenum was found. It was closed by two rows of simple catgut suture. A tubular drain was placed in the lower abdomen. There was recovery without any particular difficulty, the patient being discharged on the thirty-second day.

In the case of the second patient, a man 47 years of age, there was a fall of about 10 feet, the abdomen striking a piece of timber. There was immediate severe pain in the epigastrium. He was seen by a physician, and soon after that went to his home. The pain became worse and the physician was called again. He was sent to a hospital where it was found that the pulse was 88, temperature 96.3, blood pressure 134/95. There was board-like rigidity of the abdomen. The respiration was thoracic in type and shallow. Digital examination per rectum was painful. There was a diagnosis of probable rupture of the intestinal tract, and immediate operation advised. There was an escape of serous-like liquid with a little bile when the abdomen was opened. There was slight

congestion of the visceral peritoneum. After a laborious exploration a perforation about the size of a 10-cent piece was found about two fingers breadths from the duodenum. The perforation was closed by three layers of catgut sutures. A tubular drain was placed in the pelvis. The article states that the postoperative course was normal, but it indicates that the patient was discharged 72 days after admission.

COMMENTS: (1) We do not believe that there should always be an immediate operation in the presence of what appears to be hemorrhage due to damage of a solid organ, like the liver, spleen, etc. We believe that our experience and the experience of others would indicate that one must be extremely careful about immediate operative procedures in the presence of profound shock. If it is decided to do an operation in such a situation, there should, of course, be the intravenous introduction of material, like saline and glucose solutions to hold the patient up temporarily, with an immediate transfusion of blood as soon as the hemorrhage has been controlled. The difficulty, however, in some of these patients is that it is extremely hard to do an operative procedure that will control hemorrhage satisfactorily, especially in the case of wounds of the liver.

(2) The procedures in the two cases of rupture of the intestinal tract reported were, in our judgment, ideal. When there is strong reason to believe that there is a rupture of the intestinal tract, operation must not be delayed because if it is, there will be a fatal peritonitis.

(3) I wish to call particular attention to the employment of tubular drainage of the lower abdomen. For some years there has been a tendency to close the abdomen without drainage. We believe that in the case of rupture of the intestinal tract it is a mistake not to drain. If drainage is employed, it ought to be of such a character that drainage will be free, and we know of no better method than the employment of a suitable rubber tube. One other word: If a drain is employed, it should be permitted to remain for a week or 10 days. Regardless of the oft-repeated statement that drainage ceases within a short time after the introduction of a drainage tube, careful clinicians know that clinical results do not bear out that statement.

LeRoy Long.

Traumatic Rupture of the Bile Ducts; Kenneth M. Lewis, New York, N. Y.; Annals of Surgery; August, 1938.

In a review of the literature the author finds only 47 reported cases of traumatic rupture of the bile ducts. Since 1921 he is able to find only six reported cases, one of them being our case published in Southern Medical Journal, March, 1929. The conclusion is that the accident is very rare. The author adds an additional case treated by him at Bellevue Hospital, New York, in 1931.

In the case reported by the author the patient was a truckman 49 years of age. He was admitted to hospital July 30, 1931. He had been crushed between two trucks a short time before examination. "The trauma involved the right upper quadrant of the abdomen in the region of the costal margin." There was a history of moderate shock but it had subsided by the time he entered hospital. There was "considerable pain in the region of the right costal margin." Patient declining to remain in hospital, he was permitted to go home after strapping right chest with adhesive plaster.

Two days later he returned complaining of progressive pain in right upper abdomen, of cough, of having vomited one time. The temperature was 101. "He appeared acutely ill, was quite weak, and was in a profuse perspiration." Abdomen was distended. There was tenderness and rigidity in right upper quadrant. There were evidences of consolidation lower lobe right lung. The diagnosis was pneumonia.

There was progressive distention abdomen. "On the fourth day it was noted that there was a large amount of fluid in the abdomen." There was some jaundice. There was bile in the urine.

Seven days after the injury jaundice was very marked, the stools clay-colored and great distention of the abdomen. "There was persistent localized tenderness over the right upper quadrant of the abdomen, and the pneumonia in the right chest showed signs of resolution. Diagnosis of rupture of one of the bile ducts was made."

Surgical operation was done through a right upper rectus incision August 9, 1931, 11 days after the injury. There was a large amount of bile in the abdomen (about seven quarts). All intra-abdominal structures were deeply bile-stained. "A constant stream of bile was seen to be seeping from the region of one of the hepatic ducts, but the actual tear in the duct could not be identified." After placing a cigarette drain in Morrison's pouch the abdomen was closed.

The early postoperative course was stormy. There was profuse drainage of bile for 10 days. The jaundice gradually disappeared, but stools remained clay-colored. Bile gradually disappeared from the urine. A sinus (fistula?) with draining bile persisted. He was discharged in this condition September 4, 1931, 27 days after operation. One month after discharge the sinus (fistula?) was healed. Stools were of normal color.

In November, 1931—about two months after discharge—"the patient was again admitted to the hospital with a history that during the preceding month he had become gradually more and more jaundiced and that the stools had again become very light in color." He was kept under observation for a month, "during which time repeated biliary drainages would produce a temporary flow of bile into the duodenum, but at no time did the jaundice entirely disappear."

A second surgical operation was done January 16, 1932. There were dense adhesions fusing structures in upper abdomen. "The common bile duct was finally exposed, and was followed upwards beyond its junction with the cystic duct into the sulcus in the liver. Scar tissue could then be felt in the common hepatic duct, high up under the liver, but it was impossible to expose the stricture so that it could be seen." It was decided to discontinue operation. A cigarette drain was placed and the abdomen closed.

A duodenal fistula developed five days after operation. It healed after continuous suction for five weeks. By April, 1932, the jaundice had subsided, but there was an incisional hernia for which a third operation was done in May, 1932.

Patient has been under observation for six years, during which time "there is always a residual jaundice," for which "duodenal drainage" is done about twice a week and "if these are persisted in, the patient remains quite comfortable." However, about once every six months there is an attack of severe pain in right upper abdomen associated with sudden increase of jaundice, light colored stools and fever from 102 to 103. Morphine gives relief and "the attacks are always over within a day or two."

COMMENTS: In our case, to which the author kindly refers, the patient was an unmarried white woman of 40 years. There was a crushing injury of upper right abdomen and lower right chest by being caught between two automobiles on March 3, 1928. At the same time there were fractures of right scapula and right patella. She fainted while she was being held between the two cars, but was unconscious for only a few minutes. There was pain in right upper abdomen, and pronounced shock.

There was slight jaundice three days after injury, but no acute abdominal distress. There was comparative comfort until nine days after injury when it was noticed that the abdomen was enlarged, and the enlargement increased progressively. The jaundice was a little more pronounced, but was never extreme. There was increasing weakness. There was no nausea.

We first saw patient when she was admitted to our service at University Hospital, Oklahoma City, March 22, 1928, 19 days after injury. There was a greatly distended abdomen, slight jaundice and general weakness. The percussion note over abdomen was flat throughout. There was but little tenderness. There was no definite rigidity. There was a little yellowish staining of sclerae. The skin was sallow, with slight yellowish tinge. Pulse 110, blood pressure 110/75, direct van den Bergh 20, bile in urine, R.B.C. 3,820,000, W.B.C. 12,000, polymorphonuclears 76 per cent. The day following admission paracentesis abdominis recovered 4,500 c.c. of thin bile.

OPERATION: With a tentative diagnosis of rupture of some part of biliary tract, operation was done through a right upper rectus incision, under local novocain and general nitrous oxid-oxygen anesthesia on March 26, 1928, 23 days after injury. There was about a gallon of bile in peritoneal cavity. With the exception of gall bladder, the viscera were of a dark mahogany color. The gall bladder was pale. There were soft adhesions between and about the viscera.

After removing bile from peritoneal cavity it was observed that bile was escaping from a point in the region of hepatic duct just below the liver. No attempt was made to expose the duct because at that particular point such an attempt was regarded as futile and dangerous.

There was some question as to whether the rupture was in hepatic duct proper or in one of its radicles only. In order to determine that point, the gall bladder was opened. It did not contain a single demonstrable drop of bile. Believing that if there had not been a destructive injury of the hepatic duct proper there would be at least some bile in gall bladder, we concluded that there was a destructive injury of hepatic duct proper.

In this case there was no evidence of infection. The aspirated bile soon after admission was reported "negative" after being in culture for several days.

Remembering that tubular anatomical structures lined with mucous membrane tend to repair after injury, provided there is no infection and that there is not accumulation of material in or about them, the principal requisite appeared to be adequate drainage. We endeavored to meet this requirement by: (1) Placing a very small rubber drainage tube with the end of it at point of escaping bile, and fixing it there by a catgut suture passed through the tube before placing it in position, and then, with as much care as possible, through some loose tissue in immediate neighborhood of leak, and leaving it there for many days. We do not believe that a Penrose or a cigarette drain are comparable in efficiency to the proper kind of rubber tube. (2) Provision for escape of any material (serum, debris) from duct distal to rupture and for reduction of intraductile pressure. To meet these indications, a large rubber tube was fixed in gall bladder. Incidentally, another reason for putting tube in gall bladder was to determine time of entrance of bile into gall bladder — very important, because no bile would come out of tube in gall bladder if it had not entered hepatic duct below point of rupture. (3) Limitation of extravasation of bile, with increased drainage of peritoneal cavity at same time. This requirement was met by tucking two sheets of rubber dam under and about gall bladder, bringing the ends outside through the operative incision.

There was free drainage of bile per small tube placed at the point of rupture and about the rubber dam for seven days, after which it was intermittent, gradually decreasing.

Three days after operation bile was coming from tube placed in gall bladder. This was definite proof that bile was entering duct distal to point of rupture.

No attempt to move the bowels was made until the fourth day after operation when an enema of one pint of warm water was given, producing an evacuation of "a few small whitish fecal masses in cloudy fluid." On April 3, 1928, a small (one pint) enema of warm water was followed by the expulsion of "greenish fluid with light yellow feces." A laboratory report showed bile in the material.

The two sheets of rubber dam drainage and protective material were removed April 9, 1928 **14 days after operation.** The tube in gall bladder was removed two days later, **16 days after operation.** On April 18, 1928, drainage had ceased.

The postoperative course was satisfactory in every respect. As far as the injury to the bile duct was concerned, the patient was well on April 18, 1928—23 days after operation—but she was kept in hospital until May 3, 1928, because of the fractured right patella. The last report about her was nine years after discharge at which time she was in good health, and had been in good health all the time following operation.

Finally, we wish to stress the importance of (1) the fixation of a small rubber drainage **tube** at the point of rupture, (2) the fixation of a large rubber tube in gall bladder, if the rupture is proximal to it, in order to provide an exit for debris, to reduce intraductile pressure, and as a means of indicating when bile is entering the duct distal to rupture; and, (3) adequate drainage and protection of peritoneal cavity contiguous to the bile-tract area.

In writing these comments we have drawn heavily from our article on "Traumatic Rupture of the Bile Ducts," published in The Southern Medical Journal, March, 1929.

LeRoy Long.

Urinary Stress Incontinence, The Anatomical Defect Found and a Rational Method for Its Treatment; Davies; Surgery, Gynecology and Obstetrics; September, 1928, page 273.

This is a most excellent study of the muscles surrounding the urethra, together with the principles involved ni the surgical repair of damage to musculature, particularly at childbirth.

The following conclusions give in outline form the findings and opinions of the author:

"1. The female urethra is approximately four centimeters in length.

"2. Two layers of involuntary muscle surround its entire length.

"3. At its bladder attachment the urethra is encompassed by an additional layer of involuntary muscle called the sphincter of the vesical neck.

"4. Under resting conditions the involuntary muscles maintain a tonicity about the urethra sufficient to maintain urine within the bladder.

"5. Increased intra-abdominal pressure requires a voluntary sphincter about the urethra which contracts synergistically with the muscles causing increased intra-abdominal pressure.

"6. The voluntary muscles correspond to the three muscular layers of the abdominal wall.

"7. The deepest voluntary sphincter is derived from the levator and angulates the urethra postero-anteriorly. At times the levator supplies a voluntary coat to the entire length of the urethra.

"8. The intermediate voluntary sphincter lies between the layers of the urogenital diaphragm and is called the deep transverse perineal muscle.

"9. The superficial voluntary sphincter is due to the simultaneous contraction of the bulbocavernous muscles which lie lateral to the vagina and communicate anterior to the urethra.

"10. The involuntary sphincters are usually damaged while the head is in the midpelvis, and the damage is due to the displacement of the bladder with concomitant lacerations in the midline.

"11. The voluntary sphincters are usually damaged at the pelvic outlet.

"12. Two anatomical damages are possible: the one being due to prolonged overstretching brought about by a long labor; the other due to a midline laceration which may extend from the cervical attachment of the bladder to the external urinary meatus.

"13. Patients with stress incontinence who have no gross anatomical damages should be trained to develop the voluntary muscles of the urethra.

"14. In those having anatomical damage accurate reconstruction can be accomplished by first reapproximating the lacerated tissue at the base of the bladder, which repair when continued distally will reconstruct the involuntary sphincter a₋ the neck of the bladder and eventually, the levator and the deep transverse perineal muscles.

"15. The superficial sphincter is reconstructed as the posterior perineal body is repaired.

"16. In a series of 50 cases of stress incontinency since 1930, surgical treatment resulted in cures in all but five cases, or a successful outcome in 9₋ per cent."

COMMENTS: Urinary incontinence is very prevalent condition in women and a proper understanding of the anatomy is essential for its correction. Many operations done for this symptom are ineffective and it would be well for those doing this type of surgery to carefully read this article by Lavies, in order to increase the percentage of successful cases.

Wendell Long.

EYE, EAR, NOSE AND THROAT
Edited by Marvin D. Henley, M.D.
911 Medical Arts Building, Tulsa

Some Problems Encountered in Cataract Surgery. Watsin W. Gailey, M.D., Bloomington, Ill. American Journal of Ophthalmology, August, 1938.

This paper is a resume of the writer's experiences in dealing with the cataract problem. It is well worth while. It deals not so much with theory as with practical points learned over a period of years, some of which were gleaned in India. First is stressed the point that it is necessary for the surgeon to know what result he expects to get from the operation — eliminating the possibility of accidents and complications. Except in the case of dense hypermature cataracts the light perception and light projection tests will give this information. A history of poor vision before the formation of the cataract should make the surgeon cautious as to his prognosis—keeping in mind the fact that cataract may be a complication of glaucoma, detachment of the retina and choroiditis.

Uncompensated cardiac disease, chronic bronchitis, bronchiectasis, a s t h m a, hypertrophy of the prostate, hemorrhoids, chronic constipation, high blood pressure, infected teeth, and diabetes should be thoroughly investigated before operation and if present, corrected as much as possible, before the extraction is attempted. The author relying on experience gained in India doubts that septic teeth have any connection with inflammatory conditions following cataract removal, since practically all cases there had septic teeth (these patients may have had a high degree of resistance or have attained immunity).

Intraocular tension should be determined; the presence of a cough is important. One hundred and eighty-five is the accepted pressure (systolic) by the author for operative work on the eye. The incidence of expulsive hemorrhage is about one in a thousand. The author reports six expulsive hemorrhages. If the routine methods of reducing hypertension are not successful blood-letting is resorted to one hour before operation. Slit-lamp study helps to determine the type of operation to be done. Diabetic-cataract and senile cataract with diabetes are not inoperable if properly prepared. Postoperative iritis and iridocyclitis are apt to occur here. Caution is advised in dealing with nuclear cataracts of high myopia and nuclear cataracts with a clear posterior cortex. Wassermans are not done routinely. The lacrimal sac if infected, is removed. Prior to 1930 cultures were done routinely and an infection was expected about every two years. Since 1930 the taking of preoperative cultures has been discontinued and no infections have occurred. When the taking of cultures was discontinued, preliminary scrubbing of the skin and irrigation of the conjunctival sac was discarded. Face mask and rubber gloves are used. Which has caused the lack of infections the author is unable to state. In deciding when to operate one must consider age, visual acuity, physical status, prejudices, and occupation of patient. An important factor to the author in this decision is the state of mind or the unhappiness of the patient. Preparation for operation consists of a pad of cotton saturated with an acridine dye kept on the eye for 12 hours previous to operation. Nembutal and luminal are used to control nervousness and is used for as long as a week after operation. Five per cent euphthalmine is used for dilatation—one drop every 15 minutes for four times—first instillation two hours previous to operation.

The author attempts intracapsular extraction in patient over 40 years of age. There follows a discussion of indications for intracapsular and extracapsular extractions. A change of method may be indicated after the section is made. The author voices the opinion that elaborate preparation of the field is largely a pose but stresses the point that "instruments used within the eye be not contaminated by touching the skin or lashes." Cocaine, four per cent, is used—two minutes for six instillations, is used. O'Brien method of akinesia is used. If this is not successful then the Van Lint is used. Retrobulbar anaesthesia is produced by injection of 2 c.c. of four per cent novocaine solution. Eight minutes later the speculum is introduced.

Technique and the problems encountered in the course of the operation are gone into quite minutely. Postoperatively daily dressings are done. Postoperative complications are discussed and the method in which they should be handled. Daily dressings are continued through the fourteenth day and the shield is worn at night for another week. Patients are ordinarily hospitalized for a period of 10 days following the operation. The author's closing paragraph: "Even though we are provided with all the modern methods, problems seem to lurk at every twist and turn of the surgeon's pathway and serious complications occur all too frequently." This is an original article without bibliography.

Cholestreatoma Verum of the Right Mastoid. M. D. Friedman, M.D., and S. S. Quittner, M.D., Cleveland. Archives of Otolaryngology, August, 1938.

This case is reported because of the rarity of the condition. The patient was a male, age 25, white, American. In February, 1937, some friend commented to him that his face "seemed crooked." He was told it was Bell's palsy and would clear up in time. No improvement was noted, however, as time went on. He remembered that a year previous to this he had felt twitchings in his face at irregular intervals. General physical examination absolutely negative—no headache—no nausea—no vomiting—no olfactory disturbance and no difficulty swallowing. Neurological examination showed: peripheral type of facial paralysis, right side. The hearing was impaired right side—right external auditory lumen narrowed—membrani tympani normal and glistening—taste normal. An expanding lesion of some kind was suspected which was encroaching onto the external auditory canal.

The report of the roentgengoram taken was: "The right mastoid is densely sclerotic and entirely devoid of cellular outlines. The cortex is greatly thickened, and there is diminished density of the antrum close to the sinus, suggesting early cholesteatoma formation. The right pyramid shows a loss of continuity of the lateral portion of the superior margin but is otherwise fairly cellular. There is no thickening of the margin, and the calcium content appears to be normal. Impression: sclerosed right mastoid, with possible early cholesteatoma and involvement of the right petrosa."

A spinal puncture showed increased pressure. It was decided to approach the lesion through the right mastoid. April 26th the patient was operated. Upon removal of the cortex a white glistening membrane was seen; bone of the external canal had been absorbed; facial nerve (1.5 cm.) was brown in color and free in the debris; debris did not involve the middle ear; removal of debris in region of the lateral sinus brought a gush of blood; pressure was applied and another attempt to continue the operation was made when there was a second gush of blood; pressure pack was applied for five days; thrombosis having taken place packs were removed and the operation completed. Recovery was uneventful. Hospitalization ceased May 9th. The facial paralysis is recovering rapidly. Pathologically the tumor removed was diagnosed as an epidermoid cyst.

The Diagnosis of Nasal Allergy and Its Relation to Other Manifestations. French K. Hansel, M.D., St. Louis, Mo. The Southern Medical Journal, September, 1938.

This is quite an interesting article in which the author illustrates his various points with cases reported which do not lend themselves well to abstracting. The author's summary is as follows:

In the diagnosis of nasal allergy, the following points should be taken into consideration: (1) the nasal symptoms, (2) the changes in the mucosa, (3) the cytology of the nasal secretions, (4) the X-ray findings, (5) the histopathology and bacteriology, (6) the existence of acute or chronic infection, and (7) the influence of physical agents and endocrine factors. From the purely allergic standpoint, further investigation should consider: (1) the family history of allergy, (2) the occurrence of other manifestations in the past and present history, (3) the detailed clinical history, (4) the skin tests and other laboratory studies, and (5) the general physical examination.

These studies on the association of the various manifestations of allergy show the common occurrence of this condition in multiple rather than in single form. The patient usually presents himself for diagnosis and treatment for that manifestation which dominates the clinical picture. Associated manifestations of lesser importance, therefore, should not be overlooked. The patient with perennial nasal symptoms of allergy may have hay fever in the spring, summer, or fall. The hay fever symptoms may dominate the clinical picture while the nonseasonal symptoms may be mild or severe. If mild, attacks may be considered as acute rhinitis. Patients with perennial nasal symptoms may have asthma either with hay fever or only during the winter months. It is important to emphasize also that allergic bronchitis not infrequently accompanies nasal allergy during the winter months without any very definite evidence of true asthma. The nasal manifestations of allergy in children are frequently overlooked unless associated with asthma. The patient whose respiratory symptoms consist only of hay fever may have allergic headache or gastro-intestinal allergy or some form of skin allergy at other times of the year. Gastro-intestinal allergy or allergic headache may, on the other hand, appear as the predominating symptom. Nasal symptoms may be associated in mild degree. The diagnosis of nasal allergy is always good presumptive evidence that these other manifestations are also of an allergic nature. Such manifestations as allergic headache, gastro-intestinal allergy, and skin allergy are most frequently caused by hypersensitiveness to foods. The association of these manifestations with the respiratory types of allergy always suggests very strongly that foods also play an important part, as etiologic factors. From these studies it is evident, therefore, that most allergic patients are affected with multiple manifestations all of which must be considered in the clinical picture from the standpoint of diagnosis as well as treatment.

The Base of the Skull, With Particular Reference to Fractures. William J. Mellinger. Annals of Otology, Rhinology, and Laryngology, June, 1938.

The author's summary is as follows:

1. The base of the skull with its many foramina, their direction and the structures w h i c h pass through them, as well as the tightly adherent dura, must be carefully considered in fractures.

2. Fractures involving bones containing air cells may bring serious complications, particularly when this pneumatization is extreme. It may extend to the limits of any bone in any or all directions and the process may extend into adjoining bones.

3. The floor of the anterior fossa may consist entirely of pneumatized bone, the floor of the middle fossa almost entirely and the floor of the posterior fossa always consists partially of bone containing air cells. A basal fracture then must usually be considered compound unless proven to be otherwise.

4. The sphenoid is the "key-stone" of the skull, situated in the middle of the base and is in line of practically all basal fractures.

5. The temporal bone occupies a wide area in the base of the skull, and is unique in its connection with other bones. The arrangement is usually such that a certain amount of movement from below upward is possible.

6. Transverse fractures of the petrous pyramid usually extend through the labyrinth and seldom heal by bony union because the endochondral layer is not endowed with regenerative power. Thus in such cases there is constant danger of intracranial involvement in the event of upper respiratory infection.

7. The abducens nerve is placed in a very vulnerable position on account of its intimate relation with venous spaces throughout most of its long course, also on account of its relation with the basi-sphenoid and the petrous apex. It is very frequently involved in fractures through the middle fossa.

INTERNAL MEDICINE
Edited by Hugh Jeter, M.D., 1200 North Walker, Oklahoma City

A Broader View of Postmortem Examinations. By Alan Gregg, New York, N. Y. (Annals of Internal Medicine, August, 1938, Vol. 12, Number 2.)

In this the author in a brief and unusual manner presents a discussion on postmortem examinations and interrogates: "What advice could be given to laymen on how best to utilize a doctor's services or how can the laymen best make use of the physician's knowledge and experience?" "How can he protect himself against incompetence and selfishness? What should the layman know of the physician's professional ethics and usages? On what terms does the physician give his best service? Where lie pitfalls of misunderstanding between physician and patient? Are there any steps the layman can take to insure as well as encourage the best of medical performance?"

The author considers three factors in the solution of these questions. First: "I belong to a dinner club that plans a series of meetings at which a representative of several professions will advise the rest of us how the services of his profession can best be used by the laity. An architect, for example, will tell the rest of us how we can best make use of an architect's knowledge and experience, how to protect ourselves against incompetence or selfishness, what the layman should know of the architect's professional ethics and usages, on what terms does the architect give his best services, where lie pitfalls of misunderstanding between him and his client, what course, in short, would be wisest for the client to pursue in order to put the architect in the easiest position to give his services most effectively. And similarly we shall call upon some of the other professions; for example, an investment counselor, a newspaperman, an insurance expert, a lawyer, and—a physician. For in a society so differentiated into special callings as is the society of our times we are all laymen in everything but our own professions. And I would hold it to be wise to learn whatever possible of how to approach and maintain effective relations with other professions than one's own, and to learn this at a time divorced if not remote from the pressure of immediate need. It is probably equally wise, too, for every profession to cultivate public understanding rather than merely to court general approval."

Second: "I have realized the extraordinary fluidity of the population of the United States in contrast to the stability of residence of the Europeans. Travel by automobile has not only replaced much travel by train but it has extended the number and range of trips, excursions, visits, and it has encouraged moving and changes of residence. We think nothing of distance. We are the most restless and movable people on earth—or above it. Consequently a seriously large number of persons, separately or in families, must call an unknown physician in some unfamiliar place of residence. Now this is done usually on a basis that scarcely deserves the words choice or selection. The situation lacks the reassurance of long acquaintance with our informants or advisors. It may be hurried and urgent. It may be incredibly haphazard. Doctors are often chosen under circumstances which make it more than ever important that mutual understanding attend their relationship to patients. And so it was my second experience to realize that in Amreica especially, because of its constantly moving population, the layman needs a map of our ways. He needs to be told how we can best help him."

Third: "Lastly an experience of three years ago in the clinicopathological conference room of a well known medical school. I saw by chance a blackboard lying on its side in apparent neglect. On it were written the percentages for the preceding quarter of postmortem examinations secured on deaths (a) on the private wards and (b) on the public wards; 13 per cent of the private patients who died came to post mortem; 82 per cent of the patients on the public wards came to post mortem. Quite appropriately the table of figures on postmortems was lying on its side, for it bore evidence of neglect of one of the most enlightening and stimulating practices we physicians know—the postmortem examination. We know the postmortem can and does improve our efforts at diagnosis, we know it is the terror of the casual guesser, we know it is a reward to an eager and honest doctor even when it is a stark corrective, we know it increases our competence and knowledge—in sum, we know the postmortem serves as a merciless incentive to the best we have in us as physicians."

"But does the layman know? Let me draw these three experiences together now in the question I wish to ask you: Shall the layman be told this incentive to our best performance? Is it not true that if a layman wishes to get the best possible service from a physician he would be wise to say at the onset of an illness—'Now Doctor, there's one thing I should like to have clear: if worse comes to worst there is to be a post mortem'? I have never heard the layman's interest mentioned in discussions of postmortems. The postmortem examination has been emphasized as a way to advance scientific knowledge, or it has been thought of as a generous concession to the forgivable curiosity of a beloved doctor, or it has been urged as a method without equal in maintaining staff efficiency in hospitals—but I would inquire whether anyone unprejudiced and remote from the event has ever shown the laity where its interests lie in the matter of post mortems? Is it reasonable to tell the layman that the warning of a post mortem might urge and convert an incompetent doctor in time from proud isolation to prudent consultation? Is it reasonable to say that the mention of a post mortem would never lessen the interest of a competent and trustworthy doctor? Is it reasonable to state quite candidly that in the request for post mortems the public has a means of protecting its own interests? To have an understanding with a physician that if death comes an autopsy will follow involves, as it seems to me, no extra risk whatever to the patient. If, as the phrase goes, 'no effort is to be spared to improve the patient's chances' is it not time to have it widely known that the experience shows the practice of post mortems has improved the patient's chances?"

The author concludes: "There is real need for each profession to teach the laity how best to use its services. In America where with increasing frequency doctors' services are called in ignorance of their capacities, the ways of protecting the laity are of importance. Among other means too numerous to mention at this time one simple suggestion is then here offered for your comment: the performance of postmortem examinations, in that it has greatly improved our efforts as doctors, should be known by the laity as an advantage also within their power to demand.

So the essential point is this: do you endorse my view that one simple but powerful piece of advice in his own protection the layman could wisely be given is this—"Explain to whomever you call that if death comes a post mortem will be required"? It may be grim advice—but in the cause of good medicine we do not shirk giving grim advice. It may not be heeded—we have had that experience too. But it can be understood — and because it is in the interest of the patient, the post mortem can change gradually from being hated and feared and avoided to being used and trusted and steadily perfected. We have known

similar transitions in the past. Already, as many of you know, the clinicopathological conference is the wonder and admiration of many of our foreign visitors, who see in it a candor and fearlessness altogether to the credit of American medicine."

---o---

PLASTIC SURGERY
Edited by
GEO. H. KIMBALL, M.D., F.A.C.S.
404 Medical Arts Building, Oklahoma City

The Repair of Surface Defects of the Hand. James Barrett Brown, M.D., St. Louis, Mo. Annals of Surgery, Vol. 107, June, 1938, No. 6.

In a very well written and adequately illustrated article the author points out that most of the surface defects about the hands can be repaired by free grafts rather than by pedicle grafts.

If the initial graft is not entirely satisfactory then one may resort to a pedicle type of repair. He points out that where nerve, tendon, bone or joint is exposed or needs to be covered so that motion can take place then pedicle grafts become a necessity.

The author lays down one simple fundamental rule: that when the full thickness of the skin has been lost even over small areas, in such a kinetic region as the hand, the indication for treatment is to restore this loss as completely and as soon as possible. The author warns against methods recommended (as not leaving scars); a great many hands are allowed to heal with permanent crippling as a result.

Fresh Superficial Burns: The author favors wet packs of saline or grease gauze rather than tannic acid or plaster of paris. This allows early recognition of depth and amount of loss of skin. If there has been no full thickness loss of skin early healing usually takes place. The hand should be kept in a position of maximum function during the healing period.

Fresh Deep Burns: The author advises open wet dressings, debridement and later skin graft (free thick split graft).

Late Unhealed Burns: The first problem here is to obtain a clean wound and graft as early as possible. Secondary operations for releasing contractures often are necessary in this type of work.

Late Deformities Repaired with Free, Thick Split-Grafts:

By using about one-half to three-fourths the thickness of the skin, it is possible to remove the scar and supply a suitable graft. In cases where ulceration is present the author employs wet dressings with irrigating tubes incorporated for about four days.

Partial Restoration of Function: Some cases show deformities that are discouraging from the standpoint of satisfactory repair. Improvement in some of these cases is accomplished by restoring position of fingers or thumb and thereby increasing function.

Healed Deformities Repaired with Free Full-Thickness Grafts:

Dorsal surface loss can in many instances be successfully replaced with thick split grafts. The full thickness graft is often relied upon where widespread clean dissection and removal of the binding scar can be accomplished.

Palmar surface losses can nearly always be repaired with free grafts. Some areas may require thick grafts. The author has learned that the single contracted finger in a child with keloid formation, with its probable deep inflammation may be one of the hardest to repair and careful attention must be given this apparently simple lesion. The author points out the details of using the full thickness graft, the sutures used and the splinting necessary. He also mentions the manner of cutting the graft to pattern and the application of the graft.

Roentgen Ray Burns: The author has had most satisfactory results with excision and immediate grafts with thick split-skin grafts in repairing roentgen ray burns. If ulceration is present or if there is bone or tendon exposed in the fingers, amputations may have to be performed, or a pocket flap resorted to, but with the promise of success by early widespread free-skin grafting, most patients should fall short of this degree of neglect.

Complete Amputation of Finger Tips: The author has had experience in suturing a completely severed finger tip and has found that it lives.

Web Fingers: The author advises preparation for skin graft when dividing these webs. He has found that there is always need for skin to cover the defect.

Discussion: It is a principle that one should bear in mind that Dr. Brown has so often pointed out, viz: Immediate and early replacement of skin loss about the hands. This type of work often requires a long operative time and each detail must be carefully observed, otherwise the whole plan is upset. One must observe strict asepsis, adequate fixation, good splinting, and an early return to function in these cases.

I think most every surgeon has had the experience of suturing an amputated finger tip and finding that it remains viable and functions. I have had such cases in children but never a complete amputation of a finger tip in an adult which survived.

The above article is wholly instructive, thoroughly illustrated and very timely.

--------o--------

ORTHOPAEDIC SURGERY
Edited by Earl D. McBride, M.D., F.A.C.S.
717 North Robinson Street, Oklahoma City

The Treatment of Acute Infectious Arthritis of Undetermined Origin with Artificial Fever. Robert M. Stecher and Walter M. Solomon. Amer. J. of Medical Sciences, CXCIV, 485, 1937.

Acute non-specific infectious arthritis is a relatively common syndrome which has received scant attention in the literature and may be regarded as an acute form of atrophic, rheumatoid, or chronic infectious arthritis.

Of 20 patients, ranging in age from 14 to 51 years, treated with artificial fever therapy, 12 (60 per cent) received prompt relief and apparent cure while eight (40 per cent) were partially relieved. The course of the disease was favorably modified in every case. These results compare favorably with those observed in the treatment of acute gonorrheal arthritis with artificial fever.

Treatment consisted in induced fever (about 105 degrees Fahrenheit) by means of the Kettering hypertherm, maintained usually for four or five hours. The patients who recovered completely received this treatment for from two to 25 hours, averaging seven and three-tenths hours.

Increased circulation, with an increase in phagocytosis, occurs, but the complete mechanism which produces benefit is not fully known. Herpes labialis has been found to occur as a complication of this form of therapy in one-third of the cases after the first treatment only.

Fracturas Supracondileas Infantiles (Supracondylar Fractures in Children). F. Jimeno Vidal. Anales del Servicio de Traumatologia, Cirugia Orotopedica y Accidentes del Trabajo del Hospital Provincial de Valencia, Febrero, 1936.

The great osteogenetic capacity of the infantile periosteum and its tendency to bone proliferation when it is irritated are the chief reasons for the use of gentle manipulations, the postponement of any kind of surgical operation, and the establishment of after-treatment on the lines of uninterrupted rest until bony union takes place. The author warns against removing the splint every two days in order to see "how things are going on," moving the joint, or employing any form of massage.

The fracture is reduced under a local anaesthetic (20 cubic centimeters of a 2 per cent novocain solution). The patient is placed on a table, and the surgeon exerts traction, pulling the forearm flexed at a right angle. Countertraction through a sling, or obtained by placing the surgeon's knee on the patient's axilla, is effective. This causes the shortening to disappear. Digital pressure reduces the forward position of the proximal fragment. The forearm should be held in forced pronation to counteract the varus position and to prevent radial palsy. Fixation is by means of a non-padded plaster-of-Paris splint.

--------o--------

UROLOGY
Edited by D. W. Branham, M.D.
514 Medical Arts Building, Oklahoma City

Present Aspects of Stone Problem by Linwood D. Keyser, Roanoke, Virginia. Urological Correspondence Club. September 5, 1938.

The author of this letter has achieved distinction in his work on urinary calculi. This communication is an admirable criticism of the present day concept of calculosis of the urinary tract by an authority on this disease. It is well worth reading.

"We still possess an insufficient tangible knowledge of the cause and prevention of calculous disease in the urinary tract. This is true in spite of numerous interesting and brilliant endeavors on the part of investigators during the 20-year period which has elapsed since Osborne, Mendel and Ferry reported their epoch making observation of lithiasis in rats fed on diets deficient in vitamin A.

It is really remarkable what a variety of methods have been successful in producing calculi in experimental animals. Noteworthy are artificial hyperexcretion of stone forming crystalline material, infection and vitamin deficiency. It is equally remarkable and altogether disappointing that we cannot in a practical manner carry the fruits of these experimental efforts more intelligently to the clinical field.

For instance, artificial hyperexcretion of calcium oxalate and carbonate will produce calculosis in animals. Clinically hyperparathyroidism with its concomitant excessive urinary calcium excretion is found frequently associated with stone. In hyperthyroidism, however, while the calcium excretion is again excessive, the incidence of stone is insignificant. Why the difference? Similarly urinary tract infections and malnutrition states of vitamin deficiency type are very inconsistent in their association with lithiasis. The same type of infection and of malnutrition are found far more often without calculous disease than with it.

Much has been written on the geographic incidence of lithiasis and its bearing on the malnutrition factor. Enthusiastic research workers in vitamin insufficiency have drawn quick and far reaching conclusions. Let us remember, however, that in the stone areas of India, China and Dalmatia, it is bladder stones chiefly in male children that are being considered. No figures exist to show that renal or ureteral lithiasis in such areas is excessive, while children in neighboring communities on a similar dietary and in a similar climatic environment may be strangely free from bladder stone.

Little has been added to our knowledge of the dissolution of calculus, or prevention of recurrence beyond what we knew years ago. Methods of dissolution relying on changing the urinary reaction, administration of vitamins and drugs have not been successful in the hands of the great majority of workers. It is true that dissolution may occur not infrequently with soft calcareous masses, recently formed and in which secondary internal crystallization, i.e., the compaction of the colloid-crystalline framework into laminated areas with consequent increased density, has not taken place. The effort at dissolution has no place in vesical calculi. Indeed, small stones in calyces or ureter, non-obstructing and subsequently found to be composed of phosphate or carbonate, have almost consistently refused to yield to urinary acidification over many months. When we set out to dissolve a stone, the chances are very, very greatly in favor of failure. There is a reason for this. In the test tube I have found that stones of varying density exposed to concentration of various acids not tolerated by the urinary mucosa, suffer only slight disintegration on the surface. The colloid-crystalloid framework is unyielding and we must look for further measures to cause its breakdown.

In preventing recurrence, the change of urinary reaction and perhaps the forcing of vitamins may be of great value, but is in general secondary to the attack to be made on infection, especially of proteus and coccal types. The oxalate stone remains an enigma. Prevention of hyperexcretion of uric acid by dietary means, the occasional recognition of hyperparathyroidism and its surgical treatment are noteworthy procedures. Intense eradication of focal infection and of urostasis are emphasized as all important.

A newer line of approach suggested by Snapper, Bendein and Polak of Amsterday is worthy of recording. These observers produced calculi in rats by feeding calcium carbonate and later found that such calculosis was prevented when excessive hippuric acid in the urine was produced by concomitantly feeding sodium benzoate and glycocoll. Hippuric acid has a hydrotrophic action on the labile urinary colloids, keeping them in solution. Without precipitation or gelling of these colloids, stone will not form, regardless of vitamin deficiency or of H-ion concentration.

My experience with these drugs is limited. Three cases of phosphaturia and small gravel have cleared up shortly after administration of 45 to 60 grains of sodium benzoate and 1 to 2 oz. of Elixir of Glycocoll daily.

Similarly a patient with mixed streptococcus and proteus infection who had been afflicted with frequent passage of phosphatic ureteral calculi over a 16-year period has been free from recurrence over seven months with a crystal free urine and a slowly but definitely subsiding infection. An autogenous bacterial antigen made from the proteus was used and has seemed of great value in reducing the infection. Little effort has been made at changing the urinary reaction in this case. Sulfanilamide and di-sulfanilamide both have resulted in diminishing the proteus infection, but only temporarily if used alone. Ureteral and urethral dilatations and prostatic massage are being carried out. By such a "therapeutic barrage" we are whipping the infection down to a minimum, keeping the urinary tract well drained, and apparently

inhibiting further formation of stone. The possible role of the benzoate and glycocoll regimen is not clear but is mentioned as a suggestion that these drugs may be used in conjunction with other measures in instances of rapidly recurrent stone, which have proved obstinate.

In resume, our clinical methods of dealing with stone are based largely on empirical methods. What we have learned from experimental sources leads us to believe that the process is intimately bound up with the deposition of calcium or other urinary crystalloids in necrobiotic epithelium on the one hand with a disturbance of colloid-crystalloid solution equilibrium on the other. The tangible details of these processes themselves are obscure. Evidence, however, is gradually accumulating which is suggestive of a better understanding of the problem in the future. An excellent survey of the subject of lithiasis, etiologic factors and blood chemistry relationships is recounted in the current article by Griffin, Osterberg and Braasch (Jr. A.M.A.)."

———————o———————

Air Filtration

According to Tell Nelson, Chicago (Journal A. M. A., Oct. 1, 1938), air filtration implies the removal of impurities, usually in the form of dust, from the air. The benefits derived from such treatment of the air are of great importance in industry as well as in the control of many respiratory diseases. No air is free from dust. The concentration of dust particles in the air depends on the conditions operative in the locality in which samples are taken. The direct effect of dusts on health depends to a large extent on their chemical composition and the size of the particles. In persons who are sensitized to pollens, inhalation of air impurities precipitates symptoms of hay fever and pollen asthma. The concentration of pollen in the air varies greatly in different localities and is often enormous. In Chicago, for example, it has been shown that hundreds of tons of ragweed pollen are liberated each season. Many mechanical devices have been built for removing dusts from the air. However, because of the large variety of dusts, their difference in size and chemical composition and the varying conditions under which they are found, there is no single filtration method which is applicable to all. The main object is to remove as nearly 100 per cent of the dust as is possible. Air cleansing may be accomplished in numerous ways. In general the methods can be roughly grouped into five main divisions: air washers (water sprays), dry filters, viscous coated filters, electrical precipitators and dynamic precipitators. Each method has a definite field of usefulness and when used within its own limitations attains its maximal efficiency. In industry, the dynamic and electrical precipitators are perhaps the most efficient for the removal of the smaller particles of dust, whereas for home and hospital use dry filters are most efficient. The air washer for the removal of dust and pollen from air does not have as high a degree of efficiency as other methods. The greatest field of usefulness of the air washer is as a primary cleaner in a system in which there is a secondary filter of greater efficiency. In this capacity it will remove the larger particles and thus give a longer life to the secondary filter in addition to maintaining or increasing the humidity. Dry filters are well adapted for installation in hospitals and homes where filtration is required. Their efficiency is at its maximum when the filter is new. When properly cared for under ordinary operating conditions, the loss in efficiency of dry filters is very slight. Viscous coated filters have their lowest efficiency for dust arrestment when new, but as the filter fills with dust the efficiency increases. Electrical precipitators have lately been advocated for use in the removal of dust and pollen from the air. They maintain a high degree of efficiency for dust removal. This method is efficient for particles smaller than 0.5 micron. Its disadvantages for home and hospital use are that it may liberate ozone, which at times may produce secondary effects, and it requires constant operation to maintain its efficiency. Dynamic precipitators usually combine an exhauster and dust collector in a single unit. The dynamic precipitator has a very high degree of efficiency for dust removal as the result of the magnitude of the centrifugal and dynamic forces imparted to the dust particles by the impeller. Within the past ten years, filtration of air for the removal of particulate matter has received a great deal of attention from the medical profession. This has been particularly true in the field of allergy. Its usefulness in the relief of symptoms of hay fever and pollen asthma and in other inhalant allergies as well as its value as an aid in diagnosis has been amply demonstrated.

Physical Therapy In Treatment of Fractures

In order that physical therapy may be intelligently used in the treatment of fractures, Frank D. Dickson, Kansas City, Mo. (Journal A.M.A., Sept. 10, 1938), defines its purposes and aims to be: (1) promoting the early absorption of hemorrhage and traumatic exudate, (2) relaxation of muscular spasm to relieve pain and discomfort, (3) the reestablishment of normal circulatory conditions in the affected extremity, blood stream and lymphatics, which insures a more rapid and complete healing of the fracture and (4) building up in the muscles of the extremity that tone and flexibility so necessary to normal use. Broadly speaking, there are four basic forms of physical therapy which may be employed in the treatment of fractures to accomplish the purposes catalogued; these are heat, massage, exercise and muscular stimulation. The first two of these secure their effect by bringing about muscular and vascular relaxation; the third and fourth are of chief importance in promoting venous and lymphatic flow and preparing the muscles to resume their normal active role as soon as use may be safely permitted. Physical therapy plays but a minor role in the reduction period. However, when for any reason it is impossible to proceed with the immediate reduction of a fracture, even if the delay is but a few hours, heat and gentle massage may be used to advantage. In the postreduction period physical therapy should assume an important role in fracture treatment, but unfortunately it is durnig this period that it is most neglected. It is in the immediate postreduction period that exudate and hemorrhage which will become organized into scar tissue about the muscles, tendons, vessels and nerves and interfere with muscle action, normal circulation and joint movement can largely be removed by restoring as early as possible normal circulatory efficiency to the part. The stiffness, soreness and impaired function following a fracture are due in large part to such scar tissue and its removal or at least reduction to a minimum lessens the discomfort incident to restoring function and materially shortens the period of convalescence. Delayed union and nonunion are in the main traceable to interference with circulation at the site of the fracture so that early restoration of circulatory efficiency is the best safeguard against these catastrophes. So-called open splinting has in recent years been used more and more in the fixation of fractures; this permits the employment of physical therapy to a satisfactory extent. If a circular plaster dressing is used, it may be bivalved and the halves removed alternately for the application of physical therapy. In addition to "setting" muscles in this postreduction period, active muscle contraction may be encouraged in several ways. Even with the forearm and arm encased in a plaster cast, if the fingers are free, the patient by squeezing and relaxing the grip on a rubber sponge can exercise the forearm and arm muscles extensively. It is in the period of after-care that physical therapy is most generally used in fracture treatment. In seeking to help a patient to regain voluntary control of the muscles and joints following a fracture, heat and massage should be used to loosen up and render more pliable muscles and so reduce the stiffness and pain incident to attempts at movement. The movements which are used should be designed to bring about normal action of the joint in the most natural manner. Having the patient go through the motions of brushing the hair in elbow fractures, driving nails with a light hammer in fractures of the wrist, turning a door handle in fractures of the forearm, and reaching for objects placed at a gradually increased height in shoulder fractures illustrate the methods which may be used to encourage the patient to use the extremity in a normal manner. Physical measures may be used up to the point of pain tolerance provided the painful reaction subsides within an hour or two. Physical therapy which produces painful reaction and muscular spasm that persist until the next treatment indicates too forceful or too prolonged treatment and both amount and duration must be reduced; persistence can lead only to resistance on the part of the patient, slowing up of recovery, and a disappointing result.

Osteomas of Paranasal Sinuses and The Mastoid Process: Report of Cases

Bert E. Hempstead, Rochester, Minn. (Journal A.M.A., Oct. 1, 1938), points out that osteomas that arise in the paranasal sinuses are not common. Occasionally they are discovered in routine roentgenologic examination of the sinuses. They are not diagnosed clinically or even suspected of being present until either evidence of intracranial complications becomes manifest or external deformities appear. Most osteomas can be removed through the fronto-ethmoidal incision. If osteomas do not involve the dura or cribriform plate, removing them by the method of Cushing is illogical. Pyocele or mucocele of the sinuses can be handled best through the fronto-ethmoidal incision. Osteomas associated with intracranial complications are cared for best through the transfrontal approach. If osteomas are associated with intracranial complications and with definite infection of the sinuses, operation might be done in two stages with advantage.

Vitamin C: Methods of Assay and Dietary Sources

The facts and comments presented by Otto A. Bessey, Boston (Journal A.M.A., Oct. 1, 1938), in this review on the methods of assaying vitamin C serve to give a general idea of the present state of the subject. Chemical methods have rapidly replaced vitamin C determinations by bio-assay for many types of investigations. However, the more specific animal tests continue to be necessary in order to avoid the risk of misinterpretations of the chemical tests. Guinea pigs kept on certain purified diets fail to gain weight, and the specific pathologic changes of scurvy develop. The degree of protection or cure of the deficiency bears a quantitative relation to the amount of vitamin administered. This principle forms the basis for biologic methods of vitamin C analyses. The dietary sources of vitamin C are discussed, a table of various foods with their vitamin C content is presented and the effect on the retention, diminution or loss of vitamin C by the different methods of preparing and preserving food is also discussed.

Human Requirements For Vitamin B-1

For the ideal type of information needed to answer the question of the human requirement for Vitamin B-1 it was of course necessary to await isolation of the factor in pure form and tests of it on the human species, something accomplished only recently. It has not as yet been possible to make as many tests with the pure vitamin as might be desired, but these may reasonably be expected in the near future. George R. Cowgill, New Haven, Conn. (Journal A.M.A., Sept. 10, 1938), presents a formula which indicates that the value of the vitamin B-1:calory ratio increases with increase in body weight. Estimates of the human requirement for vitamin B derived from his formula pertain to the minimum or beriberi-preventing level; the optimal intake is undoubtedly much greater. The vitamin B-1 requirements for th enormal adult, the mother and the infant and the child are discussed and computed. Heightened metabolism and loss through excretory channels are some of the clinical factors that influence the vitamin B-1 requirement.

Relation of Drug Therapy To Neutropenic States: Chairman's Address

In 1931 the first evidence was presented that agranulocytosis was caused by the administration of certain drugs. Since that time there have accumulated a large amount of confirmatory data and reports of experiments that this concept is correct. Roy R. Kracke, Emory University, Ga. (Journal A.M.A., Oct. 1, 1938), summarizes this evidence and makes further suggestions concerning the use of some of these drugs, particularly since new preparations are benig introduced constantly and at least one of them (sulfanilamide) can be definitely added to the list of offenders. The drugs known to have produced agranulocytosis are aminopyrine, dinitrophenol, antipyrine, derivative of aminopyrine (novaldin) and sulfanilamide; acetanilid, acetophenetidin (Phenacetin), cinchophen (atophan), antimony compound (neostibosan) and quinine are suspected of causing agranulocytosis; arsphenamine depresses the granulocytes, and gold salts depress the hematologic system and they are thought to produce agranulocytosis. The disease has practically disappeared from Denmark because aminopyrine is no longer used in that country. Approximately 80 per cent of the drug-produced agranulocytosis is caused by the administration of aminopyrine or one of its compounds, with a lesser percentage being caused by the other drugs. The disease is decreasing in incidence in the United States, probably because of the more cautious use of aminopyrine by the medical profession. The number of cases of agranulocytosis from the use of sulfanilamide will probably increase ni the future, particularly if this drug is incorporated in patented remedies and indiscriminatingly sold to the public under nonrevealing names. Physicians should attempt to prevent this disease by caution in the use of these drugs, by instruction of patients concerning their purchase in drug stores and by programs of public instruction.

Apnea of The Newborn and Associated Cerebral Injury: Clinical and Statistical Study

According to Frederic Schreiber, Detroit (Journal A.M.A., Oct. 1, 1938), from January 1, 1928, to Decembre 31, 1937, 685 patients were seen in whom a relationship was suspected between the manner of birth and the later neurologic manifestations of damage to the brain. Most of these patients were seen at the Children's Hospital of Michigan, Detroit. Of the 685 children, 131 were seen because of convulsions, 69 because of spasticity, 130 for mental retardation, 248 because of combinations of these symptoms and the remaining 107 for miscellaneous neurologic conditions. Cases subject to suspicion of postnatal infection or trauma were excluded from the group, as were those in which congenital or familial factors might have significance in cerebral symptomatology. Finally, the group was limited to those infants born in one county during the ten year period. These restrictions left 500 cases. Approximately 70 per cent of these patients, whose birth records were available, had a history of apnea. There was a history of precipitate, brech, twin or premature delivery for 155 of the 500 infants; 345 were full term infants. In those of the group of 155 about whom data were obtainable, approximately 64 per cent had apnea at bithr, 11 per cent had late apnea only and 18 per cent had both early and late apnea. The total incidence of apnea in this group was 72 per cent. In the group of 345 full term infants, the incidence of apnea in the cases presenting a known history was at birth, 62 per cent; late, 9 per cent; early and late, 17 per cent, and total, 69 per cent. The depressing effect, on the respiratory center, of birth analgesics given in greater than pharmacologic doses bears a direct relationship to the degree of apnea. The extent of the apnea has a direct relationship with the severity of the cerebral symptoms after birth. The severity of the cerebral symptoms is in direct relation to the amount of damage to the brain tissue. From these relationships it apeanrs that analgesics given in greater amounts than the pharmacologic dosage may in many instances be the causative factor of fetal anoxemia, with resultant cerebral damage in the infant.

Index to Advertisers

OFFICERS OKLAHOMA STATE MEDICAL ASSOCIATION

President, Dr. H. K. Speed, Sayre.

President-Elect, Dr. W. A. Howard, Chelsea.

Secretary-Treasurer-Editor, Dr. L. S. Willour, McAlester.

Speaker, House of Delegates, Dr. J. D. Osborn, Jr., Frederick.

Vice Speaker, House of Delegates, Dr. P. P. Nesbitt, Medical Arts Building, Tulsa.

Delegates to the A. M. A., Dr. W. Albert Cook, Medical Arts Building, Tulsa, 1938-39; Dr. McLain Rogers, Clinton, 1937-1938.

Meeting Place, Oklahoma City, May 15-16-17, 1939.

SPECIAL COMMITTEES 1938-39

Annual Meeting: Dr. H. K. Speed, Sayre; Dr. W. A. Howard, Chelsea; Dr. L. S. Willour, McAlester.

Conservation of Hearing: Dr. H. F. Vandever, Chairman, Enid; Dr. J. B. Hollis, Mangum; Dr. Chester McHenry, Oklahoma City.

Conservation of Vision: Dr. W. M. Gallaher, Chairman, Shawnee; Dr. Frank R. Vieregg, Clinton; Dr. Pauline Barker, Guthrie.

Crippled Children: Dr. Earl McBride, Chairman, Oklahoma City; Dr. Roy L. Fisher, Frederick; Dr. M. B. Glismann, Okmulgee.

Industrial Service and Traumatic Surgery: Dr. Cyril C. Clymer, Medical Arts Bldg., Oklahoma City; Dr. J. Wm. Finch, Hobart; Dr. J. A. Rutledge, Ada.

Maternity and Infancy: Dr. George R. Osborn, Chairman, Tulsa; Dr. P. J. DeVanney, Sayre; Dr. Leila E. Andrews, Oklahoma City.

Necrology: Dr. G. H. Stagner, Chairman, Erick; Dr. James L. Shuler, Durant; Dr. S. D. Neely, Muskogee.

Post Graduate Medical Teaching: Dr. Henry H. Turner, Chairman, Oklahoma City; Dr. H. C. Weber, Bartlesville; Dr. Ned R. Smith, Tulsa.

Study and Control of Cancer: Dr. Wendell Long, Chairman, Oklahoma City; Dr. Paul B. Champlin, Enid; Dr. Ralph McGill, Tulsa.

Study and Control of Tuberculosis: Dr. Carl Puckett, Chairman, Oklahoma City; Dr. W. C. Tisdal, Clinton; Dr. F. P. Baker, Talihina.

ADVISORY COUNCIL FOR AUXILIARY

Dr. H. K. Speed, Chairman .... Sayre
Dr. C. J. Fishman .... Oklahoma City
Dr. W. S. Larrabee .... Tulsa
Dr. J. M. Watson .... Enid
Dr. T. H. McCarley .... McAlester

STANDING COMMITTEES 1938-39

Medical Defense: Dr. O. E. Templin, Chairman, Alva; Dr. L. C. Kuyrkendall, McAlester; Dr. E. Albert Aisenstadt, Picher.

Medical Economics: Dr. C. B. Sullivan, Cordell, Chairman; Dr. J. L. Patterson, Duncan; Dr. W. M. Browning, Waurika.

Medical Education and Hospital: Dr. V. C. Tisdal, Chairman, Elk City; Dr. Robert U. Patterson, Oklahoma City; Dr. H. M. McClure, Chickasha.

Public Policy and Legislation: Dr. Finis W. Ewing, Surety Bldg., Chairman, Muskogee; Dr. Tom Lowry, 1200 North Walker, Oklahoma City; Dr. O. C. Newman, Shattuck.

(The above committee co-ordinated by the following, selected from each councilor district.)

District No. 1.—Arthur E. Hale, Alva.
District No. 2.—McLain Rogers, Clinton.
District No. 3.—Thomas McElroy, Ponca City.
District No. 4.—L. H. Ritzhaupt, Guthrie.
District No. 5.—P. V. Annadown, Sulphur.
District No. 6.—R. M. Shepard, Tulsa.
District No. 7.—Sam A. McKeel, Ada.
District No. 8.—J. A. Morrow, Sallisaw.
District No. 9.—W. A. Tolleson, Eufaula.
District No. 10.—J. L. Holland, Madill.

Scientific Exhibits: Dr. E. Rankin Denny, Chairman, Tulsa; Dr. Robert H. Akin, Oklahoma City; Dr. R. C. Pigford, Tulsa.

Scientific Work: Dr. W. G. Husband, Chairman, Hollis; Dr. J. S. Rollins, Prague; Dr. J. L. Day, Supply.

Public Health:

Chairman—Dr. G. S. Baxter, Shawnee.
District No. 1.—C. W. Tedrowe, Woodward.
District No. 2.—E. W. Mabry, Altus.
District No. 3.—L. A. Mitchell, Stillwater.
District No. 4.—J. J. Gable, Norman.
District No. 5.—Geo. S. Barber, Lawton.
District No. 6.—C. E. Bradley, Tulsa.
District No. 7.—G. S. Baxter, Shawnee.
District No. 8.—M. M. De Arman, Miami.
District No. 9.—T. H. McCarley, McAlester.
District No. 10.—J. B. Clark, Coalgate.

SCIENTIFIC SECTIONS

General Surgery: Dr. F. L. Flack, Chairman, Nat'l Bank of Tulsa Bldg., Tulsa; Dr. John E. McDonald, Vice-Chairman, Medical Arts Bldg., Tulsa; Dr. John F. Burton, Secretary, Osler Building, Oklahoma City.

General Medicine: Dr. Frank Nelson, Chairman, 603 Medical Arts Bldg., Tulsa; Dr. E. R. Musick, Vice-Chairman, Medical Arts Bldg., Oklahoma City; Dr. Milam McKinney, Medical Arts Bldg., Oklahoma City.

Eye, Ear, Nose & Throat: Dr. E. H. Coachman, Chairman, Manhattan Bldg., Muskogee; Dr. F. M. Cooper, Vice-President, Medical Arts Bldg., Oklahoma City; Dr. James R. Reed, Secretary, Medical Arts Bldg., Oklahoma City.

Obstetrics and Pediatrics: Dr. C. W. Arrendell, Chairman, Ponca City; Dr. Carl F. Simpson, Vice-Chairman, Medical Arts Bldg., Tulsa; Dr. Ben H. Nicholson, Secretary, 300 West Twelfth Street, Oklahoma City.

Genito-Urinary Diseases and Syphilology: Dr. Elijah Sullivan, Chairman, Medical Arts Bldg., Oklahoma City; Dr. Henry Browne, Vice-Chairman, Medical Arts Bldg., Tulsa; Dr. Robert Akin, Secretary, 400 West Tenth, Oklahoma City.

Dermatology and Radiology: Dr. W. A. Showman, Chairman, Medical Arts Bldg., Tulsa; Dr. E. D. Greenberger, Vice-Chairman, McAlester; Dr. Hervey A. Foerster, Secretary, Medical Arts Bldg., Oklahoma City.

STATE BOARD OF MEDICAL EXAMINERS

Dr. Thos. McElroy, Ponca City, President; Dr. C. E. Bradley, Tulsa, Vice-President; Dr. J. D. Osborn, Jr., Frederick, Secretary; Dr. L. E. Emanuel, Chickasha; Dr. W. T. Ray, Gould; Dr. G. L. Johnson, Pauls Valley; Dr. W. W. Osgood, Muskogee.

STATE COMMISSIONER OF HEALTH

Dr. Chas. M. Pearce, Oklahoma City.

COUNCILORS AND THEIR COUNTIES

District No. 1: Texas, Beaver, Cimarron, Harper, Ellis, Woods, Woodward, Alfalfa, Major, Dewey—Dr. O. E. Templin, Alva. (Term expires 1940.)

District No. 2: Roger Mills, Beckham, Greer, Harmon, Washita, Kiowa, Custer, Jackson, Tillman—Dr. V. C. Tisdal, Elk City. (Term expires 1939.)

District No. 3: Grant, Kay, Garfield, Noble, Payne, Pawnee—Dr. A. S. Risser, Blackwell. (Term expires 1938.)

District No. 4: Blaine, Kingfisher, Canadian, Logan, Oklahoma, Cleveland—Dr. Philip M. McNeill, Oklahoma City. (Term expires 1938.)

District No. 5: Caddo, Comanche, Cotton, Grady, Love, Stephens, Jefferson, Carter, Murray—Dr. W. H. Livermore, Chickasha. (Term expires 1938.)

District No. 6: Osage, Creek, Washington, Nowata, Rogers, Tulsa—Dr. James Stevenson, Medical Arts Bldg., Tulsa. (Term expires, 1938.)

District No. 7: Lincoln, Pontotoc, Pottawatomie, Okfuskee, Seminole, McClain, Garvin, Hughes—Dr. J. A. Walker, Shawnee. (Term expires 1939.)

District No. 8: Craig, Ottawa, Mayes, Delaware, Wagoner, Adair, Cherokee, Sequoyah, Okmulgee, Muskogee—Dr. E. A. Aisenstadt, Picher. (Term expires 1938.)

District No. 9: Pittsburg, Haskell, Latimer, LeFlore, McIntosh—Dr. L. C. Kuyrkendall, McAlester. (Term expires 1939.)

District No. 10: Johnson, Marshall, Coal, Atoka, Bryan, Choctaw, Pushmataha, McCurtain—Dr. J. S. Fulton, Atoka. (Term expires 1939.)

THE JOURNAL
OF THE
OKLAHOMA STATE MEDICAL ASSOCIATION

| VOLUME XXXI | McALESTER, OKLAHOMA, NOVEMBER, 1938 | Number 11 |

Bronchoscopy in Oklaohoma*

L. C. McHENRY, M.D.
OKLAHOMA CITY, OKLAHOMA

"Bronchoscopy," the word, is used to include all forms of peroral endoscopy. In this section of the country it is very definitely a special field within the field of otolaryngology. There are a very few general surgeons within our state who, with minimum of equipment, still attempt some endoscopic procedures but this work is predominately in the hands of the otolaryngologists. This is partly because it was developed within the ranks of the laryngologists and partly because in their everyday work rhinologists and laryngologists are accustomed to working through narrow apertures and are of necessity trained to judge distance and depth by the aid of vision of but one eye at a time.

There is an increasing number of surgeons in our state who have a d e q u a t e training and equipment for the performance of bronchoscopic procedures. Bronchoscopy has become a routine part of the curriculum in all the long organized graduate courses in otolaryngology. This field of work, when viewed in the large hospitals where training in its technique may be obtained, is peculiarly inviting to the y o u n g graduate student. In such surroundings it is almost commonplace surgery and also highly spectacular. There are comparatively few men with a large experience in it. They are apt to be looked upon as ultraspecialists and able to command large fees. Too, in the large clinics equipment is easily available, assistants

*Chairman's Address, Section on Eye, Ear, Nose and Throat, Annual Meeting of the Oklahoma State Medical Association, Muskogee, Oklahoma, May 10. 1938.

are plenteous and well trained and the work does not appear to be particularly dificult. What then is more attractive to the beginning otolaryngologist than to be able to undertake bronchoscopy when entering practice in his chosen community.

Let us consider some of the difficulties that may beset the young otolaryngologist when entering upon a bronchoscopic career. First of all the cost of an adequate instrumentarium is apt to equal that of all the remainder of his professional equipment. Then he discovers that those cases which are so satisfactory and spectacular in that lives are saved by skillful surgery in dire emergencies are few and far between. Then also the economic returns from such cases are apt to be meager indeed. Even Chevalier Jackson states that 91.9 per cent of his foreign body cases were charity or part charity cases. The young bronchoscopist is discouraged too by the seeming fact that cases are referred to his care only after everything else has been tried in an effort to avoid his manipulations. Cancer of the larynx is apt to appear only when it has become so extensive t h a t an emergency tracheotomy is needed. He can then refer them, only at t i m e s hopefully, to the roentgenologist. There are also technical difficulties. In the hospital where training in bronchoscopy was obtained there were instantly available trained or partially trained assistants, the operating room facilities and instruments were quickly set up and available on order and there were nurses at least sufficiently trained to keep the instruments in working order. Without all of these things he finds himself seriously handicapped in e f f i c i e n t bronchoscopic performance. He has perhaps been taught that general anesthesia, especially ether, is not only not necessary but adds greatly to the danger of endoscopic procedures. He finds, however, that it is the only available substitute for trained assistants in a great deal of his work.

There are members of this section who have successfully practiced bronchoscopy under all the above difficulties for many years. Those years have comprised the period when the only bronchoscopic cases were those of foreign bodies, lye burns of the esophagus and advanced obstructive lesions of the larynx. Theirs has been the arduous labor of pioneers in any field of endeavor. Several of these men have relegated bronchoscopy to younger men and we have been deprived of their wisdom and skill gained in the school of experience.

Those essentials for efficient performance, technical skill and manual dexterity are gained only through experience. In our state bronchoscopic cases have been too few for experience to be gained by many. This situation is gradually but definitely changing. The everwidening field of usefulness of the bronchoscope is becoming more widely recognized. Those of us who engage in bronchoscopy have had and are obtaining better training before starting it. The bronchoscopist is being recognized as a necessary consultant to the internist, the surgeon, and the roentgenologist in the proper diagnosis and treatment of many difficult cases.

In the clinic at the Crippled Children's and University Hospitals each succeeding year shows an increase in the proportionate number of cases treated by bronchoscopy for conditions other than foreign bodies. More cases are being referred for diagnostic procedures and for treatment. This condition is of course more easily obtained in institutions where medical, surgical, and other consultative services are definitely organized. In private practice the development of wider bronchoscopic usage is coming more slowly. We who are practicing bronchoscopy can aid in this by

more widely publicising our work among the members of the medical profession.

The intensive campaign for earlier diagnosis and treatment of cancer in general is a very large factor in the increasing number of cases which are being referred for bronchoscopic procedures. A positive diagnosis of primary carcinoma of the lung can be made sufficiently early and with sufficient exactness to warrant hopeful therapy only by bronchoscopic visualization and biopsy. Carcinoma of the larynx is among the most curable of malignancies if it is diagnosed and properly treated when it is still early. The only early symptom is usually merely a persistent hoarseness. Entirely too many cases are being treated for laryngitis or not treated at all until laryngeal obstruction occurs. Biopsy of suspicious laryngeal lesions is a minor procedure with no operative risk and with but small inconvenience to the patients. Its importance in indicated c a s e s far outweighs that inconvenience. Tonsillectomy is performed by each of us almost every day with much less important indications, with much more inconvenience to the patient and with a higher operative risk.

Each of the last several years has added one or more new members to the group who are practicing bronchoscopy in Oklahoma. As our field of work is enlarged well trained hands are being a d d e d to those who do that work. To these men I would speak a word of encouragement. May they each year find themselves increasingly able to take better care of more patients. I would praise those who have labored in this field under the handicaps of past years and I implore them not to deprive us of the hardwon wisdom of their years of experience.

* * *

DISCUSSION

Millard F. Arbuckle, M.D.: Mr. Chairman and gentlemen, I cannot allow this opportunity to pass without thanking Dr. McHenry for his paper on this subject and to commend his stand on the matter of Bronchoscopy. This of course is the accepted m e t h o d of dealing with foreign b o d i e s lodged in the trachea-bronchial tree but in addition there is a much wider field of use, namely, the diagnosis and treatment of d i s e a s e s of the tracehobronchial tree. This is a most important adjunct and in some cases the only method in which the diagnosis may be definitely established. I refer particularly to tumors of the bronchus. By visual examination and guidance, i.e., bronchoscopy, we may also establish the etiological f a c t o r in bronchiectasis or lung abscess in many cases and localize the lesion. Many cases of lung abscess are improved and some cured by bronchoscopic drainage and medication. Patients with bronchiectasis are benefited by bronchoscopic examination and treatment, not only from the standpoint of improved drainage but also by the help which exact localization affords. The value of bronchoscopic study of pulmonary disorders of more or less obscure nature are appreciated more than previously but there still is much to be said concerning the matter of educating the medical profession as to the value of this important therapeutic procedure as well as the general public. Some medical men are fearful of having their patients bronchoscoped because of the possible harm to the patient. After a rather considerable experience in the study of diseases of all types, we have found that with proper procedure all patients may be bronchoscoped safely.

* * * *

PRESENTATION OF POST-OPERATIVE CANCER
OF THE LARYNX

This patient, Captain C. A., age 44 years, came to me four years ago with a history of hoarseness and the usual experience of having had his throat sprayed and treated and given cold expectorants for a long period and being told to return in a day or so, without any relief. Finally at the suggestion of Dr. Nowlin Holcomb he came in for laryngeal examination. He had a mass on the free surface of the cord in the middle third. Fortunately for him this was still localized to the true vocal cord, and it is now well recognized that cancer of the vocal cord still limited to the cord can be cured by surgical removal in over 82 per cent of the cases and at the same time the patient may be left with a larynx serviceable for phonation and respiration as is true in this case. Neck dissection is not required in this type of case because of the poor lymphatic supply and lack of invasion of the glands while the tumor is still localized to the vocal cords. Once the tumor has invaded the external portion of the larynx, glandular, involvement is almost certain to be found and the rate of curability is considerably decreased. My reason for mentioning the type of treatment given this man for the first few months and the delay in diagnoses is that we have found by experience that many cases of cancer of the l a r y n x are thus treated until it is too late. Unless one realizes that cancer of the vocal cord is free of pain and that the only symptom is continued hoarseness, and that early diagnosis and treatment means cure and late treatment means doubtful cure, he will not understand the importance of insisting that patients with continued hoarseness have at l e a s t one competent laryngeal examination. Apparently the Captain is cured and is able to carry on with his normal duties with the National Guard.

―――――o―――――

The Present Status of The Serum Therapy of Lobar Pneumonia

M. A. Blenkenhorn, Cincinnati (Journal A.M.A., Oct. 1, 1938), states that complete typing of all cases, through the entire 32 types, is the keystone of serum treatment and may provide the necessary information leading to the prevention of pneumonia. In parts of the United States in which typing has been practiced, treatable types comprise more than 50 per cent of all cases of pneumonia, save only in certain districts in the South. Now that other therapeutic serums (V. VII, VIII and probably many more by the device of rabbit serum) have been developed, the percentage will be higher. Neufeld typing of the sputum and cultures of various body fluids is a rapid and accurate method of bacteriologic diagnosis of pneumococcus types. The selection of patients for efficient and satisfactory treatment requires early diagnoses by the physician and intimate consultation with the bacteriologist. Serum must be given in adequate dosage by vein, and a double dose must be given when blood cultures are positive. Serum must be injected slowly after sensitivity tests are found negative, but the entire dose should be given during the first 24 hours. Serum accidents have been extremely uncommon and the danger of reactions should rarely preclude treatment. Refined and concentrated horse serum for type I and type II pneumonia when given during the first 24 hours is a specific comparable to the best specific biologic remedy, save only diphtheria antitoxin. When given within the first four days of the disease, the mortality rate of pneumonia may generally be reduced more than 50 per cent. In the author's experience of three years the mortality was reduced 76 per cent. In 1937 approximatiey 20 per cent of patients with type I and type II pneumonia in the United States were treated with serum.

―――――o―――――

Important Notice on Editorial Page

Observation From the Current Year's Experience With Medical Cases in a Children's Hospital*

FRANK C. NEFF, M.D.

KANSAS CITY. MISSOURI

Let us begin with the mention of the feature of the year which was the epidemic of poliomyelitis in the four months of July, August, September and October. As usual the public showed great fear, in some cases amounting to hysteria. The collapse of vaccine immunization which was attempted in 1936, as well as the failure of convalescent serum to prove itself effective, left the profession without any protective or curative treatment. In the early months of 1937 reports were published in the Journal of the American Medical Association of the recent use of zinc sulphate spray of the olfactory tract for the blocking of virus entrance to the central nervous system. You are familiar with these reports. No coordinated effort was made in our community to use a standardized procedure or to recommend it. It was too soon to learn whether this treatment immunized or was practical on any scale.

TORONTO'S RECENT EXPERIENCE WITH POLIOMYELITIS

In October, 1937, I had the privilege of visiting the Children's Hospital in Toronto to learn something about the current Toronto epidemic of this disease affecting about one person in each one thousand of the population and totaling a b o u t 2,000 cases in the province of Ontario. The epidemic brought response on the part of the University, newspapers, citizens, hospitals, and physicians to provide quarters for afflicted children, to manufacture braces and respirators, above all to make a careful investigation of the zinc-sulphate nasal spray as a preventive of poliomyelitis. The latter was managed in this fashion: advertisements in the daily papers that parents bring children to special clinics for receiving the spray at the hands of laryngolo-

gists, resulted in nearly 5,000 children being given two such treatments. From corresponding sections of the city came approximately 6,000 other children who were used as controls, not being given the nasal spray. The two treatments were spaced at 12 days. About 25 per cent lost temporarily the sense of smell, but all children were regarded as equally well sprayed.

The Toronto findings:

Of 4,713 children sprayed—11 developed poliomyelitis.

Of 6,300 children of control group—18 acquired the disease.

The attack rate for identical periods in both groups:

2.1 per 1,000 sprayed children.

2.9 per 1,000 of control group.

The committee reports in the Canadian Public Health Journal for November, 1937, that the study shows no evidence of protective value from nasal spray of one per cent zinc sulphate mixture, given with suitable equipment, on two occasions, with 12-day intervals and done by trained laryngologists; it is not a practical public-health measure.

A Few Incidents of the Small Epidemic in the Kansas City Area. In the Kansas City area there were four children who contracted poliomyelitis within two weeks following operation for removal of adenoids and tonsils. This discouraged some of us from recommending tonsillectomy in the presence of epidemic poliomyelitis; the traumatizing of the naso-pharynx may interfere with whatever protective barrier there may be in the naso-pharynx.

Kansas City, Kansas, kept open the public s c h o o l s throughout September and thereafter. Kansas City, Missouri, did not open them during this period which was in the decline of the epidemic. There was no evidence in either community that these

*Read at the Annual Meeting of the Oklahoma State Medical Association, Muskogee, Oklahoma, May 11, 1938. From the Department of Pediatrics, School of Medicine, University of Kansas, Kansas City, Kansas.

methods had any influence upon the disease. The public health authorities in certain crowded cities, London, New York and elsewhere have stated that nothing is gained by closing the schools. In Kansas City the children continued going to the movie theater. One child was admitted to our hospital directly from the movie theater in w h i c h she became paralyzed. She walked into the theater, but was unable to walk out.

A mother brought her child to our hospital for tonsillectomy; the mother herself was at the time found to be in the acute stage of poliomyelitis, involving the deltoid of one arm.

One infant, age 11 months, was brought from across the state because of supposed paralysis of the intercostal muscles and diaphragm on one side. The family was greatly p l e a s e d when the disease was found to be a one-sided pleuropneumonia and not infantile paralysis.

It is apparent that the d i s e a s e is not highly contagious, as is measles, for poliomyelitis often appears as an isolated case, while measles is never sporadic.

MEASLES

Our winter and spring epidemic has been measles. Hospitals for children have their troubles during measles epidemics. The whole personnel of the institution must become measles-conscious. One innocent little girl of two years entered our wards for correction of cross eyes; within two or three days she began to have fever, and operation was deferred because of the appearance of fever. A consultation revealed the catarrhal invasion of measles. All the other susceptible children in the same room contracted the disease from her. Hospital admissions of children will ordinarily be stopped during an epidemic except for immunes or emergencies. This little girl however did us a good turn in providing several three to five c.c. doses of blood which we citrated and gave later to contacts in the hospital. Her blood was taken six days following the measles crisis. If given a few days after exposure, the disease will usually be modified. We used adult immune blood in 10 to 15 c.c. doses intramuscularly or Dr. McKhan's Placental Immune Extract in some cases for these purposes. One child with active purpura hemorrhagica who developed measles in

our hospital was apparently improved temporarily by the disease.

Encephalitis Secondary to M e a s l e s. About one case in 200 children with measles develop n e r v o u s symptoms on the fourth to sixth day, when the rash is beginning to fade. In our hospital we took care of three such cases of post-measles encephalitis. One child was five years old, the other two were six years.*

The first child was lethargic for about one week, and soon recovered without incident, but remained somewhat more excitable than before the measles. The second child was profoundly somnolent, and had fever notably 107.5° F. on one of the early days. The duration of his unconscious state was five days. The temperature came gradually to the normal, complicated by a mild otitis media. One would expect behavior abnormalities from such a lethargic case, but as yet there seems to be none. The third child had no fever, no somnolence but throughout was irritable, irrational, had hallucinations; she had to be restrained. The administration of large doses of phenobarbital soluble had no effect. The use of chloral hydrate, 10 grains, combined with bromide, 15 grains was effective given every four hours when needed. The rectal injection of avertin to produce narcosis was necessary and successfully used for spinal puncture or when any u n u s u a l examination or treatment was undertaken. For one week this child was given progressive daily doses of typhoid vaccine to produce shock and fever, which it did, apparently with good results and surely without bad ones. She had made a complete recovery in one month from beginning of her disease which we designated post-measles toxic psychosis[1], but which we believe had a basis of encephalitis. The number of spinal fluid cells at the beginning was 23 per cmm.

Discussion: The development of encephalitis after the fever of measles has subsided is difficult to explain. It may be caused by the toxins which are left from the active infection; neurological sequellae may be produced by a secondary invader, as is sometimes the case with cardiac disease and nephritis after the acute febrile

---

*Hospital Case Numbers 71003, 71012, 71046.
1. Toxic Psychosis Following Measles; H. R. Bathurst Norman, The Lancet, London, p. 684, September 19, 1936.

period of scarlet fever has passed. It has been suggested that certain cases of measles may have a strain of the virus which is neurotropic.

Use of Repeated Blood Transufsions in Bronchopneumonia Complicating Measles and Pertussis. There were several children with the much dreaded bronchopneumonia secondary to measles, and one complicating pertussis. In protracted cases of secondary pneumonia the pathology is now known to involve the entire framework of the lung, and is known as interstitial pneumonia. It is evident that repeated blood transfusions may save life in these instances if given early. Therefore wherever possible, and especially early, we transfused the children about every other day for a few times, giving small amounts in the neighborhood of 100 to 200 cc. Secondary anemia is common in bronchopneumonia of the secondary type; early transfusion may prevent this or bring about an early recovery through the increased oxygen-carrying p o w e r of the augmented blood volume and hemoglobin.

The interstitial type of pneumonia which accompanies or follows measles is usually serious, often fatal, and any case that gets well is memorable. The following case received two transfusions, the e f f e c t of which upon the course is shown from the data below:

Dorothy, Age 4, Hospital Number 70,695,
Secondary Bronchopneumonia

	rbc	wbc	pmn	hb
Feb. 4, 1938	3,720,00	21,000	81	65%
Feb. 5, Transfusion 225 c.c. blood				
Feb. 6, Transfusion 125 c.c. blood				
Feb. 7, Oxygen by nasal catheter	4,150,00	28,200	95	76%
Feb. 9, Critical drop in fever.				
Feb. 12,	4,580,00	16,600	69	81%

This child was in a serious condition on admission but recovered on the eighth day and left the hospital in a good state of convalescence.

Low Urinary Threshold for Sugar in a Case of Diabetes

We are accustomed to regard the presence of a small amount of sugar in the urine of the treated diabetic child as a safeguard so that shock may be more easily avoided following the administration of insulin. With the s i m p l e apparatus now available for every physician and for every home the percentage of urinary sugar is easily estimated. In certain children the renal threshold is high; no sugar may appear in the urine until the blood sugar is far above the normal range of 80 to 130 mg. It sometimes happens that there may be no glycosuria until there is a glycemia 160, 200 or even higher. In such instances the child could suddenly and insidiously go into coma.

One of our cases this winter, a 13-year-old boy (Hospital No. 69869), with diabetes of only a few weeks came in with acidosis, 14 per cent CO-2 combining power and a blood sugar of 600 mg. With immediate insulin treatment of 45 units and clysis of 800 c.c. of 2½ per cent glucose in saline solution, he made immediate improvement, and his vomiting was stopped by lavage.

He was prescribed a daily diet of carbohydrate 240 grams; protein 90 grams; fat 90 grams; on this his body weight increased rapidly. The total calories provided by this diet are roughly 2,100, distributed as follows:

Calories as carbohydrate	50%
Fat	35%
Protein	15%
TOTAL	100%

This proportion of food factors is now widely recommended for juvenile diabetes.

On one occasion blood sugar came down to as low as 80 mg. but the patient was still passing sugar, as much as an ounce (30 grams) in 24 hours. This urinary sugar would mislead the physician into the belief that the patient had a dangerously high blood sugar. The patient soon got along well on 25 units of protamine-zinc insulin once daily, showing only a trace of sugar. He is a very intelligent boy, can weigh out his own diet, estimate it in grams of carbohydrate, protein and fat, and inject himself with the prescribed dosage of insulin.

Clinical Disturbance From Unrecognized Fracture of the Skull in Young Children

Case Number 1. Bilateral Subperiostal Hematomata: Infant three months of age, Hospital No. 69581. This infant fell out of bed a distance of 18 to 20 inches, and was noticed to develop a hematoma on each side of the h e a d overlying the parietal bones. These lesions were entirely similar in appearance to the cephalhematomata of the newly born. The periosteum of both b o n e s was elevated by the hemorrhage underneath. We thought we had to deal with simple hematomata but as a matter of precaution we made a roentgen film. This showed a s i m p l e fracture of each parietal bone. The recovery was without incident, and the line of fractures became indistinct in a film taken several months later.

Case 2. Clinical Resemblance to Prevertebral Abscess. Hospital No. 71282. The school teacher reported that this five-year-old boy had begun to get sleepy in school; he continued to be drowsy, he began to be feverish, cyanotic, to vomit and show difficult swallowing. Finally a hemorrhage occurred from the ear. He was brought into the hospital three weeks after the beginning of symptoms. His striking appearance was that of the cellulitis of left side of neck, also a bulging left side of the pharynx. The lateral roentgenogram of the neck showed a prevertebral swelling with forward displacement of the trachea. Through an oversight a requested film of the skull was not made. The breathing and swallowing were becoming more difficult. The whole picture seemed to make out a good case for retropharyngeal prevertebral abscess. The case was referred to the nose and throat department for operation. On the operating table a large amount of blood escaped from the incision made in the bulging pharynx, following which the boy suddenly died. The f a m i l y then recalled that the boy had fallen on his head three weeks before, but no importance was placed by them on that incident.

The autopsy findings were a fracture of the temporal bone on the left side; the formation and infection of a retropharyngeal hematoma; extension of a streptococcus cellulitis from the jugular vein thrombosis. The sudden death was probably due to the edema present, found in the midbrain and medulla. The opinion was expressed at the autopsy that an X-ray film of the skull would not have revealed this basilar fracture.

TREATMENT OF PYURIA IN CHILDREN

Those physicians who have practiced for several years know the former unsatisfactory treatment of some types of pyuria included under the name of pyelitis. Almost within the past two years, more effective bactericidal agents have become available and practical, which are used with success, marking one of the greatest advances in drug therapy. Usually the most desirable is mandelic acid, which is available in several forms, under the name of ammonium mandelate, offered in a vehicle of syrup. Cure is rapid and spectacular, both in acute and chronic cases. The safeguards and limitations are that the fluid intake of the child shall be considerably less than 1,200 c.c. in 24 hours in case there is no fever, and the function of the kidney must be normal enough to permit the excretion of s u f f i c i e n t acid phosphates to prevent throwing the child into acidosis.

Among our pyuria cases this year I would like to report the handling of one acute, one subacute, and one chronic.

1. Pyelitis in the Newborn. Boy, Hospital No. 71144. On the second day of life the infant manifested fever which in the newborn is m o s t commonly due to dehydration. A routine examination of the urine showed 140 pus cells per cmm. in centrifuged specimen. Fluids were forced by mouth, and during 18 hours, clysis of 75 c.c. of salt solution was repeated three times. In treatment begun at the onset of mild acute cases, fluids and alkaline — forming fruit juices such as grape and orange may cure, due to flushing out the urinary tract by the diuresis.

2. Subacute Pyelitis. Betty Ann, age 2½ years, Hospital No. 65214. Admitted February 22, 1937. This girl had a colipyuria. For the first seven days there was a high septic fever, with nearly 2,000 pus cells per cmm. of urine on the day elixir of mandelic acid (dr. 2) was begun. Ammonium nitrate gr. v was added to make the urine more acid, both drugs being given at four hour intervals day and night. The pH of the urine dropped from the alkaline level of 8.6 before beginning of treatment to 5.5 and 5.1 within a day and remained there. On the ninth day the pus cells had entirely disappeared. A leucocytosis of 20,000 and a polymorphonuclear percentage of 80 was found during the acute inflammatory s t a g e, which is a common finding in pyelitis.

After discontinuing the mandelic acid a relapse occurred so that treatment was again b e g u n, and the pus disappeared within two d a y s. Treatment was continued for a week longer when culture of the urine gave no growth of B. coli.

The mandelic acid should be given in conjunction with other acidifiers of the urine to reduce promptly the pH to 5.5 or lower. The size of the dose of mandelic acid will probably be smaller when ammonium chloride or nitrate is used as an adjuvant. A ketogenic high fat diet, along with juices such as cranberry, prune or plum will assist in the acid concentration of the urine. At present there are many preparations of mandelic acid and its salts. It is well to remember that most of the liquid preparations are unpleasant to the taste. A child old enough to swallow a tablet will escape the disagreeable flavor of the liquid preparations.

3. Chronic C a s e Complicated by Contamination from Colostomy O p e n i n g. Olive Jean, Hospital No. 65335. Admitted January 18, 1938. This unfortunate little girl born with imperforate anus, vaginal fecal fistula, had been operated upon to produce an artificial anus in the perineum by colostomy. Finally, possibly through contamination of the urethral meatus, there developed a severe colon bacillus pyuria. The child came into the hospital prostrated by the infection. Sulfanilamide was given but was not well tolerated nor effective. She was put on mandelic acid in the form of syrup amdelate, the dosage being one teaspoon four times in 24 hours for eight days. At the beginning of the treatment there were 16,000 pus cells per cmm. of urine; on dismissal the 10th day of the treatment there were only 10 or 12 cells per high power. She has now been well for months.

It has been advised that mandelic acid should be used only when the patient has good kidney function without severe abnormality or damage, or high blood pressure due to nephritis. A recent report* of 51 children with acute and chronic pyuria credits this drug with 39 cures of the infection. It is necessary to separate cases into acute and chronic and simple or complicated before one can assess the value of

any treatment. The f i g u r e s just mentioned would not be so impressive as a result in acute cases; they would be excellent where there is no malformation or gross abnormality in the urinary tract. This much can be said, however, that many acute cases have not been cured by previous methods of treatment; that periodic examination for pus and for negative cultures is essential; it may be that the thorough treatment of acute cases by recent methods will soon result in almost complete prevention of c h r o n i c pyelitis in children.

ATROPHY IN FRONTAL LOBE OF CEREBRUM

Jimmy F., age nine years, Hospital No. 69713. Admitted December 1, 1937. There had been convulsions with increasing frequency throughout childhood. He weighed 3½ pounds at birth. At present he falls frequently, walks with a wide base, is unsteady, knee jerks are absent, a Rhomberg is present, the head circumference normal. The boy is pleasing in appearance but he is anti-social in behavior, being very incorrigible. He has delayed speech. It is our present custom in cases of long-continued recurring convulsions to include a spinal puncture and introduction of air for the purpose of making encephalograms of the head.

The encephalogram in this case shows cortical atrophy, with much lack of development in the frontal area. In some cases of petit mal improvement may occur from injection of air.

TWO CASES OF ACUTE MENINGITIS FROM
UNDETERMINED MICRO-ORGANISM

1. Charles S., age 12, Hospital No. 70140, admitted December 31, 1937. Discharged well January 6, 1938. This boy had been sick one week with low fever and some vomiting. The day before admission he became worse and it was thought that he had a brain tumor. By the time he reached the hospital the temperature was 105° F. with all symptoms of meningitis present; spinal fluid contained 5,000 cells, mostly polymorphonuclear, the globulin t e s t positive. Organisms were not found in the spinal fluid on smear nor in culture using brain broth and blood agar plates innoculated by allowing the spinal fluid to drip directly from the needle to the culture medium. The failure to find bacteria does not warrant the neglect of serum admin-

---

*Indications for the Use of Ammonium Mandelate in Pyuria in Children; W. E. Wheeler, N. E. Jour. of Med. 217; 643; October 21, 1937.

In children 12 grams of the salt are frequently used for the 24 hours' quantity. In children the following quantities have been generally used.

Age	Ammon. mandel.	Fluid intake
Under 1 year	3 gm.	450 c.c.
1 to 2 years	4 gm.	500 c.c.
3 to 6 years	5 gm.	500 c.c.
7 to 9 years	6 gm.	600 c.c.
10 to 12 years	8 gm.	800 c.c.

istration, so 20,000 u n i t s meningococcus antitoxin were given intravenously diluted with 400 c.c. of saline solutions. This was done within 16 hours after admission. Because of the obscurity of the type of meningitis and its severity prontosil was administered intraspinally and intramuscularly, and by mouth also. The prontosil was repeated on the fourth day. He was given no serum intraspinally. The 5 c.c. of 2½ per cent prontosil was diluted by adding 10 c.c. of saline, making an 0.8 per cent solution for the intraspinal injection; the intramuscular injection of a 5 c.c. ampule of 2½ per cent solution was not further diluted. The boy walked out of the hospital cured on the seventh day, at which time his photograph was taken.

2. Douglas K., 13 months, Hospital No. 69613. Admitted November 24, 1937. He had been sick one month. His symptoms were those of meningitis in the acute stage with 1,900 cells mostly lymphocytes at the first puncture. The culture of the spinal fluid showed a growth resembling meningococcus but the diplococci were gram negative. The bacteriological laboratory was unable to identify this type of micro-organism.

The child was given no serum. His treatment was sulfanilamide grains v 3 times daily; prontosil 4.5 c.c. (2½ per cent) diluted in 10 c.c. of normal saline intraspinally. He was given also a blood transfusion. As a result of examining blood for donors both the father and mother were found to have a four-plus Wassermann; the child likewise had a similar reaction. The child made a prompt and complete recovery from the meningitis. However, we sent him home with the recommendation that stovarsol be given, although no symptom of syphillis other than a positive Wassermann was present.

FACIAL LIPODYSTROPHY IN TWO BOYS

Hospital No. 56254 and 71615. This year we have had the opportunity to hospitalize at the same time two cases of this rare but striking disease. It is only within the past 15 years that this wasting of the facial fat has become clinically known. It has been called progressive lipodystrophy, but one who has watched the course in such individuals feels that the disease is not progressive nor does it produce sickness nor death. The atrophy of the facial fat begins at the fifth to eighth years of childhood with the characteristic hollowing of the cheeks. This is so obvious that the diagnosis may be made by inspection of the face alone.

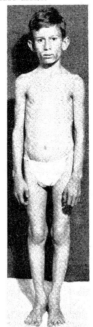

Facial Lipodystrophy in Boy of 11 Years.
(Notice also some wasting of the fat in upper part of the torso.)

There is in some cases the loss also of some subcutaneous fat of the neck, arms, chest, and abdomen. In girls there seems to be an increase in fat in the region of the abdomen and pelvis; in fact the contrast between the thin face and the well-developed body is grotesque. Parkes-Weber of England likens the body of a girl with facial lipodystrophy to the witch in Macbeth as characterized by Shakespeare. Coates[2] has enumerated 63 cases of this disease. Fat dystrophy can be differentiated from muscular dystrophy by the latter's tendency to produce muscular weakness and paralysis of the facio-scapulo-hemeral regions (Duchenne), a striking evidence being the inability of the patient with muscular dystrophy to whistle. In fat dystrophy the disturbance is purely cosmetic. There is apparently nothing to be done in the way of treatment though we tried in one of these boys the injections of Mead-Johnson's emulsified fat, 5 c.c. doses, intramuscularly, and later 20 c.c. in 250 c.c. salt solution intravenously as suggested by Dr. L. Emmett Holt, Jr. We did not find that there was any deposition of subcutaneous fat by these injections or by any sort of dietary. These boys had an insatiable appetite. One of the

2. Coates, Vincent; Idiopathic Lipodystrophy, Brit. Journal of Children's Disease. 21, p. 194, 1924.

boys, now 14 years old, is beginning to improve spontaneously in the filling out of the facies.

IN CONCLUSION

Looking back over the past year's experience in a children's hospital, I have selected features of interest to my associates and me. I hope that the narration of t h e s e histories and therapeutic procedures may be of value to you. Allow me to again express my thanks for the honor of the invitation and the kind treatment accorded me at the meeting of the Oklahoma State Medical Association.

------------o------------

Acute Appendicitis*

HORACE REED, M.D.
OKLAHOMA CITY, OKLAHOMA

Dr. Horace Reed: Mr. Chairman and Gentlemen. Dr. Kernodle is to be commended on his idea that we should give annually some time to the consideration of this disease. There are two main reasons why we should keep on talking about appendicitis, a disease which is still taking away many of us. I say "us" for the reason that if you will look in the records of deaths in the Journal of the American Medical Association, you will see that quite a number of doctors are dying from acute appendicitis annually. Then there is another reason why we should keep on talking about it. We are always going to have it with us. By its very nature there is no such thing as the prevention of appendicitis. Two or three years ago I prepared a paper in which I discussed the complications of appendicitis, and stressed the fact that the diseased appendix should be recognized while the process is still limited to the appendix, to the end that the diseased structure could be removed and thus prevent the complications which are usually the cause of death. Inflammation of the appendix, or appendicitis, is nearly always caused by an obstruction of the lumen. As long as the process is limited to the appendix there are no local signs such as pain in the region of the appendix, but the signs are referred to the abdomen as a whole, and are most always described as "indigestion." If we understand the anatomical picture, we may get a better understanding of what takes place.

The appendix is an offshoot of the gastro-

intestinal tract. It has in it no sensory nerve fibers. When there is trouble in the appendix the symptoms are transmitted through the nerves of the meso-appendix to the epigastrium, or to the abdomen as a whole. Many years ago, before we used spinal anesthesia, we occasionally operated for appendicitis in patients with lung trouble by means of local anesthesia in the line of the incision. Without the use of any anesthetic whatsoever in the appendix it could be picked up, crushed, or even removed without causing any distress to the patient unless traction was made on the meso-appendix. If such traction was made, the patient invariably complained of pain in the epigastrium. We find that this corresponds exactly to what takes place when a patient is seized with acute appendicitis. If the history of every patient with acute appendicitis is thoroughly taken, and if the story rings true to what actually takes place, the first symptom is abdominal distress which is usually described as centering in the epigastric region. This is the sign which is usually misinterpreted and is called "indigestion." That word is a very unfortunate word. It has been used through the years, how long we do not know, to designate an entity which did not exist except in the imagination. Even physicians with this earlier sign are satisfied in thinking that they have just "indigestion." We should get this through our heads that there is no such thing as "indigestion" except as a symptom. There is always a cause, and it is usually outside the stomach. It may have any location, as in the pelvis, the liver,

*Read Before the Surgical Section, Annual Meeting Oklahoma State Medical Association, Muskogee, Okla., May, 1938.

caecum, etc. The first sign of appendicitis is always the same. It is epigastric or abdominal distress. I say distress in contradistinction to what we call pain. The distress of the early signs of appendicitis, when we compare it to other causes of distress in the abdomen that are painful, as for instance, gall bladder or uretral colic, it is so much less in severity. Gall bladder and uretral colic are so painul as to require two or three times the ordinary dose of morphine to give comfort. The same is true of perforating ulcer of the stomach. I have never seen a patient with acute unruptured appendicitis who could ` not be made comfortable with a single 1/4 grain of morphine. In other words, the pain is not terrible as many seem to think it should be, but there is distress, and a better word still is "bellyache."

Now if doctors will get themselves informed as to the initial symptoms of appendicitis, there would be fewer physicians losing their lives. There would also be fewer patients treated for so-called "indigestion" when first seen by the physician. The m e d i c a l profession should be the guardian of the health and welfare, physically speaking, of the people. If in every physical examination the examiner would, in the absence of an abdominal scar, inform the patient of what he should expect in case he should have an attack of appendicitis, and stress the earliest symptoms, there would be fewer cases of ruptured appendicitis. But unless the physician knows, and knows accurately, what the earliest signs are, he cannot give the proper instructions. Since the days of Murphy who first emphasized the signs of acute appendicitis, we have been guided by four diagnostic points, namely: abdominal pain or distress which is always present; nausea, which is not always present but is in about 75 per cent of cases; toxemia, usually causing slight temperature elevation, and, finally, localization of tenderness in region of the appendix. This last sign should be called in question as to its being necessary to the making of the diagnosis. This is due to the fact that sometimes the appendix is so situated and covered by intestinal loops or omentum, or other intra-abdominal structures, the products of inflammation which usually precede perforation, or gangrene, do not reach

the parietal peritoneum. The omentum and the visceral peritoneum are like the appendix itself, devoid of sensory nerve fibers. In the second place, when there is localized tenderness and rigidity of muscle, either there is spilling of the products of infection outside the appendix sufficient to contact the parietal peritoneum, or there is a c t u a l leakage of infectious material causing actual peritonitis. The sign of localization of tenderness is of considerable value to the surgeon in his approach to the appendix. We must remember that the appendix may be found anywhere in the right side of the abdomen from the subcostal region to the pelvis, and in very rare instances it may even be on the left side, so if the diseased appendix has progressed to that point to where there is localization, it should be looked upon as a guide to the manner of approach rather than as a diagnostic sign of appendicitis. The o t h e r three diagnostic signs mentioned, namely abdominal distress, toxemia and usually nausea, should be sufficient to make a clinical diagnosis. If there is room for doubt, a blood count may be helpful. The first sign in this triad which leads to most errors is that of abdominal distress plus nausea and vomiting. If a patient has partaken of something out of the ordinary, such as a hamburger, following which he has abdominal distress and vomits the hamburger, he is quite convinced, until he is otherwise informed, that it is the hamburger that caused his "indigestion." Even doctors are not immune from such conclusions in their own cases. Let it be stressed that the indigestion which is synonymous w i t h abdominal distress and nausea, is a sign of an inflamed appendix, and it matters not what one has been eating previous to the onset of acute appendicitis, the digestive process in the stomach will be interrupted.

As to treatment we will all agree that the diseased appendix should be removed, certainly when it is acutely diseased. There has been much in recent literature in the last year or two on appendicitis, most of which has been devoted to the technical part of the operation and management. It seems that most surgeons prefer the McBurney incision, first, because it usually is the shortest and most accessible route, and, second, because such an incision will not weaken the supporting structures of the abdomen. Spinal anesthesia has rendered the operation much easier because, first, it produces relaxation of the muscles, and, second, the operator is not bothered with extrusion of the viscera through the incision while operating. As to generalized peritonitis I have very little to say. I know of no royal road, no sure method to cure generalized peritonitis when it is the result of appendicitis. Since this brief discussion is on appendicitis with a plea for treatment before it ruptures, there is no need to undertake an extended discussion of the complications that arise after inflammation has spread to the peritoneal cavity. I will say this, however, that it is my opinion after the appendix ruptures it becomes a problem which in each case the decision must be made on the basis of all the circumstances.

Dr. M. M. DeArman, Miami: I have read a recent review by Dr. McClency of Rochester on this subject. I think it is well to classify the involvement of the appendix into three groups. First, acute inflammatory without perforation. Second, with perforation and abscess formation. Third, with generalized peritonitis. Each of these three groups is a different proposition and there is a different method of attack.

There is no question in the mind of any surgeon as to the handling of acute, even gangrenous, conditions of the a p p e n d i x prior to perforation, the method of handling by operation, and the results are the same everywhere, and that those patients who are operated within 24 hours practically have a 100 per cent chance of recovery. The one with abscess formation possibly should be operated immediately if there is

localization of the appendicitis. Dr. McClency is of the opinion that with perforation and localization of the abscess, operation is much better than the conservative treatment; those with abscess formation without general peritonitis.

As to the method of handling general peritonitis, unfortunately this is where we get our mortality, and unfortunately this condition is hard to visualize and handle. Individualization of each patient requires a vast experience the majority of surgeons have not had the opportunity to have. To say that no patient with general peritonitis following perforation should have immediate operation would not be just to that patient. To evaluate the condition and symptoms that causes one to have an opinion whether this man should have an immediate operation or conservative treatment, certainly tests the ability of the majority of men who do not have a very wide range of experience. I am sorry that I did not get all of Dr. Reed's talk.

In a great many instances the symptoms do not stand out prominently. In a certain per cent there is absence of referred pain. Possibly t h e re is generalized abdominal distress, but a referred pain in the lower right abdomen is absent in quite a majority of patients. They won't all have vomiting. The great majority have nausea, but many do not have vomiting. The blood count is not to be depended upon; it is likely to be deceptive. You possibly have in general peritonitis a lower blood count at times than you have in an acute inflammatory condition. So it requires individualization. That is hard to conceive of except with men who have a great number of cases.

———o———

Cavernous Sinus Thrombosis With Case Reports*

THEODORE G. WAILS, M.D.
OKLAHOMA CITY, OKLAHOMA

Examination of the records of the hospitals in Oklahoma City shows there has been during the past 15 years 28 cases of

*Read Before the Section on Eye, Ear, Nose and Throat, Annual Meeting, Oklahoma State Medical Association, Muskogee, Oklahoma, May 10, 1938.

cavernous sinus thrombosis recorded as such. There are also about this many more that have been signed out as sinusitis, meningitis and septicemia.

A brief review of the anatomy of this

region is interesting since it is a hot spot if one contemplates surgery of the sinus. Lying on the lateral wall of the sphenoid it comes in contact with the inner wall of the orbit, the posterior portion of the ethmoid labyrinth, the anterior portion of the pituitary and has the optic nerve crossing it above to form the chiasm. The ophthalmic veins draining the orbits, nose and upper lip flow backward into these sinuses making this area dangerous for carrying emboli backward into the cavernous sinus.

There are some peculiarities of the sinus itself that adds to the hazard of thrombosis; it is trabeculated and is tranversed by the internal carotid artery. The 3rd, 4th and 6th nerves also pass through the sinus on its lateral walls.

It is connected to the sigmoid sinus by the superior and inferior petrosal sinuses and to the opposite cavernous sinus by the circular sinus, this last making bilateral infection a certainty.

Thrombosis results c h i e f l y from two sources; a small infection on the upper lip, nose, cheek or eye lids may result in emboli being carried backward through the ophthalmic veins; or thrombosis may result from nasal sinus infection with secondary osteomyelitis of the face or frontal bone carrying infection backward into the cavernous sinus.

Of the 50 or more cases examined all died but one. One more recovered of the thrombosis and succumbed later to a pneumonia of a different organism. I believe these two cases are worthy of report in detail.

A colored boy, about 15 years of age, came into University Hospital because of swelling of his left eye lids. Two days later, the right eye lids became swollen. There was marked chemosis of the conjunctiva of both eyes and marked proptosis of both eyes.

Fundus examination showed huge engorgement of retinal veins with hemorrhages into the fundus and oedema of the optic nerves. Spinal puncture showed increased pressure and an increase in spinal cell count, globulin, etc., but no bacteria. Repeated blood cultures were negative; white blood counts were only moderately raised and temperature was not high. Patient was not unconscious.

Over a period of three months and many spinal punctures, decompression was done because of the oedema of the optic nerve. He finally recovered, the proptosis and the chemosis subsided and he left the hospital with a marked impairment of vision due to the long standing passive congestion and pressure on the optic nerves. This case was reported in the A.M.A. Journal, by Dr. H. Coulter Todd, as a "Sterile Thrombosis of the Cavernous Sinus with Recovery."

The second case is not so rare a type and offers some hope of recovery of infected cavernous s i n u s thrombosis. A young girl, about 15 years of age, had a sty on the left eye lid which she opened and squeezed afterwards.

The child went to school, having headaches which neither she nor the mother considered important until one morning after the father had gone to work and the child was getting ready for school, she became irrational and the mother allowed her to go to bed. About three hours later, a p h y s i c i a n was called. Examination showed both eyelids swollen, left worse than right and considerable chemosis of the conjunctiva beginning to appear. She was irrational, had temperature about 102° and showed marked engorgement of the retinal veins.

Thinking this was most likely a streptococcic infection on account of the viciousness of the complication, she was sent to the hospital, given prontosyl by hypo, in 10 c.c. doses and typing was made for transfusions. Hot, moist packs were kept on the eyes to protect the corneae. After 48 hours staphylococcus was recovered f r o m the blood cultures and spinal fluid, so prontosyl was discontinued. The spinal cell count gradually rose from 1,000 cells and 98 per cent polys to a high of 50,000 cells and so much clumping it was impossible to accurately count them.

With staphylococcic cavernous s i n u s thrombosis, septecemia and m e n i n g i t i s diagnosed, she was started on Lederle's staphylococcic antitoxin, a new preparation then on the market only about three months. Since we had carte blanche on expenses, we gave her 20 c.c. every four hours, using it intraspinously, intravenously and subcutaneously at $20 per dose.

This amount of antitoxin kept her entirely free of toxic symptoms. Her cerebration cleared until she carried on an intelligent conversation, had no headache that she would admit and the pulse rate dropped from 160 to 110 with a corresponding decrease in temperature in spite of a spinal cell count of 50,000. After about four days of antitoxin, the spinal cell count began dropping and gradually came down from 50,000 to 2,000, with a decrease in percentage of polys. The chemosis of the eyelids and conjunctiva had meantime been gradually going down so that finally after about 10 days of transfusion and antitoxin it had practically disappeared from the eye lids. She became rational, e a t i n g her meals, turning on the radio for her favorite program and could count fingers across the room.

The transfusions had been discontinued when her blood count reached 6,000,000 and hemoglobin was 120. The donors in these cases were given typhoid vaccine intravenously to produce leucocytosis, and the blood then used at the height of the reaction; i.e. nonspecific immunized blood therapy. The cross matching seemed to change at the height of the reaction but we found it did not produce a reaction in the patient.

We also considered putting in a catheter into the lower lumbar region to give continuous drainage. However, since this would produce a current from the choroid plexus backward through the aqua duct 4th ventricle, foramen of Luschha and Magendie and the outside of the cord, it would not drain the cerebral and cerebella cisterns and would therefore not be of any material benefit.

The remarkable feature of the use of staph antitoxin, was that with a proven staph septicemia and meningitis the patient was cheerful and alert and did not look more sick than one with a bad "cold." This proves that it is not the bacteria but their toxins that kill the patients in septicemia and meningitis.

The results are not so spectacular as with diphtheria antitoxin, but after about four days of feeling better, the clinical signs began to improve, the spinal cell count decreased, temperature and pulse rate decreased, cerebration became more a l e r t and the oedema and chemosis around the eyes subsided. This last showing the clot

had been recanaliculated and the flow reestablished through the sinus. On about the twelfth day with all clinical evidences of the thrombosis about clear she contracted a lobar pneumonia, with first one and then both sides consolidated. This typed Nos. 2, 3, 4, 5 and 8 pneumococcus and not staphylococcus. Antitoxin was immediately given but the patient died next day, of a pneumonia not of the same type as her thrombosis, so it was not due to embolus in the lung.

It has been only lately that a staph antitoxin has been developed. It had always been supposed that since staph developed an endotoxin, instead of an exotoxin like diphtheria, tetanus and B. Welchi, that an antitoxin could not be developed for it. It has undoubtedly been tried many times before, but has only lately been successful of production.

It has not been so long ago that lateral sinus thrombosis was considered practically beyond surgical help, yet we now open a lateral sinus, take out the clot and pack it, or strip out the jugular vein as readily as we do a mastoid, when the need arises.

Since the cavernous sinus is trabeculated and also transfixed with nerves and the internal carotid artery, it does not lend itself readily to surgery.

I have thought that if in the Clinic I should ever get a case favorable enough it might be worth while to take out the eye, exenterate the orbit, take off the medial orbital wall, slit the cavernous sinus and put in a drain.

Tying the common carotid has been advocated as a means of lessening the movement in the sinus and thus lessening the spread of the clot to the other side.

One other surgical approach has been mentioned; i.e. taking out the middle turbinate, removing the lateral wall of the spenoid sinus and opening the cavernous sinus from its nasal side. This offers complications in that it would be hard to stop bad bleeding and would also be hard to keep a drain in the opened sinus.

Blocking of this sinus has occasionally arisen from a clot extending forward from a thrombosed lateral sinus through the petrosal sinus to the cavernous sinus.

In the last analysis treatment of this condition is the treatment of the attending meningitis and septicemia. With the coming of sulfanilimide one stands a fair chance of clearing up streptococcic septiceminas and meningitis, and with this staphylococcic antitoxin one has a fair chance with a staphylococcic infection. In addition to these specific medications one should also use nonspecific immunized transfusions, spinal punctures, subcutaneous and intra-venous saline, then treat any other complications as they arise.

It is my prediction that the next few years will see medical and surgical treatment of this c o n d i t i o n improved until cavernous sinus thrombosis will not offer the hopeless prognosis which it at the present enjoys.

---------------o---------------

Lateral Sinus Thrombosis*

D. L. MISHLER, M.D.
TULSA, OKLAHOMA

This presentation deals with the general points of diagnosis, treatment, and complications, of thrombophlebitis of the sigmoid sinus, based upon three cases which have recently been under my observation.

In the general consideration of the symptomatology of thrombosis of the lateral sinus, there are four distinct temperature charts as outlined by Dr. Tobey[1]. My three cases may be placed in two of these groups:

Type A. The accepted picture of acute sepsis with very sudden remissions to normal, or even sub-normal. This may occur several times within a few hours, or but once or twice during the 24.

Type B. The temperature at no time shows an elevation of more than one or two degrees, but a persistent irregularity, with a usual evening rise, although it may vary several times during the 24 hours.

Type C. An elevation of two or three degrees, which does not return to normal but shows slight remissions and elevations from 100° as a minimum. This type nearly always recurs after remaining at normal for a few days.

Type D. A normal temperature. At the time of mastoid operation, one may find a definite sinus thrombosis, or occasionally a broken down sinus wall and fistula, the patient having at no time shown a fever. Dr. Tobey states in a series of 73 cases, this occurred 11 times, and the sinus wall was completely necrosed in three of these.

Chills are very common and in my experience are present in about 75 per cent of the cases. They were present in all three of the cases at hand.

Care must be used in the differentiation of malarial chills and the chills and fever of a thrombophlebitis of the sigmoid sinus.

The blood culture is usually positive and should be taken just after the chill, as it is much more apt to be positive at that time. Usually after the first chill a positive culture will be obtained. Serial blood s t u d i e s are often used to demonstrate progressive loss of hemoglobin as we are usually dealing with a hemolytic type of infection. Thus, the destruction of hemoglobin even in the absence of a positive blood culture allows one to proceed with the operation without the loss of valuable time waiting for a positive blood culture.

Changes in the fundi were noted in none of my three cases preoperatively, although in one case marked fundus change was noted post-operatively. Most authorities note a change in approximately 25 per cent of the cases. The changes noted are fullness of the retinal veins, blurring of the disc margins and the entire disc, even to a marked papilledema.

Spinal puncture with the examination of the fluid and pressure variations by compression of the internal jugular vein is very important. A spinal subarachmoid block, an important and early sign in spinal cord

*Read Before the Section on Eye, Ear, Nose and Throat, Annual Meeting, Oklahoma State Medical Association, Muskogee, Oklahoma, May 10, 1938.

tumor, will cause an absence of the rise in pressure on compression of the jugular vein and it has been shown that the presence of a tumor in the cerebellar fossa may produce this same result. However, in thrombosis of the lateral sinus we are concerned chiefly with the comparison of the effects on each vein separately.

The incidence of sinus thrombosis in mastoiditis varies. Lillie[2] reports 3.8 per cent in 500 mastoidectomies. In a series of 1,257 mastoidectomies, Greenfield[3] reports 1.7 per cent of cases developing sinus thrombosis.

The mortality rate is usually below 40 per cent; Coates, Ersner and Persky[4] report 35.7 per cent. Heine[5] reported a mortality rate of 57 per cent in 1913.

It is interesting to note, especially further north, that different winters produce more sinus thrombosis cases. Some winters, the incidence of lateral sinus thrombosis will be high and the following winter the incidence is low. This runs in line, also, with the number of patients who develop mastoiditis following acute middle ear infections.

Case 1

J. R., age 10, schoolgirl in good general condition, complained of a sore throat one week previous to admission. The last three days has had a fever, chills, restless and yesterday was, apparently, delirious, vomiting severely. Ears began discharging yesterday and now complaining of double vision.

Physical examination—essentially negative, except marked discharge left ear canal and marked tenderness over left mastoid process. Throat moderately reddened with large and cryptic faucial tonsils.

X-ray—Increased density with destruction of cellular markings in region of antrum of left mastoid.

Temperature—101°; pulse 100; resp. 25; urine, negative; blood RBC 4,200,000; WBC 19,400; 86 per cent polymorphonuclear leukocytes.

Simple mastoidectomy left performed—large cellular type mastoid with pus under pressure. Small sinus exposure posterior to knee. Culture showed long chain streptococci. Patient got along nicely until the seventh postoperative day and her temperature went to 101.8° after about four days of normal temperature, also diplopia developed, then the temperature gradually rose with remissions to 104.8° with chills of marked severity and diplopia disappeared. Spinal puncture and after compression of both jugular veins the difference in increase between the right and the left was three mm. of mercury. I waited until the eleventh postoperative day, waiting for positive blood culture, which never came, and at that time reopened the mastoid cavity and exposed the knee of the sinus. Its wall was necrotic and its lumen filled with a large septic thrombus. The thrombus was removed with gentle suction and free bleeding obtained and the sinus was blocked. The internal jugular vein was then tied.

Three transfusions were given at two day intervals. The temperature practically subsided on the sixth postoperative day. Partial paralysis of the left sixth nerve developed on the fifteenth day following the ligation of the jugular vein and blocking of the sinus. This gradually cleared up after about eight months postoperative and the wearing of corrective lenses.

This case falls into Dr. Tobey's group A, as far as the febrile septic course ran.

I wish to point out the important and common complication of paralysis of the external rectus muscle on the side of the lesion, which may have been a result of a petrositis which cleared up by itself, or an increased pressure phenomena which I will discuss later.

Case 2

P. D., age 18, schoolgirl in good general condition. This patient became ill two weeks ago, with a sore throat and immediately developed earache and a discharge from the left ear. Three days ago she developed swelling and tenderness over the left mastoid area.

Physical examination—essentially negative, marked discharge purulent from left ear canal with moderate swelling and marked tenderness over left mastoid process.

X-ray—Shows marked increase density in left mastoid process with breaking down of cellular structure.

Temperature 102°, pulse 100, resp. 25; urine, negative; WBC 20,400; 92 per cent polymorphoneuclear leukocytes.

Simple mastoidectomy was done and a markedly suppurative process found with a large cellular mastoid cavity. No sinus or dural exposure.

The postoperative course which followed was not smooth; every day the temperature would exceed 101°, and some days it would go to 102°. There were no chills and generally the patient felt good, which is often characteristic of a septicemia of this nature. Then on the eleventh postoperative day the temperature went to 106° axillary following a severe chill. Blood culture showed a short chain streptococci of the hemolytic type. The diagnosis of lateral sinus thrombosis was made and permission for operation was not granted until five days later. During this time the temperature remained nearly constantly around 106° axillary with one remission daily.

On operation the sinus was exposed and it appeared grayish white below the knee; it was incised and a thrombus was disclosed and removed by suction and the sinus blocked. The internal jugular was then ligated. Three blood transfusions were given before operation and three afterward. The patient died on her sixth postoperative day.

This case had an overwhelming septicemia which was uncontrollable with the methods used. If the operation had been performed when the diagnosis was made, it might have made a great deal of difference, or if we had been using sulphanilamide at that time the patient might have never developed the thrombophlebitis and thrombus. This was a very fulminating case, and characteristic of a severe sinus thrombosis.

CASE 3

Mrs. F. S., age 30, housewife. The patient had a child three weeks previous to admission and had been having headaches with intermittent chills and fever. Her right ear ached and had discharged a small amount. Her home doctor felt she had puerperal sepsis.

Physical exhmination—revealed nothing significant. Right ear canal contains minute amount of serum — no perforation seen. Temperature 100°; pulse 100, resp. 20. Urine — essentially negative; WBC—19,500; 91 per cent polymorphoneuclear leukocytes.

Mastoid X-rays — slight clouding and suggestive loss of detail right mastoid. On the third day after admittance to the hospital a sudden temperature rise to 103°, following a moderate severe chill, occurred, and sudden drop of temperature and severe right sided headache. The following day the right ear drum was opened and moderate discharge resulted. The following day the headache was improved and she remained afebrile. The second day temperature reoccurred with severe right temporal headache. Blood culture at the time of the myringotomy showed long chain streptococcus of the hemolytic type. Because the headache continued, slight tenderness over mastoid process, moderate discharge from the ear and questionable X-ray evidence, I felt that mastoidectomy was indicated. On her sixth hospital day a mastoidectomy was done and it showed a large cellular mastoid cavity with moderate granulations and very little pus. On currettting deeply at the sinus dural angle and on exposing the dura, a large amount of pus revealed an epi-dural abscess. This was adequately drained and sinus exposed, showing an abnormal wall and a thrombus could be felt.

Two days later, as we felt we had better stop the first operation because of the patient's condition, we reopened the mastoid wound and uncovered the sinus to the bulb and posteriorly for several centimeters. The sinus was tightly thrombosed and we were unable to obtain free bleeding. Because of the recurring temperature, the jugular vein was ligated, and the thrombus did not extend to the neck. The patient recovered remarkably, being practically afebrile and symptom free until the tenth day and a paralysis of the right external rectus was noted, on the eighteenth day beginning papillodema developed and progressively became worse and by the twenty-first day she had full choked discs and right temporal headaches but no fever.

She was referred to a neuro-surgeon. Dr. Keegan, who searched for an abscess through the mastoid wound, he found nothing. Then a spinal puncture and the pressure 30 mm. with no response on right, but a fair on the left with jugular compression. He allowed the fluid to drain off very slowly to reduce the pressure to 15 mm. The patient obtained considerable relief for about 12 hours. This was repeated with the same result, but produced some sub-occipital pain, which caused concern as to the danger of further spinal puncture.

At this time it was decided to venture a puncture into cerebellum as had been done in the temporal lobe to rule out cerebellar abscess. Nothing was found. A trephine was then performed in the left frontal region and the i n s e r t i o n of a continuous drainage needle into the anterior horn of the left anterior ventricle. The ventricle was not dilated, but the needle was left in place, allowing the escape of fluid for two days. The flow of fluid stopped and the needle was removed. The patient was markedly improved as to headaches and sixth nerve paralysis. She continued to run a low grade temperature and another positive blood culture was found. She was given another transfusion. I neglected to state that three transfusions were given at the time and shortly following the early operations. Her condition steadily improved and about 14 months after her illness she seemed in perfect physical condition.

I place this case in Type C of Dr. Tobey's classification.

In summing up the three cases, we have two with sixth nerve paralysis, one with overwhelming septicemia, and one with epi-dural abscess.

In explanation of the sixth nerve paralysis, this is thought to be due to localized infection at the petrosal tip or pressure. This nerve, as you know, is a long slender filament which crosses the b a s a l subarachnoid space and is easily subject to inflammatory or pressure disturbances. Intracranial pressure commonly causes sixth n e r v e weakness by pressing the brain tightly downwards over the free border of the t e n t o r i u m where the sixth nerve crosses to enter the cavernous sinus wall. Cushing has shown that occasionally the sixth nerve lies under the inferior cerebellar artery and sometimes over. If it lies under the artery, increased pressure has more effect.

The increased intra-cranial pressure is caused by the inflammatory process and also the venous congestion following the ligation of the internal jugular vein. There is considerable difference in size and communication of the two transverse sinuses at the torcular herophili and in some cases practically all of the blood from the superior sagittal sinus goes down one side. This would account for the absence of venous congestion in some cases and marked in others.

The epi-dural abscess was merely an extension of the infection through the sinus wall.

Dr. Hartman[6] has shown with a series of two c a s e s that sulphanilamide given previous to operation for a period of three to five days, seems to mitigate the gravity of the outlook, and minimizes the chance of continued progressive septicemia. In case number two, had sulphanilamide been available during the time we were waiting for operation, the streptococcus might not have gained such a foothold.

SUMMARY

1. Sinus thrombosis following middle ear and mastoid infections carries a mortality of about 33 to 35 per cent.

2. It is recognized by recurrence of chills and fever following middle ear infections; the temperature curve falling in one of our groups as discussed.

3. Diagnosis is further established by a positive blood culture or by rapid fall in hemoglobin, characteristic of hemolytic streptococcus infections.

4. Neurologic signs consist chiefly in sixth nerve palsy, as a rule the same side.

5. Spinal puncture shows internal jugular block on same side, partial or complete.

6. Treatment consists: Medically of sulphanilamide (this has not been used personally to date) and supportive treatment. Surgical treatment consists of open operation, removal of septic thrombus and ligation or resection of the corresponding internal jugular vein.

BIBLIOGRAPHY

1. Tobey, Geo. L., Jr. Panel Discussion, Septic, Thrombophlebitis of the Sigmoid Sinus; Transactions of the Academy of Ophth. & Otol., 1937.

2. Lillie, H. I.: Infection of Sigmoid and Lateral Sinus; Surg. Gynec. & Obst. 35:418, 1922.

3. Greenfield, Samuel D.: Thrombophlebitis of the Lateral Sinus; Archive Otolaryng. 25:662, 1937.

4. Coates, G. M.; Ernsner, M. S., and Persky, A. H.: Lateral Sinus Thrombosis with Review of Literature, Ann. Otol.; Rhin. & Laryng. 43:419, 1934.

5. Heine, B. Operationen am Obr. Die operationen bei Mittelohreiterungen und ihren intrakraniellen Komplikationen, Berlin, S. Karger, 1913.

6. Hartmann, Alexis F. Septic thrombophlebitis of the Sigmoid Sinus, Medical Treatment. Panel discussion; Transactions of the Academy of Ophth. and Otol, 1937.

THE JOURNAL
OF THE
Oklahoma State Medical Association

Issued Monthly at McAlester, Oklahoma, under direction of the Council.

Copyright, 1938, by Oklahoma State Medical Association, McAlester, Oklahoma.

Vol. XXXI	NOVEMBER	Number 11

DR. L. S. WILLOUR_____Editor-in-Chief
McAlester, Oklahoma

DR. T. H. McCARLEY_____Associate Editor
McAlester, Oklahoma

Entered at the Post Office at McAlester, Oklahoma, as second-class matter under the act of March 3rd, 1879.

This is the official Journal of the Oklahoma State Medical Association. All communications should be addressed to The Journal of the Oklahoma State Medical Association, McAlester Clinic, McAlester, Oklahoma. $4.00 per year; 40c per copy.

The editorial department is not responsible for the opinions expressed in the original articles of contributors.

Reprints of original articles will be supplied at actual cost provided request for them is attached to manuscripts or made in sufficient time before publication.

Articles sent this Journal for publication and all those read at the annual meetings of the State Association are the sole property of this Journal. The Journal relies on each individual contributor's strict adherence to this well-known rule of medical journalism. In the event an article sent this Journal for publication is published before appearance in The Journal the manuscript will be returned to the writer.

Failure to receive The Journal should call for immediate notification of the Editor, McAlester Clinic, McAlester, Oklahoma.

Local news of possible interest to the medical profession, notes on removals, changes of addresses, births, deaths and weddings will be gratefully received.

Advertising of articles, drugs or compounds unapproved by the Council on Pharmacy of the A. M. A., will not be accepted.

Advertising rates will be supplied on application.

It is suggested that wherever possible members of the State Association should patronize our advertisers in preference to others as a matter of fair reciprocity.

Printed by News-Capital Company, McAlester.

EDITORIAL

IMPORTANT NOTICE

The dues of the Oklahoma State Medical Association for 1939 will be twelve dollars ($12.00) in compliance with the action of the House of Delegates at the meeting held in Muskogee.

The following is an abstract from the minutes of the House of Delegates, May 10, 1938:

"On motion of Dr. Ned R. Smith, seconded by Dr. J. S. Fulton, unanimously carrying, the annual dues will be twelve dollars ($12.00), beginning January 1, 1939."

Secretaries will please take notice when they collect the annual dues so that there will be no necessity to return checks for insufficient remittance.

WASHINGTON CONFERENCE

Immediately following a called meeting of the House of Delegates of the American Medical Association the President of the United States and the chairman of the Interdepartmental Committee to Coordinate Health and Welfare Activities were advised by a Committee (appointed by the Speaker of the House) to confer with governmental agencies. Both the President and Miss Josephine Roche, Chairman, replied very graciously to the communications. They advised they would be glad to have an early discussion of the matter with the Committee, and this meeting was scheduled to be held in Washington, October 31st.

This Committee will go to Washington with much valuable information as to the need of expansion of medical care. However, they will have no information from Oklahoma as the Survey which was requested by the American Medical Association has not been made in this State, although the material has b e e n in the hands of the committee on Economics since our meeting last May.

This Interdepartmental Committee was in possession of so much mis-information that its conclusions, at their former meeting predicated on t h i s mis-information, were far from being accurate. It is these inaccurate conclusions which have reached the lay press and been the basis of much discussion by the laity.

Organized medicine will be ably represented at this meeting as the Committee is composed of Dr. Irvin Abel, Chairman; Dr. Walter F. Donaldson, Dr. Walter E. Vest, Dr. Henry A. Luce, Dr. Fred W. Rankin, Dr. Frederic E. Sondern, Dr. E. H. Cary, and ex officio Dr. Rock Sleyster, and Dr. Olin West.

This Committee, meeting with an open minded delegation representing the Government, will be able to develop a plan under the direction of Organized Medicine, that will accomplish much toward the solution of the existing problem.

ANNUAL MEETING MAY 1, 2, 3

The Committee on Arrangements has decided on the dates of May 1, 2, 3, 1939, for the Annual Meeting. Headquarters will be Skirvin Hotel, Oklahoma City.

Editorial Notes—Personal and General

DR. WILLIAM H. KAEISER, McAlester, has been appointed County Health Superintendent of Pittsburg County.

DR. PATRICK NAGLE announces the removal of his offices from the Medical Arts Building, Oklahoma City, and the opening of a Surgical Facility, at 1021 North Lee, for the practice of general surgery, plastic surgery and industrial surgery.

DR. and MRS. JOHNNY BLUE, Guymon, spent two weeks in Colorado, vacationing, in October.

DR. REED WOLFE, Hugo, has taken over the offices of the late Dr. W. N. John, where he will continue the practice of medicine.

DR. and MRS. O. ALTON WATSON, DR. and MRS. WM. H. BONHAM, DR. and MRS. L. CHESTER McHENRY, and DR. JOSEPH C. MacDONALD, Oklahoma City, spent ten days in Washington and New York, in October, attending the national convention of Ophthalmology and Otolaryngology in Washington, and the American College of Surgeons meetings in New York.

THE SOUTHWEST CLINICAL CONFERENCE, Kansas City, was attended by the following Oklahoma doctors: L. E. Emanuel, Chickasha; Parkey H. Anderson, Anadarko; Glenn J. Collins, McAlester.

DR. and MRS. KENNETH J. WILSON, Oklahoma City, spent two weeks in New York City and Baltimore, in October. They visited their son, Dr. Chas. Hugh Wilson, who is a resident surgeon at the New Rochelle Hospital, New Rochelle, N. Y. Dr. Wilson also attended the sessions of the American Birth Control League in New York, and clinics at the Johns Hopkins Hospital, Baltimore.

DR. ELTON LEHEW, Pawnee, announces the removal of his office from the First National Bank Building to the LeHew Building.

DR. E. B. THOMASSON, Duncan, is reported ill at his home.

DR. A. C. ABERNETHY, Altus, has accepted an assignment with the United States navy as head of the Urology department of the Canacao Hospital, Philippine Islands, and sailed October 17, from Norfolk, Va.

DR. J. R. HINSHAW, Major Med.-Res., Butler, Oklahoma, spent the first two weeks of October, 3-15, attending the Medical Military Conference, Mayo Clinic, Rochester Minnesota, where some 85 physicians and surgeons of both army and navy were in conference on pertinent Medical Military problems.

DR. GEORGE A. KILPATRICK, McAlester, attended the meeting of the American College of Surgeons which met in New York City, in October.

DR. ALLAN R. RUSSELL, McAlester, attended the Sectional Meeting of the American Urological Association which met in Dallas, October 19-21.

DR. GEORGE H. KIMBALL, Oklahoma City, has returned from New York City where he attended the meeting of the American College of Surgeons in October.

DR. J. F. PARK, McAlester, attended the meeting of the International College of Surgeons at New York City; he also attended Clinics at Johns Hopkins Hospital, at Baltimore.

News of the County Medical Societies

CARTER County Medical Society met in Ardmore, Monday, October 17, with the following program: "General Consideration of Fractures," Dr. L. S. Willour, McAlester; "Electrocardiograph as an Aid in Diagnosis," Dr. Glenn J. Collins, McAlester; "Psychiatry in Medicine," Dr. Lyman C. Veazey, Ardmore.

GRADY, STEPHENS and CADDO County Medical Societies met at Anadarko, September 29th. Two Oklahoma County doctors were guest speakers for the evening, Dr. Henry H. Turner speaking on "Practical Endocrinology" and Dr. W. M. Taylor on "Acute Respiratory Diseases of Childhood." This program followed a banquet at which 19 members were present. These three societies will meet in Chickasha in November.

LINCOLN County Medical Society met October 5th with Dr. C. H. Bailey, Stroud, as host. Mrs. Bailey was hostess to the wives of those doctors attending. DR. JOHN F. BURTON, Oklahoma City, was the principal speaker.

---o---

OBITUARIES

LEALON EDWARD LAMB

Lealon Edward Lamb was born at Paragould, Arkansas, on March 23rd, 1901, and died at Kansas City, Missouri, on October 7, 1938, at the age of 37 years, 6 months and 14 days.

He came to Clinton with his parents in January, 1908, and resided here from that time until his death. He received his elementary education in the public schools of Clinton, and was graduated from the class of 1920. He continued his education at the University of Oklahoma and Medical Department of Washington & Lee, and received his B.S. degree from the University of Oklahoma in the year 1926 and his M.D. degree from the University of Oklahoma Medical school in 1928. After graduation from the University of Oklahoma he entered the Kansas City General Hospital and served one year as an intern, and during his intership at the Kansas City General Hospital he was president of the interns. Upon completion of his internship in 1929, he returned to practice his profession in Clinton, and associated himself with his father, Dr. Ellis Lamb, and in 1936 Dr. Ross Deputy joined the firm and the firm continued from that time to the date of his death as: Drs. Lamb, Lamb & Deputy.

Dr. Lamb was married to Miss Margaret Waddell, of Yukon, Oklahoma, on September 25, 1933. They established their home at 512 South 9th street in Clinton where they have since lived.

He was a member of the County, State and National Medical Societies, Fellow of A.M.A., was past president of the Custer County Society and was president of the Western Oklahoma Medical Society at the time of his death. He was a member of the Masonic Lodge and a member and past president of the Kiwanis Club of Clinton. A member of the University of Oklahoma Chapter of Beta Theta Pi fraternity and a member of Phi Bate medical fraternity.

He is survived by his widow; his father and mother, Dr. and Mrs. Ellis Lamb, of Clinton; one sister, Mrs. R. H. Dunn of Clinton, and one nephew, Bobby Ellis Dunn of Clinton, and other relatives.

---o---

DEATH NOTICES

DR. J. H. COLBY, Purcell, October 12, 1938.
DR. W. L. KENDALL, Enid, October 12, 1938.
DR. A. F. PADBERG, Canton, October 12, 1938.
DR. W. L. KNIGHT, Wewoka, October 18, 1938.

Books Received and Reviewed

OUTLINE OF ROENTGEN DIAGNOSIS, An Orientation in the Basic Principles of Diagnosis By the Roentgen Method. Leo G. Rigler, B.S., M.B., M.D., Professor of Radiology, University of Minnesota, Minneapolis, Minnesota. Atlas Edition, 254 Illustrations show in 227 Figures, presented in Drawings and Reproductions of Roentgenograms. Figures 6 to 51 and 55 to 72 are drawings in an original technic by Jean E. Hirsch. J. B. Lippincott Co., Philadelphia.

This is a compact, fairly comprehensive manual or a synopsis on Roentgen diagnosis, written in a clear diadactic style by a well recognized teacher and radiologist. This book is really the revised and expanded lectures that Dr. Rigler presents to his undergraduates and post graduate students.

The subjects are presented in outline style, each paragraph is packed with facts. Discussion on physics, details of technique, and detail discussion of the rarer lesions are omitted in an attempt to make the manual practical. The photographs and sketches that comprise the atlas are well selected and adequately labeled.

This manual is recommended to both students and physicians who desire a well planned outline study of roentgen diagnosis.

THE PRACTICE OF MEDICINE, by Jonathan Campbell Meakins, M.D., LL.D., Professor of Medicine and Director of the Department of Medicine, McGill University; Physician-in-Chief, Royal Victoria Hospital, Montreal; Formerly Professor of Therapeutics and Clinical Medicine, University of Edinburgh. Fellow of the Royal Society of Edinburgh; Fellow of the Royal Society of Canada; Fellow of the Royal College of Physicians, London; Fellow of the Royal College of Physicians, Edinburgh; Honorary Fellow of the Royal College of Surgeons, Edinburgh; Fellow of the Royal College of Physicians, Canada; Fellow of the American College of Physicians. Second Edition. With 521 illustrations including 43 in color. The C. V. Mosby Company, St. Louis, 1938. (He recommends himself highly!!)

This second edition of a work on internal medicine has been practically universally accepted. There have been many additions and amplifications including local and constitutional conditions, blood dyscrasias, protamine zinc insulin, vascular renal failure, uremic state, sulphanilamide therapy, et cetera. The regional classification of material presented makes it very convenient for ready references. There are nearly 50 color plates that are beautifully illustrated. The color makes possible accurate differentiation of certain pathological processes. As each subject is thoroughly complete in this review it would be impracticable to go into the various chapters except to say that in each instance an entire description of the subject can be expected.

ESSENTIALS OF OBSTETRICAL AND GYNECOLOGICAL PATHOLOGY WITH CLINICAL CORRELATION, by Marion Douglass, M.D., F.A.C.S. Assistant Professor of Gynecology Western Reserve University, and Robert L. Faulkner, M.D., Senior Clinical Instructor in Gynecology Western Reserve University. 148 Illustrations. The C. V. Mosby Company, St. Louis, 1938.

This work by Douglass and Faulkner is essentially for the obstetrician and gynecologist. As applied to these branches this work is covered in detail and elaborately illustrated. There appears in this small volume 108 illustrations, micro-photographs, sketches and plates, thereby in the most complete way, illustrating practically all of the printed material. Histological pathology of the organs of reproduction is elaborately covered and will be found of great value to the student and specialist in these branches.

HUMAN PATHOLOGY, A Textbook, by Howard T. Karsner, M.D., Professor of Pathology, Western Reserve University, Cleveland, Ohio, with an Introduction by Simon Flexner, M.D. Eighteen illustrations in color and 443 black and white. Fifth Edition, Revised. J. B. Lippincott Company, Philadelphia.

Dr. Karsner's book on Human Pathology has been accepted for many years as the standard text and we are now presented with the fifth edition in which you will find retained all of the worthwhile material from the former editions and the result of recent rapid advance in biological and medical research. The work covers the fields of general pathology, pathological or morbid anatomy, pathological histology, functional or pathological physiology, and the general subjects of bacteriology and immunology. It contains discussion of debated and intricate subjects serving to give the reader definite understanding of points at issue. The book is divided into two parts, one General Pathology and two Systemic Pathology, and the whole material is divided into 22 chapters, making a complete text for the student as well as the general practitioner.

MEDICAL WRITING, The Technic and The Art, By Morris Fishbein, M.D., Editor, The Journal of the American Medical Association, Chicago. With the assistance of Jewel F. Whelan, Assistant to the Editor.

The work by Dr. Morris Fishbein, who has probably had more experience with medical writing and the editing of scientific papers written by other physicians, might well be in the hands of any physician who attempts writing for publication.

The editors of all medical journals would be glad if the authors could familiarize themselves with the proper way of preparing their material and it would also be well for the editors to familiarize themselves with this book. The art of medical writing is thoroughly discussed as is the preparation of manuscript, charts, tables, illustrations, capitalization, abbreviations, style of writing, et cetera.

If you would be a better writer familiarize yourself with this publication by the American Medical Association Press.

A HISTORICAL CHRONOLOGY OF TUBERCULOSIS, by Richard M. Burke, M.D., State Veterans Hospital, Sulphur, Oklahoma.

This small book will be of interest to those who may give of their time to the study and treatment of tuberculosis. It is very interesting reading to the general practitioner as the development of the recognition and treatment of this disease is chronologically described and the progress in both treatment and prevention is shown in an orderly manner.

This being the work of an Oklahoma author should particularly appeal to the doctors of this state.

UROLOGY, By Daniel N. Eisendrath, M.D., Consulting Urologist to the American Hospital, Paris, France; Formerly Attending Urologist, Michael Reese and Cook County Hospitals; Assistant Professor of Surgery (Genito-Urinary) Rush Medical College of the University of Chicago. And Harry C. Rolnick, M.D., Attending Urologist, Michael Reese, Mt. Sini, and Cook County Hospitals, Chicago; Formerly Clinical Professor of Urology, Loyola University Medical School. A total of 750 black and white illustrations and 12 in color. Fourth Edition, Entirely Revised and Reset. J. B. Lippincott Co., Philadelphia, 1938.

This is the fourth edition of a well known book

on Urology. This edition having been revised, making it more complete in every way. It deals with every phase of urology, beginning with embryology and taking up every phase, being especially complete in the treatise of pathology, symptoms, diagnosis and treatment of urological conditions.

It is well arranged in that it deals with the various phases and anatomical sections of the genitourinary tract separately and completely which greatly clarifies the reading as well as the information.

It includes practically all of the latest information on diagnosis and treatment of urological conditions. It takes up many of the medical aspects of urology not included in other books on urology.

This is one of the better books on urology and would be very instructive to the medical man in any type of practice but especially so to the urologist.

WORKBOOK IN ELEMENTARY DIAGNOSIS FOR TEACHING CLINICAL HISTORY RECORDING AND PHYSICAL DIAGNOSIS, by Logan Clendening, Professor of Clinical Medicine, University of Kansas. Illustrated. The C. V. Mosby Company, St. Louis, 1938.

This book is an expanded arrangement of "The Laboratory Notebook Method in Teaching Physical Diagnosis and Clinical History Recording" published in 1934. In it are instructions in history taking and physical examinations together with specific outline for the purpose of recording these findings.

There are brief explicit instructions for the method of doing inspection, palpation, auscultation manipulation, et cetera, with many illustrated plates for demonstration. It also gives instruction and demonstration in examination of excretions and secretions, et cetera.

Apparently the purpose of this book is to teach not only the student but also men in clinical practice a routine of doing history taking and physical examination and making record of same. It should be very beneficial to students who are beginning their work in elementary diagnosis.

CANCER, WITH S P E C I A L REFERENCE TO CANCER OF THE BREAST, by R. J. Behan, M.D., Dr. Med. (Berlin), F.A.C.S., Co-founder and Formerly Director of the Cancer Department of the Pittsburgh Skin and Cancer Foundation, Pittsburgh, Pa. Illustrated. The C. V. Mosby Company, St. Louis, 1938.

Cancer of the breast would be the more appropriate title for this book, as Dr. Behan intimates in his preface. This presentation of breast tumors is most thorough and complete. The author has abstracted the world literature on this subject and compiled the facts and plausible theories about etiology, physiology, and diagnosis of breast tumors into this book. One-third of the book is devoted to treatment by surgery, irradiation, organ-therapy and general measures. Several chapters are devoted to a general discussion of X-ray and radium in cancer therapy. Malignancy, other than breast tumors, is discussed in general terms in scattered paragraphs in various chapters on breast tumors.

The innumerable references, quotations and abstracts make this a valuable reference book on cancer of the breast. The reading is necessarily slow and interrupted because of the style and the strong desire of the author for completeness.

This book is recommended to physicians who desire detailed reading on breast tumors and a general discussion on some cancer principles or theories to discuss.

———o———

Important Notice on Editorial Page

The School-Child's Breakfast

Many a child is scolded for dullness when he should be treated for undernourishment. In hundreds of homes a "continental" breakfast of a roll and coffee is the rule. If, day after day, a child breaks the night's fast of 12 hours on this scant fare, small wonder that he is listless, nervous, or stupid at school. A happy solution to the problem is Pablum, Mead's Cereal cooked and dried. Six times richer than fluid milk in calcium, ten times higher than spinach in iron, and abundant in vitamins B-1 and G, Pablum furnishes protective factors especially needed by the school-child. The ease with which Pablum can be prepared enlists the mother's co-operation in serving a nutritious breakfast. This palatable cereal requires no further cooking and can be prepared simply by adding milk or water of any desired temperature. Its nutritional value is attested in studies by Crimm et al who found that tuberculous children receiving supplements of Pablum showed greater weight-gain, greater increase in hemoglobin, and higher serum-calcium values than a control group fed farina.

Mead Johnson & Company, Evansville, Indiana, will supply reprints on request of physicians.

———o———

Electrolysis Controlling Factor In Use of Metals In Treating Fractures

Charles S. Venable and Walter G. Stuck, San Antonio, Texas (Journal A.M.A., October 8, 1938), point out that in order to avoid corrosion of the metals used in the direct fixation of fractures electrolysis must be eliminated, because electrolysis precedes corrosion. The physician's interest is in some metal that will be passive (electrically neutral) in the fluids of the human body. In their studies of electrolysis the authors deliberately set out to create batteries in the bones of living animals by using screws of mixed metals of different potentials which were not coupled. At necropsy biochemical examinations of the tissues about the screws revealed that ions of one metal had migrated to the neighborhood of another metal in accordance with the law of electromotive force of metals. This probed the presence of the effects of electrolysis. They then tried a number of the so-called rustless and noncorrosive steels in combination with baser metals and in each instance found changes in tissue, necrosis of bone and other electrolytic effects. They found, however, that there were no such effects when one alloy, vitallium, made of cobalt, chromium and molybdenum, was used. Their experiments were repeated several times to check and recheck the apparent fact that this singular alloy seemed consistently to remain inert. With the inherent characteristic of constant passivity of this strange alloy, vitallium, shown in all their experiments, with or without couple, in physiologic solution of sodium chloride, in blood serum and in vivo, they naturally turned to its application in human osteosynthesis. At this time they know of no other metal or alloy except vitallium which is so completely electrically neutral and sufficiently strong to meet the needs of fracture fixation but they believe that, with the recognition of electrolysis as the controlling factor, metallurgists may develop others. Fifty-seven cases, including the authors' and those of five other surgeons, are listed in which vitallium appliances were retained for three months or more. End results as to healing of the fracture were analyzed and the tolerance of this metal by healing bone was observed. There has been neither overstimulation of bone growth, with excessive callus, nor demineralization of bone at the fracture sites or about the screws or nails inserted in the bone. The use of vitallium or any equally inert nonelectrolytic alloy in the fixation of old ununited or malunited fractures or even fresh fractures opens a new approach to this problem.

ABSTRACTS : REVIEWS : COMMENTS
and CORRESPONDENCE

SURGERY AND GYNECOLOGY

Abstracts, Reviews and Comments from
LeRoy Long Clinic
714 Medical Arts Building, Oklahoma City

Five Hundred Thyroidectomies, Some Practical Reflections (Cinq Cents Thyroidectomies, Quelques Reflexions d'ordre Pratique). R. E. Valin, Ottawa, Canada; L'Union Medicale du Canada; October, 1938; Volume 67, No. 10, page 1070.

Reporting 500 thyroidectomies during the last 10 years, the author directs attention to the prevalence of goiter in the Ottawa Valley which he believes is largely due to the drinking of water of low iodine content, most of the drinking water coming from a range of mountains north of the valley.

With the exception of goiter of adolescence, it appears that surgical operations were done for practically all types of disease of the thyroid gland. The reason given is the belief that goiter, of whatever type, with the exception of adolescent goiter, is, potentially, a goiter that can be relieved best by surgical operation. In this connection, there is a reference to the well-known fact that an apparently quiescent goiter may become dangerously and suddenly active after unusual physical or mental stress and strain. Attention is directed to the fact, too, that, under such circumstances, a quiescent goiter may become very active and dangerous in the advanced period of life. Again, one must consider the danger of malignancy in apparent goiter without any subjective symptoms, such change making ·the surgical removal of the goiter justifiable.

There is a reference to the erroneous belief that cysts of the thyroid gland are without danger, and in that conenction the reader is very pertinently reminded that all cysts of the thyroid gland originate from fetal adenomas with which practically all malignancies of the thyroid are associated.

An interesting table of statistics touching the 500 thyroidectomies reported is presented as follows:

Hyperplastic goiters of the Basedow type	151
Toxic adenomas	111
Non-toxic adenomas, including cystic adenomas and colloid adenomas	207
Malignant tumors	6
Acute thyroiditis	3
Thyroiditis with suppuration	2
Thyro-cardiac goiters	8
Supernumerary thyroids	2
Intra-thoracic goiters(Goitres plongants)	12
Preliminary ligation of poles	2
Mortality	2
Recurrencies	6
Myxoedema	0
Tetany	0
Traumatism of the recurrent laryngeal nerves	2

The belief is expressed that the basal metabolic rate is of great importance. In the group of hyperplastic goiters of the Basedow type there was a B.M.R. of from plus 25 to plus 95, and it was found that generally the B.M.R. is in proportion to the severity of the symptoms.. However, this was not always true, because patients were seen who presented a visible enlargement of the thyroid, but without subjective symptoms. And a number of those patients showed a relatively high B.M.R. Such patients should be properly prepared for surgical operation just as if they had definite clinical symptoms, and when they are not so prepared the results may not be good.

There is another group of patients in which there is no visible enlargement of the thyroid, but who have subjective symptoms indicative of thyroid disease. In such cases the B.M.R. is of great importance, but it must not be forgotten that the B.M.R. is not the only important factor, the rapidity of the pulse being still more important. It is believed that a rapid pulse and an elevated B.M.R. are parallel conditions in the case of a patient suffering from hyperthyroidism.

In the series reported there were subtotal thyroidectomies, bilateral, in all, with the exception of two, and all in a single seance. In the two exceptions there were preliminary ligations of the superior poles. With the modern method of preparation, including particularly the administration of Lugol's solution, it is rarelv necessary to resort to surgical operations in series. If the operations are to be divided into stages, it is the opinion of the author that after a unilateral thyroidectomy there should be an interval of six weeks before performing a thyroidectomy on the opposite side.

It is advised that in all cases of toxic adenoma of the thyroid there should be a subtotal thyroidectomy, and not the simple removal of the adenoma, because in such a situation there frequently exists small, invisible adenomas, that are toxic. Recurrencies in such cases are usually attributable to defective technique of the operator.

The author does not practice the intracapsular enucleation, but does a complete extracapsular dissection. The extracapsular procedure is more radical, and the concomitant hemorrhage is less and very much easier to control. There is less shock, and at all stages of the operation one is able to observe the anatomical relation of the structures of the neck.

Attention is directed to the symptoms of intrathoracic goiter, the most frequent being a sensation of smothering during sleep, or in a change of posture; an incapacity to stoop, like the attitude in lacing the shoes; a chronic cough; dyspnoea during effort; respiratory spasm simulating acute attacks of asthma. Frequently there is no ocular evidence of goiter, but an X-ray examination of the contiguous chest will reveal the shadow indicating an intra-thoracic enlarged thyroid.

The two fatalities following operation were associated with symptoms of acute hyperthyroidism. One of the patients died on the second day and the other on the fourth day. Notwithstanding the extreme low mortality (two out of 500 patients), the author remarks that there are symptoms which ought to restrain the surgeon from doing an operation (Il y a des indices qui doivent determiner chez les patients tres intoxiques l'opportunite d'une intervention).

The B.M.R. is not regarded as the sole index of the ability of the patient to undergo an operation. Of even more importance is the age of the patient; the patient who has had thyroid disease for many years usually having an hypertrophied heart in poor condition. The pulse is of great importance, the patient whose pulse does not become slower under appropriate treatment, including iodine and rest, usually being a very poor risk patient. It is believed that a persistent tachycardia, independent of exterior emotive causes, is a very bad sign, and is an index of a tumultuous and difficult convalescence. The duration of hyperthyroidism must be considered with great care in connection with the risk, because the longer the hyperthyroidism has existed the more will cardiac reserve be lost.

The psychological attitude of the patient is of extreme importance in connection with prognosis, and it is not wise to undertake a surgical operation when there is great psychological distress. This is particularly true when the patient has had iodine for a long time, because then it is not possible to secure the good results that usually come after the relatively short period of administration of iodine, and in such a situation an operation should be approached with great care.

Speaking again of recurrencies, the author expresses himself as believing that a surgical operation done in the proper way and under proper conditions is a cure for hyperthyroidism, but one must be careful to make a distinction between typical symptoms of true hyperthyroidism, such as the loss of weight, tachycardia, cardiac fibrillation, hypertrophy of the gland, exophthalmus, and elevated B.M.R., and those conditions simulating disease of the thyroid, such as nervous exhaustion, general physical decline, menopause, psychoses, infected tonsils neuro-vegetative dystonia.

It is insisted that the operative incision should be of ample length so that all the anatomical structures of the neck are exposed. It is remarked that a scar of the neck is a scar regardless of its length, but that a few inches more are of extreme importance for the surgeon in connection with the security of the surgical operation.

Anesthesia in all the patients of the series was produced by the local infiltration of the operative area with one per cent novocain, preceded, in the earlier years, by the hypodermatic administration of ¼ grain morphine and 1/100 grain hyoscin about half an hour before patient was taken to the operating room. In recent years avertin has been substituted for the morphine and hyoscin. The author now prefers avertin because it is less toxic and there is a profound and durable sleep.

Remarking that it was observed in several surgical clinics that patients presenting a marked hyperthyroidism, and who had had a normal or subnormal blood iodine after the administration of Lugol's solution, were those who presented greater risk of recurrence of the hyperthyroidism after subtotal thyroidectomies, it is advised that in such patients a more considerable quantity of thyroid tissue should be removed at operation, and in that connection the statement is made that now the percentage of blood iodine is determined in all patients during the period of preoperative investigation.

Finally, there is a short reference to the comparative results of X-ray therapy, and a surgical operation for the removal of the proper amount of thyroid tissue. It is the definite conclusion of the author that a properly performed surgical operation produces results very much superior to those produced by X-ray therapy.

COMMENTS: Dr. Valin, the author of this article, is Director-General de L'Association des Medecins de Langue Francaise de l'Amerique du Nord, and is one of the well-knewn French Canadian surgeons. The article is written in a systematic, logical manner. We consider it a very important contribution touching the treatment of diseases of the thyroid gland.

LeRoy Long and LeRoy D. Long.

The Treatment of Postoperative Tetany with Dihydrotachysterol; Pickhardt and Bernhard; Annals of Surgery; September, 1938; Volume 108, No. 3, page 362.

Holtz and his coworkers were among the first to observe that very large doses of "Vigantol," a German preparation of irradiated ergosterol, led to a series of toxic symptoms, designated by some authors as hypervitaminosis D. Hypervitaminosis D has as one of its characteristic features a hypercalcemia. The main symptoms of this condition include headache, nausea, vomiting, hematuria, and a moderate elevation of blood pressure. An abnormally high calcium level in the serum, over a relatively long period of time, results in the deposition of calcium salts in the heart, blood vessels, kidneys, and other organs of the body.

Holtz searched for a toxic factor as a possible cause of the hypervitaminosis and found that by prolonging the irradiation of ergosterol under certain conditions he could destroy, in large part, the antirachitic factor, vitamin D, but that the "calcinose" factor was still present. Extensive investigation of the action of the "calcinose" factor by Holtz and his associates was undertaken on both normal and parathyroidectomized animals. The results indicated that this "calcinose" factor caused a marked increase in the amount of calcium in the serum of normal animals with a deposition of calcium in the organs of the body; in the parathyroidectomized animals appropriate amounts of this "calcinose" factor elevated the serum calcium to normal and prevented the symptoms of parathyroid insufficiency. Similar results have been obtained in the author's series of patients following the development of postoperative hypoparathyroidism.

Holtz and his coworkers described this preparation which they call "A. T. 10" and which is now designated chemically as dihydrotachysterol. This compound, although derived from irradiated ergosterol, differs from the parent substance in that it is almost devoid of any antirachitic action, while the calcium mobilizing factor persists and exceeds that of viosterol.

The authors conclude that the new therapeutic agent, dihydrotachysterol ("A. T. 10"),, has great value in the control of postoperative tetany, and the symptoms can be alleviated within 42 to 72 hours after instituting treatment. These patients are usually irritable, extremely nervous, and physically played out, and certainly the removal of these symptoms, as soon as possible, is of the utmost necessity.

Therapy with dihydrotachysterol must be strictly individualized, that is, the blood calcium level must be carefully checked at intervals before and after medication has been instituted. Until the maintenance dose has been determined, the amount of "A. T. 10" given by mouth, may vary from 1 to 3 cc. every other day to 1 to 2 cc. per week, depending on the severity of the deficiency. The authors have on occasion administered dosages as high as 10 cc. daily for a period of several days, but during this period they kept a careful check on the patients' serum calcium findings. The product is not harmless and excessive dosage may well induce symptoms of hypercalcemia.

They make a plea for the routine determination of serum calcium both pre- and postoperatively in all thyroid surgery.

This new substance, in their hands, has been of definite value, both from a subjective point of view and in the control of tetany. Their observations, taken in conjunction with those of Holtz and his coworkers, suggest that dihydrotachysterol merits further chemical study and is recommended for the treatment of postoperative hypoparathyroid tetany.

LeRoy D. Long.

A Comparison of the End-Results of Treatment of Endocervicitis by Electrophysical Methods: Cautery Coagulation, and Conization; Jacoby; American Journal of Obstetrics and Gynecology; October, 1938; Volume 36, No. 4, page 656.

This investigation was employed to determine the comparative estimate of end-results in patients treated by the three methods of cautery, coagulation, and coning of the cervix. One hundred and fifty cases were used, 50 each treated with cautery, coagulation, and coning.

The technique for the three types of procedure have been adequately described and are not repeated but the author feels that the simplest of the procedures is coagulation, then cauterization, and the most difficult is conization.

Of the 150 cases 138 were followed to a point of complete cure which was determined as freedom from symptoms and eradication of pelvic pathology. Fifty of those completely followed were of the group treated by coagulation and 44 each in the groups treated by cauterization and conization.

"The average length of time required to cure patients treated by cauterization was four months. The average length of time required to cure patients treated by coagulation was seven months. The average length of time required to cure patients treated by conization was 7.3 months."

"Repetition of the same or one of the other methods was necessary in one case originally cauterized, in five cases originally coned, and in six cases originally coagulated." The author has also tabulated the number of patients who formed cysts of Nabothian character in the different groups and there were four patients treated for this difficulty who had been originally cauterized, nine who had been originally coagulated, and 17 who had been originally coned.

There was moderate stenosis of the cervical canal in six patients treated by coagulation.

"Acute inflammation of the tubes and ovaries developed in four patients treated by coagulation and in three treated by conization."

It is the author's conclusion that all three methods are satisfactory for removing the diseased cervical mucosa. However, from his study, the patients treated by cauterization were cured more quickly and with fewer complications than by the other two methods.

He also feels that in all instances Nabothian cysts and cervical erosion are best treated by cauterization.

It is also his contention that the cautery is superior to the other two electrophysical methods for treating chronic cervical inflammation.

COMMENTS: In the abstracts submitted for this column last month an article by Dr. Norman Miller on the advantages and disadvantages of conization was summarized.

It is extremely interesting to get this carefully controlled group by Jacoby employing the three different methods in an equal number of patients. It was Miller's contention that the simpler cervical lesions could be well treated by cauterization, whereas the more serious and extensive lesions were better treated by conization. It is herewith Jacoby's opinion that cautery is the superior method in all of the chronic cervical inflammatory lesions that he sees.

From these two careful studies, one is able to draw the conclusion, when combined with one's own practical experience, that all three of these methods of treating chronic cervical lesions can be recommended in particular types with the actual cautery being superior for all erosion and Nabothian cysts and being almost equal, if not equal, in advantage to the other three methods for the treatment of the chronic endocervicitis group.

It is an interesting fact that in this group, at least, and in others the complications were slightly more frequent and more severe in the coagulation group.

Wendell Long.

Supravaginal Hysterectomy, A Review of 535 Consecutive Personal Cases; Walter T. Dannreuther, New York City; The American Journal of Surgery; September, 1938; Volume 41, page 373.

In this series careful attention was paid to the condition of the cervix and supravaginal hysterectomy and not performed unless the cervix was an innocent one or had received preliminary treatment.

Very careful attention was paid to the preoperative preparation of the patients with particular emphasis placed upon blood transfusions in anemia, proper correction of diabetic condition and of cardiovascular disease.

The technique employed by Dannreuther is given in considerable detail.

The postoperative complications occurred in 65 of the 535 patients and are carefully broken down into tables for study.

There were nine deaths with a mortality of 1.7 per cent.

It will be interesting to read the conclusions of the author which follow:

"1. Supravaginal hysterectomy is the most popular and widely practiced method of uterine extirpation.

"2. Its selection in individual cases should depend more upon the condition of the cervix than the convenience of the operator.

"3. Extensive cervical disease, malignancy, and potentially malignant lesions are absolute contraindications.

"4. The vaginal surface of the portio must be completely epithelialized and the endocervical canal free from infection and inflammatory products, to justify cervical retention.

"5. Many damaged cervices can be reconverted to a healthy state before operation.

"6. The incidence of subsequent carcinoma of the cervix is no higher after a supravaginal hysterectomy in properly selected cases than in women who have never been operated upon.

"7. Adequate preoperative preparation of the patient is important.

"8. Hysterectomy can be done more rapidly with clamps than with primary ligatures and the use of clamps does not predispose to postoperative embolism.

"9. When there are raw areas that cannot be satisfactorily peritonealized, sheets of gutta-percha tissue are useful to prevent visceral agglutination.

"10. In a series of 535 consecutive personal cases the morbidity was 11.0 per cent and the mortality 1.7 per cent.

"11. Eliminating one death which was due to a diagnostic error, and two others which might have been obviated by an earlier appreciation of the necessity of interference to relieve intestinal obstruction, the mortality should have been 1.1 per cent."

COMMENTS: This is a very sound review of a constructive series of patients. It is not remarkable for a particularly low mortality or complication percentage. However, there is an excellent discussion of the proper preliminary treatment of the cervix and the instances in which Dr. Dannreuther feels the cervix may safely remain.

While vaginal hysterectomy and c o m p l e t e abdominal hysterectomy have a definite and invaluable field of usefulness, supravaginal hysterectomy will certainly be found to satisfy the criteria more satisfactorily in the average instance where the uterine body should be removed because of disease of that organ. It naturally should be employed only after very careful consideration of the pathology and limited to individuals where there is a clear indication for operation. In the event that it is employed, the cervix should be most carefully examined, biopsies taken where necessary, and mild disease corrected if the cervix is to be left in situ.

Wendell Long.

The Miller-Abbott Double Lumen Tube in Intestinal Obstruction; Robert A. Wise; American Journal of Surgery; September, 1938; Volume 41, No. 3, page 412.

Treatment of intestinal obstruction (paralytic or mechanical) is always difficult. These seriously ill patients will not survive an exploratory operation. Simple enterostomy often fails to alleviate. The method described is an elaboration of the so-called Wangensteen method of decompression of upper intestinal tract. The author reports striking results.

The double lumen rubber tube (ten feet long and 16 French in diameter) was devised by Dr. T. Grier Miller and Dr. W. Osler Abbott, who have made studies concerning secretion and absorption in small intestine. They with Dr. I. S. Ravdin suggested this tube be used in the treatment and diagnosis of intestinal obstruction at a joint meeting of the New York and Philadelphia Surgical Societies on February 9, 1938.

The tube is described as follows: "A rubber septum extends throughout its length, making it into a double lumen tube. The inflation tube opens into a soft rubber balloon; the suction tube has several openings at its distal end and terminates in a metal tip. When the tube has passed the pylorus and the balloon is inflated, it will be carried, by peristalsis, down the entire length of the intestine. As it traverses the intestinal tract, suction is applied which removes fluid and gas from each distended loop. It is possible with this tube to deflate the entire gastrointestinal tract in patients with intestinal obstruction from whatever cause—mechanical or paralytic."

The patient is placed on the right side where he is kept from two to six hours. The tube is introduced through the nose. Technique of passage of the tube so that it will go through the pylorus into duodenum is described. It is important that one know when the tube has passed into the duodenum.

Once the tube is in the duodenum, 30 cc. of air is injected into the balloon, the balloon tube clamped and constant Wangensteen suction applied to the suction tube. Each hour six inches more of the tube is inserted until the eight-foot mark is reached. The suction tube is irrigated each hour with 20 cc. of water.

The author reports three cases which illustrate the use of the tube in: (1) paralytic ileus, (2) mechanical obstruction, and (3) as an aid in the diagnosis and location of an obstructive lesion in the small intestine.

The case of paralytic ileus followed a severe trauma to the hip with fracture. All usual measures to deflate the abdomen had failed and the patient's condition was becoming progressively worse. The relief afforded in this case by the tube was most rapid and within 48 hours the patient was cured of his ileus. No operative procedure could have accomplished this.

The second case reported had a partial mechanical obstruction of the small intestine (probably associated with umbilical hernia) which rapidly became complete. The benefit afforded by the tube in this case was stated to be miraculous, the distention being relieved and the obstruction disappearing. The patient took fluids and semisolids within 48 hours.

One agrees with the author that "had the obstruction remained even after deflation of the abdomen, and operation been necessary, the tube would have been a great aid in locating the point of obstruction.

The third case reported was due to adhesions following several operations but the site of obstruction of small bowel was unknown. It was possible by using this tube to locate the site of the obstructive lesion in the lower ileum. This greatly facilitated the ease and dispatch with which the patient was relieved at a subsequent operation.

LeRoy D. Long.

---o---

EYE, EAR, NOSE AND THROAT
Edited by Marvin D. Henley, M.D.
911 Medical Arts Building, Tulsa

Applied Mechanics of Cataract Extraction. Edward Jackson, M.D., D.Sc., Denver, Colorado. American Journal of Ophthalmology, September, 1938.

The function of the different coats of the eyeball is discussed in detail. One is reminded of the fact that the cornea extends under the scleral margin and that it is thicker at the margin than in its center. Jackson says; "Operations throughout must be planned and carried out with the least possible damage to tissue nutrition and function, consistent with the removal of the opacity obstructing vision.

Beer's, Graefe's and Jaeger's cataract knives are discussed. The Graefe seems to be the most popular. The corneoscleral incision is discussed with an accompanying diagram. The author says the placing of this incision has much to do with the subsequent healing of the wound. He tries to place the corneal incision exactly in the corneal margin, getting the conjunctival flap, when it was considered necessary, by turning back the cutting edge as the incision is completed.

The opening of the lens capsule is next discussed. Jackson is of the opinion that the posterior capsule takes little or no part in the formation of a secondary cataract. Of 49 cases examined for end results it was found that only eight required a secondary operation for capsular opacity. Blood in the anterior chamber or the exudate of a severe uveitis usually preceded these opacities. The making of the puncture and counter-puncture in the sclera divides the corneal ring and so lessens the ability of the tissue around the incision to retain its shape and apposition.

The capsulotomy does not require removal of the lens as a whole, but only the removal of the firm nucleus. The remaining cortex in the capsule disintegrates without causing uveal inflammation. Jackson does not think there is a justification for the so-called "Indian intramuscular extraction" except in cases where the patient comes a long distance and can stay only a few days (as in India). He maintains that the removal of the capsule breaks down the normal division between the anterior and posterior contents of the eyeball.

Corneal section causes or increases astigmatism, usually against the rule. This gradually diminishes, being greatest soon after operation. Even after the astigmatism has ceased to decrease as time goes on, hyperopia may still show a slow increase. This may indicate that it takes a long time for the eye to become adjusted following an operation. Conjunctival sutures and fixation of the rectus tendon by a stitch are frowned upon by Jackson. He says the uncut corneal ring is a better guarantee of healing. The paper is original without bibliography.

The Management of Intra-Ocular Foreign Bodies.
William H. Evans, M.D., Youngstown, Ohio. The
Eye, Ear, Nose and Throat Monthly, September,
1938.

This is a resume of the experiences of an ophthalmologist who is located in an industrial community. From a patient with history of an eye injury routine examination should consist of: checking vision of both eyes, an external examination for abrasions or wounds of the cornea, conjunctiva, sclera, iris and lens, (fluorescin stain should be used), note pupillary reaction, ophthalmoscopic examination, translumination, and the slit lamp should be used in all cases. After this preliminary examination is made a temporary dressing is applied and the patient is hospitalized. Atropine and bichloride ointment are used before the dressing is applied.

X-ray should be done, not necessarily before removal of the foreign body—if it is easily located and removed—but surely afterwards as there have been instances where one foreign body has been removed successfully and the second one present overlooked because of failure to take a picture. Very soon after seeing the patient the author routinely gives some form of foreign protein. He uses one of the following: 20 million of triple typhoid vaccine intravenously, 5 c.c. of boiled milk or of lactigen intramuscularly, or 20,000 units of diphtheria antitoxin subcutaneously. This is done every three or four days following. Acetyl salicylic acid or sodium salicylate, gr x, is given every three hours. Sulfanilimide, gr xv, is given every four hours for the first few days.

Extrusion of foreign bodies spontaneously have been reported. Migration of the body backward has never been reported. Probable causes of an extrusion are: Contraction of a fibrinous band that extends from the foreign body to the point of perforation; suppuration at the point of perforation weakens the body wall; compression of the globe by extraocular muscles; pull on the choroid by the ciliary muscle in accomodation, through action of currents in the intra-ocular fluids. Okaoe's report of the action of common metals on the retaina of rabbits is given. The metals mentioned are: Copper, nickel, lead, brass and iron.

Before any procedure is instigated it is essential to know: whether or not the foreign body is magnetic, location in the globe and its size. The author in discussing the procedure to be carried out divides the discussion under the following heads and gives the method of removal:

A. Magnetic foreign bodies:
   1. Magnetic foreign bodies in the anterior chamber.
   2. Magnetic foreign bodies in the lens.
   3. Magnetic foreign bodies in the vitreous.
B. Non-Magnetic Foreign bodies:
   1. Non-magnetic foreign bodies in the anterior chamber.
   2. Non-magnetic foreign bodies in the lens.
   3. Non-magnetic foreign bodies in the vitreous.

Each individual case must be studied carefully before one can decide what course will be pursued. The patient or some member of the family or both should be told of the gravity of the case. To prevent separation of the retina when there is a wound or incision of the sclera, cautery, thermophore or electrocoagulation is recommended. As soon as possible all foci of infection should be removed. Frequent consultation is advisable.

The graver complications are usually due to infection or trauma, so handle tissues carefully. Complications mentioned are: Panophthalmitis, iritis and iridocyclitis, separation of the retina, sympathetic ophthalmia, glaucoma. The patient should be kept under observation for quite some time following the removal of a foreign body to note any visual changes. A bibliography is appended.

Dietary Treatment of Chronic Sinusitis. Burt R. Shurly, M.D., Detroit Mich. The American Journal of Surgery, October, 1938.

Note: The entire October edition of this journal is devoted to an Eye, Ear, Nose and Throat Symposium; there are some 280 pages; contributors are the leading men of this speciality in the United States; this would be a valuable addition to your library.

A brief review of the history of sinus infection is given with the author's experiences during his practice. It is more of a general talk, which is characteristic of Dr. Shurly. He finally arrives at the following conclusions:

The treatment of chronic sinusitis calls for surgical intervention. Dietetic treatment should be used as a therapeutic aid.

The prophylactic treatment in early infancy may offer much in preventing bony malformations of the nose and sinuses, by a proper use of vitamin D, particularly in milk and eggs and leafy vegetables.

Vitamin A, deficiency may appear as a borderline manifestation and influence the resistance to infection, with lowered vitality of tissues, especially in the ear, nose and throat.

Vitamin C, as a preventive of scurvy, has a special influence on the mucous membranes of the gums, nose and mouth.

The value of raw vegetable juice and mineral salts lies in promoting cell growth and selection.

Special attention to endocrine balance with the use of iodine and thyroid extracts is worthwhile in establishing vasomotor tones.

Food allergy must be determined by special tests and history. The prevention of sinus infection at the time of the removal of tonsils and adenoids, may require special dietetic treatment and cod liver oil.

More than 20,000 units of vitamin D per kilogram of cod liver oil may result in intoxication with symptoms of hyperparathyroidism.

In a case of chronic sinusitis, after necessary surgery special inquiry should be made regarding the diet of the individual, so that the physician may give inteligent advice toward increasing resistance to infection.

Spontaneous Hemorrhage into the Maxillary Sinus. Sobisca S. Hall, M.D., and Harvey V. Thomas, M.D., Clarksburg, W. Va. Archives of Otolaryngology, September, 1938.

Literature of the last ten years contain only two references to this condition. Communications in 1933 with seven of the outstanding rhinologists revealed that only one of them had observed the condition in his long experience. Books published by Gradle, Bishop, Thomson, McKenzie, Hajek, Ballenger and Ballenger, Phillips, Loeb, Jackson, Coates and Jackson and Skillern make no mention of this condition. The blood supply of the antrum is discussed but the various books and authors are rather indefinite—the point of entry of the vessels into the antrum is not given.

The authors have observed 12 persons in the last ten years of their practice or about one patient in 1,400 in their practice. These were made up of five women and seven men; ages 31 to 66 years; the right antrum was involved in five cases and the left in seven; no bilateral hemorrhage occurred; hemophilia nor vicarious menstruation were present; all were American born; blood pressure in all patients was normal; there was no history of a preceding trauma, such as a direct blow or a violent blowing of the nose or any similar incident.

X-ray showed a pre-existing or coexisting, hyperplastic maxillary sinusitis in 10 of the 12 cases. In hyperplastic disease new capillaries occur but the authors are of the opinion that there must have been a gross lesion of one of the major antral vessels because the hemorrhage was too persistent and too severe to have originated from a minor capillary bed. They arrived at this conclusion from the evidence of the gross and microscopic examination. Tuberculosis, malignancy, ulcer, syphilis and a physical rent were ruled out.

The Wasserman was negative in all cases. The symptoms complained of were constant burning pain during the bleeding located in the inner canthal region of the eye of the side involved, the bleeding felt as if it were actually in the eye; there was a burning, itching and tickling sensation high in the nose of the affected side. Sudden and expulsive hemorrhage would occur of bright red blood, stopping and starting again without known reason. The authors thought that this stopping and starting could be explained possibly by a blood clot closing the ostium of the antrum until there was sufficient hemorrhage into the antrum to increase the pressure to the point to where there would be a sudden outpouring of fresh blood. Periods between bleeding varied from a few minutes to several hours.

On 10 of the 12 patients an external radical operation was done; two patients were not operated. The 10 were operated to control hemorrhage and to obtain a correct pathologic picture as the possibility of a malignancy was considered. The last two patients the hemorrhage was controlled by antral lavage. Microscopic examination of the tissue obtained in the radical operations showed nothing more than a hyperplastic mucous membrane. All patients recovered. The authors are of the opinion that had literature on this subject been available all but one of the radical operations could have been avoided and the hemorrhage controlled by antral lavage.

PLASTIC SURGERY
Edited by
GEO. H. KIMBALL, M.D., F.A.C.S.
404 Medical Arts Building, Oklahoma City

Arteriovenous Aneurysms. Mont R. Reid, M.D., and Johnson McGuire, M.D. Annals of Surgery, October, 1938, Vol. 108, No. 4.

In 1925, Reid published a series of four papers under the general title of "Studies on Abnormal Arteriovenous Communications, Acquired and Congenital." In these articles the literature of the subject was rather extensively reviewed. He put forward the thesis that there was no essential difference, except in the size and number of arteriovenous fistulae, between angiomata, cirsoid aneurysms and arteriovenous aneurysms; and this view has been rather generally confirmed.

Thirty-three cases were reported and the clinical studies of them, together with laboratory investigation, formed the basis for certain remarks concerning the effects upon the body of arteriovenous communications, and their treatment. At that time the author realized that there were many matters in connection with this subject which hadn't been solved; that further investigations of it would yield important physiologic, pathologic and therapeutic observations. This has not only proven to be true, as witnessed by the important contributions upon the subject, but has led to by-paths which give promise of yielding important observations concerning conditions which are more frequently encountered than are abnormal arteriovenous communications. We have in mind cardiac disabilities, especially aortic insufficiency and cardiac failure, the state of the capillary bed, the normal absence of capillaries in certain parts of the human body and of other animals, blood volume, circulation time, etc. Indeed, rarely has the investigation of such an infrequent clinical condition been so fruitful of important collateral

contributions. This field of investigation seems limitless for new problems always present themselves, and there are still many old ones which have not been solved.

"The purpose of this report, the authors state, 'is to present another series of 30 cases (12 in detail) to discuss our clinical observations and surgical procedures and to supplement, whenever pertinent, these clinical studies from observations made in our laboratory of experimental surgery.'

"They give a history, physical findings, and operative procedures in each case. Each case is accompanied by a clear cut photograph with explanatory legends attached.

It is impossible to abstract all of the details of this very fine article on this subject. Results of the experimental work is given in detail. The authors bring out the facts relative to damage to the heart caused both by arteriovenous and cirsoid aneuyrisms."

Author's summary:

1. An analysis of 21 cases of arteriovenous and nine cases of cirsoid aneurysms is presented, which is supplemented by observations upon experimentally produced arteriovenous aneurysms in dogs.

2. Sixteen of the arteriovenous aneurysms were operated upon and all except one case of pulsating exophthalmos, were cured. In two instances the aneurysms healed spontaneously without operation. Four patients failed to return and could not be traced. All nine cirsoid aneurysms were operated; three cured and six improved. No deaths in all 30 cases. Total of 39 operations upon the 24 patients who were subjected to surgical treatment.

3. Clinical and experimental observations were discussed in detail which may throw some light on the physiologic and pathologic effects of arteriovenous fistulae.

4. In our limited clinical and experimental observations we could not confirm Holman's findings of a marked increase of the total circulating blood.

5. A Venturi meter was used in some of the experiments to measure the flow of blood in a segment of the vena cava. An easy method of making an arteriovenous fistula which can be alternately closed and opened is illustrated.

6. The time to operate and the standard curative operative procedures, are discussed. Two new operative procedures are illustrated and described in the case reports.

COMMENT: There is very little to add to such a complete report as the authors have presented.

I should like to call the attention of anyone interested in this subject to this particular article. The entire essay cannot be abstracted conveniently.

Some Observations on the Repair of Cleft Lip, by Neal Owens, New Orleans, La. From Southern Medical Journal, September, 1938.

The author has a well written article concerning various phases of harelip surgery. He mentions that authors in general are not satisfied entirely with the final result. He quotes Blair as saying that "with one notable exception it is doubtful that a single broad principle, advantageously applicable to the unoperated upon cleft lip or palate of the infant has been established in the past half century." He says further, "that there is reason to believe that the results obtained by some of the earlier surgeons compared favorably with those of today." The above statements reflect the feeling of most surgeons engaged in the repair of cleft lip and palate. There is one hopeful aspect regarding the management of these cases: Due to a more thorough knowledge and a greater understanding, both on the part of the medical profession and patients, individuals with facial clefts are more than ever before being referred to men who are adequately prepared to carry out their repair.

The author states that he is not offering any new principle, but merely commenting on some of the difficulties encountered in the repair of these defects.

"Historical: Operations for the repair of facial clefts are among the earliest described in the literature and according to Velpeau, Celsus and other earlier surgeons, pared and sutured the harelip and made relaxation incisions on the inner surface of the cheek. Blair, in attributing this operative procedure to Celsus, said that after his death the fine points of the art were lost, and it was not until the second quarter of the 19th century that we find the earlier practices again recommended. The first successful closure of a complete palate is attributed to LeMonnier (Kirkham), the operation being accomplished by abrading the edges of the cleft with an actual cautery. In 1825, Mannoir, of Geneva, again called attention to the recommendation of Franco in 1561 that the posterior surfaces of the two halves of the lip should be separated from the bone as far back as the cheeks prior to the closure of the lip cleft. A staphylorrhaphy was performed by Stevens, of New York, in 1827. Velpeau is given credit for recognizing that the prime requisites for the repair of harelip are abrading the border and maintenance of perfect contact. Husson in 1836 recommended that the denuding incisions, in paring the lip, should be made concave. Following this, Mirault in 1944 gave his classic description of the operation of flap formation for the repair of cleft lip. Bell recognized the necessity of extending the incision into the floor of the nostril for the correct repair of incomplete cleft of the lip. Ambroise Pare, in 1541, described obturators for the closure of clefts of the palate. Although the production of the first artificial palate is attributed to Delabarre (Blair) in 1820, Diffenback, in 1834, reported the first operation for the cure of clefts involving the hard and soft palate. This procedure included the liberation of muco-periosteal flaps through lateral incisions close to the alveolar border. These flaps were raised, approximated in the mid-line and their median borders sutured. Baizeau in 1858, and von Langenback, in 1861, claimed originality for this operation. Cases of hard and soft palate clefts were reported cured in 1842 by A. Mason Warren, of Boston, by the raising of muco-periosteal flaps which were sutured in the midline without making lateral incisions. Diffenbach, eight years prior to his description of the operation in which he raised muco-periosteal flaps for the correction of cleft palate, successfully closed a cleft palate by doing an osteotomy of the palate process, followed by suturing the pared medial borders of the cleft in the mid-line. Billroth, in 1861, abandoned cutting the tensor palati tendon by fracturing the humular process. Thiersch in 1867 successfully closed a cleft of the palate by means of a full thickness flap taken from the cheek. Following this, Rotter, in 1889, successfully closed the same type of defect by means of a forehead pedicle flap which he previously grafted on the under surface with a Thiersch graft.

The etiology of this congenital deformity is unknown, although many factors have been offered as an explanation of its cause. Heredity, disease, pressure, and chemical changes stand out as the most plausible at the present time. Fraser, Beatty, and Lyons feel that heredity plays an important role and offers the most probable explanation of the etiology of this condition. Beatty says that several writers have shown the hereditary nature of this malformation and that a cleft palate so frequently co-exists with other remote developmental deformities that it forms a rather convincing argument against the accidental etiology of the condition. Beatty, in commenting further on the etiology of this deformity, says that some breeders of small animals claim that cleft palate is much more likely to appear in the young of inbred strains. He also says that the hereditary tendencies to these defects play such an important part in many of his case histories that they cannot be ignored. Lyons is in accord with the opinion that hereditary influences are the most important factors of etiology. Based on a study of 2,000 cases, he feels that there is an abnormal condition present in the germ plasm of one or both parents. The hereditary factor has been strongly suggestive in some of our cases. In one family three sisters were born with clefts of the lip and palate, of varying degrees. Another patient operated upon was of the third generation in this family to be born with a cleft of the lip, the mother and the grandmother before her having been born with this congenital defect. J. S. Davis, in a very thorough study on the incidence of congenital clefts of the lip and palate, says that definite conclusions cannot be drawn as to the relative importance of various possible etiological factors, although in his series of negroes syphilis must be considered. He also says that it is possible that the frequency of occurrence of congenital clefts of the lip and palate may vary in different parts of the world, supporting this statement by an analysis of the statistics compiled from the draft record of the defects found in the first 2,500,000 men examined for the U. S. army in the World War. In this latter analysis he found that the ratio of occurrence of congenital clefts of the lip and palate per 1,000 men examined was 1.55 in Vermont as compared to 0.16 per 1,000 in Arkansas. Ritchie says that a definite mechanical force affecting the inactive tissue appeals to him as a reasonable basis for discussion in considering the etiology of this condition. Frazer, in noting that the fissured condition occurs only where a cleft exists normally at an earlier period in the embryo, claims that this does not exclude the possibility of mechanical intervention's figuring in the causative role. In fact, it is where the fissure would be expected to exist if intervention occurred before the closure of the palate. He apparently places little credence in the theory that amniotic or epidermal bands act as causative factors in producing fissures, saying that an epidermal band in the line of a persistent cleft might be the effect and not the cause of the condition. Ritchie feels that the embryonal development of the active tissues probably offers a reasonable basis for a discussion on the etiology of facial cleft. Social status has long been considered by some as a possible etiologic factor in the formation of facial clefts and other developmental deformities, although this is certainly not borne out in Davis' statistical analysis where social status was apparently of little importance since a smaller number of clefts (percentage) occurred among the negroes where conditions were unfavorable. This was noted, however, that clefts occurred more frequently in the public ward series of white patients (one out of every 895 deliveries) than occurred in the private ward series of white patients, where the ratio was one out of 981 deliveries. Fraser is inclined to give credence to the theory that chemical changes is the factor of importance in the etiology of this condition and says that the tendency of modern teratological work is to show that the various degrees of monstrosity and defects can be produced as the result of certain salts in compartive excess on the developing embryo are particularly striking in their production of definite and more or less localized deformities.

Mall is quoted as saying that we need no longer seek for mechanical obstruction which may compress the umbilical cord, such as amniotic bands, for it is now clear that the impairment of nutrition which naturally follows faulty implantation or the various poisons which may be in a diseased uterus can do the whole mischief. There has been little or no evidence to cause one to assume that age or race play any role of importance as predisposing causes of facial clefts. The old suggestion of prenatal influence has probably been discarded as a possibility by every one.

The author has an excellent discussion of the statistics based on reports of Proebelius in 1865 which vary greatly to those of reports of John Staige Davis of Baltimore on the Johns Hopkins Hospital Obstetrical service. He makes quite a detailed account which is very interesting and shows much time and thought, and well worth any surgeon's time who might be interested in this type of reparative surgery.

The author has some timely illustrations and photographs which are very good.

The author recommends careful study and thorough examination before any operation is undertaken. He also mentions the preliminary procedure carried out by various men.

He also recommends intra-tracheal anesthesia with cyclopropaine. He also outlines some important points in operative technique as well as postoperative care.

Conclusions: The author has given a very fine essay on the subject of cleft lip and palate. He has detailed the history somewhat as well as techniques concerning this problem. The article is accompanied by photos of end results which seem equal to plastic surgery throughout the country.

It is gratifying to note that he believes in thorough pre-operative procedure.

————————o————————

ORTHOPAEDIC SURGERY
Edited by Earl D. McBride, M.D., F.A.C.S.
717 North Robinson Street, Oklahoma City

Ambulatory Method of Treating Femoral Shaft Fractures, Utilizing Fracture Table for Reduction. Roger Anderson. Amer. Jr. of Surgery, XXXIX, 538, March, 1938.

The author gives a continuation of his well-known method of pin fixation and reduction of fractures of the femur, using two pins above and two below. He stresses the importance of spiral fractures causing difficulty due to locking of the fragments, and that overtraction is often necessary to obtain proper reduction.

A series of cases is reported which shows excellent reduction of subtrochanteric and supracondylar fractures. The advantage claimed by the method is better control of the fragments and more rapid and secure reduction, which, when properly done can be maintained by the incorporation of the upper and lower pins in a well-fitting plaster cast. Two pins are used below to prevent lateral slipping of the lower fragment. The method is claimed to give much more rapid rehabilitation, less hospitalization, freedom of hip and knee movements, minimum of aftercare and thorough maintenance of fragments in correct position.

Giant Cell Tumor of the Cervical Spine. DeForest P. Willard and Jesse Thompson Nicholson. Annals of Surgery, CVII, 298, February, 1938.

Giant-cell tumor of the cervical spine is a comparatively rare lesion. The authors estimate that the lesion occurs in the vertebrae in about 8 per cent of the cases. The cervical vertebrae are reported involved in seven instances. A decided majority of all giant-cell tumors occur in individuals over 20 years of age, but the majority of vertebral lesions are found in individuals under 20 years of age.

Giant-cell tumor is classified as non-malignant, but Coley and Meyerding reported the cases of patients who died of metastases. Geschickter and Copeland recognizes a "malignant variant which is the result and not the cause of recurrence." They

also claim that the "malignant variant" structure is primary and, if recurrence results, metastasis is apt to follow. One would infer from this that inadequate r e m o v a l is responsible for secondary changes in the tumor.

The authors conclude that the treatment of choice is curettement; if this fails resection or amputation must be performed.

The case reported by the authors was that of a white female, aged nine. When the child was first examined, it was believed that there was a forward dislocation of the right inferior facet of the third cervical vertebra. She was treated in hyperextension for two weeks without any results and then a Walton manipulation was done, followed by application of a plaster cast to the head and the torso. Several weeks later when the cast was removed, roentgenographic examination revealed the presence of a rounded cystic tumor, projecting posteriorly from the fourth cervical vertebra. The tumor was completely removed by laminectomy. Pathologically, it resembled the spindle-cell variant of giant-cell tumor recognized by Geschickter and Copeland. One year after removal the patient was free from symptoms and roentgenographic examination did not show any recurrence.

————————o————————

INTERNAL MEDICINE
Edited by Hugh Jeter, M.D., 1260 North Walker,
Oklahoma City

Relation of Drug Therapy to Neutropenic States. Chairman's Address. Roy R. Kracke, M.D., Emory University, Georgia. The Journal of the American Medical Association, October 1, 1938, Vol. III, No. 14.

In this the author, one who has been an authority on the subject of agranulocytosis particularly upon the role played by drugs in the etiology of agranulocytosis, has carried up to date data of extreme interest in this connection.

The incrimination of aminopyrine in the production of neutropenic diseases is based on geographic studies, population as related to habitual use of drugs, cases in which the administration of drug has been recorded and the occasional case in which the administration of aminopyrine has been a factor and who had recovered to have subsequent reproduction of the disease.

Evidence all seems to indicate that the occasional person who acquires the disease after the administration of the drug does so on the basis of hypersensitivity to the drug. The amount of the drug, therefore, does not play an extremely important part.

Attention is called to a recent report of Plum in which it is seen that since the restriction of the sale of aminopyrine in Denmark, the disease has disappeared. Previous to this, reaching a peak in about 1934, the incidence in Denmark paralleled that of other countries. An extremely interesting chart is given in this connection.

Reports of cases of agranulocytosis following the administration of sulfanilamide are also given. Table No. 1 lists the author's dates and other important data in this connection. Table No. 2 lists drugs reported to have caused agranulocytosis as follows:

Table 2
Drugs Reported to Have Caused Agranulocytosis[*]

	No. of Cases
Aminopyrine	Over 300
Dinitrophenol	7
Arsphenamine[**]	20
Antipyrine	2
Derivative of aminopyrine (novaldin)	2

Acetanilid? _____ 2
Acetophenetidin (phenacetin)? _____ 3
Cinchophen (atrophan)? _____ 1
Antimony compound (neostibosan)? _____ 8
Sulfanilamide _____ 11
Quinine? _____ 4
Gold salts?*** _____ (Plum) 19

* The drugs known to be capable of producing
the disease are not followed by a question
mark: for the others, followed by a question
mark, the evidence is not adequate.

** Hematologic depression limited to granulocytes only.

***Hematologic depression not limited to gran-
ulocytes.

Table No. 5 listing preparations that should be
used with caution is also interesting.

**Table 5.—Preparations That Should Be Used with
Caution Because They May Depress the Leukocytes**

Preparations Containing Aminopyrine

Allonal	Dymen
Alpnebin	Dysco
Amarbital	Eu Med
Amidol	Gardan
Amido-Neonal	Gynalgos
Amidonine	Hexin
Amidophen	Ipral-Amidopyrine
Amidopyrine	Kalms
(aminopyrine)	
Amidos	Lumodrin
Amidotal compound	Midol
Amifeine	Mylin
Aminol	Neonal compound
Am-Phen-Al	Neurodyne
Ampydin	Nod
Amytal compound	Optalidon
Analgia	Peralgia
Antabs	Phenamidal
Baramid	Phen-Amidol
Barb-Amid	Phenopyrine
Benzedo compound	Pyramidon
Cibalgine	Pyraminal
Cinchopyrine	Seequit
Compral	Yeast-Vite
Cronal	

Drugs Known to Produce Depression of the Marrow

Dinitrophenol	Antipyrine
Arsphenamine	Sulfanilamide
Novaldin	Sedormid
	(Thrombocytopenia)

The author believes that approximately 80 per
cent of drug-produced agranulocytosis is caused by
aminopyrine or one of its compounds.

There is evidence that there is decreased incidence in the United States.

COMMENT: This report continues to be a warning of tremendous importance to practitioners of
medicine and the data herein produced seems to
justify clearly the contention that agranulocytosis
in many instances follows the administration of
certain drugs. Personal experience, however, leads
me to believe that other important factors of which
infections of unusual type or of unusual circumstances, may also play a great part in the cause of
this serious disease. Within the past three years
I have had under observation a patient who is still
living, is in better health than before her first attack and who had during the course of ten and
one-half months, nine attacks of agranulocytosis
wherein the temperature reached as high as 105.2°
and the total neutrophile count zero. This patient
was carefully observed in a hospital for 15 months
and investigation continuously made as to the possibility of drugs being a cause, but no such history
could be obtained. Previous to the first attack
there had been two bone lesions, so far as Dr.
O'Donoghue, the orthopedic surgeon in the case,
and I have been able to determine, subacute osteomyelitis of first the right and a month later the
left femur.

**The Gordon Test for Hodgkin's Disease: A Reaction
to Eosinophils. James B. McNaught, M.D., San
Francisco. The Journal of the American Medical Association, October 1, 1938, Vol III, No. 14.**

The author here has given more data concerning
the Gordon test for Hodgkin's disease which was
first instituted in 1932 and concludes that the
Gordon test is of no more practical value in the
diagnosis of Hodgkin's disease than is the finding
of eosinophiles in the lymph nodes.

COMMENT: It appears that the biopsy of a
lymph gland will give as much information and
considerably more in some cases as the Gordon
test and this is in keeping with my personal experience.

————————o————————

UROLOGY

Edited by D. W. Branham, M.D.
514 Medical Arts Building, Oklahoma City

**The Steinach Operation for the Relief of Prostatic
Symptoms. J. G. Yates Bell, London, England.
Urologic & Cutaneous Review, October, 1938.**

The author reviews the experience of other investigators with this procedure in the relief of
prostatism. He details his experience in 28 cases
treated in this way. Of these 28 patients he classified 15 as deriving some therapeutic benefit from
the operation.

COMMENT: The great difficulty in evaluating
any particular procedure in the treatment of prostatic hypertrophy is the lack of constancy as far
as the symptoms are concerned. I have observed
individuals suffering from early prostatic obstruction, voiding four and five times nightly who derived marked temporary benefit by the simplest
therapeutic measures. Because of this fact, such a
small series of cases as the author presents is worthless from a scientific viewpoint.

As far as the majority of American urologists
are concerned they seem to have an unanimity of
opinion that this operation is a futile gesture in
the treatment of this disorder.

————————

**A Practical Method of Staining Treponema Pallida
by Means of Low Surface Tension Stain. Robert
D. Haire, M.D., Hobbs, N. M. Journal of Laboratory & Clinical Medicine, August, 1938.**

By making use of a low surface tension solvent
which increases the penetrating power of the
stain, satisfactory demonstration of the syphilitic
organism was possible in simple contact smears.

The stain is made by using hexylresorcinol solution as a solvent for gentian violet, making 1 per
cent solution of the stain. The secretion from the
chancre is placed on a slide and fixed by heat and
the stain is applied for 30 minutes. Twelve known
cases of syphilitic infection were successfully stained
and diagnosed by this method.

COMMENT: I have seen a few of these stains
and there is no difficulty in recognizing the organism. However, in these the typical spiral morphology is somewhat distorted and because of this
I would hesitate to make a diagnosis from the
stained smear alone for fear of confusion with
other spirrillum.

Doubtless more experience in examining such
smears will encourage confidence in this diagnostic
procedure.

————————o————————

IMPORTANT NOTICE

ON EDITORIAL PAGE

OFFICERS OKLAHOMA STATE MEDICAL ASSOCIATION

President, Dr. H. K. Speed, Sayre.

President-Elect, Dr. W. A. Howard, Chelsea.

Secretary-Treasurer-Editor, Dr. L. S. Willour, McAlester.

Speaker, House of Delegates, Dr. J. D. Osborn, Jr., Frederick.

Vice Speaker, House of Delegates, Dr. P. P. Nesbitt, Medical Arts Building, Tulsa.

Delegates to the A. M. A., Dr. W. Albert Cook, Medical Arts Building, Tulsa, 1938-39; Dr. McLain Rogers, Clinton, 1937-1938.

Meeting Place, Oklahoma City, May 15-16-17, 1939.

SPECIAL COMMITTEES 1938-39

Annual Meeting: Dr. H. K. Speed, Sayre; Dr. W. A. Howard, Chelsea; Dr. L. S. Willour, McAlester.

Conservation of Hearing: Dr. H. F. Vandever, Chairman, Enid; Dr. J. B. Hollis, Mangum; Dr. Chester McHenry, Oklahoma City.

Conservation of Vision: Dr. W. M. Gallaher, Chairman, Shawnee; Dr. Frank R. Vieregg, Clinton; Dr. Pauline Barker, Guthrie.

Crippled Children: Dr. Earl McBride, Chairman, Oklahoma City; Dr. Roy L. Fisher, Frederick; Dr. M. B. Glismann, Okmulgee.

Industrial Service and Traumatic Surgery: Dr. Cyril C. Clymer, Medical Arts Bldg., Oklahoma City; Dr. J. Wm. Finch, Hobart; Dr. J. A. Rutledge, Ada.

Maternity and Infancy: Dr. George R. Osborn, Chairman, Tulsa; Dr. P. J. DeVanney, Sayre; Dr. Leila E. Andrews, Oklahoma City.

Necrology: Dr. G. H. Stagner, Chairman, Erick; Dr. James L. Shuler, Durant; Dr. S. D. Neely, Muskogee.

Post Graduate Medical Teaching: Dr. Henry H. Turner, Chairman, Oklahoma City; Dr. H. C. Weber, Bartlesville; Dr. Ned R. Smith, Tulsa.

Study and Control of Cancer: Dr. Wendell Long, Chairman, Oklahoma City; Dr. Paul B. Champlin, Enid; Dr. Ralph McGill, Tulsa.

Study and Control of Tuberculosis: Dr. Carl Puckett, Chairman, Oklahoma City; Dr. W. C. Tisdal, Clinton; Dr. F. P. Baker, Talihina.

ADVISORY COUNCIL FOR AUXILIARY

Dr. H. K. Speed, Chairman......................................Sayre

Dr. C. J. Fishman.......................................Oklahoma City

Dr. W. S. Larrabee..Tulsa

Dr. J. M. Watson...Enid

Dr. T. H. McCarley..McAlester

STANDING COMMITTEES 1938-39

Medical Defense: Dr. O. E. Templin, Chairman, Alva; Dr. L. C. Kuyrkendall, McAlester; Dr. E. Albert Aisenstadt, Picher.

Medical Economics: Dr. C. B. Sullivan, Cordell, Chairman; Dr. J. L. Patterson, Duncan; Dr. W. M. Browning, Waurika.

Medical Education and Hospital: Dr. V. C. Tisdal, Chairman, Elk City; Dr. Robert U. Patterson, Oklahoma City; Dr. H. M. McClure, Chickasha.

Public Policy and Legislation: Dr. Finis W. Ewing, Surety Bldg., Chairman, Muskogee; Dr. Tom Lowry, 1200 North Walker, Oklahoma City; Dr. O. C. Newman, Shattuck.

(The above committee co-ordinated by the following, selected from each councilor district.)

District No. 1.—Arthur E. Hale, Alva.

District No. 2.—McLain Rogers, Clinton.

District No. 3.—Thomas McElroy, Ponca City.

District No. 4.—L. H. Ritzhaupt, Guthrie.

District No. 5.—P. V. Annadown, Sulphur.

District No. 6.—R. M. Shepard, Tulsa.

District No. 7.—Sam A. McKeel, Ada.

District No. 8.—J. A. Morrow, Sallisaw.

District No. 9.—W. A. Tolleson, Eufaula.

District No. 10.—J. L. Holland, Madill.

Scientific Exhibits: Dr. E. Rankin Denny, Chairman, Tulsa; Dr. Robert H. Akin, Oklahoma City; Dr. R. C. Pigford, Tulsa.

Scientific Work: Dr. W. G. Husband, Chairman, Hollis; Dr. J. S. Rollins, Prague; Dr. J. L. Day, Supply.

Public Health:

Chairman—Dr. G. S. Baxter, Shawnee.

District No. 1.—C. W. Tedrowe, Woodward.

District No. 2.—E. W. Mabry, Altus.

District No. 3.—L. A. Mitchell, Stillwater.

District No. 4.—J. J. Gable, Norman.

District No. 5.—Geo. S. Barber, Lawton.

District No. 6.—C. E. Bradley, Tulsa.

District No. 7.—G. S. Baxter, Shawnee.

District No. 8.—M. M. De Arman, Miami.

District No. 9.—T. H. McCarley, McAlester.

District No. 10.—J. B. Clark, Coalgate.

SCIENTIFIC SECTIONS

General Surgery: Dr. F. L. Flack, Chairman, Nat'l Bank of Tulsa Bldg., Tulsa; Dr. John E. McDonald, Vice-Chairman, Medical Arts Bldg., Tulsa; Dr. John F. Burton, Secretary, Osler Building, Oklahoma City.

General Medicine: Dr. Frank Nelson, Chairman, 603 Medical Arts Bldg., Tulsa; Dr. E. R. Musick, Vice-Chairman, Medical Arts Bldg., Oklahoma City; Dr. Milam McKinney, Medical Arts Bldg., Oklahoma City.

Eye, Ear, Nose & Throat: Dr. E. H. Coachman, Chairman, Manhattan Bldg., Muskogee; Dr. F. M. Cooper, Vice-President, Medical Arts Bldg., Oklahoma City; Dr. James R. Reed, Secretary, Medical Arts Bldg., Oklahoma City.

Obstetrics and Pediatrics: Dr. C. W. Arrendell, Chairman, Ponca City; Dr. Carl F. Simpson, Vice-Chairman, Medical Arts Bldg., Tulsa; Dr. Ben H. Nicholson, Secretary, 300 West Twelfth Street, Oklahoma City.

Genito-Urinary Diseases and Syphilology: Dr. Elijah Sullivan, Chairman, Medical Arts Bldg., Oklahoma City; Dr. Henry Browne, Vice-Chairman, Medical Arts Bldg., Tulsa; Dr. Robert Akin, Secretary, 400 West Tenth, Oklahoma City.

Dermatology and Radiology: Dr. W. A. Showman, Chairman, Medical Arts Bldg., Tulsa; Dr. E. D. Greenberger, Vice-Chairman, McAlester; Dr. Hervey A. Foerster, Secretary, Medical Arts Bldg., Oklahoma City.

STATE BOARD OF MEDICAL EXAMINERS

Dr. Thos. McElroy, Ponca City, President; Dr. C. E. Bradley, Tulsa, Vice-President; Dr. J. D. Osborn, Jr., Frederick, Secretary; Dr. L. E. Emanuel, Oklahoma City; Dr. W. T. Ray, Gould; Dr. G. L. Johnson, Pauls Valley; Dr. W. W. Osgood, Muskogee.

STATE COMMISSIONER OF HEALTH

Dr. Chas. M. Pearce, Oklahoma City.

COUNCILORS AND THEIR COUNTIES

District No. 1: Texas, Beaver, Cimarron, Harper, Ellis, Woods, Woodward, Alfalfa, Major, Dewey—Dr. O. E. Templin, Alva. (Term expires 1940.)

District No. 2: Roger Mills, Beckham, Greer, Harmon, Washita, Kiowa, Custer, Jackson, Tillman—Dr. V. C. Tisdal, Elk City. (Term expires 1939.)

District No. 3: Grant, Kay, Garfield, Noble, Payne, Pawnee—Dr. A. S. Risser, Blackwell. (Term expires 1938.)

District No. 4: Blaine, Kingfisher, Canadian, Logan, Oklahoma, Cleveland—Dr. Philip M. McNeill, Oklahoma City. (Term expires 1938.)

District No. 5: Caddo, Comanche, Cotton, Grady, Love, Stephens, Jefferson, Carter, Murray—Dr. W. H. Livermore, Chickasha. (Term expires 1938.)

District No. 6: Osage, Creek, Washington, Nowata, Rogers, Tulsa—Dr. James Stevenson, Medical Arts Bldg., Tulsa. (Term expires, 1938.)

District No. 7: Lincoln, Pontotoc, Pottawatomie, Okfuskee, Seminole, McClain, Garvin, Hughes—Dr. J. A. Walker, Shawnee. (Term expires 1939.)

District No. 8: Craig, Ottawa, Mayes, Delaware, Wagoner, Adair, Cherokee, Sequoyah, Okmulgee, Muskogee—Dr. E. A. Aisenstadt, Picher. (Term expires 1939.)

District No. 9: Pittsburg, Haskell, Latimer, LeFlore, McIntosh—Dr. L. C. Kuyrkendall, McAlester. (Term expires 1939.)

District No. 10: Johnson, Marshall, Coal, Atoka, Bryan, Choctaw, Pushmataha, McCurtain—Dr. J. S. Fulton, Atoka. (Term expires 1939.)

THE JOURNAL
OF THE
OKLAHOMA STATE MEDICAL ASSOCIATION

| VOLUME XXXI | McALESTER, OKLAHOMA, DECEMBER, 1938 | Number 12 |

Factors of Safety in Surgery of Toxic Goiter*

R. M. HOWARD, M.D.
OKLAHOMA CITY, OKLAHOMA

In surgery of goiter there are numerous factors which, if carefully considered, will add to the safety of the operation.

To fully appreciate these factors and before approaching work of this kind one should have a thorough knowledge of the anatomy, and physiology of the thyroid gland, as well as the various pathological changes which may be encountered. In addition to this, one's work in this field is g r e a t l y simplified by having a definite clinical classification of goiter. The following classification was adopted by the American Association for the S t u d y of Goiter.

1. Diffuse non-toxic goiter.
2. Diffuse toxic goiter.
3. Nodular non-toxic goiter.
4. Nodular toxic goiter.

Our modern conception of the subject not only makes quite easy the recognition of these various types, and their various manifestations, but gives us a pretty clear picture of the kind of treatment needed for their cure.

Factors of safety in surgery of t o x i c goiter can be considered under the following headings:

1. Proper evaluation of the condition of the patient when first seen.
2. Response to preoperative preparation.
3. Technic of operation.
4. Postoperative care.

In discussing this subject I wish to deal with it from the standpoint of the relief afforded the patient as well as the safety to life of the operative procedure.

The diagnosis of the typical diffuse toxic goiter affords no particular problem. The h i s t o r y and physical findings are quite characteristic. Many patients, however, are seen who present some of the symptoms of hyperthyroidism, but in whom the picture is far from being complete. It is in this type of case, unless extreme care is exercised, that not only will results be far from satisfactory if operation is done, but in which cases that can be relieved by operation are overlooked.

In the first group in which no operation should be done are those so-called neuro-circulatory asthenias or chronic nervous exhaustion, n e u r o a s t h e n i a s, menopausal disturbances, hypertension, leukemias, diabetes and tuberculosis w i t h o u t hyperthyroidism; while in the latter group will be those early cases; cases in remission from iodine; and the low grade cases of hyperthyroidism that may go on for years, finally resulting in severe nervous, and circulatory disturbances. Most of these cases by a careful history and physical examination can be properly classified; others must be kept under close observation for a considerable time without the administration of iodine before arriving at a conclusion. None of the patients should be operated until a certain diagnosis can be made. Unless hyperthyroidism exists they not only will not be benefited by operation

*Read Before the Surgical Section, Annual Meeting, Oklahoma State Medical Association, Muskogee, Oklahoma, May, 1938,

but will be a constant source of worry to the operator.

Factors to be considered in evaluation of the patient's condition when first seen are: Age, duration of disease, weight loss, severity of the hyperthyroidism, condition of the heart, complicating conditions and has the patient had iodine.

Age undoubtedly affects the operative mortality. Those of advanced age have not the reserve of the younger individual. Into this group fall many cases of nodular toxic goiter, as well as neglected cases of diffuse toxic goiter. The mortality rate will be higher in the upper age group. In nearly all cases in this group there will be a marked w e i g h t loss, great muscular weakness and cardiac complications. Hyperthyroidism in people of advanced age is not unusual.

The duration of the disease must be carefully considered. Those of long duration may have developed organic changes of grave importance. These particularly apply to the circulatory s y s t e m, and the liver, whereas in those of short duration we have only to consider the severity of the process. Mortality will be definitely higher in those cases giving a history of long duration. They are more difficult to prepare, and respond poorly to the preoperative preparation with iodine.

Excessive weight loss always places the patient in the hazardous group. This is usually accompanied by an increased food intake. Due to the intensity of the disease one always expects organic changes. Extreme debility and emaciation are an index to the severity of the disease. Operation must not be done on these cases until a remission is secured.

The degree of hyperthyroidism must be estimated when the patient is first seen. In the younger and earlier cases this is usually obvious. The increased activation of every cell in the body, in the severe case, is startling. This is due to the increased metabolic activity induced by the excessive secretion of the thyroid gland. It is only by having a clear and complete picture of the patient's history, and the condition of the patient when first seen, that progress during the time of preoperative preparation can be determined. This estimation must not be based entirely on the height of the basal metabolism. While high rates are expected in severe hyperthyroidism, low rates do not always indicate a lower rate of intoxication. Not all cases of severe hyperthyroidism are accompanied by a high rate, and an extremely rapid pulse. Lahey has called attention to a group which he terms "apathetic hyperthyroidism." Many of these patients are in the elderly group, and while they fail to show typical activation of hyperthyroidism they usually have a moist warm skin, loss of weight, rapid pulse, tremor, a stare, a rather firm gland and an elevated metabolism, which makes diagnosis quite certain. Because of the apparent mildness of the symptoms these patients are often not properly prepared, nor the risk correctly estimated. These are very dangerous cases.

There are certain serious thyroid states including the above which must be realized from the history and examination when the patient is first seen. Any patient who has had a rapid increase in all the symptoms of hyperthyroidism with marked increase of weight loss may be said to be on the verge of a thyroid crisis. In addition to the progressively increasing intensity of the symptoms they have had, they develop delirium, high temperature, v o m i t i n g, diarrhea and at times jaundice. If this condition persists for a few days it usually results in a fatality. This state is explained on the basis of liver failure. The severely stimulated metabolism has burned up the protective glycogen in the liver. Surgery is not permissible in the patient in crisis, or in one approaching a crisis. All patients with hyperthyroidism should be prepared and submitted to surgery in order to avoid these critical states. The treatment of the patient in crisis is immediate administration of large doses of iodine, and continual intravenous glucose and s a l i n e solution. Once the patient is over the crisis he should be prepared as any other patient and operated. A patient who has had one crisis, is likely to have another unless this procedure is followed.

Some of these patients on first examination will have auricular fibrillation, some congestive heart failure with or without fibrillation. Many of these on investigation will be found to be neglected, often undiagnosed cases of hyperthyroidism. To these the term "Thyrocardiacs" has been applied. While o f t e n the symptoms of hyperthyroidism may be mild, a certain diagnosis can u s u a l l y be made. After preparation surgery should be done. The results are excellent, they carry on with comfort although most will of course have severely damaged hearts. Fibrillation may persist, but in the majority entirely disappear.

Complications should be found or excluded by a careful physical examination. Surgery, except that directed at the relief of the toxic thyroid, should be avoided except in extreme emergency. Complicating conditions requiring surgery should be left until the toxic thyroid has been removed. Hyperthyroidism with complicating conditions, as tuberculosis and diabetes require special preparation and special operative technic. The occurrence of an acute infection, such as tonsillitis, may convert in a few days a mild case of hyperthyroidism into one that is very severe.

An important point to determine in the history is, whether the patient has, or has not had, iodine. If he has this will enable one to determine the influence this may have had on his present condition, and tell how difficult the preoperative preparation may be. If he has had goiter medicine he has had iodine. Too many of our patients today have had iodine, either on their own initiative, on the advice of friends, or given in treatment of the condition by s o m e physician.

In the preoperative preparation of these patients iodine plays an important part. In the toxic goiter patient, either diffuse or nodular, who has previously not had iodine, its administration for, on the average of, ten days brings about a remission of symptoms which makes surgery safe in most of them. In the diffuse type the improvement in all symptoms will be most marked. This with rest, plenty of food, predominant in carbohydrates, and p l e n t y of fluids, changes the entire picture in the most severe case. The heart slows, the nervous system becomes s t a b l e, the metabolism drops and the patient gains weight. When this has reached its maximum, operation should be done. The degree of improvement the patient makes during preoperative preparation will determine the type and degree of operation to be done. The patient who fails to improve must be con-

sidered a grave risk. The patient who has had iodine will not improve to the same degree, and in some the gland has become so iodine fast that but little improvement is noted. These patients should be thoroughly saturated with iodine over a longer period of time before operation. This in some way affords protection from postoperative hyperthyroidism, but this type of case will always be one which will afford considerable worry. The introduction by Plummer of iodine, in the preoperative preparation, has resulted in one of the greatest advances in surgery of the thyroid. It has resulted in an easier operation, a smoother convalescence, a decreased mortality and fewer multi-stage operations. During preparation all elderly patients, and all patients with cardiac changes, receive digitalis. Prior to operation every patient should have a laryngoscopic examination to determine the condition of the vocal cords.

The operation for goiter is pretty well standardized. There are a few points in the technic which for me are important factors in this work, not only from the standpoint of safety from technical errors, but from the standpoint of results.

Each operation must be planned so that a proper amount of gland is removed to effect a cure, yet sufficient gland left to carry on function. The parathyroid glands and recurrent laryngeal nerves must be safeguarded, hemorrhage controlled and the wound closed so as to leave the least possible scar. How much gland to remove will depend on the character of the gland encountered. In the diffuse type, rich in cells, all that can be safely removed should be removed, while in the gland which is poorer in cells with much fibrosis, more gland must be left. These are problems which must usually be decided during the course of the operation. In nodular goiter the problem of saving all good gland possible should be kept in mind, and it should be remembered that the two types may coexist in the same thyroid. Recurrences are undesirable, so are cases of postoperative myxedema. The latter has given me more trouble than the former.

Proper handling of the upper pole, mobilization of the lobe, marking the lateral aspects of the gland with haemostats and division of the i s t h m u s with dissection lateral from the trachea, are points which if carried out consecutively add much to the ease and safety of the operation in diffuse toxic goiter. In nodular goiter all adenomas must be removed but the operation done in such a way as to save any good thyroid tissue. Operation must be done with dispatch, but never at the expense of technical safety.

Lahey's plan of grading patients when first seen and during preparation is an excellent one. Grade one, good risk; grade two, doubtful risk; grade three, dangerous risk; grade four, risk in which fatality will result if operation is done. Unless some such plan is followed, errors in type, and extent of operation may be made. Since the introduction of iodine in the preoperative preparation of these cases, ligations and multi-stage operations a r e n o t frequent, but should be used in the severer grades. The operation should be so conducted that if during its course indications arise it can be quickly terminated, and at a later date completed. There is no question that multi-stage operations save many lives. Parathyroid glands should be looked for and avoided, if found after removal they s h o u l d be transplanted under the muscle.

A competent anesthetist is an important part of the operative team. His judgment must be accepted many times as to the advisability of doing a stage operation. Local anesthesia should be used in many of the elderly patients. All patients under general anesthesia, at the completion of the operation, should be allowed to awake before closure of the wound. Coughing and straining will disclose many times bleeding v e s s e l s which might cause serious trouble if not ligated. To have the patient talk and see how well he breathes while out of the anesthetic will be a great satisfaction to the surgeon.

Postoperative care is of extreme importance. Patients must be kept under the closest observation. Our immediate postoperative orders consist of plenty of morphine, plenty of iodine, fluids intravenously and the use of ice to control the temperature. Our most frequent complication is tracheitis for which we use benzoin inhalations, and codeine. O x y g e n inhalations, or the oxygen tent is used in the more s e v e r e cases. Any complication

should be noted as soon as it occurs, particularly respiratory embarrassment which requires widely opening of the wound and at times tracheotomy. There should be no d e l a y in carrying out these procedures. Any indications of tetany requires prompt administration of large doses of calcium. A dry wound at the completion of the operation for goiter prevents many of the minor postoperative complications. The use of fine catgut in tying of the many small vessels is also of importance.

When the patient leaves the hospital the surgeon's work is not completed. These patients must be kept under observation for many months. A great many of these patients, as a result of their past hyperthyroidism, have an irritable nervous system. Many of their minor postoperative discomforts will assume grave proportions unless explained. Much can be done to relieve most of them. Following thyroidectomy for hyperthyroidism nearly all of these patients, if we cure them, are going to have a mild hypothyroidism. This persists for a few months. It is during this time that adjustment of possibly the underlying cause of the disturbance takes place, and is, I believe, an essential part of the cure. Care should be exercise in giving thyroid extract to these people unless the condition becomes extreme.

It is only by reviewing carefully and impartially the records of those submitted to operation that our results can be determined. Such a review of our cases is now being made, with particular reference to the hazardous cases. These statistics are not yet complete except in part.

We have determined the following:

In a recent review of 1,000 cases submitted to operation, excluding thyroiditis and malignancy, there were: diffuse nontoxic goiter 16, diffuse toxic goiter 516, nodular goiter 144, nodular toxic goiter 324.

In these cases the following postoperative complications were encountered: postoperative hemorrhage one, cases requiring tracheotomy five, postoperative t e t a n y five, severe wound infections two, pneumonia 4.

There were 16 with persistence or recurrence of symptoms requiring further operative procedure.

There were 21 requiring thyroid extract

for postoperative myxedema. Of this number seven are now taking thyroid extract and will probably have to continue to do so. Mortality in the 1,000 operated cases was 12. Causes of death were: postoperative hyperthyroidism six, pneumonia with multimple abscesses of l u n g one, recurrent nerve injury and its complications two, air embolism one, cerebral embolism two.

The mortality prior to 1922, when no iodine was used preoperatively was 4.3 per cent. The total mortality of the 1,000 operative cases reviewed was 1.2 per cent. Two hundred of these c a s e s were done prior to 1925 when iodine was introduced in the preoperative preparation in all cases. During this time it was used only in the diffuse cases, and its use was but little understood. The mortality in these cases was 2.5 per cent. The mortality since preoperative preparation with iodine in all cases is .5 per cent. We now have up to the p r e s e n t date 487 consecutive cases without a death. In the pre-iodine days multi-stage operations w e r e extremely common. Now we reserve them for the grave cases.

Statistics such as these while low, correspond to those reported from l a r g e r clinics over the country. Only by close attention to the factors I have tried to discuss will one be able to keep mortality in goiter surgery at a minimum. Credit for the present low mortality can go to no one group of individuals, it must be shared with all the workers and clinicians in this field who have been so generous in their teachings of the many intricate problems involved in surgery of the thyroid gland.

CONCLUSIONS

1. Extreme care should be used in the differential diagnosis of mild hyperthyroidism, and those conditions simulating hyperthyroidism.

2. Evaluation of the patient's condition when first seen is of extreme importance in estimating the risk involved at operation.

3. In the presence of certain grave thyroid states serious consideration must be given to the type of the operative procedure.

4. The use of iodine in the preoperative preparation of goiter patients has not only greatly reduced the mortality but has also

reduced the number of multi-stage operations.

5. A brief report is submitted of 1,000 cases operated for goiter with special reference to complications and mortality.

REFERENCES

1. Percy, Nelson M. Transactions American Association for the Study of Goiter. 1 to 12, 1937.

2. Lahey, Frank H. Surgical Clinics of North America. 16-96-152. ecember, 1937.

3. Dinsmore, Robert S. Diagnosis and Treatment of Diseases of the Thyroid Gland; Crile and Associates. Chapter 32-377.

4. Pemberton, John de J. Mayo Clinic 28-509. 1936.

5. Clute, Howard M. Transaction American Association for the Study of Goiter, 78. 1937.

6. Jackson, Arnold. Goiter and Other Diseases of the Thyroid Gland. 9-153.

7. Hertzler, Arthur E. Surgical Pathology of the Thyroid Gland. 9-171.

* * * *

DISCUSSION

S. A. Risser, M.D.
Blackwell, Oklahoma

Dr. Howard's paper is really an encyclopedia in brief on the surgery of toxic goiter. He has outlined the major factors which make for the safe and successful treatment of toxic goiter. There is very little to add to what he has so well stated in his paper, and the brief time allotted to discussion can be perhaps best utilized in merely emphasizing some of the points he made, restating them for the sake of emphasis for those of us who are not specialists in this line of work but who necessarily must do some.

It goes without saying that a thorough knowledge of the anatomy and physiology of the thyroid is essential. There is perhaps no other gland the functions of which are so closely interrelated with the other e n d o c r i n e glands and with the entire physiologic and metabolic processes of the body as is the thyroid, and unless the physician is cognizant of these facts, and can evaluate the relative responsibility of the various organs in the symptom-complex, the results of his treatment — to put it mildly — will not be satisfactory.

Before a proper classification of the patient or his disease can be made it is necessary to secure a careful history of his disease, to reconstruct the onset and progress of the pathologic process and to measure its influence on the vital tissues and forces. Careful questioning very often proves the disease to have existed much longer than was recognized by the patient, and so to have exercised wide reaching damage to the heart and circulatory system generally. At best it is frequently very difficult to estimate the reserve power of the heart and other vital organs, and the good workman will exercise great care in getting clear in his mind the whole picture of the patient. To this end the history, time of onset, loss of weight, extent of digestive disturbances, muscle tone and nerve balance, and the basal metabolic rate must be determined, with a careful study of the heart, liver and kidney functions, the determination as to whether and for how long iodine (which can be both a blessing and a bane) has been taken.

All these are questions which must be answered before the disease can be classified or the patient "typed" as to the character of the pathologic process, or his need of or probable reaction to any particular type of operation. After all attempts to make a classification of goiter types, and the one Dr. Howard has quoted is as simple and workable as any, each patient is a separate and distinct pathological entity, and types and averages hold for him only up to a certain point. It is for the goiter surgeon to predetermine so far as possible in what respects the particular patient corresponds to or differs from the average and the type, so to prepare his patient and plan his operative procedure that the patient will be cured.

Careful examination, perhaps with extended observation and treatment, will disclose those types which should not be operated, as Dr. Howard listed in his paper.

Rest with sedatives if necessary, forcing of a high carbohydrate diet, plenty of fluids, digitalis if indicated, and the administration of iodine will convert otherwise apparently hopeless risks into operable cases. The essayist has rightly stressed the need of attention to the previous iodine intake of these patients. The indiscriminate use of iodine can greatly hinder the satisfactory preoperative preparation of our patients, as previous X-ray treatment may complicate the operative removal of the offending gland.

Given the proper preoperative preparation of the patient, it is my preference to employ local anesthesia in practically all cases. The extent of anesthesia may be made sufficient for wide exposure and efficient mobolization of the poles, and complete hemostasis. Also, the patient's reply to questions is a most satisfactory index to possible encroachment of the dissection on the recurrent laryngeal nerves.

The aftercare is merely a continuation of the preoperative care — rest, sedation, fluids and food, iodine, plus the care of complications if and when they arise—and the continued observance of these patients after they leave the hospital.

Dr. Howard's operative statistics rank well with those of other operators and goiter clinics, and the future progress of goiter surgery will continue to be advanced by the painstaking and careful work which is evidenced in his paper. I have profited by reading it.

Masked Intermittent Malaria, A Study*

DAVID W. GILLICK, M.D., F.A.C.P.
Superintendent and Medical Officer,
Shawnee Indian Sanatorium
SHAWNEE, OKLAHOMA

During the past two years it has become increasingly noticeable to some of those interested in the fact, that malaria is still a public health problem in Oklahoma. Not

*Read Before the Section on General Medicine, Annual Meeting, Oklahoma State Medical Association, Muskogee, Oklahoma, May 11, 1938.

so much, of course, the disease that manifests the typical or classical symptoms of the malady, but rather the atypical or what was formerly called the masked intermittent form of the disease.

It might be well to refresh our minds on

some features of malarial cachexia. The symptoms are varied both in character and intensity. There is fever at intervals but chills do not occur and the temperature-curve is typical neither of remittent nor intermittent f e v e r although it may approximate e i t h e r the one or the other. Again the fever is sometimes wholly irregular though its range is not high, and it seldom exceeds 103 degrees Fahrenheit. The skin often presents a rather dirty, yellowish-brown complexion to a marked degree. The spleen may or may not be enlarged, but there is always a marked anemia. Many of the local and general symptoms are dependent upon the well marked anemia. Among the general features may be mentioned debility, frequent sweatings and a certain amount of edema. Nervous symptoms may also be noticeable. Chief among these are tremors, neuralgia, palsies, vertigo, wakefulness and nervous palpitation of the heart. Among the rarest concomitants of this condition is paraplegia. Malarial neuritis is met with and presents most·of the features common to other toxic forms of neuritis. Slight cough and dyspnea evidence the presence of a mild bronchitis; and anorexia, n a u s e a, diarrhea and other symptoms of chronic gastro-intestinal catarrh are observed. The j o i n t s and voluntary muscles may and often are quite painful. Hemorrhages from the various mucous surfaces and into the rectum are not uncommon.

The foregoing, of course, p r e s e n t s a rather typical picture of malarial cachexia, however the true masked intermittent type is s o m e w h a t different. This presents itself in much the same form as chronic malarial cachexia but with the important difference that there is no fever. This type comprises the long list of conditions at the head of which stands neuralgia, most frequently involving the supra orbital branch of the trigeminus. Often a striking periodicity is observed, the painful paroxysms u s u a l l y beginning in the morning and terminating in the late afternoon hours, the patient's suffering increasing steadily in intensity until just before the close of the attack when they s u d d e n l y abate. Among the nerves implicated with relative frequency are the occipital, the intercostal and the sciatic. Except what a p p e a r s to be characteristic, of course, or unless the

attacks yield promptly to a specific, a certain diagnosis of malarial neuralgia should not be entertained.

The masked intermittent type may assume the forms of paraesthesia, anesthesia, convulsion or paralysis. They may also appear under the guise of edema, hemorrhages from the various mucous outlets of the body or into the skin, diarrhea, dysentery, dyspepsia, bronchitis, pneumonia, appendicitis, etc.

Again let me emphasize that since infections such as these may all obey the law of periodicity one would not be justified in pronouncing in favor of malarial infections unless they yield readily to a therapeutic specific or the parasite is found. In most cases of this type of the disease we were able to find the estivo-autumnal parasites. The organism appeared as a small hyaline disk, a ring form within the red blood corpuscle, often very few in number. Other features of the hematological study of these cases was the marked leukopenia ranging down sometimes as low as 3,000 and in the differential a marked monocytosis which seems to be characteristic of chronic malarial infection in the afebrile period. This was not noted in any of the active fresh infections that were having paroxysms at the time or close to the time of examination.

THE ANEMIA OF MALARIA

In long standing cases of malaria, anemia is a predominant part of the picture. Although the patient may present the febrile reactions characteristic of the disease there may also exist a marked pallor and other signs and symptoms referable to the long standing a n e m i a. Examination of the blood reveals usually only a moderately reduced erythrocytic count and markedly reduced hemoglobin content. The volume index is below 1 and the red cells show a central pallor, the extent of which is dependent upon the degree of hemoglobin reduction. In cases of masked intermittent malaria there usually are signs of basophilic degeneration in m a n y of the red cells. These changes include varying degrees of polychromatophilia and extensive basophilic stippling so much so that one may suspect lead-poisoning in some instances and a moderate degree of anisocytosis and poikilocytosis. The l e u k o c y-tic count is usually normal or decreased and actual leukopenia existing at the expense of the granulocytic cells. Therefore, there is a relative but not an absolute lymphocytosis.

To distinguish this state from that which is produced by acute and quickly developing malaria, one should appreciate that in the rapidly developing disease there does not present an appreciable degree of hyperchromic a n e m i a. We have studied many cases of the estivo-autumnal malaria that have been characterized by relatively sudden onsets and by a rather widespread parasitic invasion of the red cells, and in these cases there seldom existed any considerable anemia. Also it should be pointed out that in this type of malaria the leukopenic index is not present but there is more often a leukocytosis caused by an increased number of granulocytes with a moderate cellular shift to immaturity. One of the characteristics of the Schilling Differential made on the cases to which I refer was the fact of the existence, in practically all of them, of a monocytosis running as high as 25 per cent in some instances and I believe that I would be safe in pointing out that one could surely expect to find an increase in monocytes in all cases of chronic malaria in the afebrile stage.

It might be well at this point to make some mention of the method used in making differentials as well as examining the blood film for the parasite. It is absolutely essential that if the slide method is used in preference to the thick drop, over which it has many advantages, that a truly thin film is secured. This can only be accomplished by repeated effort and practice on the part of the technician. To secure a slide that has the erythrocytes piled up in great numbers upon each other and expect to find the parasites in it is obviously foolish. The film must be extremely thin so that the red cells are separated from one another and distinct, and each cell can be examined as to its various characteristics independent of its neighbor. Then, and only then, and with the aid of the proper stain, will one be able to determine whether or not an individual has an infection. We have found for our purpose that the best stain to use in making such an examination is Giemsa's stain made fresh as needed, leaving it on the slide sufficiently long to produce the necessary contrast. The use of properly prepared water for the washing of the slide is absolutely essential and no results worthwhile can be obtained without attention being paid to this fact.

It is not my purpose to make any recommendations as to treatment or as to methods of control of this situation. Those who are far more skilled in the matter are making an earnest effort to control the situation, however a few thoughts along the line of an appraisal of the extent of malaria I will attempt.

Sizing up a malaria situation by the eye is clearly to i n v i t e trouble. It is somewhat like the matching of cases by medical students in a clinical amphitheatre. As each patient is wheeled in they look attentively for outward signs of disease resembling those of patients they have seen before and often become very skilled in d i a g n o s i s at a distance. They miss, of course, all a t y p i c a l cases. Carried into practice, the method is dangerous enough in clinical medicine, but in malaria it is disastrous, and for the same reason; a large proportion of the cases depart from the supposed rule. The truth of the matter is not that there are a great many exceptions, but that there is no rule. In every field of malariology matching cases leads nowhere but to confusion. A mosquito harmless in Java is found to be the chief infector in the interior of Sumatra. A m e t h o d of treatment unusually successful in India is almost without effect in Sardinia. The half of mile radius sufficient for larva control in the Malaya has to be quintupled in the Mediterranean B a s i n. A village in Spain in which half the population is in bed with chills and fever in August turns out to be less infected than a village in Africa where virtually no one has to abandon work on account of malaria at any time. This is elementary knowledge to students of malaria but not to all of those who are somewhat acquainted with the disease. The health officer must be able to c o n v i n c e the authorities that time, money and lives can be saved by pausing to obtain a thorough knowledge of each individual problem before acting, as the physician takes time to make an accurate diagnosis before proceeding to treatment.

The first thing a health officer wants to know about his problem is how much malaria there is, afterwards he can determine his course and consider how to deal with it. He can do nothing, however, until he has established a base line with which to measure progress and is in a position to contrast this malaria situation with some other which he may have chosen for comparison. To do this he will have to find some way of measuring malaria, of expressing the result in numbers.

Now malaria marks its victims in four different ways—it produces a very characteristic fever; it causes anemia by blood destruction; it fills the blood stream with easily recognized parasites; and it enlarges the spleen, an organ so placed that when swollen it can be felt and its size estimated t h r o u g h the abdominal wall. With all these signs to go by, it would seem that no malaria case could escape recognition. With a little effort the total amount of malaria in any community could be determined and the health officer would know where he stood at any moment.   .

Unfortunately, as soon as we begin to put this method into practice we run into an absurd difficulty. The four tests do not divide the population neatly into two groups, the malarious and the non-malarious, as we should like. They unexpectedly produce four different groups of people which partially overlap but somehow do not seem very homogeneous. Some have parasites but no fever; some spleens but no parasites, and I have personally seen a number of apparently healthy infected persons looking quite out of place. Let us examine these four groups to see what they mean and how they differ from one another.

First, the group with clinical symptoms. Counting the sick is the statistical method usually applied to infectious diseases and m a l a r i a with its characteristic attacks would seem to make such a census anything but difficult. In infantile paralysis it is possible that only one in a thousand infected children actually develop the unmistakable paralytic signs of the disease, but with malaria, even if the symptoms are occasionally puzzling, the parasites can always be found during the acute stage in any drop of blood. Now while this is perfectly true of acute malaria, the chronic cases carry their infections with less ostentation. They may present a general pic-

ture of poor health but they will be up and a b o u t most of the time and for a long period show no parasites in the blood. In epidemics of malaria the number of actually ill people can be counted rather easily ·but when the disease is more intense, when a large portion of the population is infected so often that they never have time to recover from the disease, then in other words, the situation becomes e n d e m i c. When this happens, curiously enough, the amount of obvious illness decreases. A growing tolerance tends to suppress clinical manifestations and acute attacks become infrequent. Let us always remember that the amount of malaria, that is, its incidence as measured by the number of infected people, is one thing and its intensity or transmission rate as determined by the frequency of inoculation is quite another. It is like money, the amount of which economists tell us, is far less important to business than the velocity of circulation.

The group with anemia. But if the clinical picture of malaria does not correspond with the intensity of infection neither does the anemia which it causes. In the individual the blood picture is modified as time goes on by growing tolerance to the effects of the disease and in the community it is influenced by so many factors not connected with malaria, that a n o r m a l standard hardly exists. As an index of malaria it receives little attention for its implications are uncertain and r e q u i r e elaborate analysis. A trained miscroscopist can pick up indications of the degree of anemia from the blood preparation which he is examining for parasites and such a study could be included more often than it is in population surveys. The principal objection is that anemia is a condition not specific from malaria and cannot stand alone as a mark of the disease. Like the death rate and the birth rate, the hemoglobin rate can be used, as Boyd suggested, "to present completely the general physical impairment of the community," but for all the epidemiological information it gives it is hardly worth the trouble and expense of investigating.   .

The group with parasites. We have now arrived at the third group of malaria victims — those who have parasites in their circulating blood. Here we have to make a distinction at once. Some will be having active a t t a c k s and we understand why their blood should be full of parasites; but the others will be the so-called apparently healthy carriers — people without symptoms whose activities are unrestricted by their latent infection but who quite unknown to themselves have numbers of organisms in their blood at the time of the examination. How this comes about we have to admit we do not understand at all. The acute attack ends with the removal of all the parasites from the circulation by the sensitized g i a n t phagocytes of the spleen and other tissues. It is true that the parasites have r e f u g e s in the body where they are free from attacks but when they venture into the circulation they are at once mopped up by the watchful defenders, or if they succeed in making some headway the fight is on again with chills and fever and the patient has a relapse. Fairly frequently the parasites are allowed to circulate freely in the body for a period and even to increase their numbers up to a certain limit without molestation. It seems to take place almost by agreement, the dogs are called off as it were, and no symptoms whatever result. This happens very often to individuals with enlarged spleens so that it is evident that the reticulo-endothelial system is ready but not functioning. Then one day the parasites are all gone again, slaughtered or bottled up somewhere out of sight and discipline is restored in the body. Such recurring invasions of the parasites have been called h a e m i c relapses which does not, of course, explain them but it is these which we pick up in a general b l o o d examination of a malarious population. They are the results of previous infection and if we could interpret them aright might give some useful information as to the past experiences of the community with malaria. To avoid complications of an acute clinical attack, which are always an inexplicable mixture of new infections, reinfections and relapses, it is better to look for the healthy carrier in winter or at a time when no transmission of malaria is taking place.

The percentage of population which has parasites in the circulation at any given moment is known as the parasitic rate but of course, it can never be accurately determined even by the most careful microscopic s e a r c h. Ross drew a distinction

therefore, between a rate and an index. The rate refers to the true situation as it exists in the population and should be confined to data which gives us the whole truth, such as the exact death rate or birth rate. But where we judge by sample of the population or by the inexact methods or indirectly by some correlated phenomenon the figure we obtain is an index, such as index prosperity or a parasitic index obtained from the examination of children only.

Now it is generally considered that the relative number of parasitic carriers depends upon the recent prevalence or diffusion of malaria. Thus the annual wave of new infection this summer will be reflected in the parasitic rate of the following winter and a great epidemic will leave its traces in the blood of the population for four or five years.

The group with enlarged spleens. The oldest method of measuring malaria is by counting the enlarged spleens. Dempster hit on the idea in 1847: "The spleen test," he wrote, "forms an accurate method of estimating the salubrity of different localities and its degree of enlargement is most probably indicative of the intensity of the remote cause of the disease." What this remote cause was, no one was destined to know for another 50 years but the test proved a sound one.

There are two kinds of enlarged spleens, as Christophers has pointed out. The soft, turgid with blood, acute and transitory; and the hard spleen caused by the mobilization of phagocytic tissue slow to return to normal. The spleen index may be 50 per cent in July and four per cent in December. This is epidemic malaria and these would be soft spleens. But in endemic areas there is a mixture of hard and soft spleens. The soft spleens will be found in the early age group and in those persons protected by fortune or by screens from multiple infection. Hence the spleen rate itself is a complex phenomenon and to simplify our indices as much as possible we tried to keep the chronic and acute spleens apart. It is not easy to distinguish them while new infections are taking place, nor are we so much interested in acute spleens if our object is to obtain an idea of the intensity of malaria. It is the spleens which persist in winter in apparently well individuals which measure the extent of a new reaction to infection. They do not measure the immunity itself, for a spleen may diminish in size with the establishment of a polyvalent immunity. They indicate en masse precisely what we wish to know—namely the intensity of malaria to which the population has been previously exposed. The winter spleen then, and not the summer, is the best measure of previous malaria intensity or transmission rate.

At this point I should like to add a word about the overlapping of infection. There will be overlapping of infection even with low endemicity and relatively infrequent inoculations for infected b i t e s are never e v e n l y distributed. Christophers has pointed out that if 100 infections were distributed completely at random among 100 individuals you would get the following r e s u l t s : 37 would escape infection; 37 would got one infection; 18 would get two infections; six would get three infections; two would get four or more infections. The infection rate is only 63 per cent but there will already be a nucleus of individuals who have been infected two or more times in rapid succession and will be building up a hard spleen. The incidence of malaria can go no higher of course, than 100 per cent, but the intensity of infection may still incrase almost indefinitely bringing about what is known as a hyperendemic situation.

The infectivity of a community is shown by the acute infection and it is correspondingly high if the endemicity is low. Epidemic malaria then, is the malaria of nonimmuned, and endemic m a l a r i a is that which is of sufficient intensity to create and maintain an effective continuous immunity from year to year, as revealed in the splenic index.

LATENCY IN MALARIA

The latent period represents a precarious equilibrium between the p a r a s i t e and what Taliafero called "the killing mechanism of the host." The parasites out of reach go on dividing at normal rate but any increase is prevented by the watchful phagocytes. In fact the parasites are reduced to such a low level that the spleen begins to diminish in size having not very much to do. T h i s infection-immunity balance is

subject at first to irregular wide oscillations before coming to a provisional stability. A case of falciparum malaria may recrudesce time after time with only the briefest intermittencies, whereas the curve of vivax resistant shows long waves of quite a different order. In any event, latency once established may terminate theoretically in one of two ways; cure with eradication of the parasites or an upsetting of the balance followed by a relapse. The word "theoretically" is used because we never know when anyone is cured. Our only proof is a renewed susceptibility to reinfection by the same strain of parasite (a test impossible of application, of course, in nature). If it is true that immunity can exist for some time after the disappearance of the last plasmodium, even such evidence would leave us in doubt as to when the event took place.

The suggestion has been made that the body rarely or never succeeds in completely eradicating a malaria infection. It is well known that canaries after inoculation with malaria, usually remain infected all the rest of their lives, although Sergent reports that occasionally an infected bird after several years may again become susceptible to reinfection. He believes that there is no true immunity to malaria but only a state of "premunition" sustained by living parasites in the body.

During a long latency the control of the body over the parasites may relax to such an extent that the peripheral blood becomes thronged with parasites as in a clinical attack, although no symptoms whatever are produced and the infected individual remains completely unaware of the event. Thus he becomes an "apparently healthy carrier"; the sort of person we look for when we take the parasitic index of a population. Important as this phenomenon is to malarial epidemiology we have no satisfactory explanation of it. Claus Schilling believed that immunization in malaria is a reciprocal reaction between organism and host in which each is protected from the other as in ordinary "carrier" diseases. The truce in malaria must be a little different than that in other "carrier" diseases being transitory and apt to end unexpectedly in a renewal of hostilities.

CONCLUSION

If there is any conclusion to be drawn from these few remarks it is that we should hold our mind open to the progress that is being made and the effort on the part of earnest workers in trying to untangle some of the baffling and apparently insoluble problems of the malaria situation. Let us always remember that ignorance, poverty and disease constitute the vicious triangle of human social inadequacies. An attack on any one of them helps to dissipate the other two. It is astonishing at this day and age to see those whose minds are completely closed to the possibility of malarious infection manifesting itself in anything but a frank syndrome of chills, fever and sweats.

REFERENCES

Anders, James M.: Practice of Medicine, Fourteenth Edition.

Magner, William: Hematology, 1938.

Osgood and Ashworth: Atlas of Hematology, 1937.

Kracke and Garver: Diseases of the Blood and Atlas of Hematology, 1937.

Hackett, L. W.: Malaria in Europe, 1937.

Manson and Bahr: Manson's Tropical Diseases, Tenth Edition, 1936.

Beckman, Harry: Treatment in General Practice, 1930.

Amy and Boyd: J. Roy. Army Med. Corps, 67; 1936.

Briercliffe: The Ceylon Malaria Epidemic 1934-35. Colombo, 1935.

Collins: Am. J. Trop. Med., 14; 1934.

Hasselmann; J. Philip. Isl. M. Assoc., 14; 1934.

Rogers and Megaw: Tropical Medicine. London, 1935.

The Therapeutics of Malaria. Quart. Bull. Health Org. L of N., Geneva, 2; 1933.

Treatment of Malaria. Fourth general report of the Malaria Commission. Bull. Health Organization, L. of N., 6; 1937.

Watson: Some pages from the history of the prevention of malaria. Lecture Roy. Faculty of Physicians & Surgeons, Glasgow, 1934.

---o---

The Treatment of Acute Empyema

H. DALE COLLINS, M.D.
OKLAHOMA CITY, OKLAHOMA

The treatment of acute empyema has been f a i r l y well standardized, but the methods of application of these standards have not been well understood by all physicians who are called upon to apply them. This question is of considerable interest to many branches of our profession. It is especially interesting to the general practitioner, the internist, the pediatrician and finally the surgeon. We must seek the co-operation of all these specialties in evolving an effective method of therapy for this condition. It may be said that there are many methods of treatment advocated in acute empyema. Most of these proposed methods are not new, but are modifications of principles that have long been known. For practical purposes there are only two methods of treatment, namely, closed and open drainage. Closed drainage has had many variations from its original principle; some of these variations have been useful while o t h e r s are so complicated that their routine or universal applications would be difficult for most of us. Suffice it to say, any advocated method must be tried over a period of several y e a r s in order to establish its merit, because the incidence of empyema varies from year to year, the virulency and type of organism also vary, and these in turn dominate the mortality rate. If you were to judge your method of t h e r a p y by the empyemata treated in years when the pneumonic infections were mild you could o b t a i n a rather false impression of your skill and your particular method. In checking the records in the Oklahoma University and Crippled Children's Hospitals for the past ten years I found that our mortality rate up until 1933 was low enough to compare with the lowest published statistics. But in 1933 we received a large number of cases suffering from a virulent strain of organisms. Our mortality promptly raised far above the average figure and elevated our exceedingly low figure to an average percentage. Even so, our figures over a 10 year period compare favorably with like statistics from other institutions and much better than many that have been reported. One of the surprising things about this review of the cases from these two hospitals was the great incidence of chronic empyemata which were being admitted. When an empyema becomes chronic it is an admission of failure with our therapy. We must adopt some effective method of treatment which will prevent this high incidence of chronic empyemata.

The method of treatment of acute empyemata which is advocated in this paper has been used over a p e r i o d of several years and has been effective in saving life and preventing chronicity. Nevertheless, it is not a perfect method, else we would have had no chronicity and no mortality; but in comparison to other methods it has given us the best results. In order to present the problem of treatment it will be necessary to briefly review the etiology, physiology, pathology and the diagnosis of acute empyema.

In this discussion I have eliminated the tuberculous empyema from any consideration, and will confine my remarks to the non-tuberculous t y p e s of pleural infections.

Empyema has a number of causes. The most frequent cause is pneumonia, and this may be divided into two main types, namely, the pneumococcic and the streptococcic. The next most frequent cause is an empyema following a penetrating injury of the pleural cavity. In our series there were about an equal number due to stab wounds and gun shot wounds. The next most common causes are the rupture of a lung abscess and the extension of infection from a suppurative process in the peritoneal cavity. There is a distinct difference in the two types of pneumonia. In the pneumococcic empyemata the purulent exudate occurs after the pneumonia has subsided, when the vital capacity of the patient has increased. The exudate thickens rapidly and contains an abundance of fibrin; it can only be aspirated with a large sized needle. There is an early formation of pleural adhesions and when these adhesions have formed they prevent a shifting of the mediastinum. When the pus is placed in a test tube very little, if any, serum settles out. We find pneumococci in the smears and cultures from the exudate.

In comparison, the streptococcic empyema occurs at the height of the pneumonic process, the exudate forms rapidly and in greater quantity, and unfortunately this pleural effusion occurs when the vital capacity has already been lowered by the existing pneumonia. The exudate tends to be serous and thickens slowly, adhesions form more tardily and the mediastinum becomes rather late in the disease. Complications are much more common in the streptococcic infections. It has often been said that a patient rarely dies of an uncomplicated empyema; the fatalities are due to complications e x i s t i n g with the pleural infection.

Prior to the World War the incidence, severity and method of treatment of the streptococcic pleural infections were little known to the medical profession. Most of the army surgeons were men who were taken from civil life and had not dealt with empyemata other than the type which followed l o b a r pneumonia. The standard method of treatment for these cases had been open drainage. The influenza epidemic descended upon us with the virulent streptococcic pneumonias. The death rate f r o m the pneumonias was exceedingly high, but the death rate in those cases complicated by empyemata with open operation was m u c h higher. Ordinarily the mortality in the empyemata will compare with the mortality of the pneumonias and will be in about the same proportion. The Empyema Commission was created, headed by Dr. Evarts A. Graham of St. Louis. They reported that the empyemata were due to hemolytic streptococci and were very different in character from the pneumococcic empyemata, a n d, furthermore, these cases would not tolerate early open drainage. Repeated aspirations with delayed open drainage was advocated. Closed drainage became widely used and received its greatest impetus during this epidemic. When the recommendations of the commission became known and their methods applied the mortality promptly fell to an appreciable degree. In one case it dropped from 40 per cent to four per cent. This proves how necessary it is for us to understand the difference in these two distinct and different pathological processes affecting the pleural cavity. In our series of 264 cases we still see cases that are subjected to early open drainage. These cases develop a pneumothorax producing a massive collapse of the lung and a shifting of the mediastinum. This either leads to a fatality or produces chronicity. The operative procedure in the treatment of acute empyema is rarely an emergency procedure and an elective time may be selected when the patient and the local conditions are most favorable.

The pathologists have been of invaluable aid. They have e x p l a i n e d conditions w h i c h have not been well understood. Most pathologists agree that the immediate or direct cause for an empyema is the actual rupture of a peripheral subpleural lung abscess into the pleural cavity; in fact, it has been proved that there is generally a rupture of many of these superficial abscesses in the majority of cases.

There are two principal types of empyemata. The most common type is the massive empyema, those cases w h i c h have fluid throughout the entire pleural cavity. However, we do see a considerable number of encapsulated empyemata in which the pus is localized to a p o r t i o n of the p l e u r a l cavity. The type of empyema which develops depends upon the type of organism, its virulence and the multiplicity of subpleural abscesses, as well as the resistance of the patient. If one has a small abscess which ruptures slowly near the base of the pleural cavity when the organisms are not too virulent you can well imagine that the patient will have a small encapsulated collection of fluid, but if the abscesses are multiple, d e v e l o p rapidly from virulent organisms and rupture from many different areas this patient will suffer a massive collection of fluid. The pathologist has also taught us the manner in which the pleural cavity closes, and this is of extreme importance. Pleural adhesions form along the entire border of the abscess; these adhere and close the space by advancing from the periphery of the abscess; the cavity is finally closed by the formation of sufficient adhesions to pull the. visceral pleura to the chest wall. It is questionable whether the positive intrapulmonary pressure or an increased negative intrapleural pressure developed by closed drainage has any material effect in closing an empyemic cavity.

It would be well to say a few words about the diagnosis of acute empyema. The physical findings of a massive empyema are so clear cut that they need no elaboration. But the encapsulated variety may test the diagnostic ingenuity of the most capable physician. In these cases the X-ray is the most valuable aid. We advise a stereoscopic A P and a lateral of the chest. In this manner the fluid may be located w i t h accuracy and certainly will aid in making a differential diagnosis. The interlobar collections of fluid may be identified by the appearance of an elliptical shadow between the lobes of the lung. The shadow is best seen on the lateral view. The diagnostic puncture is a procedure to definitely confirm the preliminary diagnosis and informs us as to the character of the fluid, its location and the amount of fluid. We have smears and cultures made from the aspirated fluid. In encapsulated collections of pus it is absolutely necessary to locate the fluid accurately enough that one will not t r a v e r s e an uninfected pleural surface in puncturing the abscess. This is important; otherwise there is danger of spreading the infection.

The treatment of any case must be more or less individualized and the findings at any given time must govern the choice of your surgical procedure. Our choice of treatment in the majority of cases is repeated aspirations until the patient has a true pleural abscess, then open drainage. A true pleural abscess may be described as a collection of well formed pus with sufficient pleural adhesions to prevent a compression of the lung when open drainage is established.

I feel very definitely that the choice of an anesthetic is a decision of importance. A general anesthetic is to be avoided if possible. L o c a l anesthetic can be used easily with little pain or discomfort to the patient. However, at times we do use a light gas anesthetic, preferably cyclopropane, in those cases that cannot be subjected to a local anesthetic.

The preoperative preparations are essential and vital in the proper treatment. In preoperative medication the use of large doses of morphine is to be discouraged. A moderate sized dose of morphine is well tolerated, but certainly a dose of morphine sufficient to perceptibly slow respiration is to be avoided. The same statement may be made with reference to the barbiturates. Any drug which lessens the already limited respiratory volume and thus further impairs the vital capacity is a very definite contraindication. Preoperatively we encourage a liberal carbohydrate diet and, in addition, we give a surplus of sugars either by mouth or more often by the intravenous route, in the form of 10 per cent glucose. It is very necessary that they have as large a reserve supply of glycogen as possible. Occasionally in patients who have had a very septic condition or a prolonged illness it is well to give a blood transfusion in order to build up their resistance. However, in my experience this has been rarely necessary in the a c u t e cases.

There are a few points about the technical procedures relative to pleural drainage that demand some emphasis. In those cases of massive empyemata that have had repeated a s p i r a t i o n s of considerable amounts of fluid, and particularly in the encapsulated type, it is absolutely necessary that aspiration be done immediately b e f o r e operation. Otherwise, in a few cases one will be embarrassed by finding no fluid at the site chosen for operation, either because the pleural cavity has partially closed or you have missed the site of the encapsulated fluid. When a rib is resected unless the freshly cut rib ends are protected they will soon be bathed in a pool of pus. They may be protected by applying bone wax over the cut ends. This will prevent bone infection to some extent. Before opening the pleura all subcutaneous and muscle bleeders are tied and the sutures for closure are placed in the tissues so that the operative procedure is near completion before the incision is made into the pleural cavity. If one waits until the pleura is opened before taking these steps it is a disagreeable task with added danger of further spread of infection.

The choice of drainage tubes is a factor in the proper treatment. We have almost entirely dispensed with the ordinary rubber tubing and have substituted the Wilson flange tube drain. These tubes come in various lengths and widths and we try to adjust the size of the tube to the size of the patient so that it will fit firmly and offer adequate drainage. The flange will prevent losing a tube in the pleural cavity. This accident has occurred to many surgeons and is annoying as well as embarrassing. The tubes are short enough

that they can be easily cleansed and thus insure proper drainage. The only objection to the flange tubes is that with a wide flange it acts as a foreign body and prevents healing about the site of the flange and leaves a rather large defect; but to overcome this objection we cut off a portion of the inner flange so that its diameter is not more than one inch, and this is found to be sufficient to prevent the tube slipping out. Needless to say it is imperative that the drainage tube be placed at the most dependent portion of the abscess cavity. It is not an uncommon error to find the drainage tube above the level of the fluid, and this is a potent factor in the production of chronicity.

If the proper time has been chosen for the operative treatment the next most important phase is the postoperative care. It is absolutely necessary to dress the wound with moist dressings. Dry dressings dam the drainage tube and prevent drainage. A high caloric diet, 3,000 calories or above, is encouraged. One may read many diversified opinions about the advisability of pleural irrigations. I am convinced that one of the greatest aids to sterilization of the pleural cavity, re-expansion of the lung and rapid healing is the irrigation of the pleural cavity with fresh Dakin's solution. The Dakin's solution dissolves the fibrinous exudate, decorticizes the pleura (thus aiding expansion of the lung) and acts as an antiseptic. We routinely irrigate the cavity with Dakin's every two to three hours. The only contraindication to its use is a broncho-pleural fistula. When the pleural cavity is irrigated if there is any fibrinous plug in the tube it can be removed with tissue forceps. It is rather surprising at times the quantity of fibrin to be found in the pleural exudate. One of the disadvantages of closed drainage is that this fibrin cannot be removed and if allowed to remain will delay healing. We continue to use the blow bottles. It is a rather debatable question whether the use of this apparatus aids materially the re-expansion of the lung. The only good reason I have for continuing its use is an experience which occurred several years ago. A young child one and a half years of age, with a pneumococcic e m p y e m a, was operated. Postoperatively the child cried long and lustily throughout the waking period, and within eight days after the drainage of a massive empyema the cavity had entirely closed. This convinced me that the deep respiratory movements, repeated o f t e n enough, were a distinct aid.

When is empyema cured? This is a fundamental question which is not well understood. An empyema may be said to be cured when the cavity has been entirely obliterated. For that reason we continue the above mentioned routine treatment until the cavity holds less than 15 cubic centimeters; the flange tube is removed and a small soft rubber tube is substituted. This tube is gradually shortened until the cavity is entirely closed.

The above mentioned outline of treatment must be altered in children under two years of age. Our greatest mortality occurs in young infants because they lack resistance to infection, their vital capacity is easily impaired and the simple operative procedures are sometimes shocking. Something must be done to prevent these serious complications. We are prone to continue aspiration over a longer period of time before operation. In many cases I feel that the fatal outcome was hastened by a rib resection, and if we are willing to do a simple thoracotomy without rib resection I b e l i e v e our mortality will be lessened. Occasionally drainage will not be adequate and will necessitate a rib resection later, but this operation will come when the infection is less acute and the resistance has improved.

To summarize, I feel that the most effective and most fool proof method of treatment of an acute empyema is repeated aspiration followed by rib resection. We have used all methods and our results will prove the statement above. It is true that about 10 per cent of all cases will be cured by aspiration alone, but this is not a method to be relied upon for a cure. Danna and Elias report excellent results with aspiration and air injection. We have used this method and found it to be as effective as aspiration alone and is best suited for a trial in the encapsulated types. Closed drainage has its merits and it must be a worthy method, otherwise it would not have such a widespread use. As I see the situation the big disadvantage to its use is the fact that very few hospitals have adequate trained personnel for the accurate care which must be given this method. If it is to be used it should be used early before a true abscess has formed. Failures with its use lead to serious complications and may produce a fatality or chronicity. In a well formed abscess it does not seem to me to be a logical procedure any more than draining a boil by inserting an aspirating needle instead of an incision with adequate drainage. I believe that open operation performed at the proper time with dependent drainage will be the most effective method of treatment because it can be used in any locality and every hospital is equipped adequately for the procedure.

---------------0---------------

The Sinus Problem*

WILLIAM L. BONHAM, M.D.
OKLAHOMA CITY, OKLAHOMA

The subject of sinus disease has been the object of so much discussion, commercial advertising and unmitigated criticism that I feel a brief review of the problem should be of interest at this time. We have all had

the experience, I am sure, of seeing a patient with his first attack of sinus infection, who, when informed of the diagnosis would exclaim with horror that he had heard that there was no cure for this condition. At s o c i a l functions, pink teas, bridge parties and over the back fence it

*Read Before the Section on Eye, Ear, Nose and Throat, Annual Meeting, Oklahoma State Medical Association, Muskogee, Oklahoma, May 10, 1938.

is not unusual to hear fanciful discussions of the sufferings of some friend or acquaintance who is having treatments or has had an operation for sinus disease. To the majority of people any abnormal condition in the nose is roughly classified as "sinus trouble," the sinus often taking the blame for headaches which are caused by o t h e r abnormalities. The information gleaned by the layman is usually then from purely social discussion with uninformed individuals or f r o m commercial advertisements urging these sufferers to purchase some particular medicine for relief.

When a patient presents himself at your office for relief from an acute sinus infection, the problem is, as a rule, not baffling and recovery takes place along lines wholly satisfactory to the patient. But when a patient presents himself with a chronic sinus infection of several or many years standing and having run the gauntlet of remedial measures suggested by g r a n d-mother, neighbors and commercial advertising, he still is likely to expect a cure with no more extensive procedures than would be used in the treatment of an acute infection. If clinical examination and X-ray studies show chronic pathological changes have taken place in the sinuses which make an operation necessary the patient or relatives are likely to interpose the objection that once an operation is performed he will continue having operations the rest of his life and therefore insist either on conservative treatment or some m i n o r operative procedure from which complete relief cannot be expected. Consequently, it is not upon our shoulders but rather upon the shoulders of the dissenting patients and relatives that there rests much of the responsibility for the phrase—"Once a sinus, always a sinus."

There seems to be one monkey-wrench in the machinery as far as permanence of cure from the patient's point of view is concerned. This is due to the fact that with each attack of head cold following the operation it is quite likely that there will be some purulent discharge from the sinuses and the patient still looks on this as a continuation of his old trouble rather than as a new infection. Our problem, therefore, seems to be to study each in-dividual case from the s t a n d p o i n t of e t i o l o g y, symptomology, pathology and type of treatment to be instituted which is most likely to provide a cure and then to acquaint the patient as far as possible with what to expect in the future.

PATHOLOGY

The pathological change in the sinuses may be c l a s s i f i e d[1] as either acute or c h r o n i c. The acute infections may be either catarrhal or purulent w h i l e the chronic infections may be purulent, hypertrophic, polypoid or fibrotic.

The pathological change involved in the acute catarrhal stage is similar to that of acute rhinitis. There is first a constriction of the blood vessels followed by relaxation of the vessels with an extravasation of lymph into the soft tissues causing them to swell. A thick mucoid discharge follows and the stratified ciliated epithelium is infiltrated with lymphocytes and polymorphonuclear leukocytes. The connective tissue and fibers of the mucosa are widely separated by coagulated serum resulting in edema and into these connective tissue spaces there occurs leukocytic infiltration. There is marked enlargement of the blood vessels.

In the acute purulent stage there is the same pathological c h a n g e as described above except that the reaction is somewhat less marked and pus is present on the surface of the mucosa. Scattered hemorrhages may be present in the tissues. The interstitial tissues show a greater cellular infiltration composed almost exclusively of polymorphonuclear leukocytes.

Repeated infections of the type described above ultimately produce chronic changes which are strikingly similar in all the sinuses. A m o n g the most noted of the changes are those of the vascular channels, the pathological changes of the contiguous soft and bony tissues being secondary to these changes. Hypertrophic sinusitis is characterized by thickened and edematous mucosa and periosteum and is usually associated with polypoid masses of the soft tissue and rarefaction and osteo-porosis of the bone. This is perhaps the most common variety. The vascular changes consist of inflammatory infiltration of the veins and lymphatics followed by an increase in the fibrous tissue which replaces the smooth muscle and elastic tissue. The resiliency and contractibility of the vessels is impaired, resulting in stasis and interference with drainage of the s i n u s e s. This increased stagnation of fluids results in further extravasation into the fibrous tissues, increasing the tendency to polypoid hyperplasia. Changes in the soft tissues and involvement of the periosteum and bone result from the lymphatic and venus obstruction. There is leukocytic infiltration chiefly with lymphocytes, plasma cells and an occasional eosinophile. The cellular reaction is most marked in the walls of the veins and lymphatics and adjacent stroma presenting the p i c t u r e of phlebitis and some peri-phlebitis as well as lymphangitis with s o m e peri-lymphangitis. Polypoid masses result from continued turgescence of the tissues. Thinning of the surface epithelium occurs from continued pressure while the mucous glands show cystic degeneration due to the obstruction of the excretory ducts by edema of the stroma. The bony structures ultimately show signs of absorption and osteo-porosis. Necrosis and sequestration may result.

In fibrotic sinusitis, which is also called atrophic sinusitis, there is an atrophy of the tissue which is very slight in the early stages but in the later stages results in a marked reduction of soft tissue and bony structure. Mild cases of fibrosis show no necrosis, crust formation or putrefactive odor. Some areas of the epithelium of the mucosa may be thickened with the formation of papillae while other areas are thin and the epithelium is squamous in character. The secretory g l a n d s are usually small, atrophic, and inactive but if the efferent ducts are obstructed, they become cystic. The stroma becomes infiltrated with lymphocytes and plasma cells. In this fibrotic type of sinusitis the vascular changes consist in arterial involvement in contrast to the changes in the veins and lymphatics in the hypertrophic type. One can usually demonstrate endarteritis, arteritis or peri-arteritis. There occurs an early cellular reaction around the vessels, and an increase in the fibrous tissue and partial or complete occlusion of the lumen of the arteries and arterioles due to the thickening of the vessel walls is seen later.

The veins and lymphatics show decreased fluid content and in some instances are collapsed. The bone and cartilage show alternating a r e a s of cartilage and bone formation interspersed with areas of absorption. In advanced atrophic cases there is ozena, loss of secretion and crust formation with possible necrosis.

There may be a combination of these types with involvement of both the afferent and the efferent blood vessels and the surface of the mucosa is nodular or trabeculated and p r o d u c e d by alternating areas of edema and hypertrophy interspersed by fibrotic or atrophic zones. The bony changes are likewise irregular with areas of osteo-porosis in some parts and exostosis and osteitis in other parts.

SYMPTOMATOLOGY

In general the symptoms causing the sinus patient to seek relief are nasal discharge, nasal obstruction which varies with the amount of discharge and headaches which may increase in severity at different times of the day and which are usually frontal in type. In acute sinusitis the discharge is at first serous but later becomes mucopurulent and in the acute cases there is usually no odor while in chronic cases a foul odor may be present. The nasal obstruction is alternating, intermittent, and usually more marked on the diseased side. Involvement of the a n t e r i o r group of sinuses most often produces frontal headache while involvement of the posterior group most often produces occipital headache. Morning frontal headache decreasing in intensity toward the afternoon usually indicates involvement of the frontal or ethmoid sinuses, w h i l e morning frontal headaches increasing in intensity toward the afternoon suggests maxillary involvement. M o r n i n g occipital headache increasing in intensity toward the afternoon suggests the possibility of sphenoid involvement. In chronic sinusitis nasal discharge may be the only s y m p t o m, and headache when present usually means interference with drainage.

DIAGNOSIS

The diagnosis may be made by a careful h i s t o r y and examination, including transillumination and X-ray. By the time the history is completed we know whether or not we are dealing with an acute or chronic infection and we often have some idea as to the group of sinuses involved. On first inspection the finding of pus in any one particular area is no indication of its origin, because blowing of the nose and snuffing may cause the pus to be located in any position. However, on removal of this pus and shrinking of the nasal mucosa and waiting for some time, the reappearance of pus in the middle meatus points to involvement of the anterior group while pus coming from above the middle turbinate points to involvement of the posterior group of sinuses. However, the absence of discharges does not rule out the possibility of infection and careful shrinkage of the nasal mucosa together with careful investigation of the middle meatus and the spheno-ethmoid recess, combined with suction, transillumination and X-ray, irrigation of the antra and possibly probing the frontal may be necessary before the diagnosis is made.

A. R. Sohval and M. L. Som[2] r e p o r t masked sinusitis as a cause of obscure fever in nine cases. The patients were generally young and the duration of f e v e r varied from one week to two-and-one-half years. Previous tentative diagnosis included infectuous mononucleosis, rheumatic fever, bacterial invasion of the blood stream, subacute bacterial endocarditis, carbuncle of the kidney, epidemic encephalitis and endemic t y p h u s fever. They recommend that all patients with fever of unknown etiology and especially those with headache should have a routine X-ray examination of the sinuses, intra-nasal examination and diagnostic irrigation of the antra and sphenoid sinuses. They advise the irrigation routinely despite negative findings even by X-ray.

TREATMENT

Having arrived at a diagnosis one then proceeds to select the type of treatment most suited to the individual case. In general the treatment of acute sinusitis is the same as that for acute rhinitis and consists of rest in bed, the usual supportive medication, hot fluids, shrinking agents to the nasal mucosa, heat and suction or the well known displacement treatment. Surgical treatment in the acute stage is rarely indicated. The middle turbinate may have to be refracted or the antrum irrigated. External incision and drainage is rarely indicated and the less surgical intervention the better in the acute stage.

Since the introduction of the displacement method of introducing fluids into the accessory nasal sinuses, this procedure has become rather widely used for both diagnosis and treatment. Arthur Proetz[3] in his resume suggests that four conditions are indispensable to proper displacement filling: (1) the ostium must be in proper position relative to the sinus, (2) the ostium must be covered with fluid, (3) negative pressure must exist at the ostium, and (4) the ostium must be patent. In order to fulfill the first two requisites the head hangs over the edge of a table so that the chin and external auditory canals lie in the same vertical plane. Some prefer propping the patients' shoulders on a pillow and suspending the head laterally with the patient lying on the side. The suction may be applied by any device which will deliver approximately 150 mm Hg. of negative pressure with a nasal suction tip which contains a thumb release opening sufficiently large to p e r m i t equalization of pressure when not closed. Proetz now routinely uses a 1:3 dilution of iodized oil for diagnostic purposes and a ¼ per cent solution of ephedrine sulphate in physiological saline solution for treatment. An extremely useful procedure in prognosis is called by Proetz "washing through." Immediately after completion of the displacement treatment and before the patient moves, continuous suction is applied to one nostril while a syringefull of the solution is poured into the other. The nasal contents with whatever pus has been washed out of the sinuses is thus drawn into the suction tip receptacle for study. It is suggested that this form of treatment is so effective for emptying the antrum that it may replace the canula or trocar.

The treatment of chronic infection requires careful consideration of the extent and probable character of the pathological change present within the sinuses as well as the consideration of the previous degree of incapacitation of the patient and the probable progression of the disease and future incapacitation. It is indeed rare that these cases may be classed as emergencies. Consequently they s h o u l d be under observation for some time before a final decision is made as to the type of operation to be performed. In those cases where the disease has not been present too long and the pathological change is not too great it is advisable to use intra-nasal operative procedures. However, in those· cases in which intra-nasal procedures have failed or in which one is able to demonstrate by clinical examination and X-ray that the pathological change has produced chronic hyperplasia or polypoid degeneration of the sinus mucosa with suppuration or involvement of bone, the external route should be employed.

SINUSITIS AS A FOCUS OF INFECTION

Some authorities are of the opinion that the sinuses rarely act as a focus of infection while other equally capable authorities are of the opinion that the sinuses very frequently act as a focus of infection. Some of the diseases which it is suggested may be secondary to a primary infection in the sinuses are acute and chronic infectious arthritis, myositis, neuritis, bronchitis, numerous ocular diseases, kidney disease, chorea, lymphadenitis, acute rheumatic fever, myocarditis, pericarditis, and endocarditis. Without entering into any controversial discussion of the subject I feel that one is justified in including the sinuses in a search for a focus of infection and in the event that infection is found the usual steps should be taken to eradicate the disease just as would be done if the sinus infection were the primary complaint.

SUMMARY

This is a problem which requires careful study of each patient as an individual pathological entity.

The diagnosis and mode of treatment, whether medical or surgical, should be based upon the apparent pathological change present in the sinuses as determined by the usual diagnostic procedures.

The patient should be informed regarding the severity of his condition, his chances of complete relief from symptoms, and also regarding the possibility of recurrence of at least some of his symptoms with each future head cold.

BIBLIOGRAPHY

1. "Diseases of the Nose and Throat." Imperatori and Burman.
2. "Masked Sinusitis," A. R. Sohval and M. L. Som: Archives Otolaryngology. 25:37-47, January, 1937.
3. "Evaluation of the Displacement Method," Arthur W. Proetz. Annals Otolaryngology Rhinology and Laryng. 46: 699-734, September, 1937.

Surgical Treatment of Ectropion and Entropion*

C. B. BARKER, A.B., M.D., F.A.C.S.
GUTHRIE, OKLAHOMA

The average life is too short and one's practice is insufficient to try out all operations, therefore we must compare experiences and from these select the best operations for the various conditions, thereby eliminating many failures.

From the many operations for the correction of ectropion and entropion, we have selected those which have given us the best results.

The results of the operation often depends upon the placing of a certain stitch, and if tension is desired, a mattress suture should be used.

*Read Before the Section on Eye-Ear, Annual Meeting, Oklahoma State Medical Association, Tulsa, Oklahoma, May, 1937.

First, we will start with the deformities of the upper lid.

The patient comes to the physician because of irritation of the lids to the eyes, and impaired vision, as in trichiasis and entropion following trachoma.

The operation which will best relieve the irritation caused by a thickened and rough lid on the eye ball, is the operation of choice.

Ectropion and entropion can be relieved by one of five ways.

1. Evert the lashes from the eye ball.

2. Lift the irritating edge of the lid away from the eye by a mucous graft.

3. Remove the irritating portion of the lid, as tarsectomy.

4. Take up the slack when the lid falls away from the eye ball (ectropion).

5. Narrow the palpebral f i s s u r e by stitching the lower lid to the upper lid at the external angle, the opposite of a canthoplasty.

The various stitches and electric cautery have been disappointing to us.

However, if the case is not very far advanced, the electric cautery will suffice, but one must cut a grove wide and deep so the gap will result in a scar which will contract and turn the lid margin outward.

If we have entropion of the upper lid, and the lid is thin and not due to trachoma, the David operation will give very good results.

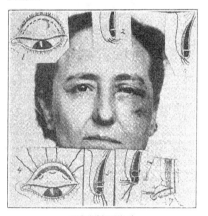

PICTURE NO. 1
In picture No. 1 it was necessary for the patient to keep every eye lash removed from both upper lids for 20 years.
She was completely relieved when the lid margin was turned away from the eye ball.

In a small percentage of c a s e s which have a tarsus, that is, two or three times its normal thickness and distorted, associated with trichiasis, and the e y e b a l l shows a chronic and continuous irritation usually associated with entropion, viz., the tarsus seems to be poisonous to the cornea. We do a partial tarsectomy with a canthoplasty.

When doing a tarsectomy, dissect the conjunctiva well down onto the eye ball, and place mattress sutures so the lid margin will be everted.

When a canthoplasty is done, the conjunctiva and skin is brought between the cut ends of the severed ligament by a mattress suture. This will lengthen the palpebral fissure and prevent the union of the cut ends of the severed ligaments, and the scar will not contract and produce the opposite condition from that desired.

In ectropion of the lower lid, the Kuntz operation is very good. This operation displaces the skin of the lower lid laterally at the external angle and the m a r g i n bearing cilia should be excised, a "V" cut from the center of the tarsus. If this operation is done carefully and the calipers are used to insure accuracy, the results will be very satisfactory.

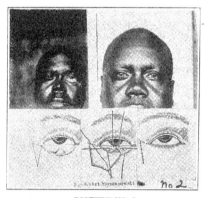

PICTURE NO. 2
In this patient there was a constant irritation of the eye, due to exposure.
Was completely relieved after the lid was placed in the proper position.

In senile ectropion we stitch the lower lid to the upper. Fuch's operation narrows the palpebral fissure.

A mucous graft will give an excellent result.

Split the conjunctiva from the skin about five to eight mm. deep, the whole length of the lid, and then stitch the skin edge over a small rubber tube. This will convert the trough into a flat surface, then remove a strip of mucous m e m b r a n e from the mouth and stitch into place.

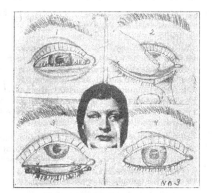

PICTURE NO. 3

The eye lashes of all four lids were
turned inward so there was a constant irritation of the eye ball. This was relieved
by a mucous membrane graft from the
mouth.

If the upper lid is thickened and entropion is present, a Beard's modification of
the Hotz operation is a very good one. The
result depends upon the placing of the
sutures and canthoplasty.

(See picture No. 4. This patient's vision
was hand motions at time of operation,
January 1, 1914.)

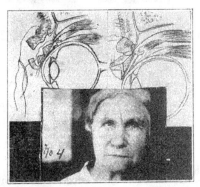

PICTURE NO. 4

This patient had chronic trachoma and
the eye lashes rubbed the cornea until it
was very hazy. The eye cleared after a
Beard's operation and she has had 20
years of good sight and of much comfort.

This picture was taken 20 years after
the operation.

Decompression of Small Intestine in Treatment of Intestinal Obstruction

Intestinal intubation as an adjunct to the treatment of intestinal obstruction has proved successful
in the hands of Charles G. Johnston, Grover Cleveland Penberthy, R. J. Noer and J. C. Kenning, Detroit (Journal A.M.A., October 9, 1938), in 54 cases.
That alone it cannot be depended on is obvious
from the fact that intestinal obstruction is protean
in its manifestations and causes. Each case must
be individualized and the obstruction treated as to
its specific requirements. Intubation does not exclude operative means of handling obstruction but
rather facilitates any operative procedure which
may be necessary. The advantages of the method
in properly selected cases are: 1. It carries the patient past the period when operation is most dangerous. 2. It prepares the patient for operation by
control of distention, thus making operation less
traumatic for the patient and easier for the surgeon. 3. It affords a means of localizing the site
of obstruction and frequently indicates its nature.
4. It permits oral feeding of the patient during a
period when food and fluid are so essential and
frequently permits one to improve the patient's
nutritional state during the period of treatment.
5. It releases the tension above the site of obstruction and frequently reestablishes the normal passage of intestinal contents, thus permitting the
patient to be operated on in the interval stage if
advisable. 6. In the treatment of paralytic ileus
this is the only method which can uniformly be depended on to relieve the distention of the small
intestine, which is not uncommonly fatal. The disadvantages of the method are: 1. It necessitates
careful selection and evaluation of cases. It is not
suitable for treatment of strangulated types of
obstruction. 2. It requires hard work on the part
of the surgeon and his associates. Passage of the
tube and attention to details with regard to the
patient and the equipment require continued attention. 3. It is not suitable for obstruction of the
large intestine, since, despite the fact that the tube
frequently traverses the entire intestinal tract, it
cannot be depended on to reach the large intestine
quickly enough to be of value. Of the 54 patients
treated by intubation, 14 died. Of these, five died
as a result of intestinal obstruction. In the remaining nine who died, intestinal intubation was
carried out to relieve distention associated with
other conditions which caused the death. The
number of cases presented is small, and conclusions regarding mortality are difficult. The data
do, however, indicate that intubation of the small
intestine in selected cases has a definite place in
the care of patients suffering from intestinal obstruction.

----o----

Pathology of Vitamin C Deficiency

After discussing the pathologic changes that occur in the bones, teeth, gingiva, muscles, eyes and
skin consequent to a deficiency of vitamin C, Gilbert Dalldorf, Valhalla, N. Y. (Journal A.M.A., October 8, 1938), concludes that the anatomic effects
of vitamin C deficiency are prompt to appear, certainly in the young, and that they occur, if the
vascular changes are included, even in the mildest
degrees of deficiency. Since clinical reports agree
that subclinical scurvy, whether on the basis of
c h e m i c a l tests or measurements of capillary
strength, is common, it may be assumed that mor-
phologic stigmas due to the same deficiency are
likewise common. However, both clinical and anatomic identification of scurvy remains, as it always has been, a matter of alertness on the part
of the physician. The recently acquired understanding of the scorbutic process affords pathologists and biologists a useful tool in the study of disturbances of intercellular materials. It should be
of value also in the study of similar changes in
senility.

THE JOURNAL
OF THE
Oklahoma State Medical Association

Issued Monthly at McAlester, Oklahoma, under direction of the Council.

Copyright, 1938, by Oklahoma State Medical Association, McAlester, Oklahoma.

| Vol. XXXI | DECEMBER | Number 12 |

DR. L. S. WILLOUR............................Editor-in-Chief
McAlester, Oklahoma

DR. T. H. McCARLEY............................Associate Editor
McAlester, Oklahoma

Entered at the Post Office at McAlester, Oklahoma, as second-class matter under the act of March 3rd, 1879.

This is the official Journal of the Oklahoma State Medical Association. All communications should be addressed to The Journal of the Oklahoma State Medical Association, McAlester Clinic, McAlester, Oklahoma. $4.00 per year; 40c per copy.

The editorial department is not responsible for the opinions expressed in the original articles of contributors.

Reprints of original articles will be supplied at actual cost provided request for them is attached to manuscripts or made in sufficient time before publication.

Articles sent this Journal for publication and all those read at the annual meetings of the State Association are the sole property of this Journal. The Journal relies on each individual contributor's strict adherence to this well-known rule of medical journalism. In the event an article sent this Journal for publication is published before appearance in The Journal the manuscript will be returned to the writer.

Failure to receive The Journal should call for immediate notification of the Editor, McAlester Clinic, McAlester, Oklahoma.

Local news of possible interest to the medical profession, notes on removals, changes of addresses, births, deaths and weddings will be gratefully received.

Advertising of articles, drugs or compounds unapproved by the Council on Pharmacy of the A. M. A., will not be accepted.

Advertising rates will be supplied on application.

It is suggested that wherever possible members of the State Association should patronize our advertisers in preference to others as a matter of fair reciprocity.

Printed by News-Capital Company, McAlester.

EDITORIAL

CAN HE REVOLUTIONIZE THE FAITH OF OUR FATHERS?

Assistant Attorney General, Mr. Thurmond Arnold, in a speech over a national hookup on October 26th, had the following to say relative to our religion:

" . . . Every organized state must have its established church, or as I h a v e expressed it elsewhere, its *folklore*. T h a t church must e m b o d y the fundamental truths and principles which give a state its greatness. At the same time that church must not impose *ridiculous* and unnecessary material sacrifices on the great mass of the people. The fact that today the established church of the modern state is legal and economic, promising security for this life rather than hereafter, distinguishes us from the Middle Ages. The *future life* can no longer be offered as a substitute for economic misery in the living world. . . ."

This is the same Mr. Arnold who instituted and is conducting the grand jury investigation of the American Medical Association to ascertain whether or not Organized Medicine is now conducting itself as to infringe upon the anti-trust laws. It is apparently his policy to not only destroy the methods of the practice of medicine as has been carried out the past 150 years but *now* he would ridicule and revolutionize, if possible, the f o u n d a t i o n s of the Christian religion upon which this nation has lived and progressed for many generations.

An attack upon the method of the practice of medicine may be excusable, but when he tries to r i d i c u l e the Christian faith and say that it is more important to carry out their present economic programs against our existing misery than prepare ourselves for eternal life he will probably receive the deserved b i t t e r criticism of American Christianity.

Those who would foster communism or Hitlerism always attempt destruction of the religion of the country in which they operate, as religion and communism are incompatible.

————o————

SOUTHERN MEDICAL ASSOCIATION

Oklahoma City did themselves proud in entertaining the Southern Medical Association and appeared to furnish everything that was necessary to make the meeting a decided success.

The General Chairman, Dr. Henry H. Turner, was honored by being elected First Vice President.

The Oklahoma physicians took advantage of this excellent program, 552 having registered during the meeting. There was a total registration of 2,260 physicians and with the ladies, students, nurses, exhibitors, et cetera there was a total of 3,832.

Both the Commercial and Scientific Exhibits were extensive and of a very high character and well patronized by the visiting doctors. The Scientific Sections were all well attended and presented excellent programs.

The entertainment offered by the Oklahoma physicians was much enjoyed by the many visitors and certainly our capitol city has shown its ability to handle so large a meeting in a satisfactory manner.

--------o--------

"RENDER UNTO CAESAR"

In the September, 1938, issue, the Journal published an article entitled "Investigate Before You Buy." The article pointed out that certain physicians had been swindled on the pretense of buying a listing to be used by Insurance Companies. This article indicated that the swindling was done by an organization known as the Underwriters Service Bureau of Philadelphia.

This article came to the attention of the President and General Manager of Underwriters Service Bureau, Inc., of Drexel Building, Philadelphia, Pennsylvania. Under date of October 3rd they wrote the Journal, protesting vigorously against the imputation in this article that his company was morally or legally guilty and respectfully urged that a retraction be printed. They were immediately advised that the case would be investigated and that they would be further informed.

With the realization that the Journal is to be of service to the Medical Profession and at the same time be fair to others, we were confronted with a serious proposition. An unwarranted retraction might result in damage to the physicians and surgeons of Oklahoma.

With this in view, the Journal instituted a most thorough investigation. Complaints from Tulsa, Oklahoma City, Duncan, and elsewhere, were investigated. It was determined that a certain alleged agent or agents of Underwriters Service Bureau had taken listings from physicians and garages, and collected money, and cashed drafts which were not honored. Underwriters Service Bureau claimed not to have received the remittances. Investigation was then conducted through two sources in Philadelphia and it was determined that the parties who had committed these "indiscretions" in Oklahoma were discharged former employees of Underwriters Service Bureau, Inc.; that therefore the Underwriters Service Bureau was not responsible either legally or morally.

In fairness to the organizers and managers of Underwriters Service Bureau, Inc., we feel constrained to state that our confidential and reliable reports show them to be men of experience, integrity and morality. The company was greatly embarrassed, as were we, by the imposition on Oklahoma physicians and garages.

We asked them to advise us the names of their true representatives should they again attempt to open the field in Oklahoma. This they kindly consented to do, stating that for the time being his company intended to do nothing further towards covering this state and that when such a time does arrive, the manager personally will cover the state. This assurance from them, recommended as they are, was highly pleasing to us.

This situation demonstrates how easily a company can be maligned by former commission salesmen. It demonstrates how physicians and surgeons can be imposed upon. We can only recommend that all physicians, contemplating buying such a listing, investigate, first, the reliability of the listing company; and second, the authority of the alleged salesman. Under no circumstances should drafts be cashed for such purported salesmen.

The Journal stands ready and willing at all times to investigate the responsibility of listing companies. We might copy after the State Bar of Oklahoma, which organization, through its Board of Governors, investigates such listing companies and publishes the names of those on the approved list. Until such a step is taken by the State Medical Association, we believe it advisable for all physicians to communicate with either the Journal or the officers of the State Medical Association. They should further communicate with responsible civic associations.

If such a procedure had been followed in this case, our doctors would not have been defrauded and the Underwriters Service Bureau would not have been so criticized.

In publishing this letter we have a twofold purpose; that of clearing the name of the Underwriters Service Bureau, Inc.; and that of cautioning physicians and surgeons about the purchase of such listings.

FOR THE DOCTOR

A "Tentative E d i t i o n of Diagnostic Standards," for tuberculosis of the lungs and related lymph nodes, has just been issued in pamphlet form by the National Tuberculosis Association through its Committee on Diagnostic Standards, appointed in 1936 and headed by Dr. Fred H. Heise, medical director of Trudeau Sanatorium, Saranac Lake, New York.

Both primary and reinfection tuberculosis are described u n d e r the heading, "Pathogenic Development of Pulmonary Tuberculosis."

"It is not always possible on clinical and roentgenological evidence to differentiate primary and reinfection tuberculosis," says the committee. "It is important, however, to recognize the pathogenic phase in which a given lesion presents itself, since such knowledge is, within strict limitations, the safest available prognostic criterion."

The committee d e a l s with the clinical c o u r s e of tuberculosis correlated with pathological conceptions. It continues: "The e a r l y pulmonary infiltration, the most common early lesion of reinfection, and the precursor of most of the chronic and fatal tuberculosis in adults may appear at any age, but most frequently between 18 and 30 or 35 (in negroes, a few years earlier). The onset may be symptomless, d e v o i d of abnormal physical signs, and denoted only by the appearance in the roentgenogram of a soft mottled or cloudy patch. Symptoms, when present, are constitutional—mainly fatigue, loss of energy and a small loss of weight; when more severe, they suggest grippe and the lesion may resemble grippal pneumonia."

Failure to find tubercle bacilli in the sputum does not rule out cavity, the report states. Excavation usually is the beginning of progressive pulmonary tuberculosis and prevention or c l o s u r e of the cavity is the most important single feature of clinical recovery. Otherwise, contamination of other parts is inevitable.

The tuberculin test, X-ray evidence, the history of exposure, symptoms and clinical manifestations, physical signs and laboratory methods are included under the section, "Diagnosis of Tuberculosis." Constitutional and local symptoms are explained in detail. The extent of pulmonary lesions is explained in a descriptive summary, as are observations bearing on cases considered arrested, quiescent, etc.

A form for the description and classification of common thoracic lesions is included in the pamphlet. There are no important changes from former diagnostic standards in the sections on location and extent of lesions.

"An ideal nation-wide program for detecting active and potential human sources of contagion with a reasonable degree of promptness and before they have infected many of their associates requires repeated application of tuberculin tests to the entire population, followed by periodic clinical, roentgenologic and laboratory examinations of each infected patient," the committee says.

The National Tuberculosis Association offers the pamphlet tentatively "in order that it may be tried out by clinicians and public h e a l t h administrators." It welcomes comments from both specialist and general practitioner. This is the eleventh i s s u e of "Diagnostic Standards." The publication does not attempt to formulate new or original principles, but only to incorporate those w h i c h are already well established.

The committee includes, b e s i d e s Dr. Heise, Dr. H. E. Kleinschmidt, director of health education of the National Tuberculosis Association, who served as secretary; Dr. J. Burns Amberson, Jr., Tuberculosis Division, Bellevue Hospital, New York, N. Y.; Dr. G. Burton Gilbert, secretary of the Colorado School of Tuberculosis, Colorado Springs, Colo.; Dr. R. H. Kanable, superintendent of the Wyoming State Tuberculosis Sanatorium, Basin, Wyo.; Dr. John H. Korns, Bureau of Tuberculosis, Department of H e a l t h, Cattaraugus County, Olean, N. Y.; Dr. F. M. McPhedran, Research Department, Germantown Hospital, Germantown, Pa.; Dr. Max Pinner, chief of the Division of Pulmonary Disease, Montefiore Hospital, New York, N. Y.; Dr. C. A. Stewart, University of Minnesota Medical School, Minneapolis, Minn., and Dr. P. A. Yoder, superintendent of the Forsyth County Sanatorium, Winston-Salem, N. C.

The cost of this booklet of 32 pages is financed by the annual Christmas Seal sales. A copy will be mailed, free on request, to any physician in the state by the

Oklahoma Tuberculosis and Health Association, 22 West 6th Street, Oklahoma City. Due to improved methods of early diagnosis the family doctor becomes of prime importance to the tuberculosis eradication campaign. Physicians should welcome the opportunity to expand their field of usefulness. "Diagnostic Standards" is an important aid to this end.

---o---

Editorial Notes—Personal and General

DR. FINNEY, of Baltimore, Md., lost his hat to some Oklahoman at the Dr. Curt von Wedel home during the Southern Medical meeting in Oklahoma City in November. The Oklahoman is urged to get in touch with Dr. von Wedel, return the Baltimore hat to him, and re-claim his own.

DR. ED. D. GREENBERGER, McAlester, spent two weeks in November in New York attending the meeting of the American Academy of Roentgenology.

DR. and MRS. K. D. GOSSOM, Custer City, are spending the winter months in Florida.

---o---

OBITUARIES

Doctor Thomas M. Haskins

The rolling tide of destiny, on its onward way to eternity, called home over the waters of eternal rest, a true son and scholar in the profession of which he dearly loved, lived and exemplified, in the person of Doctor Thomas M. Haskins. The solace and consolation in the hour of bereavement to the family of such a worthy one is found in recalling to a sad memory the honor of being the sons and daughters or descendants of such a worthy man while the Creator of all things worthy and great extended to him a long and useful life, as well as a compassionate and worthy father. A gentleman, a man—and after all what is man?—but one of God's greatest handiworks. To have known one good man—one man who, through the chances and mischances of a long life has carried his heart in his hand, like a palm branch, waving all discords into peace—helps our faith in God, in ourselves, and in each other, more than many sermons.

The Tulsa County Medical Society and its members wish to extend to the family its heart-felt sympathies in their hour of sadness in the loss of their loved one and our loss to our society and the public in general of so worthy a character.

JOHN C. PERRY, M.D., Committee Chairman.

---o---

Books Received and Reviewed

"DOCTORS, I SALUTE!" by Emilie Chamberlin Conklin. Light & Life Press, Winona Lake, Indiana, 1938.

An autographed copy of this book has been received by the Editor and is greatly appreciated. It is beautifully constructed, mechanically, and includes 72 poems dedicated to The Healers of The World, whose lives are dedicated to the relief of pain and distress.

The poems evidence a very beautiful interpretation of the healing art and in some instances are so lavish in their praise that they make a doctor reader blush when he realizes his inability to meet the high standard evidenced by the writer.

I am glad to recommend this work of verse to our physicians and believe that they will receive some very refreshing relaxation in the reading of this volume.

---o---

Scientific Exhibit American Medical Association

Application blanks are now available for space in the Scientific Exhbit at the St. Louis Session of the American Medical Association, May 15-19, 1939. Attention is called to the fact that the meeting is a month earlier than usual, and applications close January 15, 1939. Blanks will be sent on request to the Director, Scientific Exhibit, American Medical Association, 535 North Dearborn street, Chicago, Ill.

---o---

"Stone Walls Do Not a Prison Make Nor Iron Bars a Cage."

Winter is a jailer who shuts us all in from the fullest vitamin D value of sunlight. The baby becomes virtually a prisoner, in several senses: First of all meteorologic observations prove that winter sunshine in most sections of the country averages 10 to 50 per cent less than summer sunshine. Secondly, the quality of the available sunshine is inferior due to the shorter distance of the sun from the earth altering the angle of the sun's rays. Again, the hour of the day has an important bearing: At 8:30 a.m. there is an average loss of over 31 per cent, and at 3:30 p.m., over 21 per cent.

Furthermore, at this season, the mother is likely to bundle her baby to keep it warm, shutting out the sun from baby's skin; and in turning the carriage away from the wind, she may also turn the child's face away from the sun.

Moreover, as Dr. Alfred F. Hess has pointed out, "it has never been determined whether the skin of individuals varies in its content of ergosterol" (synthesized by the sun's rays into vitamin D) "or, again, whether this factor is equally distributed throughout the surface of the body."

While neither Mead's Oleum Percomorphum nor Mead's Cod Liver Oil Fortified With Percomorph Liver Oil constitute a substitute for sunshine, they do offer an effective, controllable supplement especially important because the only natural foodstuff that contains appreciable quantities of vitamin D is egg-yolk. Unlike winter sunshine, the vitamin D value of Mead's antiricketic products does not vary from day to day or from hour to hour.

---o---

Etiology of Nausea and Vomiting of Pregnancy: Preliminary Report

J. William Finch, Hobart, Okla. (Journal A.M.A., October 8, 1938), states that nausea and vomiting of pregnancy develop at the same time at which the corpus luteum of pregnancy reaches an appreciable size. The symptoms disappear at about the time the gland is known to begin retrogressive changes. In a series of patients with nausea and vomiting of pregnancy in varying degrees when injected intradermally with from 0.02 to 0.03 cc. of progestin in oil a cutaneous reaction developed directly proportional to the severity of the symptoms. A control series of patients who were not nauseated and in the pregnant state gave negative cutaneous reactions when tested in the same manner. Patients treated with subcutaneous corpus luteum extract and progestin along the lines of allergic desensitization were gradually relieved of their symptoms. A high percentage of the patients with nausea and vomiting of pregnancy either had other diseases of allergy or gave a family history of allergy. Intradermal testing may determine, even before pregnancy, whether a patient will or will not be nauseated when pregnant by determining whether or not she is sensitive to progestin.

ABSTRACTS : REVIEWS : COMMENTS
and CORRESPONDENCE

SURGERY AND GYNECOLOGY
Abstracts, Reviews and Comments from
LeRoy Long Clinic
714 Medical Arts Building, Oklahoma City

Infections of the Hand; Three Years' Experience in a Clinic for Study of Whitlow. By E. A. Devenish, M.S., F.R.C.S., London, England. Archives of Surgery, November, 1938, page 726.

The discussion in this contribution includes both whitlow (usually called felon in the United States) and paronychia.

Incidence: In about one per cent of all casualties there is either injury or infection, or both injury and infection of the fingers. There were 388 patients in this group out of a total of 41,474 patients who reported to the casualty service of University College Hospital during three years.

Of the 388 patients 61 were cases of injury, and apparently not considered in the report. This leaves 327 patients with infection of the digits.

In 58.7 per cent of this group of 327 there was a definite history of injury, and previous injury suspected in an uncertain number of others.

Age: 60 per cent in the second or third decade, 40 per cent being distributed from childhood to 60 years and more. The youngest was one year, the oldest 75.

Occupation: Children 18 per cent. Manual laborers, craftsmen, housewives and domestic servants made up most of the others. There were but few clerical workers.

Sex: Injury nearly twice as frequent in men. Paronychia nearly twice as frequent in women.

Injury in most cases comparatively slight. Only three had received first aid treatment. A common complication is the entrance of a foreign body, often not suspected by patient.

The index and middle finger and the thumb most often affected.

The well-known association of trivial injury with infection is emphasized. This has been proven in a practical way. For example, a large engineering firm arranged for the application of strict prophylactic measures in trivial cuts and scratches, the result being "a material reduction in the incidence of infection."

Management: Early operative treatment, before suppuration, is deprecated. The author makes this very pertinent statement: "The function of operation is the evacuation of pus, and it is as important to avoid undue haste in operating as to avoid undue delay."

Here is a most significant statement: "In the early stages treatment must be directed to helping the tissues in their struggle with the infection. The most important elements in this are elevation and absolute immobilization of the limb."

"Immobilization is secured by means of light metal or plaster splints."

It is believed that elevation of the limb reduces swelling and congestion of the inflamed area.

When operation for the evacuation of pus is necessary, hot fomentations are applied twice daily after operation to prevent formation of crusts, thus keeping the opening patent.

After the cessation of drainage, the hand and fingers should be used as soon as possible, beginning in a gradual way, in order to relieve and prevent stiffness. This is emphasized by the author in the following concise remarks: "There is one important point which remains, that is, the relation of disuse to the function of the hand. The hand seems to be dependent for efficiency on constant use. Complete disuse, whether produced by therapeutic immobilization or a tender scar, is followed by atrophic changes in the fingers, which result in their disablement."

Finally, "after the wound has healed, every patient is examined to determine the mobility of the fingers before he is finally discharged."

COMMENTS: Bearing in mind that the pathology of the average felon (whitlow) is a deep cellulitis **outside** of the tendon sheath or bone; and that the distinct tendency is for it to localize in that situation, it is easy to understand the advice that one should refrain from doing an early, illadvised operation, because such a blunder, as stated by the author, is often followed by sloughing, and frequently by invasion of the tendon sheath and even the bone, producing an osteomyelitis.

In our judgment, the old-time dictum that in the case of a felon one should "cut to the bone" is a grievous error.

We believe that when operation is done for the evacuation of pus the digit should be anesthetized. Generally this can be done by injecting a one per cent or two per cent solution of novocain deeply on each side of the digit at the base. A small rubber band wound tightly about the base of the digit just proximal to the point of injection is of service in localizing the solution. Then the incision should be made slowly and with care, **stopping when pus escapes**. No felon should be incised, helter skelter, by making a quick, blind, slashing incision.

The advice about the benefits from immobilization and elevation while awaiting either spontaneous cessation or the liquification of the exudate (pus formation) is of tremendous importance, but too often neglected.

LeRoy Long.

The Effect of the Direct Application of Cod Liver Oil Upon the Healing of Ulcers of the Feet in Patients with Diabetes Mellitus: Harold Brandaleone; Annals of Surgery, July, 1938, page 141.

In a previous study the author found that careful care of the feet of patients with diabetes mellitus decreased the incidence of infection of the feet, improved the condition of the skin, and helped in healing the ulcers. In many cases, however, in spite of this treatment, the ulcers failed to heal and constant foot care was necessary to avoid serious infection. It occurred to the author that as the tissues in many of these patients were not in an optimum state of nutrition and since vitamin A stimulates the growth of epithelial tissue, that the direct application of cod liver oil might be an effective method of treatment. The healing action of cod liver oil has been reported by several observers who used it in the treatment of wounds, burns, crushing injuries, superficial sores and carbuncles. Cod liver oil has also been reported to have a bactericidal power.

The author studied two groups of diabetic patients, one a controlled group of 11 patients who received routine foot care, consisting of daily foot soaks, thorough drying, and the application of lanolin. This routine foot care was carried out for a period of from one to 32 weeks. The second group consisted of 21 patients who had received routine foot care for a period of from one to 136 weeks when cod liver oil was applied locally to the lesions.

When cod liver oil treatment was instituted the routine foot care was continued, but after drying the feet, gauze saturated with cod liver oil was applied directly to the ulcer and this was kept in place by a noncompressing bandage.

In the 11 diabetic patients with ulcers of the feet who were treated with routine care three lesions remained unhealed, nine were improved, one healed completely and eight recurred.

Of the 21 diabetic patients with ulcers of the feet, which had existed for previous periods varying from one to 136 weeks, having been treated with routine foot care prior to cod liver oil therapy, 20 of these patients had complete healing of the ulcers following the local application of cod liver oil. The average time required for healing to take place was about 10 weeks.

The average duration of these ulcers prior to this cod liver oil therapy was 24 weeks.

The results in the second group suggest that cod liver oil will increase the rate of healing of ulcers in patients with diabetes mellitus. The factor in cod liver oil which is responsible for this remains open to discussion. It is possible that the vitamin content is the responsible agent. On the other hand, cod liver oil contains some highly unsaturated fatty acids—arachidonic, with an iodine number of 334, and clupanidonic with an iodine number of 368. Unsaturated fatty acids apparently have a stimulating effect on the growth of hair and may also have a stimulating effect on epithelial tissue.

LeRoy D. Long

The Influence of Long-Continued Injections of Estrogen on Mammary Tissue. By Ludwig A. Emge and K. M. Murphy, San Francisco, Calif. American Journal of Obstetrics and Gynecology, Vol. 36, November, 1938, page 750.

These authors have studied a large group of transplantable mammary adeno-fibromas known to possess malignant potentialities after the rats in which they were located had been subjected to long continued injections of estrogen. It was hoped that in this way the effect of such estrogen administration upon the production of carcinoma of the breast could be somewhat clarified.

They have found that the carcinogenic potentiality of the sex hormones is apparently extremely variable. They have also found that this quality is limited by biological circumstances. For example, there is no doubt that estrogen plays some role in the production of cancerous states of the mammary gland and uterus in mice susceptible to cancer. However, in mice refractory to cancer there is little or no influence, and in large rodents, particularly the rat, there is far less susceptibility to estrogen while in larger animals the susceptibility is practically nil.

In consideration of this problem of the carcinogenic potentiality of sex hormones it is evident that the effect is limited by species differentials as well as individual characteristics.

The authors feel, therefore, that they have obtained no knowledge of the effects of estrogenic hormones in higher mammals, particularly man, but that the carcinogenic potentiality of estrogen administration is probably smaller in human beings than in experimental animals and that it is certainly smaller in the individual not susceptible to malignant disease.

The conclusions drawn from their work follow:

"1. Transplantable mammary adenofibromas known to possess malignant potentialities were refractory to the influence of estrogen with the exception of one tumor, in which a carcinoid state occurred.

"2. Estrogen did not prevent the loss of glandular tissue in mammary adenofibromas known to do so in the process of continued transplantation.

"3. Tumors known to u n d e r g o sarcomatous changes did not show an increased sarcomatous tendency when exposed to continued estrogen administration.

"4. Various dosages of estrogen administered to rats of different ages over long periods of time did not produce breast tissue changes beyond those expected for long estrogen stimulation."

In discussion Dr. J. Mason Hundley, Jr., of Baltimore, reviewed the work of Lacassagne and others in this same field of investigation using mice. He, too, calls attention to the fact that most experimental work has been done in mice and there is very little positive information as to the carcinogenic activities of estrogen in the human being. In relation to the possible danger of increasing the probability of cancer by estrogenic therapy in the human being, he feels that the deductions drawn from the experimental work are illogical because the dosages were tremendous and prolonged, over practically the entire life of the experimental animal. For example, in Lacassagne's experience the equivalent dosage in an average human female would have been crystaline estrogen 3,000,000 international units at one dose, begun early in childhood and continued for several years.

It is Dr. Hundley's feeling, therefore, that no comparable dosage over such a long fraction of the human being's life is employed in practice and that in the therapeutic application of estrogen in the human being there is little or no danger of carcinogenic properties in the drug.

In discussion, Dr. Howard C. Taylor, Jr., of New York, reported investigation in another direction using estrogen in two contrasting strains of mice, one with a high tumor incidence and one with a low incidence. The strain susceptible to tumor formation showed a relatively low reaction to the injections of estrogen. "From these experiments which we have repeated with many animals, we can draw certain tentative conclusions. By all odds the most important factor in the development of mammary carcinoma in mice is this inherent constitutional factor. The addition of estrogenic substance simply emphasizes this difference. If one may make any inference as to the risk of giving estrogenic substances to women, one might expect that, if there is already a constitutional predisposition to mammary carcinoma in a certain woman, there may be a slight increase in the risk by giving her estrogenic therapy, whereas the woman who has no such constitutional predisposition is unaffected."

Comment: There are essentially three problems to be carefully considered in the prolonged use of large dosages of estrogens in the human female.

In the first place one must evaluate the influence of such estrogen therapy in the average individual with no particular constitutional tendency to malignancy of the breast or uterus. While estrogen should be employed carefully in such patients, there is probably practically no danger of producing a malignancy of the breast or uterus.

The second problem is concerned with the use of estrogens in individuals who have had malignant tumors of the breast or uterus and who have had recognized treatment for them. It is probable that the reasonably cautious use of estrogens for the relief of vasomotor symptoms will have little or no influence upon the incidence of recurrence or extension but effort should be made to reduce the dosage to the lowest possible effective level and to limit the time of application to as short a period as possible.

The third problem concerns itself with the use of estrogenic substances in patients who have had endometriosis wherein it was necessary to remove both ovaries and leave ectopic endometrial tissue in place, for example in the bowel wall or in the culdesac. Theoretically, estrogen administration would activate such endometrial remnants but actually it apparently has little influence, probably because of the absence of progestin and estrogens can be used safely in moderate dosages for the relief of vasomotor symptoms incident with the castration.

It is very well to state again that the carcinogenic properties of estrogen as demonstrated in experimental animals does not apply to human beings. However, in individuals susceptible to malignancy and in individuals who have had malignancies of the breast and uterus caution should be employed in the administration of estrogens, both as to dosage and the length of time of treatment.

Wendell Long

---o---

EYE, EAR, NOSE AND THROAT
Edited by Marvin D. Henley, M.D.
911 Medical Arts Building, Tulsa

Secondary Mastoid Infections. Harold Hays, M.D., F.A.C.S., New York. The Eye, Ear, Nose and Throat Monthly, November, 1938.

The author gives his views of a much discussed question. Before the simple mastoid was so thoroughly standardized, a second operation was sometimes necessary to finish removing the infected cells—in such cases, however, there was a continuous discharge from the middle ear.

Hays states: "In secondary mastoid infections we have a clinical entity which may occur in any individual who has been operated upon for mastoiditis, a condition which cannot be avoided, a condition purely accidental and which may take place even after the most perfect original operation has been performed."

The changed anatomy of the region is discussed following a simple mastoidectomy. The history of the secondary infection is almost uniform. An acute cold, sore throat or upper respiratory infection is precipitated that allows the infection to travel through the Eustachian tube into the middle ear and the operated area. This may occur from year to year, particularly in children. There is pain in the ear and tenderness over the mastoid wound. Mucopus or pus may discharge spontaneously from the ear canal. Most of these cases are not serious and a simple incision through the old mastoid wound into the antrum and middle ear will alleviate the signs and symptoms. Hays does this many times under ethyl chloride anaesthesia in the office. Bulging of the old mastoid scar does not necessarily need to be waited for, as an incision will relieve the tension and provide drainage and shorten the time of recovery.

Two cases are reported. One a man age 55 in which an incision was made and drain installed without encountering pus but giving a recovery period of three days. The second case was that of a boy that had had a double mastoid performed some years before. This boy ran a high temperature and a high blood count. He also had an acute throat infection which complicated the case making the blood count and temperature useless as a diagnostic aid. His chief complaint was pain in and behind the right ear. There was a seromucoid discharge from an old drum perforation. He was given sulfanilimide and mercurochrome nose drops for the throat infection which proved to be streptococcus. There was not any improvement in 24 hours so the original incision was opened and a drain inserted. No pus was encountered but improvement was noted immediately and in a few days he was able to visit the office. The packing was removed. The third day following the temperature rose and he was taken to the hospital. Under general anaesthesia the wound was opened widely without finding any evidence of bone infection. A drain was inserted and he recovered uneventfully. The three problems considered in this case were: 1. Was this a continuance of the streptococcus infection in the throat? 2. Was it an infection in the middle ear which could be relieved by again re-opening the mastoid wound? 3. Or was it some deep-seated complication as yet undiscovered?

The Problem of Intranasal Medication. Original paper by Theodore E. Walsh, M.D., and Paul R. Cannon, M.D., Chicago, Ill. Published in the Annals of Otology, Rhinology and Laryngology, September, 1938. This Digest from The Digest of Ophthalmology and Otolaryngology, Vol I, No. I, November, 1938.

As the result of the interest in the common cold inspired by the health columns in popular literature, the public has become aware of the dangers and the necessity of early treatments of this disease and physicians are often asked for an opinion as to the merits of various preparations or so-called "cures." Although the proper treatment is not always known, physicians have often assumed that even if certain preparations did little if any good, they did at least no harm.

"Recent observations of the effects of various drugs on the nasal mucosa and in the lungs following nasal applications, however, have proved this idea to be erroneous. It therefore seems important at this time to review the problem of nasal medication and to point out some of the effects of commonly used drugs, both on the nasal mucosa and on the lungs."

The effects on the nasal mucosa of materials used as vehicles for intranasal medications:

"Oils: Perhaps the most commonly used vehicle for intranasal medication at the present time is mineral oil. Its popularity is due, no doubt, to the belief that it is bland and does no harm to nasal tissues, and because it causes no discomfort even in the presence of acute infections. Stark, however, observed that the mucous glands of the rabbit's nose became hyperactive after intranasal use of plain mineral oil. Fox later found in rabbits treated for periods as long as nine months with intranasal sprays of mineral oil that liquid petrolatum apparently exerts a deleterious effect on the nasal mucosa of a rabbit. Even more marked changes were found when menthol, eucalyptol and camphor were used similarly, dissolved in mineral oil." Other investigators "found that although liquid petrolatum had no immediate effect on the activity of the ciliary beat, it did cause slowing down or loss of mucous streaming." It has been "suggested that oily mixtures are to be avoided where ciliary streaming still functions, because they interfere not only with the ciliary beat but with its effectiveness, by lying on the mucous blanket and by being propelled with great difficulty by it. It is apparent that, insofar as their effects on the nasal passages are concerned, oily solutions effect both the mucosa and the cilia deleteriously and that drugs dissolved in them act less effectively than in saline solutions."

Aqueous Solutions: If oily solutions affect the nasal tissues and cilia adversely, do aqueous solutions act similarly? "This question has been studied by both Stark and Proetz. The former irrigated the nasal mucous membrane with 0.9 per cent saline, 2.0 per cent saline, and plain tap water and found, that although the effect was harmful in every case, isotonic saline solution caused less harm than did either of the other two. Proetz ascertained the effects of various salt solutions on ciliary beat and found that the cilia of both man and animals remained active for long periods in 0.9 per cent solution of sodium chloride, but lost their activity when more concentrated solutions of sodium chloride were used. When the saline solutions were made hypotonic the outlines of the cilia were gradually lost and the surfaces became cloudy. These experiments indicate quite definitely, therefore, that isotonic saline is the vehicle of choice for drugs to be used in the nose.

Antiseptics: Ever since the bacterial nature of disease became known, various chemical substances have been used in the attempt to stop bacterial growth in tissues. This has been particularly true of respiratory disease, and many kinds of drugs have been used in the nose and throat because of their presumed bactericidal effects. In recent years the silver salts, for example argyrol and neosilvol, have been especially popular, the thymol and merthiolate have also been widely used.

"Evaluation of the rationale of such medications requires consideration of several factors: first, are such drugs actually bactericidal; second, do they remain in the nose long enough and in proper concentration to exert an effect; and third, to they injure nasal mucosa, mucous glands or cilia? In order to ascertain to what extent these drugs are bactericidal for micro-organisms commonly found in respiratory infections, we performed a number of experiments. Put from a patient with bronchiectasis was mixed thoroughly with solutions of the drugs to be tested and the mixtures were allowed to stand at room temperature. At varying intervals of time, 0.1 cc. of the mixture was mixed with melted blood agar, plates were poured, and after 24 hours' incubation, colony counts were made. The results showed that the only drug with any appreciable bactericidal effect was 1 per cent thymol. When one considers that in an upper respiratory infection the causative organisms are not lying free on the surface of the mucous membrane, but are in the epithelial or subepithelial tissues, and furthermore, that in all probability drugs placed in the nose remain there for no longer than from 10 to 15 minutes, it is improbable that even such drugs as thymol can exert bactericidal effect in the upper respiratory tract.

Lierle and Moore, and Proetz agree that thymol causes immediate cessation of the ciliary beat, and that merthiolate causes an initial slowing of ciliary action with cessation after a few minutes. Lierle and Moore state that the silver proteins cause initial increase of ciliary activity followed by marked slowing, although they suggest that this latter effect may have been due to the fact that the drugs were used in watery (not isotonic) solution.

Astringents: Astringents are also frequently used in nasal therapy, and their use has become more general in recent months because of the experimental work done on poliomyelitis of monkeys, but in view of the uncertainty at the present time that the nose is actually the portal of entry in poliomyelitis, the use of such astringents seems questionable. Lierle and Moore found that 2 per cent sulphate caused almost immediate cessation of ciliary activity in the rabbit's nose and that resuscitation was not effected.

"Vasoconstrictors: Probably the most common complaint of patients suffering from upper respiratory disease is nasal obstruction, and nearly all of the solutions prescribed for use in the nose contain a vasoconstrictor. The most widely used drugs for this purpose are adrenalin, ephedrine, benzedrine and Neosynepherin. It is important, therefore, to know what effect these drugs may have on the mucous membrane and the ciliary activity. All observers who have worked with adrenalin agree that this drug in 1:1,000 dilution causes immediate cessation of ciliary action. Weak solutions of ephedrine, on the other hand, cause an initial speeding of the ciliary beat at times, but this is in no way detrimental to ciliary activity. Fitzhugh reports that Neosynepherin hydrochloride causes no apparent harm to the nasal mucosa, and states that this drug has a slightly longer vasoconstrictive effect than adrenalin or ephedrine and is less toxic than either."

The passage of nasal medicaments from nose to lungs:

"Of more importance than the effects of nasal medicaments upon the tissues of the upper respiratory tract is the problem of their effect on the lungs. All doubt as to the ease with which medicinal solutions placed in the nose can directly go to the lungs has been removed by the observations within recent years of the widespread occurrence of lipoid pneumonia secondary to the use of nasal oil drops and sprays."

The intranasal use of medicated oils has proved that such light fluids may go directly to the lungs and cause serious irritation, the severity depending upon the kind and quantity of material aspired and the length of time during which it has been used.

Effects upon lungs from intranasal administration of watery solutions of commonly used medicaments:

"In view of the ease with which the nasal oils may pass from the nose to the lungs, the question arises, do watery solutions of drugs applied in the nose reach the lungs, and if so, do they cause harm?

"Antiseptics: It is generally assumed that silver salts, Neosilvol and argyrol, which are so widely used in nasal therapy, are non-toxic and non-irritating. The following observations, however, suggest that they may be potentially dangerous when so employed. Healthy rabbits were treated with these drugs and were studied histologically and by roentgenogram. The extensive edema, necrosis and desquamation of septal cells, all demonstrate the toxic effect of such materials when they enter the lungs under the conditions of these experiments.

The effect upon the lungs of vasoconstrictive agents in watery solutions:

"In the course of our studies we have tested aqueous solutions of some of the commonly used vasoconstrictive agents, instilled intranasally into normal rabbits. In no instance have we found any evidence of severe pulmonary irritation or necrosis such as we have seen so constantly after the use of nasal oils, antiseptic solutions or astringents."

COMMENT: "These studies emphasize particularly the potential dangers from the use of medicated oils and also antiseptic and astringent solutions, because of the chance that such materials may go directly from the upper respiratory passages to the lungs and there cause serious damage to pulmonary tissues. It is reasonable to assume, therefore, that aqueous solutions of antiseptics, when similarly used in the nose, may also reach the lungs. It would seem more important to prove that they do not enter the lungs when used in humans, than to assume that they do not.

Corneal Reaction to Weed Pollen. A. Reas Anneberg, M.D., Carroll, Iowa. The American Journal of Ophthalmology, November, 1938.

This is a short article reporting six interesting cases—occurring in a period of four weeks—apparently resulting from contact with massive quantities of pollen. The eyes were red, painful, had an itching sensation and remained painful even when closed. A sensation of a foreign body was produced, even though not present. Both palpebral and bulbar conjunctiva were inflamed. In some cases an iris spasm was present with an accompanying small pupil. At first the cornea was clear but in from two to four days there appeared areas of grayish infiltration. These areas were from one-half to one millimeter in diameter. When the inflammation was at its height there was a diffuse haziness and a stippling of the whole cornea in two cases. Fluorescin failed to stain any of the corneas. The infiltration lasted a week or ten days with no impairment of vision resulting. Pig-weed-redroot appeared to be the predominating pollinating plant in all cases.

There was one of the six patients who gave a previous history of allergy. About the seventh day his infiltration broke down into a marginal ulcer. Other patients' eyes were kept patched after the use of butyn and bichloride ointment. The allergic individual did not return between the third and sixth days. The ulcer became secondarily infected and healed with difficulty, only after some infected teeth were, extracted. The treatment on all included daily intramuscular injections of 10 c.c. of lactigen (Abbott).

COMMENT: It has been my unpleasant experience during the season just passed to have had two patients who were very allergic. The eye complications were ulcerations-violent-painful-fulminating. Various procedures were instigated but none would keep the condition under control in the presence of an acute exacerbation of the allergic condition. Both patients were elderly females, white.

----------o----------

ORTHOPAEDIC SURGERY
Edited by Earl D. McBride, M.D., F.A.C.S.
717 North Robinson Street, Oklahoma City

"An Evaluation of Excision in the Treatment of Ununited F r a c t u r e of the Carpal Scaphoid (Navicular) Bone." Arthur J. Davidson and M. Thomas Horwitz. Annals of Surgery, CVIII, 291, August, 1938.

A small but very definite percentage of the cases of ununited fractures of the carpal scaphoid fail to unite despite the progress which has been made in their treatment.

The authors realize that good results have been attained in cases of delayed or early non-union by prolonged fixation in a non-padded plaster cast as recommended by Bohler; also by the method of multiple drilling and by the use of an autogenous bone peg.

However, they feel that total excision still has a very definite place in the treatment of these cases and is the treatment of choice in irreducible fractures, in badly comminuted fractures of the scaphoid (especially those associated with other carpal injuries such as a dislocated semilunar bone), and in neglected cases of non-union with marked and irreparable degeneration of the fragments. In cases where early return to work is essential, and which show obvious non-union and persistent disability, they also advise total excision following a fair but not too prolonged conservative regimen.

They state that early excision will result in a normally functioning and painless wrist with little or no deformity. The efficiency of the procedure diminishes, however, with delay because of the development of arthritis and periarthritic changes in the wrist. They advise against partial excision, as the disability is liable to persist after the procedure.

The authors use a dorsal incision, two, inches long, lateral and parallel to the tendon of the extensor pollicis longus. The wrist is immobilized from seven to ten days, and thereafter motion is encouraged.

They analyze eight cases, all in males between the ages of 21 and 49 years. Seven cases had total excision and one had partial excision. Results were very good or excellent in five cases, good in two cases, and poor in one case. The latter case was one of seven years' duration with marked osteoarthritic changes.

The authors conclude that "total excision must be considered in the rational therapy of ununited fracture of the carpal scaphoid. When utilized early before secondary arthritic and periarthritic changes take place, a very satisfactory result with regard to anatomic, functional and economic recovery may be anticipated."

----------o----------

"Tumors of the Spine. With a Consideration of Ewing's Sarcoma." Robert R. Rix and Charles F. Geschickter. Archives of Surgery, XXXVI, 890, June, 1938.

Two hundred and ninety-one tumors affecting the bone structure of the spinal column, available for study in the Surgical Pathological Laboratory of the Johns Hopkins Hospital, are analyzed. All of these tumors were demonstrable roentgenographically.

In the order of their frequency they are; metastatic carcinoma, primary tumors of the spinal column, glial tumors, tumors of the pleural sheath of the spinal cord, tumors of generalized distribution, tumors of the sympathetic nervous system, and tumors of teratological origin.

The metastatic carcinoma is the most common neoplasy of the vertebral column and usually originates either in the breast, when it is multiple and destructive, or in the prostate, when it usually involves the lower spine and has osteogenetic characteristics.

Of the primary tumors of the spine, the malignant sarcomata are found to include chondrosarcoma, osteolytic sarcoma, and sclerosing sarcoma. These may be secondary to multiple exostoses or to Paget's disease. Chordoma affects the upper and the lower ends of the spine of the adult and produces a destructive lesion.

The benign growths include the giant-cell tumor and the osteochondroma. Hemangioma is rare. There were 12 neuroblastic tumors. No typical Ewing's sarcoma of the spine was found. The differential diagnosis is discussed, and there are numerous illustrations.

----------o----------

PLASTIC SURGERY
Edited by
GEO. H. KIMBALL, M.D., F.A.C.S.
404 Medical Arts Building, Oklahoma City

Ectropion and Entropion of the Eyelids. Webb W. Weeks, M.D., N. Y. University School of Medicine. From American Journal of Surgery, October, 1938, page 78.

The author gives in detail the method used for correction of ectropion and entropion of the eyelids. He uses local anesthesia of one per cent of pontocaine for the conjunctiva instilled locally with two per cent novocaine with adrenalin added infiltrated into the eyelid.

Cautery punctures are advised for ectropion of recent origin when local non-surgical measures fail. Also twisted black silk No. 5 sutures are used in some cases for correcting ectropion. In the atonic and atrophic cases and in the paralytic cases the Kuhnt-Szymanowski operation is used.

The author gives diagrams and a detailed description of the technique employed. If the ectropion is due to a scar either from a burn, infection or trauma, the area is divided and a graft supplied in the defect. The author prefers skin from the opposite eyelid for this purpose. A graft from the upper arm, thigh, scrotum or the prepuce may be used.

Entropion: The author uses ·cautery punctures as in ectropion applying the needles to the skin side going down into but not through the tarsus. The Celsus operation is used in some cases. In others the Birch-Hirschfield is employed.

If the entropion is partial and at the outer one-third of the eye-lid the Spenser Watson procedure relieves the rolling in and the trichiasis as well. When the condition is due to cicatricial contracture with tarsal deformity and trichiasis, the Streatfield-Snellen procedure is used.

Summary: Surgical experience dealing with spastic ectropion or entropion where early eyelid structural changes have set in, has shown that the simpler operative procedures are quite uniformly successful; and that where permanent damage has occurred the plastic operative procedures described gives excellent cosmetic and functional results.

Comment: The plastic procedure employed about the eyelids demand considerable detailed study. Neglect in any one step may result in a poor result. All infection must be obliterated before any grafting is considered. Co-operation between ophthalmologist and plastic surgeons is essential. Ideally to do this work probably a man should be a competent ophthalmologist plus a highly trained technician in plastic repair.

The Effect of Local Antiseptic Agents on Infected Wounds. David P. Anderson, Jr., M.D., Philadelphia. From Annals of Surgery, November, 1938.

The author has carried out some experimental work to determine the rate of healing in infected wounds. Agents used:

1. Dry gauze. 2. Moist saline dressing. 3. Alcohol dressing. 4. Iodoform gauze. 5. Azochloramide in normal saline. . 6. Merthiolate 1/1,000. 7. Katadyn silver. 8. Dakin's solution and zinc peroxide cream.

Two cases were given sulfanilamide by mouth.

Conclusions: The group of local agents considered in this study had little or no beneficial effect upon the healing of infected wounds, except for the action of zinc peroxide in specific cases.

The few antiseptic agents which had definite bactericidal action on surface organisms in normal granulating wounds were ineffective in the presence of tissue necrosis, and it is only under the latter circumstances that the existing infection is likely to retard healing.

1. Healing of granulating wounds under normal conditions as determined by precise volume measurements, occurs according to a regular geometric curve which may be expressed, in function of area and time.

2. The presence of a large number of organisms on the surface of wounds does not ordinarily retard healing.

3. A quantitative study has been made of the effect of local agents, particularly antiseptic substances, on the rate of healing and the bacterial flora of infected wounds.

In the management of infected wounds, less attention should be given to the selection of a potent local antiseptic agent. It is of more importance to consider the problem of increasing local tissue immunity, which may be influenced by factors of a general nature remote from the site of the wound, and aiding the sequestration of necrotic tissues rich in bacteria by mechanical or chemical debridement and adequate surgical drainage.

UROLOGY
Edited by D. W. Branham, M.D.
514 Medical Arts Building, Oklahoma City

Why Does the Trichomonas Vaginalis Recur? Report of 38 cases. Earl John Karnaky, Houston, Texas. The Urologic and Cutaneous Review, November, 1938.

The author is of the opinion that trichomonas infection is curable in a high percentage of cases, 70 to 80 per cent. Those that fail to improve or tend to recur do so because of infection in the sexual partner. In an examination of 150 husbands in whose wives trichomonas vaginalis recurred, he found 38 cases of these to have the organism either in the urethra, the prostate or under the prepuce. Most of these men had no complaints as far as disease of these structures was concerned.

Therapeutic attention to the male and careful personal hygiene, particularly in sexual intercourse, produced excellent results in these refractory cases. The use of a rubber cundrom and instillation of argyrol into the urethra are effective measures to prevent infection.

He feels that trichomonas vaginalis infection in the male is self-limited disease, disappearing usually in two or three months. As far as the treatment of the infection in the female is concerned, the ordinary antiseptic drug will be found effective providing the P-H of the mucous membrane of the vagina is lowered to a sufficient acidity. A P-H of 4.0 to 4.4 is necessary to obtain a high percentage of cures. By the addition of hydrolysed glucose and lactose to the ordinary antiseptic drugs he has been able to raise the percentage of permanent cures to 93 per cent.

Metastases From Occult Carcinoma of the Prostate. Ormond S. Culp, Baltimore, Maryland. Journal of Urology, October, 1938.

The purpose of this report is first, to remind practitioners of the startling incidence of prostatic carcinoma. Second, to show that metastases occur not infrequently from microscopic tumors found only at autopsy. Third, to record an unusual case of occult carcinoma of the prostate with metastases.

A brief review of the literature by the author emphasizes the prevalence of this disease and the author details a case report in which the dominant clinical finding was the neurological disorder manifest in a transverse myelitis due to vertebral metastasis.

He summarizes his impression in the following statements:

1. Carcinoma of the prostate is the most common type of cancer in men, occurring in more than 14 per cent of those over 50 years of age.

2. Prostatic cancers frequently metastasize to the vertebral column and usually do so only when far advanced.

3. Occult carcinoma found only on serial sections of the prostate may metastasize extensively, producing severe neurological manifestations without any urinary symptoms.

4. Any unexplained spinal cord lesion should suggest early prostatic carcinoma even though rectal examinations are negative.

XXXI   INDEX TO CONTENTS   1938

SCIENTIFIC PAPERS

AUTHORS

BOOK REVIEWS

COMMITTEE REPORTS

OBITUARIES

EDITORIALS

EDITORIAL NOTES

22, 54, 55, 129, 130, 174, 175, 202, 250, 353, 423

ABSTRACTS

MISCELLANEOUS

OFFICERS OKLAHOMA STATE MEDICAL ASSOCIATION

President, Dr. H. K. Speed, Sayre.

President-Elect, Dr. W. A. Howard, Chelsea.

Secretary-Treasurer-Editor, Dr. L. S. Willour, McAlester.

Speaker, House of Delegates, Dr. J. D. Osborn, Jr., Frederick.

Vice Speaker, House of Delegates, Dr. P. P. Nesbitt, Medical Arts Building, Tulsa.

Delegates to the A. M. A., Dr. W. Albert Cook, Medical Arts Building, Tulsa, 1938-39; Dr. McLain Rogers, Clinton, 1937-1938.

Meeting Place, Oklahoma City, May 15-16-17, 1939.

SPECIAL COMMITTEES 1938-39

Annual Meeting: Dr. H. K. Speed, Sayre; Dr. W. A. Howard, Chelsea; Dr. L. S. Willour, McAlester.

Conservation of Hearing: Dr. H. F. Vandever, Chairman, Enid; Dr. J. B. Hollis, Mangum; Dr. Chester McHenry, Oklahoma City.

Conservation of Vision: Dr. W. M. Gallaher, Chairman, Shawnee; Dr. Frank R. Vieregg, Clinton; Dr. Pauline Barker, Guthrie.

Crippled Children: Dr. Earl McBride, Chairman, Oklahoma City; Dr. Roy L. Fisher, Frederick; Dr. M. B. Glismann, Okmulgee.

Industrial Service and Traumatic Surgery: Dr. Cyril C. Clymer, Medical Arts Bldg., Oklahoma City; Dr. J. Wm. Finch, Hobart; Dr. J. A. Rutledge, Ada.

Maternity and Infancy: Dr. George R. Osborn, Chairman, Tulsa; Dr. P. J. DeVanney, Sayre; Dr. Leila E. Andrews, Oklahoma City.

Necrology: Dr. G. H. Stagner, Chairman, Erick; Dr. James L. Shuler, Durant; Dr. S. D. Neely, Muskogee.

Post Graduate Medical Teaching: Dr. Henry H. Turner, Chairman, Oklahoma City; Dr. H. C. Weber, Bartlesville; Dr. Ned R. Smith, Tulsa.

Study and Control of Cancer: Dr. Wendell Long, Chairman, Oklahoma City; Dr. Paul B. Champlin, Enid; Dr. Ralph McGill, Tulsa.

Study and Control of Tuberculosis: Dr. Carl Puckett, Chairman, Oklahoma City; Dr. W. C. Tisdal, Clinton; Dr. F. P. Baker, Talihina.

ADVISORY COUNCIL FOR AUXILIARY

Dr. H. K. Speed, Chairman..Sayre

Dr. C. J. Fishman...Oklahoma City

Dr. W. S. Larrabee..Tulsa

Dr. J. M. Watson..Enid

Dr. T. H. McCarley...McAlester

STANDING COMMITTEES 1938-39

Medical Defense: Dr. O. E. Templin, Chairman, Alva; Dr. L. C. Kuyrkendall, McAlester; Dr. E. Albert Aisenstadt, Picher.

Medical Economics: Dr. C. B. Sullivan, Cordell, Chairman; Dr. J. L. Patterson, Duncan; Dr. W. M. Browning, Waurika.

Medical Education and Hospital: Dr. V. C. Tisdal, Chairman, Elk City; Dr. Robert U. Patterson, Oklahoma City; Dr. H. M. McClure, Chickasha.

Public Policy and Legislation: Dr. Finis W. Ewing, Surety Bldg., Chairman, Muskogee; Dr. Tom Lowry, 1200 North Walker, Oklahoma City; Dr. O. C. Newman, Shattuck.

(The above committee co-ordinated by the following, selected from each councilor district.)

District No. 1.—Arthur E. Hale, Alva.

District No. 2.—McLain Rogers, Clinton.

District No. 3.—Thomas McElroy, Ponca City.

District No. 4.—L. H. Ritzhaupt, Guthrie.

District No. 5.—P. V. Annadown, Sulphur.

District No. 6.—R. M. Shepard, Tulsa.

District No. 7.—Sam A. McKeel, Tulsa.

District No. 8.—J. A. Morrow, Sallisaw.

District No. 9.—W. A. Tolleson, Eufaula.

District No. 10.—J. L. Holland, Madill.

Scientific Exhibits: Dr. E. Rankin Denny, Chairman, Tulsa; Dr. Robert H. Akin, Oklahoma City; Dr. R. C. Pigford, Tulsa.

Scientific Work: Dr. W. G. Husband, Chairman, Hollis; Dr. J. S. Rollins, Prague; Dr. J. L. Day, Supply.

Public Health:

Chairman—Dr. G. S. Baxter, Shawnee.

District No. 1.—C. W. Tedrowe, Woodward.
District No. 2.—E. W. Mabry, Altus.
District No. 3.—L. A. Mitchell, Stillwater.
District No. 4.—J. J. Gable, Norman.
District No. 5.—Geo. S. Barber, Lawton.
District No. 6.—C. E. Bradley, Tulsa.
District No. 7.—G. S. Baxter, Shawnee.
District No. 8.—M. M. De Arman, Miami.
District No. 9.—T. H. McCarley, McAlester.
District No. 10.—J. B. Clark, Coalgate.

SCIENTIFIC SECTIONS

General Surgery: Dr. F. L. Flack, Chairman, Nat'l Bank of Tulsa Bldg., Tulsa; Dr. John E. McDonald, Vice-Chairman, Medical Arts Bldg., Tulsa; Dr. John F. Burton, Secretary, Osler Building, Oklahoma City.

General Medicine: Dr. Frank Nelson, Chairman, 603 Medical Arts Bldg., Tulsa; Dr. E. R. Musick, Vice-Chairman, Medical Arts Bldg., Oklahoma City; Dr. Milam McKinney, Medical Arts Bldg., Oklahoma City.

Eye, Ear, Nose & Throat: Dr. E. H. Coachman, Chairman, Manhattan Bldg., Muskogee; Dr. F. M. Cooper, Vice-President, Medical Arts Bldg., Oklahoma City; Dr. James R. Reed, Secretary, Medical Arts Bldg., Oklahoma City.

Obstetrics and Pediatrics: Dr. C. W. Arrendell, Chairman, Ponca City; Dr. Carl F. Simpson, Vice-Chairman, Medical Arts Bldg., Tulsa; Dr. Ben H. Nicholson, Secretary, 300 West Twelfth Street, Oklahoma City.

Genito-Urinary Diseases and Syphilology: Dr. Elijah Sullivan, Chairman, Medical Arts Bldg., Oklahoma City; Dr. Henry Browne, Vice-Chairman, Medical Arts Bldg., Tulsa; Dr. Robert Akin, Secretary, 400 West Tenth, Oklahoma City.

Dermatology and Radiology: Dr. W. A. Showman, Chairman, Medical Arts Bldg., Tulsa; Dr. E. D. Greenberger, Vice-Chairman, McAlester; Dr. Hervey A. Foerster, Secretary, Medical Arts Bldg., Oklahoma City.

STATE BOARD OF MEDICAL EXAMINERS

Dr. Thos. McElroy, Ponca City, President; Dr. C. E. Bradley, Tulsa, Vice-President; Dr. J. D. Osborn, Jr., Frederick, Secretary; Dr. L. E. Emanuel, Chickasha; Dr. W. T. Ray, Gould; Dr. G. L. Johnson, Pauls Valley; Dr. W. W. Osgood, Muskogee.

STATE COMMISSIONER OF HEALTH

Dr. Chas. M. Pearce, Oklahoma City.

COUNCILORS AND THEIR COUNTIES

District No. 1: Texas, Beaver, Cimarron, Harper, Ellis, Woods, Woodward, Alfalfa, Major, Dewey—Dr. O. E. Templin, Alva. (Term expires 1940.)

District No. 2: Roger Mills, Beckham, Greer, Harmon, Washita, Kiowa, Custer, Jackson, Tillman—Dr. V. C. Tisdal, Elk City. (Term expires 1939.)

District No. 3: Grant, Kay, Garfield, Noble, Payne, Pawnee—Dr. A. S. Risser, Blackwell. (Term expires 1938.)

District No. 4: Blaine, Kingfisher, Canadian, Logan, Oklahoma, Cleveland—Dr. Philip M. McNeill, Oklahoma City. (Term expires 1938.)

District No. 5: Caddo, Comanche, Cotton, Grady, Love, Stephens, Jefferson, Carter, Murray—Dr. W. H. Livermore, Chickasha. (Term expires 1938.)

District No. 6: Osage, Creek, Washington, Nowata, Rogers, Tulsa—Dr. James Stevenson, Medical Arts Bldg., Tulsa. (Term expires, 1938.)

District No. 7: Lincoln, Pontotoc, Pottawatomie, Okfuskee, Seminole, McClain, Garvin, Hughes—Dr. J. A. Walker, Shawnee. (Term expires 1939.)

District No. 8: Craig, Ottawa, Mayes, Delaware, Wagoner, Adair, Cherokee, Sequoyah, Okmulgee, Muskogee—Dr. E. A. Aisenstadt, Picher. (Term expires 1939.)

District No. 9: Pittsburg, Haskell, Latimer, LeFlore, McIntosh—Dr. L. C. Kuyrkendall, McAlester. (Term expires 1939.)

District No. 10: Johnson, Marshall, Coal, Atoka, Bryan, Choctaw, Pushmataha, McCurtain—Dr. J. S. Fulton, Atoka. (Term expires 1939.)

OFFICERS OF COUNTY SOCIETIES, 1938

COUNTY	PRESIDENT	SECRETARY
Adair		
Alfalfa	F. K. Slaton, Helena	L. T. Lancaster, Cherokee
Atoka-Coal	J. S. Fulton, Atoka	J. B. Clark, Coalgate
Beckham	R. O. McCreery, Erick	P. J. DeVanney, Sayre
Blaine	J. S. Barnett, Hitchcock	W. F. Griffin, Watonga
Bryan	P. L. Cain, Albany	Jas. L. Shuler, Durant
Caddo	J. Worrell Henry, Anadarko	P. H. Anderson, Anadarko
Canadian	A. L. Johnson, El Reno	G. D. Funk, El Reno
Carter	T. J. Jackson, Ardmore	Emma Jean Cantrell, Wilson
Cherokee	P. H. Medearis, Tahlequah	H. A. Masters, Tahlequah
Choctaw	G. E. Harris, Hugo	F. L. Waters, Hugo
Cleveland	O. E. Howell, Norman	J. L. Haddock, Jr., Norman
Coal	(See Atoka)	
Comanche	E. B. Dunlap, Lawton	Reber M. Van Matre, Lawton
Cotton	W. W. Cotton, Walters	G. W. Baker, Walters
Craig	W. R. Marks, Vinita	F. T. Gastineau, Vinita
Creek	C. R. McDonald, Mannford	J. F. Curry, Sapulpa
Custer	Ross Deputy, Clinton	Harry Cushman, Clinton
Garfield	E. J. Wolfe, Waukomis	John R. Walker, Enid
Garvin	G. L. Johnson, Pauls Valley	John R. Callaway, Pauls Valley
Grady	L. E. Wood, Chickasha	R. F. Bazo, Chickasha
Grant	I. V. Hardy, Medford	E. E. Lawson, Medford
Greer	Leb B. Pearson, Mangum	J. B. Hollis, Mangum
Harmon	W. G. Husband, Hollis	R. H. Lynch, Hollis
Haskell	A. T. Hill, Stigler	N. K. Williams, McCurtain
Hughes	W. L. Taylor, Holdenville	Imogene Mayfield, Holdenville
Jackson	Jas. E. Ensey, Altus	J. M. Allgood, Altus
Jefferson	C. S. Maupin, Waurika	C. M. Maupin, Waurika
Kay	G. C. Moore, Ponca City	R. G. Obermiller, Ponca City
Kingfisher	John R. Taylor, Kingfisher	F. C. Lattimore, Kingfisher
Kiowa	I. M. Bonham, Hobart	J. Wm. Finch, Hobart
Latimer	R. L. Rich, Red Oak	E. B. Hamilton, Wilburton
LeFlore	E. M. Woodson, Poteau	W. L. Shippey, Poteau
Lincoln	E. F. Hurlbut, Meeker	Ned Burleson, Prague
Logan	F. R. First, Crescent	E. O. Barker, Guthrie
Marshall	J. H. Logan, Lebanon	J. F. York, Madill
Mayes	S. C. Rutherford, Locust Grove	E. H. Werling, Pryor
McClain	J. E. Cochran, Byars	R. L. Royster, Purcell
McCurtain	R. D. Williams, Idabel	R. H. Sherrill, Broken Bow
McIntosh	D. E. Little, Eufaula	Wm. A. Tolleson, Eufaula
Murray	P. V. Annadown, Sulphur	Richard M. Burke, Sulphur
Muskogee	Finis W. Ewing, Muskogee	S. D. Neely, Muskogee
Noble	J. W. Francis, Perry	T. F. Renfrow, Billings
Nowata	M. B. Scott, Delaware	H. M. Prentiss, Nowata
Okfuskee	L. J. Spickard, Okemah	C. M. Bloss, Okemah
Oklahoma	C. J. Fishman, Oklahoma City	John F. Burton, Oklahoma City
Okmulgee	V. M. Wallace, Morris	M. B. Glismann, Okmulgee
Osage	R. O. Smith, Hominy	Geo. Hemphill, Pawhuska
Ottawa	Benj. W. Ralston, Commerce	W. Jackson Sayles, Miami
Pawnee	R. E. Jones, Pawnee	M. L. Saddoris, Cleveland.
Payne	E. M. Harris, Cushing	John W. Martin, Cushing
Pittsburg	A. R. Russell, McAlester	Ed. D. Greenberger, McAlester
Pontotoc	W. F. Dean, Ada	Glen W. McDonald, Ada
Pottawatomie	E. Eugene Rice, Shawnee	F. Clinton Gallaher, Shawnee
Pushmataha	E. S. Patterson, Antlers	D. W. Connally, Antlers
Rogers	F. A. Anderson, Claremore	W. A. Howard, Chelsea
Seminole	A. N. Deaton, Wewoka	Claude B. Knight, Wewoka
Stephens	W. T. Salmon, Duncan	Fred T. Hargrove, Duncan
Texas		R. B. Hayes, Guymon
Tillman	J. E. Childers, Tipton	O. G. Bacon, Frederick
Tulsa	M. J. Searle, Tulsa	Roy L. Smith, Tulsa
Wagoner	S. R. Bates, Wagoner	Francis S. Crane, Wagoner
Washington	J. E. Crawford, Bartlesville	J. V. Athey, Bartlesville
Washita	J. Paul Jones, Dill	Gordon Livingston, Cordell
Woods	Arthur E. Hale, Alva	Oscar E. Templin, Alva
Woodward	C. W. Tedrowe, Woodward	V. M. Rutherford, Woodward

NOTE—Corrections and additions to the above list will be cheerfully accepted.

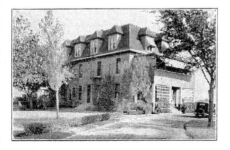

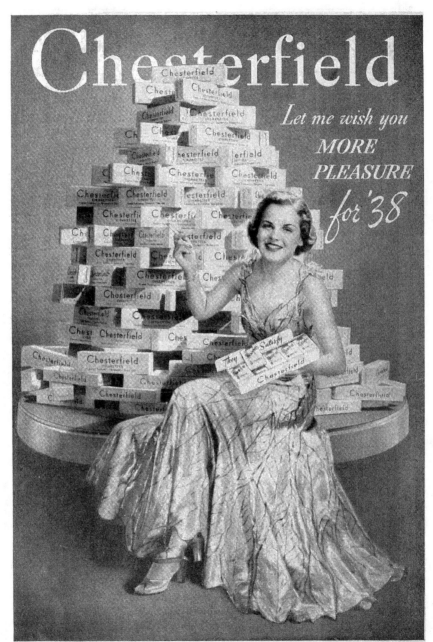

Chesterfield

Let me wish you
MORE
PLEASURE
for '38

State Dues $12, Payable January 1st

THE JOURNAL
OF THE
OKLAHOMA STATE MEDICAL ASSOCIATION

VOLUME XXXI   McALESTER, OKLAHOMA, DECEMBER, 1938   Number 12

Published Monthly at McAlester, Oklahoma, under direction of the Council.

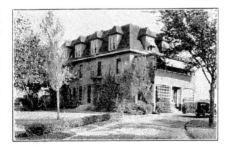
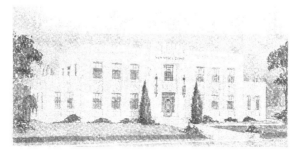

HOW MUCH SUN
Does the Baby Really Get?

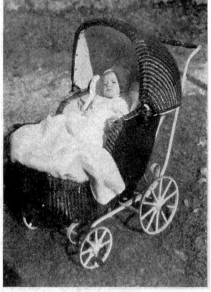

THIS BABY has been placed in the sunlight. (1) The mother discovers the baby is blinking, so she promptly shields its eyes and much of its face from the light. (2) Since the baby's body is covered, the child will then be getting only reflected light or "sky-shine" which is only 50% as effective as direct sunlight as an antiricketic agent (Tisdall). (3) Even if the baby were exposed nude, it has never been determined how much of the ergosterol of the skin is synthesized by the sun's rays (Hess). (4) Time of day also will affect the amount of sunshine or sky-shine reaching this baby's face. At 8:30 A. M., average loss of sunlight, regardless of season is over 31% and at 3:30 P. M. is over 21%. (5) Direct sunlight, moreover, is not always 100% efficient. U. S. Weather Bureau maps show that percentage of possible sunshine varies in different localities, due to differences in meteorological conditions. (6) In cities, smoke and dust, even in summer, are other factors reducing the amount of ultraviolet light.

While Oleum Percomorphum cannot replace the sun, it is a valuable supplement. Unlike the sun, it offers measurable potency in controlled dosage and does not vary from day to day or hour to hour. It is available at any hour, regardless of smoke, season, geography or clothing. Having 100 times the vitamins A and D content of U.S.P. cod liver oil (U. S. P. minimum standard), Oleum Percomorphum can be administered in *drops*, which makes it an ideal year-round antiricketic. Use the sun, too.

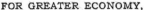

FOR GREATER ECONOMY, the 50 cc. size of Oleum Percomorphum is now supplied with Mead's patented Vacap-Dropper. It keeps out dust and light, is spill-proof, unbreakable, and delivers a uniform drop. The 10 cc. size of Oleum Percomorphum is still offered with the regulation type dropper.

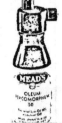

www.ingramcontent.com/pod-product-compliance
Lightning Source LLC
Chambersburg PA
CBHW071356050326
40689CB00010B/1666